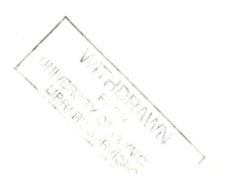

Immunology and Immunopathology of the Liver and Gastrointestinal Tract

Immunology and Immunopathology of the Liver and Gastrointestinal Tract

EDITED BY:

STEPHAN R. TARGAN, M.D.

Professor of Medicine
UCLA School of Medicine
Center for the Health Sciences
Los Angeles, California

FERGUS SHANAHAN, M.D.

Assistant Professor of Medicine
UCLA School of Medicine
Center for the Health Sciences
Los Angeles, California

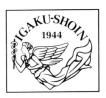

IGAKU-SHOIN   **New York · Tokyo**

Interior Design by Wanda Lubelska
Cover Design by Wanda Lubelska
Typesetting by Progressive Typographers
Printing and Binding by Arcata Graphics/Halliday

Published and distributed by

IGAKU-SHOIN Medical Publishers, Inc.
1140 Avenue of the Americas, New York, N.Y. 10036

IGAKU-SHOIN Ltd.,
5-24-3 Hongo, Bunkyo-ku, Tokyo

Library of Congress Cataloging-in-Publication Data

Immunology and immunopathology of the liver and gastrointestinal tract
  /edited by Stephan R. Targan, Fergus Shanahan.
   p.   cm.
   Includes index.
   ISBN 0-89640-168-5
  1. Gastrointestinal system — Diseases — Immunological aspects.
2. Liver — Diseases — Immunological aspects. 3. Gastrointestinal
system — Immunology. 4. Liver — Immunology. I. Targan, Stephan R.
II. Shanahan, Fergus.
  [DNLM: 1. Gastrointestinal System — immunology.
2. Gastrointestinal System — pathology. 3. Liver — immunology.
4. Liver — pathology. WI 700 I328]
RC802.9.I45 1989
616.3'3079 — dc20
DNLM/DLC
for Library of Congress   89-15446
                                                                                              CIP

ISBN: 0-89640-168-5 (New York)
ISBN: 4-260-14168-6 (Tokyo)

Printed and bound in U.S.A.

10 9 8 7 6 5 4 3 2 1

Preface

This book emphasizes the importance of the mucosal immune system in health and disease. In a single volume, an overview of normal immune function is juxtaposed with our current understanding of disease mechanisms in the gut and liver. The chapters are arranged in a fashion which establishes the macrosphere of the gastro-intestinal tract to provide a foundation to understand the cellular and molecular microsphere. This represents a departure from the traditional perspective and orientation of texts on gastrointestinal immunology. Our focus on recent advances highlights concepts that are likely to shape future approaches to research and treatment.

The participating authors are leading investigators in their disciplines. Our restrictions on content and style were few. We encouraged the authors to provide their views on the subject matter and to make intellectual forays into the future, where appropriate. We persuaded the contributors to render their information in an interpretive manner rather than encyclopedic.

It was our intent to compile a text to meet the needs of a broad audience. The authors' chapters are erudite, yet conclusions are drawn concisely and clearly. Their contributions comprise an update for the gastroenterologist, hepatologist and clinical immunologist, and provide an overview for the non-specialist. The book also answers the basic investigator's demands for a clinical framework for their pursuits. The basic scientist will find this book provides a useful reference for viewing their work within the context of several important diseases. Of course it is our personal wish that this book may stimulate ideas for future investigations that might lead to more effective treatment of immune mediated diseases of the liver and gastrointestinal tract.

We are grateful to the contributing authors who interrupted busy schedules and graciously withstood our "gentle" prodding to comply with deadlines. We thank our assistant, Loren Karp, for her editorial efforts which ensured continuity, and without whom this book would never have been completed. Finally, we thank Lila Glass Maron and her colleagues at Igaku-Shoin for their professionalism and patience.

STEPHAN R. TARGAN
FERGUS SHANAHAN

Contributors

Graeme J.M. Alexander, M.R.C.P.
Honorary Senior Lecturer
Liver Unit
King's College School of Medicine and Dentistry
London, England

Marvin E. Ament, M.D.
Chief, Division of Pediatric Gastroenterology and Nutrition
Professor of Pediatrics
UCLA Center for Health Sciences
Los Angeles, California

Vincent G. Bain, M.D., F.R.C.P.(c)
MRC Research Fellow
Liver Unit
King's College School of Medicine and Dentistry
London, England

A. Dean Befus, Ph.D.
Professor, Department of Microbiology and Infectious Diseases
Health Science Centre
University of Calgary
Calgary, Alberta, Canada

William E. Beschorner, M.D.
Immunopathology, Department of Pathology
The Johns Hopkins University School of Medicine
Baltimore, Maryland

John Bienenstock, M.D.
Chairman, Department of Pathology
McMaster University
Hamilton, Ontario, Canada

Edgar C. Boedeker, M.D.
Chief, Department of Gastroenterology
Walter Reed Army Institute of Research
Walter Reed Army Medical Center
Washington, D.C.

William R. Brown, M.D.
Head, Gastroenterology Division
Department of Medicine
University of Colorado School of Medicine
And
Medical Investigator
V.A. Medical Center
Denver, Colorado

Maureen G. Bruce, Ph.D.
Departments of Microbiology and Medicine
The University of Alabama at Birmingham
Birmingham, Alabama

Kenneth Croitoru, M.D.C.M.
Assistant Professor
Department of Medicine, Intestinal Disease Research Unit
McMaster University
Hamilton, Ontario, Canada

Christopher Cuff, Ph.D.
Research Fellow in Biology
Immunology Graduate Group
Department of Biology
University of Pennsylvania
Philadelphia, Pennsylvania

Richard H. Duerr, M.D.
Division of Gastroenterology
Department of Medicine
UCLA School of Medicine
Los Angeles, California

Adrian L.W.F. Eddleston, M.D., F.R.C.P.
Professor of Liver Immunology
Liver Unit
King's College School of Medicine and Dentistry
London, England

Charles O. Elson, M.D.
Director, Division of Gastroenterology
University of Alabama at Birmingham
Birmingham, Alabama

Peter B. Ernst, D.V.M., Ph.D.
Assistant Professor
Department of Pathology, Intestinal Disease Research Unit
McMaster University
Hamilton, Ontario, Canada

John L. Fahey, M.D.
Professor of Microbiology and Immunology
UCLA School of Medicine
Los Angeles, California

Claudio Fiocchi, M.D.
Department of Gastroenterology and Research Institute
Cleveland Clinic Foundation
Cleveland, Ohio

W. Lance George, M.D.
Associate Professor of Medicine
UCLA School of Medicine
And
Chief, Infectious Diseases Division
West Los Angeles V.A. Medical Center
Los Angeles, California

Wayne W. Grody
Assistant Professor
Department of Pathology
UCLA School of Medicine
Los Angeles, California

Gregory R. Harriman, M.D.
Mucosal Immunity Section
Laboratory of Clinical Investigation, NIAID
Clinical Center
National Institutes of Health
Bethesda, Maryland

Stephen M. Holland, M.D.
Fellow, Division of Infectious Diseases
The Johns Hopkins Hospital
Baltimore, Maryland

Steven P. James, M.D.
Mucosal Immunity Section, Laboratory of Clincal Investigation
National Institute of Allergy and Infectious Diseases
National Institutes of Health
Bethesda, Maryland

Martin F. Kagnoff, M.D.
Professor of Medicine
Laboratory of Mucosal Immunology
University of California, San Diego
La Jolla, California

Thomas M. Kloppel, Ph.D.
Cortech, Inc.
Denver, Colorado

Klaus J. Lewin, M.D., F.R.C. Path.
Professor of Pathology, Division of Surgical Pathology
and Professor of Medicine
Division of Gastroenterology
UCLA School of Medicine
Los Angeles, California

Richard P. MacDermott, M.D.
T. Grier Miller Professor of Medicine
Chief, Gastrointestinal Section
University of Pennsylvania School of Medicine
Philadelphia, Pennsylvania

Ian G. McFarlane, Ph.D., M.R.C.Path.
Consultant Biochemist and Honorary Senior Lecturer
Liver Unit
King's College Hospital and School of Medicine and Dentistry
London, England

Lloyd Mayer, M.D.
Associate Professor of Medicine
Chief, Division of Clinical Immunology
The Mount Sinai Medical Center
New York, New York

James Neuberger, D.M.
Honorary Senior Lecturer
The Liver Unit
The Queen Elizabeth Hospital
Birmingham, England

John G. O'Grady, M.D., M.R.C.P.I.
Lecturer in Medicine
Liver Unit
King's College School of Medicine and Dentistry
London, England

C.A. Ottaway, M.D., Ph.D.
Department of Medicine
St. Michael's Hospital
University of Toronto
Toronto, Ontario, Canada

Thomas C. Quinn, M.D.
Senior Investigator
Laboratory of Immunoregulation
National Institute of Allergy and Infectious Diseases
And
The Johns Hopkins University School of Medicine
Baltimore, Maryland

Donald H. Rubin, M.D.
Associate Professor of Medicine and Microbiology
University of Pennsylvania
And
Research Associate
Veteran's Administration Medical Center
Philadelphia, Pennsylvania

Gary J. Russell, M.D.
Assistant Pediatrician
Massachusetts General Hospital
And
Instructor in Pediatrics
Harvard Medical School
Boston, Massachusetts

Wolfgang H. Schraut, M.D.
Department of Surgery
The University of Pittsburgh
Pittsburgh, Pennsylvania

Fergus Shanahan, M.D.
Assistant Professor of Medicine
UCLA School of Medicine
Center for the Health Sciences
Los Angeles, California

Phillip D. Smith, M.D.
Senior Investigator
Cellular Immunology Section
Laboratory of Immunology
National Institute of Dental Research
National Institutes of Health
Bethesda, Maryland

Michael C. Sneller, M.D.
Mucosal Immunity Section
Laboratory of Clinical Investigation, NIAID
Clinical Center
National Institutes of Health
Bethesda, Maryland

Andrzej M. Stanisz, Ph.D.
Assistant Professor
Department of Pathology, Intestinal Disease Research Unit
McMaster University
Hamilton, Ontario, Canada

Ron H. Stead
Lecturer
Department of Pathology
McMaster University
Hamilton, Ontario, Canada

William F. Stenson, M.D.
Associate Professor of Medicine
Washington University
St. Louis, Missouri

Robert G. Strickland, M.D.
Professor and Chairman
Department of Medicine
University of New Mexico School of Medicine
Albuquerque, New Mexico

Warren Strober, M.D.
Head, Mucosal Immunity Section
Laboratory of Clinical Investigation, NIAID
Clinical Center
National Institutes of Health
Bethesda, Maryland

Stephan R. Targan, M.D.
Professor of Medicine
UCLA School of Medicine
Center for the Health Sciences
Los Angeles, California

Ronald P. Turnicky, D.O.
Immunopathology Fellow
Department of Pathology
The Johns Hopkins University School of Medicine
Baltimore, Maryland

W. Allan Walker, M.D.
Pediatrician
Massachusetts General Hospital
And
Professor in Pediatrics
Harvard Medical School
Boston, Massachusetts

Roger Williams, M.D.
Director and Consultant Physician
Liver Unit
King's College School of Medicine and Dentistry
London, England

Contents

xiii

CHAPTER 1

Immunology of the Liver and Gastrointestinal Tract in Health and Disease: A Perspective

FERGUS SHANAHAN

STEPHAN R. TARGAN

Interactions between the host and the external environment occur along two major surfaces — the skin and the mucosal membranes. The environmental interface at mucosal sites involves an area much larger than that covered by the skin. (The surface area of the small intestine is equivalent to that of a tennis court.) Within the intestine, only a single layer of epithelium separates the internal milieu from the external environment, and through that single layer of cells, essential nutrients must be absorbed, while infectious, toxic, and immunogenic material present in the gut lumen must be selectively excluded. This dilemma for host survival is solved by the presence of elaborate defense mechanisms, which include a precisely regulated mucosal immune system in addition to nonimmunologic defenses such as gastric acidity, digestive enzymes, peristalsis, mucus secretion, and the mutually competitive interactions of the gut flora.

The clinical imperative of mucosal defense (respiratory, intestinal, and others) can be appreciated if one considers the frequency with which mucosal infections challenge the host over a lifetime. That 5–10 million children die annually from infectious diarrhea indicates its worldwide importance as a health-care issue. The spectrum of gastrointestinal infections seen in patients with acquired immune deficiency syndrome (AIDS) is additional testimony for the critical role played by the mucosal immune system in host defense against the myriad of potentially pathogenic organisms in our environment. Indeed, it has been argued that mucosal immune defenses against enteric infections are more important for the overall survival of the species than the immunoregulatory abnormalities associated with autoimmune or malignant diseases. The anatomic and functional importance of the mucosal immune system has seldom been portrayed from this perspective in traditional textbooks of immunology or gastroenterology.

1

The mucosa-associated lymphoid tissue of the gut collectively represents the largest lymphoid organ in the body. Functionally, the mucosal immune system is distinct from the systemic immune system in several important respects. First, the effector mechanisms of mucosal immunity, both humoral and cellular, exhibit certain unique features. These include the transepithelial transport of IgA as the predominant immunoglobulin in mucosal secretions and the occurrence of cellular effectors such as mucosal mast cells, intraepithelial lymphocytes, and certain lamina propria lymphocytes, which differ functionally and phenotypically from their counterparts within the systemic immune system. A second distinguishing feature of the mucosal immune system is specific homing or migration patterns of mucosal immunocytes. Homing facilitates the retention of sensitized effector cells at specific mucosal sites and permits traffic between the different mucosal tissues so that an immune response elicited at one mucosal site may be reflected at another. This common mucosal immune system has important physiologic and potential therapeutic implications that include: transfer from mother to neonate of passive immunity to enteric or dietary antigens by breast milk; the enterohepatic circulation of IgA; and the future design of oral vaccines. Another unique feature of mucosal immunity is the phenomenon of oral tolerance, implying that a positive response by the mucosal immune system may be paralleled by a suppression or lack of responsiveness within the systemic immune system. This serves to protect the host from repeated stimulation of systemic immunity by trivial or harmless antigenic material.

Presentation of antigenic material to the mucosal immune system follows specific pathways, including the specialized M cells, which are strategically positioned overlying lymphoid follicles and are ideally adapted for sampling luminal antigens and subsequent presentation to the immune system. In addition, the nonspecialized or surface enterocytes lining the intestine are also capable of processing and presenting antigens, although the relative importance of this phenomenon in health and disease has not been established. Finally, antigens that gain entry by a paracellular route can be presented to the mucosal immune system by macrophages and dendritic cells in the intestinal lamina propria. Once antigen engages the mucosal immune system, a complex sequence of events may lead to the induction of an immune response. Specific details are still under investigation. However, the events involved include: 1) the influence of unique regulatory cells within the intestinal lymphoid follicles; 2) the migration of committed immunoblasts to the mesenteric lymph node; 3) clonal expansion; 4) maturation; and 5) preferential homing to the mucosal site where the antigen was encountered and also to other mucosal tissues. The mature effector cells, which then police the mucosa, consist of two functionally distinct populations above (intraepithelial) and below the mucosal basement membrane (lamina propria).

Regulation of the mucosal immune response occurs at several levels, including: the role of cell surface recognition molecules of the major histocompatibility complex (MHC); "switch" cells, which influence the isotype of secretory immunoglobulin; antibody feedback circuits; and regulatory cells and lymphokines mediating helper/suppressor networks. Besides these apparently autonomous control mechanisms, convincing evidence suggests that the mucosal immune system is subject to neurocrine, paracrine, and endocrine modulation. Direct innervation of mucosa-associated lymphoid tissue has been demonstrated. In addition, enteric neuropeptides and certain hormones can alter the function of several effector cells *in vitro,* and may influence cellular traffic within and between mucosal tissues *in vivo.*

Communication between the neuroendocrine system and the immune system appears to be bidirectional. The intercellular messengers produced by the immune system, which may act on nerve terminals and other local structures, include not only interleukins and other cytokines but also neuropeptides. Intercellular peptide messengers probably occurred early in evolution and are well conserved. That the immune system and nervous system should share the same messengers is not surprising. Indeed, increasing awareness of the diversity and versatility of the secretory products of the mucosal immune system has extended our concepts of the potential role of the mucosal immune system in intestinal physiology and pathophysiology. The influence of the mucosal immune system on intestinal epithelial cell and smooth muscle function might be an important area to explore for future therapeutic interventions in inflammatory disorders.

The destructive potential of the immune system is reflected by the number of chronic diseases that have an immunolgic basis. In the liver and gastrointestinal tract, both the mucosal and systemic immune systems may participate in the pathogenesis of several important disorders. In some instances, such as atrophic gastritis or chronic active hepatitis, a cellular antigen has been identified as the target of an autoimmune reaction. In others, such as inflammatory bowel disease, the immune system may mediate tissue injury in a nonspecific manner with no specific cellular target being evident. In most cases, the fundamental immunoregulatory defect(s) has not been precisely determined.

Our concepts of the underlying mechanisms in immune-mediated disorders should be sufficiently broad to accommodate evidence for genetic predisposing factors and environmental triggers. Celiac disease is probably the clearest example of how genetic susceptibility may interact with environmental agents to trigger immune-mediated tissue damage. The interaction is a complex one; two genes are probably involved, and two environmental agents (dietary gluten and a virus) have been implicated. Similar interactions may be involved in the pathogenesis of chronic active hepatitis, in which identical patterns of tissue injury may be triggered in susceptible individuals by a variety of environmental agents including drugs and viruses. Although environmental agents are generally thought to trigger an abnormal immune response by inducing some alteration to a specific target cell, the possibility that the mucosal immune system itself might be the target of a viral infection deserves attention. The immunoregulatory disturbances associated with AIDS and the existence of more than one human immune deficiency virus should alert investigators to the possible existence of other viral infections that might be specific to the mucosal immune system.

Advances in the treatment of immunologically based diseases have lagged behind improvements in our understanding of their pathophysiology. However, some therapeutic success stories are already unfolding, one being the ultimate experiment in immunology — organ transplantation. While small bowel transplantation is still under experimental investigation, the clinical success of liver transplantation is well established. Other exciting therapeutic prospects include the exploitation of functional differences between the mucosal and the systemic immune systems in the design of tissue-selective immunosuppressive drugs and mucosal-specific monoclonal antibodies, modulation of the neuroendocrine-immune axis, and the utilization of homing patterns within the common mucosal immune system for the development of oral vaccines.

Advanced technology, particularly in cell culture systems, monoclonal antibodies, and molecular biology, coupled with the vigorous research efforts prompted by the AIDS epidemic, have focused new energy on the investigation of the mucosal and systemic immune systems. It is likely that the avalanche of information recently generated in relation to the immunology and immunopathology of the gut and liver will soon pay dividends in terms of novel and effective treatments for the chronic immune-mediated diseases that affect these organs.

CHAPTER 2

Current Concepts in Immunology: An Update

JOHN L. FAHEY

INTRODUCTION

The immune system includes five major systems, the CD4 (helper/inducer) T cells and CD8 (suppressor/cytotoxic) T cells, the B cells, the NK cells, and macrophages/monocytes. Each of these systems has its own characteristics and functions, but all interact in many important ways to produce normal immune functions. Characterization of the immune system proceeds both by reduction and by assembly. Comprehension of the specific mechanisms of immune response requires highly focused studies with reduction of variables to a minimum. On the other hand, operation of the system and maintenance of health in response to disease is an extraordinary, complex array of interactions that require understanding of the most important variables as well as imagination and skill in interpretation. Much of the understanding may fall into the realm of molecular immunology and the imagination and skill into clinical immunology. Cellular immunology certainly falls in between, as it uses both in vitro and in vivo studies designed to reduce complex or obscure issues to assessable levels as well as to synthesize molecular events into sequences in order to understand the complex operations of the immune system.

For the investigator involved in specific studies, progress almost always seems painfully slow, especially if the desire is to make a significant change in understanding mechanisms or developing new therapy for disease. In the larger perspective of the decade of the 1980s, however, the advances in immunology have been enormous. A substantial base has been developed for further advances.

A great deal of attention has been devoted to growth of molecular immunology, in which the resources and issues of immunology are combined with the technology

5

and concepts of molecular biology. Parallel advances in cellular immunology have occurred with the introduction of mice with severe combined immunodeficiency (SCID), which allows introduction of human immune progenitor cells, making possible in vivo investigation of development of specific components of the immune system. Tissue culture systems that parallel many aspects of complex in vivo systems are particularly valuable in studies of growth and differentiation factors, their receptors, and the changes induced in individual cells. Developments in monoclonal antibodies, flow cytometry, and related technology have permitted better definition of functionally distinct lineages and separate stages of maturation and activation. The lengthening, complex, and arbitrary CD nomenclature for human phenotypes/antigens, provides concensus and neutral terminology. However, reagents that use numbers different from CD numbers or lab slang letter-number jumbles do present obstacles to the investigator with other major interests.

FUNDAMENTAL STRUCTURES AND GENES

Advances of the past decade have been cogently summarized by Nossal.[1] Similarities and differences between T cells and antibodies in binding antigens have been elucidated. Antigen presentation and the nature of the antigens recognized by T cells have been found to differ. T cells can react with short sequences of peptide (including those resulting from processing of native molecules) that may not normally be available for recognition by antibody.

The T-cell receptor has been defined as a heterodimer. These peptide chains are defined by V-D-J translocations in genes that are ultimately transcribed in individual mature T cells. The T-cell response is not accompanied by affinity maturation, which is a prominent feature of B-cell response to continuing antigen exposure. Furthermore, T-cell recognition takes place with a relatively low binding affinity, requiring stabilization by associated corecognition molecules, such as CD4 or CD8.

Antigen presentation, in conjunction with major histocompatibility complex (MHC) class II molecules, has been particularly important in understanding how the T-cell receptor "sees" each antigen. The interaction between antigen and MHC class II occurs at a slow association rate but also has a very low dissociation rate. Thus the MHC molecules on cell surfaces may normally be partially occupied by peptides that are self-derived or formed by enzymatic cleavage.[1]

Molecular research is detailing the splice mechanisms underlying unique translocational events leading to specific gene selection and expression. Somatic generation of antibody and T-cell receptor diversity and the programmed appearance of V-gene families in ontogeny allow for generation of a huge recognition repertoire.

The nature of the relevant regulatory DNA-binding proteins and of promoters and enhancers (and suppressors) of immune cell gene transcription and the function of nuclear proto-oncogenes such as C-myc that are transcribed during immune induction are foci of current research.

Finally, the processes of maturation in both the B- and T-cell systems, the mechanisms of proliferation and activation of distinct lymphoid cell categories, and the lymphokines and cytokines and their receptors effecting immunoregulation have been redefined.

LYMPHOKINES, CYTOKINES, AND GROWTH FACTORS

Lymphokine, cytokine, and growth factor research has expanded rapidly, and terminology that was appropriate initially may not now fit the larger emerging concepts. For example, some of the lymphokines, such as interleukin-2 (IL-2), do seem to act almost entirely within the immune system. Others, such as IL-1 and IL-6, come from and act on many different tissues. Within the context of the immune system, however, these soluble factors are tremendously important in guiding and modulating immune system development and activation.[2]

The sequential effects of individual factors at different stages of the response cascade generally are explained as a sequence of activation factors, growth factors, differentiation factors, and isotype switching factors. Although IL-1, IL-2, IL-4, IL-5, IL-6, and gamma-interferon can guide specific events, evidence is accumulating that the effect of a particular factor depends on which factors have acted before in the sequence.

Lymphoid cell signaling mechanisms can be viewed as transmembrane, cytoplasmic, and nuclear gene events. Calcium mobilization and activation of protein kinases and of phosphatidyl inositol metabolic pathways in response to antigenic stimulation are beginning to form an outline of intracellular events in the sequence of signal systems between the cell surface and cytoplasmic changes and gene response.

NATURAL KILLER CELLS

Natural killer (NK) cells are CD3$^-$, T-cell receptor (alpha, beta, gamma, delta)-negative, large granular lymphocytes. They commonly express certain cell surface markers, such as CD16 (Leu11) and NKH-1 (Leu19). They mediate cytolytic reactions that do not require expression of class I or class II MHC molecules on the target cells.[3]

A separate population of T lymphocytes that are either alpha, beta-positive or gamma, delta-positive may express, particularly upon activation, cytolytic activity that resembles that of NK cells. These T lymphocytes should not be termed NK cells. They should be termed either T lymphocytes displaying "NK-like" activity or "non-MHC-requiring" cytolytic T cells.

Lymphokine-activated killer cells (LAK) are IL-2-activated lymphocytes in either of the two above categories. The relative contribution of the respective cell type depends on the source of lymphocytes and conditions for activation. For instance, lymphocytes from peripheral blood or spleen will produce LAK cells predominantly from NK cells.[2]

The cytolytic reaction, which is a distinctive feature of the NK population, may occur because of a variety of receptor-ligand systems, rather than a specific receptor-ligand interaction. This functional heterogeneity is evident for both tumor target cells and virus-infected cells. A role for NK cells in protection against viral infections has been supported by observations by Biron et al.[3] of a young woman with complete NK cell deficiency with normal T- and B-cell responses who suffered repeated *Varicella* virus infection and severe cytomegalovirus infection. Other roles for NK cells have related to regulation of hematopoiesis and B-cell activation.

NK cells and LAK cells are being employed in clinical cancer immunotherapy trials in conjunction with simultaneous IL-2 infusions to maintain the in vivo activation and proliferation of these cells. Intravenous or transfused LAK cells, however, do not appear to localize in the tumors, suggesting that direct lysis by cell-cell interaction is unlikely and indicate some caution in direct extrapolation of in vitro observations to in vivo applications.

The NK cells are an interesting population of cells with powerful potential for therapeutic applications. Interestingly, NK cells have been shown to respond to IL-3 and IL-4, as well as to IL-2. The former two lymphokines apparently have an additive effect to that of IL-2. The NK cells present many questions for biologic, genetic, and molecular definitions, including identification of their stem cells and their full role in the normal balance of immune response.

NEURO- AND BEHAVIORAL IMMUNOLOGY

A relatively new scientific area that impinges on all of immunology, and especially the gastrointestinal tract, is variously called psychoneuroimmunology or neurobehavioral immunology. Interactions between the central nervous system and the immune system are being identified and additional questions being posed about the immunologic effects of psychological factors and personality. The issues of concern are in both directions, e.g., of the psyche and nervous system on the immune system and, in the other direction, the influence of the immune system on the CNS and the psychological state. Direct nerve distribution into lymphoid organs has been identified, and receptors for neuropeptides exist on lymphocytes.[4] Thus the potential exists for nervous system modulation of immune function.

Neural cells have receptors for lymphokines, and lymphocytes have been shown to be able, under some circumstances, to generate ACTH and beta-endorphin. Interesting preliminary data has already been obtained indicating that lymphokines (especially IL-1) produced by the immune system have an impact on the central nervous system.[4] The circumstances under which immune activation contributes to or alters CNS activity need to be better defined.

The biologic and pathologic significance of immune alterations identified with neurologic factors or psychological states are hard to assess.[5] The fact is that occurrence of infection or neoplasia is clinically demonstrated to occur only when there is drastic impairment of the immune system, as in primary or acquired immune deficiency diseases or in certain advanced neoplasia, or following immunosuppressive chemical or radiation therapy. Smaller immune changes for the most part are not associated with readily evident pathology. Immunologic methods may not be sensitive and reproducible enough to define the lesser changes that have significance in relation to disease. Also, clinical and animal studies could be refined to provide clearer evidence of the effects of lesser immune changes. Alternatively, small or moderate changes in immune function may not be relevant to disease. Indeed, changes in lymphocyte number occurring during diurnal variation (e.g., as much as 30–40% from the maximum or minimal level) is greater than most of the changes reported to occur in psychological disorders, such as depression. Too often elevation in an immune parameter is equated with better health and reduction with worse. Until the significance of such shifts associated with nervous system or psychological states are defined, however, it is much better just to describe the direction of the change without judgmental interpretations.

As the dynamics of the immune system and its interaction with other systems come to be appreciated, a better understanding of relationships between the nervous system, the immune system, and psychological factors can be better established.

CLINICAL IMMUNOLOGY: NEW THERAPIES

Identification of specific lymphokines and cytokines and the ability to produce them in quantity by recombinant technology have revolutionized the possibilities for immune therapies. Some of these possibilities will certainly be realized. Some advances will arrive in studies that are entirely rational, stepwise efforts as well as by other approaches that are more empiric. A balance between both approaches is, by and large, achieved in modern biomedical science. Single-agent intervention may be sufficient in a few situations, but combinations of agents are beginning to be evaluated. Furthermore, treatments may be targeted to specific sites by antibodies or smaller antigen recognition units.

Immune suppression advanced considerably with the introduction of agents that are active only when present at sufficient levels in body fluids. Cyclosporine is such a metabolic inhibitor of T-cell function: it interferes with the production of and response to interleukin-2. As a consequence, immunosuppression can be induced quickly and, also, immunosuppression terminated rapidly after cessation of administration. The timing of these effects contrasts, of course, with cytotoxic suppressive agents, which take some time to become effective and which have considerable persistence after stopping administration.

Clinical immunology involves understanding the normal functions of the immune system and the disorders occurring in disease and contributing to disease, as well as efforts at therapy. Thus clinical immunology is an exciting and challenging field of biology and medicine. Frustration, however, can occur with the long time and many failures that occur in bringing observations in fundamental immunology to practical benefit. The resolution of clinical immunology issues in molecular and cell biology terms is inherently difficult. One is the increasing complexity of the relevant systems as research moves from molecular to cellular to clinical. Molecular and biochemical evaluations of immunologic events are often defined in seconds and minutes. Effects revealed by cellular immunology techniques usually need hours and days. Clinical and disease effects may require days or weeks to be manifest. Linking events described in one context with events occurring in another presents major challenges to investigators. Understanding some of the problems, however, should help to shape effective studies as well as interpretation of immunologic research findings.

REFERENCES

1. Nossal GJV: Triumphs and trials of immunology in the 1980s. *Immunol Today* 9:286–91, 1988.

2. Klaus GGB: Lymphocyte receptors, signals and cytokines. *Immunol Today* 9:157–59, 1988.

3. Hercend T, Schmidt RE: Characteristics and uses of natural killer cells. *Immunol Today* 9:291–93, 1988.

4. Blalock JE: A molecular basis for bidirectional communication between the immune system and neuroendocrine systems. *Physiol Rev* 69:1–32, 1989.

5. Cohen JJ: Methodological issues in behavioral immunology. *Immunol Today* 8:33–34, 1987.

SECTION **A**

IMMUNOLOGY OF THE MUCOSAL IMMUNE SYSTEM

PART **ONE**

THE AFFERENT LIMB OF THE MUCOSAL IMMUNE SYSTEM

CHAPTER 3

Role of the Intestinal Mucosal Barrier and Antigen Uptake

GARY J. RUSSELL

W. ALLAN WALKER

INTRODUCTION

The gastrointestinal tract provides an important barrier that facilitates the absorption of necessary nutrients and excludes the penetration and uptake of microorganisms, toxins, and potentially harmful antigens. Small quantities of antigenic, intact macromolecules can be absorbed by normal intestinal mucosa and enter the systemic circulation without apparent adverse effects.[1] Maturational changes occur in the mucosal barrier that allow an increased absorption of antigenic material in the immature intestine of neonates and infants. The uptake of these macromolecules is immunologically significant and may play a role in the pathogenesis of several gastrointestinal diseases such as milk protein-induced enteropathy, celiac disease, necrotizing enterocolitis, and inflammatory bowel disease.

Research has increasingly focused on the mechanisms of intraluminal handling of antigens, the route of antigen uptake, and the role of the mucosal immune system in excluding or tolerating absorbed antigens. Additionally, there have been extensive efforts to understand the physiologic and biochemical changes that occur with mucosal maturation and how these changes relate to the uptake or exclusion of antigenic macromolecules. Knowledge of the mechanisms promoting the maturation of the mucosal barrier and prevention of antigenic macromolecular uptake might be of considerable importance in the management of certain gastrointestinal disease states.

The mechanisms of intestinal antigen uptake will be reviewed, with an emphasis on the maturational changes occurring in the developing mammalian intestine that may effect the permeability of the intestinal mucosa.

THE MUCOSAL BARRIER

The collective effects of nonimmunologic factors functioning independently or in conjunction with immunologic mechanisms to prevent the adherence and uptake of pathogens and macromolecules comprise the mucosal barrier (Table 3–1). The functional integrity of this barrier changes during maturation and in response to ingested material. Several of the nonimmunologic factors such as the bacteriocidal or bacteriostatic effect of gastric acidity, the proteolysis of large macromolecules by pancreatic enzymes, and the clearing effect of gastrointestinal peristalsis have previously been reviewed.[2,3]

Mucous Coat

The mucous coat provides a mechanical barrier against the penetration of microorganisms to the epithelial surface and may act as a vehicle to eliminate trapped microorganisms from the gastrointestinal tract. The release of mucus from goblet cells increases after exposure to antigen-antibody complexes, thus providing a thicker protective barrier.[4,5] This viscous coat contains highly glycosylated mucin glycoproteins that may be capable of interacting with microorganisms or toxins, thus preventing their attachment to the epithelial surface.[2,6] Furthermore, the mucous coat may function as a binding matrix for secretory immunoglobulins, enhancing their effectiveness by preventing rapid loss by normal peristalsis (Fig. 3–1). Maturational changes have been observed in the carbohydrate composition of purified mucous glycoproteins from rat small intestine in which a smaller amount of total carbohydrate, and less fucose and N-acetylgalactosamine was found in newborn rat mucin.[7]

The concept that the glycoconjugate composition of mucin is important for normal mucosal function is supported by the finding that specific alterations in mucin glycoproteins occur in association with ulcerative colitis.[8-10] Although the mucous coat may afford protection by entrapment of particles in a viscous blanket or by competitive binding at specific carbohydrate binding sites, a possible role in the pathogenesis of intestinal disease states is still speculative at this time.

Table 3 – 1   COMPONENTS OF THE MUSCOSAL BARRIER

Nonimmunologic
  Intraluminal
    Gastric acid
    Pancreatic proteases
    Peristalsis
  Mucosal surface
    Mucous coat
    Enterocyte membrane integrity
    Epithelial tight junctions
Immunologic
  Secretory IgA system

FACTORS IMPORTANT IN MUCUS FUNCTION

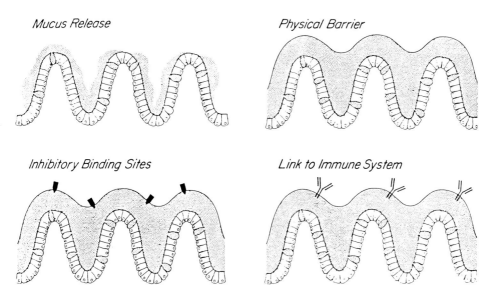

Figure 3 – 1 Four proposed mechanisms for mucous protection: rate and quantity of mucous release, viscous blanket (physical barrier), competitive binding sites, and link to the mucosal immune system. (From Snyder JD, et al: Structure and function of intestinal mucin: developmental aspects. *Int Arch Allergy Appl Immunuol* 82:351 – 356, 1987, with permission)

Membrane Composition

The apical membrane of intestinal epithelial cells is the site of most macromolecular uptake and attachment of potentially pathogenic microorganisms. Various glycoproteins on microvillus membranes are considered to be important mediators in the attachment and absorption of intraluminal substances. For example, it has been shown that *Escherichia coli* binds to mannose carbohydrate moieties of microvillus glycoproteins,[11] and fucose is the carbohydrate moiety necessary for *Vibrio cholerae* attachment.[12] Table 3 – 2 lists known associations between bacteria and toxins and their respective receptor glycoconjugates.

Table 3 – 2 BACTERIAL/TOXIN RECEPTORS OF THE INTESTINAL SURFACE

Bacteria/toxin	Carbohydrate receptor
Escherichia coli	Mannose
Vibrio cholerae	Fucose
Clostridium toxin	N-acetylgalactosamine
Shigella toxin	N-acetylglucosamine

Maturation of intestinal epithelial cell membrane occurs as the cell migrates from the crypt to the villus[13-15] and corresponds to the expression of various brush border enzymes such as sucrase-isomaltase, lactase, maltase, and alkaline phosphatase. Studies using monoclonal antibodies that identify specific cell surface components on rat intestinal epithelial cells indicate that there is a gradual change in the expression of certain cell surface epitopes as undifferentiated crypt cells mature into differentiated mature absorptive cells.[16]

Differences in membrane composition and microvillus enzyme expression are found in newborn animals, compared with adult microvillus membranes. Microvillus membrane preparations from newborn rabbits have a higher lipid-to-protein ratio and a more fluid and disorganized structure compared with those of adults.[17] The increased microvillus membrane content of lipid is also present in the newborn rat; however, there is no significant difference in the molar ratio of cholesterol to phospholipid between newborn and adult microvillus membrane.[18] Additionally, the microvillus membrane phospholipid composition shows age-related differences, with an increase in phosphatidylcholine and a decrease in phosphatidylethanolamine in newborn intestine as compared with adults. An increase in the fluidity of newborn microvillus membranes may more readily allow invagination of the membrane by macromolecules, thus facilitating increased macromolecular absorption.

Binding studies utilizing lectins have also demonstrated maturational changes in the carbohydrate moieties of glycoconjugates within the microvillus membrane. *Ulex europaeus* (fucose-specific) and concavalin (mannose- and glucose-specific) bind significantly more to microvillus membrane preparations from adult rats, and *Triticum vulgaris* (glucosamine- and sialic acid-specific) binds more to newborn microvillus membranes.[19] The differences found in the incorporation of these carbohydrates onto membrane lipids and proteins during glycosylation are due to maturational changes in the amount of specific glycosyltransferases within the enterocytes.[20] Thus a decrease in sialyltransferase activity and an increase in fucosyltransferase activity is responsible for a shift from sialylation to fucosylation during weaning (Fig. 3–2). Furthermore, these maturational changes can be induced to occur in preweanling animals by cortisone treatment.[20] As mentioned earlier, intestinal binding of some microorganisms is dependent on specific carbohydrate moieties. The maturational changes in glycosylation may be important in forming receptors for certain hormones and growth factors necessary for intestinal epithelial cell differentiation or for the colonization of luminal pathogens.[21]

Immune-Mediated Exclusion

Immunoglobulins present in the intestinal secretions are primarily derived from plasma cells in the lamina propria[22] and prevent the attachment and absorption of various microorganisms and antigens. Antibody coating of bacteria can prevent binding to epithelial cell surfaces[23,24] and intraluminal antigen-antibody complexes are capable of inducing mucous secretion by goblet cells.[6,25]

Quantitatively, the amount of IgA in secretions is significantly less than in serum, but it is the predominant immunoglobulin in secretions, due to a proportionally low level of IgG. At least 95% of the IgA in the gastrointestinal fluid is in the form of secretory IgA (SIgA) consisting of a J chain and a secretory component bound to dimeric IgA of both IgA_1 and IgA_2 subclasses.

GLYCOPROTEIN COMPOSITION OF MICROVILLUS MEMBRANE
(CARBOHYDRATE SIDE CHAIN)

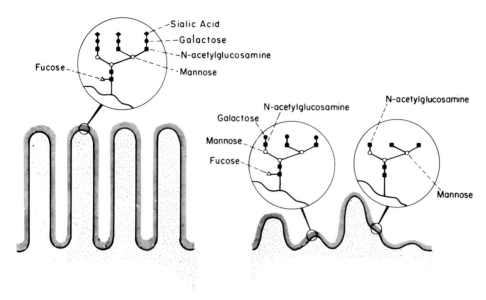

Figure 3 – 2 Diagrammatic representation of glycosylation of microvillus membrane glycoproteins and glycolipids in mature and immature animals. The addition of sugars to these molecules differs developmentally in the mature and immature animal and may explain the differences in binding of antigens and toxins to the intestinal surface. (From Israel EJ, et al: Development of intestinal mucosal barrier function to antigens and bacterial toxins. *Adv Exp Med Biol* 216A:673–784, 1987, with permission)

Plasma cells in the intestinal mucosa are predominantly dimeric IgA-secreting cells and differ from IgA-producing cells in the spleen, lymph node, and tonsil, which secrete IgA primarily in the monomeric form. Within the mucosal plasma cell, dimeric IgA is incorporated with a J-chain protein, which is also synthesized by the plasma cell. After secretion from the plasma cell, the dimeric IgA attaches to a receptor on the basolateral membrane of secretory epithelial cells and is endocytosed. The receptor molecule is then cleaved; the fragment remaining covalently bound to the immunoglobulin is the secretory component. The SIgA is transported across the epithelial cell apical membrane and released into the external environment. Immunoglobulin A that is bound to secretory component is more resistant to proteolytic degradation than monomeric IgA and thus can remain effective in bacterial agglutination[23,24] and neutralizing viruses[26] while in the intestinal lumen.

Direct evidence that the presence of immunoglobulins in intestinal secretions can prevent the attachment and uptake of pathologically significant amounts of antigens in humans is still lacking. The concentration of IgA in saliva, stool, and serum of newborn animals and humans is decreased; thus it has been hypothesized that this transient deficiency may in part be responsible for an increased transport of antigens and presumably bacterial attachment to the newborn intestinal mucosa.[27-31]

This hypothesis is supported by studies of patients with selective IgA deficiency. These patients have circulating immune complexes and precipitating antibodies to absorbed bovine milk proteins.[32] When the serum of IgA-deficient individuals was studied for the appearance of complexes after milk ingestion, three of seven subjects had increases in antibody-antigen complexes that peaked at 120–150 min.[33] In another three subjects there was a tendency toward the formation of two peak concentrations of complexes, the first at 30–60 min and the second at 120–150 min after drinking milk. Additionally, the circulating immune complexes found in some patients contained bovine milk proteins. Presumably the same process occurs in the transient IgA deficiency of the newborn, providing at least a partial explanation for an increase in antigen uptake and bacterial invasion in newborns and infants. This may also be a contributing factor in the development of necrotizing enterocolitis, a bacterial invasive disease occurring during infancy and in the increased incidence of microbial infection (giardiasis, toxogenic diarrhea) in selective IgA-deficient individuals.

Recently, further supportive evidence that intraluminal antibodies are protective against the development of necrotizing enterocolitis in low-birth-weight infants has been reported.[34] Low-birth-weight infants for whom breast milk was unavailable were randomized to evaluate the efficacy of an oral immunoglobulin preparation in the prevention of necrotizing enterocolitis. None of the 88 infants who received oral immunoglobulin supplementation with feedings developed necrotizing enterocolitis, compared with 6 of the 91 infants in the control group. The oral immunoglobulin preparation was predominantly monomeric IgA; however, significantly increased levels of IgA were recovered in the stool samples of the treated infants, which may indicate that less proteolysis of intraluminal monomeric IgA occurred in the newborns. Thus immunoglobulins provided as an oral supplement or in breast milk may be a protective factor in the prevention of bacterial invasion and development of necrotizing enterocolitis in susceptable infants.

ANTIGEN UPTAKE BY IMMATURE INTESTINE

Increased neonatal intestinal transport of intact macromolecules has been demonstrated in several animal species by measuring serum levels of radiolabeled fed proteins.[35,36] In neonatal rabbits starved for 72 hr, the amount of immunoreactive bovine serum albumin (BSA) measured in the rabbit serum following BSA feeding was significantly greater compared with controls.[37] This finding would suggest that even mild mucosal injury to the neonatal intestine may have a significant effect on mucosal barrier function.

Clinical studies on human infants have shown similar results.[38-41] Rothberg[38] found measurable quantities of BSA in the serum of premature infants following a feeding of this protein, but BSA was not detected in older children fed an equivalent amount of the protein. Similarly, Roberton[40] reported higher serum B-lactoglobulin concentrations in preterm infants fed a cow's milk-based formula than in term neonates fed similar amounts of the formula. Furthermore, children with intestinal worm infestation were found to have significantly greater serum concentrations of ovalbumin 30 min after a test meal of two eggs than that found after antihelminthic therapy.[41]

These studies indicate that immature or injured intestine has a less effective mucosal barrier than mature intestine and that it allows the passage of intact intraluminal macromolecules into the systemic circulation. The intestinal uptake of food protein antigens can be immunogenic. Eastham et al.[39] reported a larger percentage of infants under 3 months of age with serum antibodies to food antigens than the percentage of infants exposed to the tested antigen after 3 months.

Concept of Closure

The maturation of the mucosal barrier depends on the development of immunologic and nonimmunologic mechanisms to prevent microorganisms and macromolecules from reaching the epithelial surface as well. An effective mucosal barrier is also affected by the functional maturation of the intestinal epithelial cells. When these maturational changes occur, the intestinal uptake of macromolecules decreases and is referred to as "closure".[42] In rodents, closure occurs during weaning at around 20 days of age and corresponds to the loss of Fc receptors on the enterocytes (which facilitate colostral immunoglobulin uptake), the loss of the brush border lactase disaccharidase, and the emergence of brush border sucrase activity.

The time at which closure occurs in humans is less clear. Human milk contains specific growth factors and hormones that potentially play a role in intestinal maturation.[43,44] Immunoglobulins present in human milk may be protective to the neonate but have not been considered to be a source of passive immunity such as that described in ruminants and rodents. A more complete characterization of the maturational effect on neonatal intestinal development of breast milk components such as epidermal growth factor and somatomedin-C will be important to our understanding of antigen handling and closure in the human infant.

ANTIGEN UPTAKE BY MATURE ENTEROCYTES

Small but detectable amounts of potentially antigenic dietary macromolecules can gain access to the systemic circulation in normal adult animals and humans without deleterious effect.[1,45] The uptake of potentially harmful substances is increased in the newborn period and when an alteration in the mucosal integrity exists.[41] Several routes of intestinal uptake have been described for different macromolecules, toxins, and microorganisms. The route of molecular uptake often depends on size, surface charge, or the presence of specific receptors or glycoconjugates on the membrane surface.

Intestinal epithelial cells form tight junctions at their apical membranes, creating an effective barrier against intercellular uptake of intraluminal macromolecules. This does not appear to be an absolute barrier to the passage of macromolecules, since small amounts of serum proteins are normally present in the intestinal lumen of adults.[46] In certain conditions, such as intestinal anaphylaxis, a route for intestinal antigen uptake may thus be provided. This hypothesis has been supported by demonstrating that there is an increased uptake of BSA, a bystander antigen, in rats with intestinal anaphylaxis locally induced by egg albumin.[47] Although it was not proved that BSA uptake was by the paracellular route, such a pathway was suggested by the presence of intravenously injected radiolabeled rat albumin in the intestinal lumen. More recently, Phillips et al.[48] convincingly demonstrated that macromolecular uptake can occur through epithelial tight junctions during cholinergic stimulation. In these studies, horseradish peroxidase was found to pass through the tight junctions of crypt epithelial cells, with no changes observed in the crypt junctional strand network. Increased permeability did not occur in the villus epithelium. This route of antigen uptake may be most important during states of mucosal injury or inflammation.

A second route by which intraluminal antigens may cross the intestinal epithelial barrier is through the exclusion zone at the villus tip. As epithelial cells mature, they migrate from the crypt to the villus and are shed from the tip of the villus, leaving a gap between terminal epithelial cells.[49] The uptake of carageenan and particulate dietary components into rat villi has been reported to occur by this route.[49,50]

The absorptive epithelial cells of the intestine are highly specialized cells that absorb, sort, transport, and digest macromolecules (Fig. 3–3). Nonselective uptake of molecules occurs by fluid phase endocytosis or pinocytosis which are transported in smooth membrane vesicles. Selective uptake occurs when a sufficient concentration of macromolecules adhere to the surface membrane, either by receptor-mediated binding or by adherence to glycoconjugates, causing invagination and the formation of a vesicle. Clathrin-coated pits located at the bases of microvilli are the

ANTIGEN BINDING AND UPTAKE IN THE IMMATURE INTESTINE

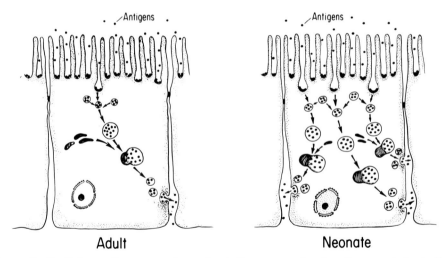

Adult   Neonate

Figure 3–3 Schematic comparison of relative amounts of antigen uptake in the adult and neonatal intestine. Molecules adherent to the surface membrane in pits between microvilli are endocytosed and transported intracellularly in vesicles that fuse with lysosomes to form phagolysosomes in which digestion occurs. The vesicles then fuse with the basolateral membrane, and the contents are released into the intercellular space by exocytosis.

usual sites for absorption. The vesicles are transported intracellularly to the supranuclear region, where they fuse with lysosomes, forming phagolysomes in which digestion occurs. Although soluble and membrane-bound macromolecules may be endocytosed simultaneously, the molecules are sorted prior to entering the tubulocisternae system and are then transported to the lysosome via separate intracellular routes.[51] The phagolysosomes migrate to the basal membrane, fuse, and release the vesicle contents into the intercellular space. Molecules that are endocytosed by receptor mediation often escape digestion by lysosomes and are released into the intercellular space intact. This has been shown to be a mechanism for providing passive immunity in neonatal rats, in which immunoglobulins from breast milk are absorbed by the intestine and enter the systemic circulation without lysosomal degredation.[52,53]

A recent report,[54] suggests that enterocytes can express class II (Ia) antigens on their basolateral surface in the postweanling state and under conditions of inflammation and that the release of mediators (interferon-γ) in the small intestine and colon may express the class II antigen on the microvillus surface. The role of class II antigen expression in antigen presentation from the gut to the mucosal lymphocyte and the role of the enterocyte as a possible antigen-presenting cell remain to be determined.

ABSORPTION BY SPECIALIZED EPITHELIAL CELLS

Peyer's patches in the intestinal mucosa are covered by a dome of epithelial cells comprised of absorptive cells and membranous epithelial cells that specialize in the absorption and transport of microorganisms, viruses, and antigens to the underlying lymphocytes and macrophages. These cells were initially characterized by the presence of luminal surface microfolds rather than microvilli[55] and thus were termed "M" for microfold cells. When microvilli were observed on these cells, the name persisted and now refers to "membranous" epithelial cells because of the very thin rim of cytoplasm, only $0.1-0.3$ μm thick, separating the intestinal lumen from the lymphoid cells below.[56,57] M cells form tight junctions with adjacent epithelial cells, thus maintaining the integrity of the intestinal epithelium. The origin of M cells remains unclear. It was first thought that they developed from mature absorptive cells[58,59]; however, more recent evidence suggests that they are derived from undifferentiated crypt cells and that this differentiation occurs via transitional cells, termed immature-appearing M cells.[60]

The absorption and intracellular transport of antigen by M cells was first demonstrated using horseradish peroxidase (HRP) that was injected into the intestinal lumen of mice[56] (Fig. 3–4). After 1 min, HRP adhered to the surfaces of columnar cells and M cells, and after 5 min HRP was found in cytoplasmic vesicles of M cells, but not in the columnar cells. After 1 hr, HRP was present in the extracellular space and the vesicles within the adjacent lymphocytes, thus providing evidence for direct antigen uptake from the intestinal lumen and delivery to the lymphoid system. Subsequently, investigators have shown that M cells are capable of endocytosing and transporting bacteria, viruses, and the protozoan *Cryptosporidium*.[61–63]

The apical membrane of M cells differs from surrounding columnar cells in other ways, besides the microvillus arrangement. M-cell apical membranes have less

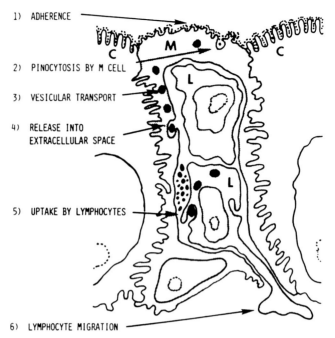

1) ADHERENCE

2) PINOCYTOSIS BY M CELL

3) VESICULAR TRANSPORT

4) RELEASE INTO
   EXTRACELLULAR SPACE

5) UPTAKE BY LYMPHOCYTES

6) LYMPHOCYTE MIGRATION

Figure 3–4 Diagram summarizing the stages observed in the transport of horserad-ish peroxidase by the M cell from the intestinal lumen to the intraepithelial lympho-cyte (columnar cells, C; lymphocytes, L). (From Owen RL: Sequential uptake of horse-radish peroxidase by lymphoid follicle epithelium of Peyer's patches in the normal unobstructed mouse intestine: an ultrastructural study. *Gastroenterology* 72:440–451, 1977, with permission)

alkaline phosphatase and more esterase activity than absorptive cells.[64] They also have an abundance of cholesterol, except in endocytotic pits, demonstrated by filipin-induced membrane lesions in thin-section and freeze-fracture replicas.[65] Reovirus type 1 preferentially adheres to the surface of M cells and is then endocy-tosed by the cell, traverses the cytoplasm in vesicles, and is released into the extracellular space.[61] The binding of reovirus type 1 to M-cell apical membrane appears to be specific, since none were found on the luminal surface of goblet cells. They were only occasionally found adjacent to the luminal surface of absorptive cells[61] and were never observed in the absorptive cell cytoplasm.[66]

The possibility that M cells possess specific surface adherence molecules that can be recognized by the reovirus type 1 is suggested by the observation that type 3 reovirus adheres to and is endocytosed by absorptive cells as well as M cells.[66] The ability of reovirus type 3 to adhere to and be endocytosed by absorptive cells has been shown to be determined by $\sigma 1$ viral hemagglutinin protein; thus adherence and transcellular transport of reovirus by M cells appears to be independent of viral surface proteins.[66]

Selectivity of antigen or microorganism attachment and uptake by absorptive cells and M cells may be facilitated by specific membrane receptors or glycopro-teins. The presence of membrane-associated glycoconjugates has been demon-strated by the binding of various lectins to the luminal surface of M cells.[64,67]

Recent studies by Neutra et al.[67] have shown that ferritin conjugated to wheat germ agglutinin and *Ricinus communis* agglutinin I and II applied to living rabbit Peyer's patches bind more avidly to M cells than the surrounding absorptive cells. These findings indicate that rabbit M cells display terminal galactose and perhaps N-acetylgalactosamine residues as well as sialic acid and/or N-acetylglucosamine

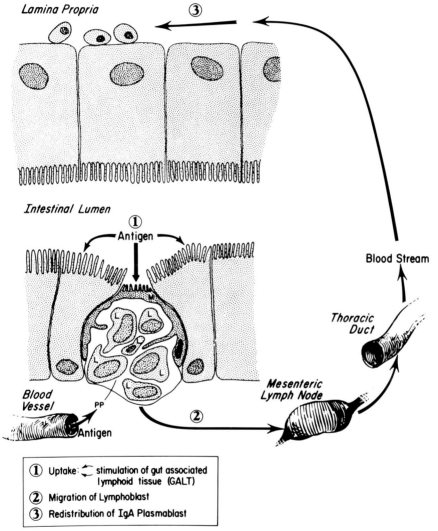

Figure 3–5 Diagram representing the migration and localization of mucosal lymphocytes after antigenic stimulation. Lymphocytes within the gut-associated lymphoid tissue are stimulated by intraluminal antigens (1) via M cells, absorptive cells or by antigens reaching the lymphoid tissue by the systemic circulation. Lymphoblasts migrate to mesenteric lymph nodes (2) and after further maturation, enter the systemic circulation and return to the mucosa (3) residing in the lamina propria as plasma cells secreting IgA in response to absorbed antigens. (From Walker WA, et al: Uptake and transport of macromolecules by the intestine: possible role in clinical disorders. *Gastroenterology* 67:531–550, 1974, with permission)

residues that are available in vivo for binding of luminal lectins. Additionally, it was shown that cationized ferritin and lectin-ferritin conjugates are endocytosed via deep clathrin-coated pits and transported in a complex system of tubulocisternae and clear vesicles. Furthermore, the transport of these adherence molecules was 50 times greater than that of soluble tracer bovine serum albumin-gold conjugate.[67]

Peyer's patches are the site of origin of antigen-specific antibody-containing cells in the lamina propria.[68] B lymphoblasts (and T lymphoblasts) arise from Peyer's patches after antigenic stimulation and migrate to mesenteric lymph nodes, thoracic duct lymph, and then to the blood before localizing to the intestinal mucosa.[69-71] Evidence currently suggests that the M cells overlying these Peyer's patches play an important role in facilitating the uptake of certain macromolecules and microorganisms and transporting these antigens to the closely associated lymphocytes and macrophages (Fig. 3–5). Further research is necessary to determine whether specific receptors are also present on the apical membrane of M cells that would enhance selective antigenic endocytosis and transport.

CURRENT RESEARCH ON MUCOSAL BARRIER FUNCTION AND ANTIGEN UPTAKE

Most of our knowledge regarding the maturation of the intestinal mucosal barrier has been gained from animal models. It has become clear that maturational changes occur in intraluminal proteolysis of foreign proteins, mucous composition, and glycosylation of enterocyte surface proteins. These factors are at least partially responsible for the increased intestinal uptake of antigens in the newborn animal. Modulation of these maturational events has been observed in rodents after treatment with cortisone, thyroxine, and epidermal growth factor.[20,71-74]

In order to better understand the *human* host defense mechanisms, investigations are now being extended to study intestinal microvillus membranes from human fetuses, infants, and adults. The activity of key glycosyltransferases in the enterocyte are essential for the incorporation of specific carbohydrate moieties on cell surface proteins that are necessary for the attachment of certain pathogenic microorganisms. These studies will be useful in determining the susceptibility of neonates and infants to infectious gastroenteritis caused by organisms such as *E. coli* and the lack of disease caused by shigellosis and *Clostridium difficile* in neonates. Preliminary studies by Israel et al.[75] have demonstrated the presence of a receptor for IgG on the surface of human fetal intestinal microvillus membranes. This observation suggests that in addition to the transplacental route of transport, an additional means of acquiring passive immunity is present in human fetuses.

Organ culture techniques have been used to study antigen uptake by normal and diseased human intestinal explants, modulation of fetal intestinal hydrolase activity and DNA synthesis.[76-78] In addition, human fetal intestine has been successfully transplanted subcutaneously into congenitally athymic mice and has been shown to have the morphologic and brush border disaccharidase characteristics of mature small intestine.[78] These experimental models utilizing human intestinal tissue are being used to evaluate the maturational effects of hormones and growth factors that have been identified in human milk. These studies may explain the observation by Bauer et al.[79] that antenatal administration of corticosteroids to

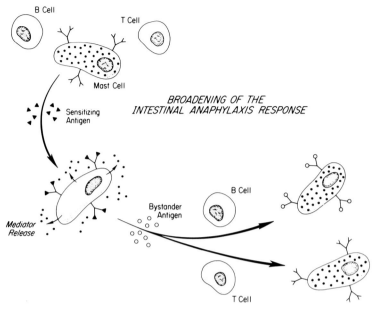

B Cell

T Cell

Mast Cell

BROADENING OF THE
INTESTINAL ANAPHYLAXIS RESPONSE

Sensitizing
Antigen

B Cell

Bystander
Antigen

Mediator
Release

T Cell

Figure 3 – 6   This diagram depicts the concept of broadening of the intestinal anaphylaxis response to include bystander antigen. When animals are rendered sensitive
to a specific allergen through T- and B-cell-mediated processes, IgE-bound mast cells
appear in the intestinal mucosa. Upon oral challenge with the sensitizing antigen,
IgE-allergen complexes on mucosal mast cells trigger the clinical manifestations of
intestinal anaphylaxis. Bystander antigens present in the lumen under these conditions cross the mucosal barrier and result in an additional IgE-mediated allergic response to this antigen, thus broadening the intestinal allergic response to include
additional antigens.

women at risk for delivering prematurely, significantly reduced the incidence of
necrotizing enterocolitis in the infants treated with steroids.

In recent work completed by Kleinman and Block, using an animal model for
intestinal anaphylaxis,[80] it was noted that IgE-sensitized animals exposed to sensitizing antigen intraluminally (resulting in intestinal anaphylaxis and protein-
losing enteropathy) also developed a broadening of the IgE-mediated response to
include bystander antigen. This new concept may help to explain the increase in
allergic responses to soy milk after milk-allergic infants have been changed to soy
formula. Figure 3 – 6 depicts this concept diagramatically.

A better understanding of the modulating factors and their mechanism in intestinal maturation may be beneficial for improved management of very premature
infants in whom there exists an extremely immature and vulnerable mucosal
barrier. These studies may influence feeding practices for neonates and infants by
showing the benefits of breast milk and the timing for introduction of solid foods.

REFERENCES

 1. Husby S, Jensenivs JC, Svehag S-E: Passage of undegraded dietary antigen into the
    blood of healthy adults. *Scand J Immunol* 22:83 – 92, 1985.

2. Walker WA: Mechanisms of antigen handling by the gut. *Clin Immunol All* 2:15–40, 1982.

3. Udall JN, Walker WA: The physiologic and pathologic basis for the transport of macromolecules across the intestinal tract. *J Pediatr Gastroenterol Clin Nutr* 1:295–301, 1982.

4. Lake AM, Bloch KJ, Neutra MR, et al: Intestinal goblet cell mucous release. II. In vivo stimulation by antigen in the immunized rat. *J Immunol* 122:834–837, 1979.

5. Lake AM, Bloch KJ, Sinclair KJ, et al: Anaphylactic release of goblet cell mucus. *Immunology* 39:173–178, 1980.

6. Snyder JD, Walker WA: Structure and function of intestinal mucin: developmental aspects. *Int Arch Allergy Appl Immunol* 82:351–356, 1987

7. Shub MD, Pang KY, Swann DA, et al: Age-related changes in chemical composition and physical properties of mucous glycoproteins from rat small intestine. *Biochem J* 215:405–411, 1983.

8. Podolsky DK, Isselbacher KJ: Glycoprotein composition of colonic mucosa: specific alterations in ulcerative colitis. *Gastroenterology* 87:991–998, 1984.

9. Podolsky DK, Fournier DA: Emergence of antigenic glycoprotein structures in ulcerative colitis detected through monoclonal antibodies. *Gastroenterology* 95:371–378, 1988.

10. Podolsky DK, Fournier DA: Alterations in mucosal content of colonic glycoconjugates in inflammatory bowel disease defined by monoclonal antibodies. *Gastroenterology* 95:379–387, 1988.

11. Boedekar EC: Enterocyte adherence of *Escherichia coli:* its relation to diarrheal disease. *Gastroenterology* 83:489–492, 1982.

12. Jones GW, Freter R: Adhesive properties of *Vibrio cholera:* nature of the interaction with isolated rabbit brush border membranes and human erythrocytes. *Infect Immunol* 14:240–245, 1976.

13. DeBoth NJ, Van der Kamp AW, Van Dongen JM: The influence of changing crypt cell kinetics on functional differentiation on the small intestine of the rat. Nucleotide and protein synthesis. *Differentiation* 4:175–182, 1975.

14. Raul F, Simon P, Kedinger M, et al: Intestinal enzyme activities in isolated villus and crypt cells during postnatal development of the rat. *Cell Tissue Res* 172:167–172, 1977.

15. Quaroni A, Kirsch K, Herscovics A, et al: Surface-membrane biogenesis in rat intestinal epithelial cells at different stages of maturation. *J Biochem* 192:133–139, 1980.

16. Quaroni A, Isselbacher KJ: Study of intestinal cell differentiation with monoclonal antibodies to intestinal cell surface components. *Dev Biol* 111:280–292, 1985.

17. Pang KY, Bresson JL, Walker WA: Development of the gastrointestinal barrier. III. Evidence for structural differences in microvillus membranes from newborn and adult rabbits. *Biochim Biophys Acta* 727:201–208, 1983.

18. Chu SW, Walker WA: Development of the gastrointestinal mucosal barrier: changes in phospholipid head groups and fatty acid composition of intestinal microvillus membranes from newborn and adult rats. *Pediatr Res* 23:439–442, 1988.

19. Pang KY, Bresson JL, Walker WA: Development of gastrointestinal surface. VIII. Lectin identification of carbohydrate differences. *Am J Physiol* 252:G685–G691, 1987.

20. Chu SW, Walker WA: Developmental changes in the activities of sialyl- and fucosyltransferases in rat small intestine. *Biochim Biophys Acta* 883:496–500, 1986.

21. Israel EJ, Walker WA: Development of intestinal mucosal barrier function to antigens and bacterial toxins. *Adv Exp Med Biol* 216A:673–784, 1987.

22. Jonard PP, Rambaud JC, Dive C, et al: Secretion of immunoglobulins and plasma proteins from the jejunal mucosa. Transport rate and origin of polymeric immunoglobulin A. *J Clin Invest* 74:525–535, 1984.

23. Lamm ME: Cellular aspects of immunoglobulin A. *Adv Immunol* 22:223–290, 1976.

24. Williams RC, Gibbons RJ: Inhibition of bacterial adherence by secretory immunoglobulin A: a mechanism of antigen disposal. *Science* 177:697–699, 1972.

25. Walker WA, Wu M, Bloch KJ: Stimulation by immune complexes of mucus release from goblet cells of the rat small intestine. *Science* 97:370–371, 1977.

26. Taylor HP, Dimmock NJ: Mechanism of neutralization of influenza virus by secretory IgA is different from that of monomeric IgA on IgG. *J Exp Med* 161:198–209, 1985.

27. Walker WA: The principle of handling intestinal antigens. *Front Gastrointest Res* 13:10–33, 1986.

28. Allansmith M, McClellan BH, Butterworth M, et al: The development of immunoglobulin levels in man. *J Pediatr* 72:276–281, 1968.

29. Selner JC, Merrill DA, Claman NH: Salivary immunoglobulins and albumin: development during the newborn period. *J Pediatr* 72:685–690, 1968.

30. Haneberg B, Aarskog D: Human fecal immunoglobulins in healthy infants and children and in some diseases affecting the intestinal tract or the immune system. *Clin Exp Immunol* 22:210–213, 1975.

31. Burgio GR, Lanzavecchia A, Plebani A, et al: Ontogeny of secretory immunity: levels of secretory IgA and natural antibodies in saliva. *Pediatr Res* 14:1111–1114, 1980.

32. Cunningham-Rundles C, Brandeis WE, Good RA, et al: Milk precipitins, circulating immune complexes and IgA deficiency. *Proc Natl Acad Sci USA* 75:3387–3389, 1978.

33. Cunningham-Rundles C, Brandeis WE, Good RA, et al: Bovine antigens and the formation of circulating immune complexes in selective immunoglobulin A deficiency. *J Clin Invest* 64:272–277, 1979.

34. Eibl MM, Wolf HM, Fürnkranz H, et al: Prevention of necrotizing enterocolitis in low-birth-weight infants by IgA-IgG feeding. *N Engl J Med* 319:1–7, 1988.

35. Walker WA, Isselbacher KJ: Uptake and transport of macromolecules by the intestine: possible role in clinical disorders. *Gastroenterology* 67:531–550, 1974.

36. Udall JN, Pan K, Fritze L, et al: Development of gastrointestinal mucosal barrier. I. The effect of age on intestinal permeability to macromolecules. *Pediatr Res* 15:241–244, 1981.

37. Rothman D, Udall JN, Pang KY, et al: The effect of short-term starvation on mucosal barrier function in the newborn rabbit. *Pediatr Res* 19:727–731, 1985.

38. Rothberg RM: Immunoglobulin and specific antibody synthesis during the first weeks of life of premature infants. *J Pediatr* 75:391–399, 1969.

39. Eastham EJ, Lichauco T, Grady MI, et al: Antigenicity of infant formulas: role of immature intestine in protein permeability. *J Pediatr* 93:561–564, 1978.

40. Roberton DM, Paganelli R, Dinwiddie R, et al: Milk antigen absorption in the preterm and term neonate. *Arch Dis Child* 57:369–372, 1982.

41. Reinhardt MC, Pagnaelli R, Levinsky RJ: Intestinal antigen handling at mucosal surfaces in health and disease: human experimental studies. *Ann Allergy* 51:311–314, 1983.

42. Walker WA: Gastrointestinal host defence: importance of gut closure in control of macromolecular transport. *Ciba Found Symp* 70:201–219, 1979.

43. Sheard NF, Walker WA: The role of breast milk in the development of the gastrointestinal tract. *Nutr Rev* 46:1–8, 1988.

44. Weaver LT, Walker WA: Epidermal growth factor and the developing human gut. *Gastroenterology* 94:845–847, 1988.

45. Paganelli R, Levinsky RJ: Solid phase radioimmunoasssay for detection of circulating food protein antigens in human serum. *J Immunol Methods* 37:333–341, 1980.

46. Plaut AG, Keonil P: Immunoglobulins in human small intestinal fluid. *Gastroenterology* 56:522–530, 1969.

47. Bloch KJ, Walker WA: Effect of locally induced intestinal anaphylaxis on the uptake of a bystander antigen. *J Allergy Clin Immunol* 67:312–316, 1981.

48. Phillips TE, Phillips TL, Neutra MR: Macromolecules can pass through occluding junction of rat ileal epithelium during cholinergic stimulation. *Cell Tissue Res* 247:547–554, 1987.

49. Nicklin S: Intestinal uptake of antigen — immunological consequences. In Miller K, Nicklin S: *Immunology of the Gastrointestinal Tract,* Vol 1. Boca Raton, CRC Press, 1987, p 87.

50. Nicklin S, Miller K: Effect of orally administered food grade carageenans on antibody-mediated and cell-mediated immunity in the inbred rat. *Food Chem Toxicol* 22:615–618, 1984.

51. Gonnella PA, Neutra MR: Membrane-bound and fluid-phase macromolecules enter separate prelysosomal compartments in absorptive cells of suckling rat ileum. *J Cell Biol* 99:909–917, 1984.

52. Rodewald R: Intestinal transport of antibodies in the newborn rat. *J Cell Biol* 58:198–211, 1973.

53. Jones RE: The selective uptake and transmission of proteins to the circulation from the small intestine of the suckling rat. *Biochim Biophys Acta* 451:151–160, 1976.

54. Bland P: MHC class II expression by the gut epithelium. *Immunol Today* 21:174–178, 1988.

55. Owen RL, Jones AL: Epithelial cell specialization within human Peyer's patches: an ultrastructural study of intestinal lymphoid follicles. *Gastroenterology* 66:189–203, 1974.

56. Owen RL: Sequential uptake of horseradish peroxidase by lymphoid follicle epithelium of Peyer's patches in the normal unobstructed mouse intestine: an ultrastructural study. *Gastroenterology* 72:440–451, 1977.

57. Wolf JL, Bye WA: The membranous epithelial (M) cell and the mucosal immune system. *Rev Med* 35:95–112, 1984.

58. Bhalla DK, Owen RL: Cell renewal and migration in lymphoid follicles of Peyer's patches and cecum — an autoradiographic study in mice. *Gastroenterology* 82:232–242, 1982.

59. Owen RL, Bhalla DK: Cytochemical analysis of alkaline phosphatase and esterase activities and of lectin-binding and anionic sites in rat and mouse Peyer's patch M cells. *Am J Anat* 168:199–212, 1983.

60. Bye WA, Allan CH, Trier JS: Structure, distribution, and origin of M cells in Peyer's patches of mouse ileum. *Gastroenterology* 86:789–801, 1984.

61. Wolf JL, Rubin DH, Finberg DH, et al: Intestinal M cells: a pathway for entry of reovirus into the host. *Science* 212:471–472, 1981.

62. Owen RL, Piece NF, Apple RT, et al: Phagocytosis and transport by M cells of intact *Vibrio cholera* into rabbit Peyer's patch follicles (abstr). *J Cell Biol* 95:446, 1982.

63. Marcial MA, Madara JL: *Cryptosporidium:* cellular localization, structural analysis of absorptive cell-parasite membrane-membrane interactions in guinea pigs, and suggestion of protozoan transport by M cells. *Gastroenterology* 90:583–594, 1986.

64. Owen RL: And now pathophysiology of M cells — good news and bad news from Peyer's patches. *Gastroenterology* 85:468–470, 1983.

65. Madara JL, Bye WA, Trier JS: Structural features of and cholesterol distribution in M-cell membranes in guinea pig, rat and mouse Peyer's patches. *Gastroenterology* 87:1091–1103, 1984.

66. Wolf JL, Kauffman RS, Finberg R, et al: Determinants of reovirus interaction with the intestinal M cells and absorptive cells of murine intestine. *Gastroenterology* 85:291–300, 1983.

67. Neutra MR, Phillips TL, Mayer EL, et al: Transport of membrane bound macromolecules by M cells in follicle-associated epithelium of rabbit Peyer's patch. *Cell Tissue Res* 247:537–546, 1987.

68. Husband AJ, Gowans JL: The origin and antigen-dependent distribution of IgA-containing cells in the intestine. *J Exp Med* 148:1146–1160, 1978.

69. Walker WA, Isselbacher KJ: Intestinal antibodies. *N Engl J Med* 297:767–773, 1977.

70. Guy-Grand D, Griscelli C, Vassalli P: The mouse gut T lymphocyte, a novel type of cell. Nature, origin, and traffic in mice in normal and graft-versus-host conditions. *J Exp Med* 148:1161–1677, 1978.

71. Pang KY, Newman AP, Udall JN, et al: Development of gastrointestinal mucosal barrier. VIII. *In utero* maturation of microvillus surface by cortisone. *Am J Physiol* 249:G85–G91, 1985.

72. Israel EJ, Pang KY, Harmatz PR, et al: Structural and functional maturation of rat gastrointestinal barrier with thyroxine. *Am J Physiol* 252:G762–G767, 1987.

73. Berseth CL: Enhancement of intestinal growth in neonatal rats by epidermal growth factor in milk. *Am J Physiol* 253:G662–G665, 1987.

74. Conteas CN, DeMorrow JM, Majumdar APN: Effect of epidermal growth factor on growth and maturation of fetal and neonatal rat intestine in organ culture. *Experientia* 42:950–952, 1986.

75. Israel EJ, Simister N, Freiberg E, et al: Immunoglobulin G binding site on the human fetal intestine. *Clin Res* 36:806A, 1988.

76. Menard D, Arsenault P, Pothier P: Biologic effects of epidermal growth factor in human fetal jejunum. *Gastroenterology* 94:656–663, 1988.

77. Jackson D, Walker-Smith JA, Phillips AD: Macromolecular absorption by histologically normal and abnormal small intestinal mucosa in childhood: an *in vitro* study using organ culture. *J Pediatr Gastroenterol Nutr* 2:235–247, 1983.

78. Winter HS, Black PR, Bhan AK, et al: A model to study development and immune function in the human small intestine. *Adv Exp Med Biol* 216A:1377–1381, 1987.

79. Bauer CR, Morrison JC, Poole K, et al: A decreased incidence of necrotizing enterocolitis after prenatal glucocorticoid therapy. *Pediatrics* 73:682–688, 1984.

80. Kleinman RE, Bloch KJ, Walker WA: Gut induced anaphylaxis and uptake of bystander protein: an amplification of anaphylactic sensitivity. *Pediatr Res* 15:598, 1981.

CHAPTER **4**

Antigen Presentation in the Intestine

LLOYD MAYER

INTRODUCTION

The intimate relationship of the external environment to the intestinal tract dictates that a unique mechanism be established for handling the myriad of foreign antigens that are continuously present. Although a series of nonimmunologic mechanisms are well recognized and provide protection from bacteria, viruses, and toxins (Table 4–1), specific immune responses are generated to maintain homeostasis. Since the nature of any immune response requires the "education" of immunoreactive cells, trafficking and processing of antigen(s) to the appropriate sites and cells is critically important. Over the past several years it has become evident that several mechanisms exist by which antigens (bacteria, viruses, toxins, and complex antigens) are processed and presented to cells of the mucosal immune system.[1-3] This relates, in part, to a number of loosely organized lymphoid structures that make up the gut-associated lymphoid tissue (GALT).[4] Still, some basic concepts predominate in the peripheral and mucosal immune systems. Antigen recognition and immune response by T lymphocytes require antigen to be degraded (processed) and presented to the T-cell antigen receptor in a complex with products of the major histocompatibility complex (MHC).[5] Thus, only cell-bound antigens can be recognized by T cells which, in turn, play a major role in regulation of B-cell activation[6] and maturation,[7] monocyte activation,[8] and T-cell differentiation.[9] B cells, in contrast, can respond to soluble antigens, yet appear to be activated more efficiently with cell-bound antigens (resulting in receptor cross-linking), especially in the presence of T cells. Thus several levels of immune response are evident within the GI tract: the "cruder" B-cell responses to bacteria and their products (i.e., multiple repeating polysaccharide subunits) and the more evolved selective T-cell responses, which can result in either an effector type of response

33

Table 4 – 1 IMMUNOLOGIC AND NONIMMUNOLOGIC DEFENSES AT MUCOSAL SURFACES

Nonimmunologic	Immunologic
Physical	Immunoglobulin (IgA)
Mucus barrier	Cell-mediated immunity
Cilia	Tissue macrophages
Tight junctions	Mast cells
Cell renewal	
Peristalsis	
Chemical	
Lysozyme	
Spermine	
Commensal organisms	
Bile salts	
Acid in stomach	
Glycoproteins	

itself or regulate other cells to generate a coordinated immune response.[10] In order to understand these issues more clearly, a basic understanding of antigen processing and presentation in peripheral lymphoid tissue is required.

As noted above, coordinated immune responses first require the organism to be able to recognize substances as foreign. The recognition of self versus non-self by cells of the immune system is at the center of an immune response, yet mechanisms involved in this system have generated considerable debate. What has evolved from these controversies is a general schema relating mechanisms by which complexes of self and non-self can be recognized by immunocompetent cells and can result in education and cellular activation. A simple model for such a schema is depicted in Figure 4 – 1. In this scenario, a foreign protein is endocytosed by a phagocytic cell (an accessory cell), degraded by a series of prepackaged enzymes, and re-expressed on the surface of the accessory cell in a complex with products of the major histocompatibility locus [HLA-D (class II) in man or I-A/I-E (class II) in mice]. In contrast proteins synthesized within the cell (i.e. viral antigens, tumor antigens) complex to class I molecules (HLA-A,-B,-C in man, H-2D or K in mouse) before being expressed on the cell surface an antigen-specific receptor on the T lymphocyte recognizing a unique protein sequence of the processed antigen as well as self MHC, will fit the processed antigen/MHC complex in a relatively low affinity lock and key interaction.[11] Evidence for this interaction has recently been strengthened by the co-isolation of a putative antigen in the antigen-binding cleft of a crystallized class I molecule.[12] Furthermore, in vitro data documenting specific peptide binding to distinct class II molecules, solidified this concept as fact.[13] Thus a large macromolecular antigen can be endocytosed by an accessory cell and degraded, or be endogenously synthesized and the resultant antigenic peptides can bind to MHC class II or I molecules, respectively. These complexes are then re-expressed on the surface of the phagocytic cell, where T-cell Ag receptors can recognize and bind to them, resulting in the activation of the T cell.

The questions of which cells can function as accessory cells and what mechanisms are involved in the processing and complexing of foreign proteins remain to be addressed.

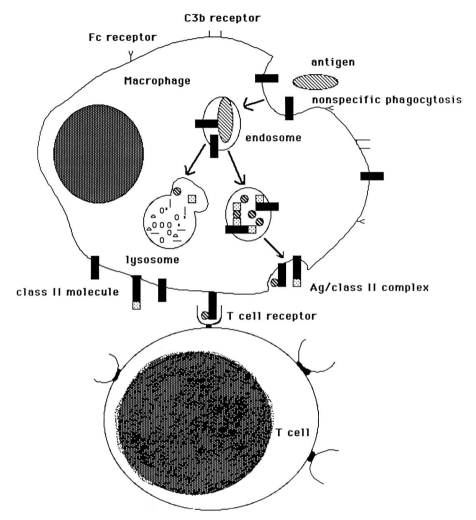

Figure 4–1 Schema for interaction of accessory cells (in this case a macrophage) and T cells. Intact antigen is endocytosed via either nonspecific phagocytosis, Fc receptor binding to immune complexes, or C3b receptor binding to immune complexes. Protein degradation occurs within the endosome with subsequent binding to class II molecules endocytosed concomitantly. The class II/Ag complex is then transported back to the cell surface, where it can be recognized by the T-cell antigen receptor (cross-linking receptors resulting in T-cell activation). An alternate pathway is via the lysosome, which fuses with the endosome and results in complete degradation of the protein. This pathway is probably used to eliminate bacteria and toxins without generating an immune response.

ACCESSORY CELLS

In order to generate a helper T-cell response, two requirements for accessory cells have been proposed: 1) interaction with an accessory cell expressing class II (HLA-D) molecules; 2) the ability to take up and process Ag;[14] and 3) the presence of cell adhesion molecules (ie. LfA-1, 1CAM-1). These requirements have become less stringent more recently, but the basic concepts are unchanged. Given the above, the only cell initially thought to function as an accessory or antigen-presenting cell was the monocyte/macrophage. Several studies have clearly demonstrated the critical role that the monocyte plays in T-cell activation.[14-17] Antigen is taken up via endocytosis either by receptor-mediated processes (e.g., Fc-γ, C3b receptors for immune complexes) or as a random event. The endocytosed protein is subjected to a series of degradative enzymes (activated by the low pH within the endosome) present in the endocytotic vesicle. At this point, there is some controversy regarding the fate of the partly degraded antigen. There is evidence to suggest that the vesicle (endosome) fuses with a primary lysosome (becoming a secondary lysosome), further degrading the protein into small antigenically distinct peptides.[18] These peptides are complexed to class II antigens either already present on the engulfed membrane, or newly synthesized, and/or travelling from the Golgi. These Ag/MHC complexes are then re-expressed on the cell surface. Alternatively, there is growing evidence to suggest that endocytosis and subsequent acidification of the endosome itself is sufficient to result in processed Ag, which can then be complexed to class II molecules.[19] In either case, the end result is the surface expression of an immunoregulatory complex that is capable of being recognized by the T-cell antigen receptor. Presumably, cross-linking the receptor results in T-cell activation, cytokine release, and clonal proliferation of antigen-specific T cells. The contribution of monokines, secreted by monocytes, to T-cell proliferation has also been well documented. Interleukin-1 (IL-1) will induce the expression of IL-2 receptor on T cells, which then allows for IL-2-induced T-cell proliferation.[20]

Thus the critical role of accessory cells is quite clear. What has become evident more recently is that several cells are capable of functioning as antigen-presenting cells provided they meet the requirements outlined earlier. B lymphocytes, by virtue of their specific antigen receptors (surface Ig molecules), are probably the most efficient antigen-presenting cells, stimulating T cells in a linked or cognate interaction (Fig. 4–2).[21-23] T cells activated in this fashion can easily regulate B-cell growth and differentiation via secretion of lymphokines that are presumably quite potent at short range (noncognate interaction).[24] In addition to expression of class II antigens, B cells can internalize immune complexes by Fc receptor-mediated endocytosis,[21] or potentially by binding to Ag via the surface Ig itself.[22] B cells can also secrete IL-1, which, as mentioned earlier, is critical for T-cell activation.[25]

In 1973, Steinman and Cohn described a novel accessory cell, the dendritic cell, which appears to be the most potent antigen-presenting cell (on a cell-per-cell basis) described.[26] Although nonphagocytic, dendritic cells are rich in class II Ag and bind T cells with great avidity (forming clusters in culture).[27] Dendritic cells are thought to be the major stimulator population in primary mixed lymphocyte reactions (MLRs),[28] and are extremely potent in antigen presentation to primed T cells.[27] Dendritic cells are found throughout the body in various forms (e.g., Langerhan's cells in the skin,[29] and in lymphoid aggregates, spleen, lymph nodes, etc).[30]

T/B cell interactions

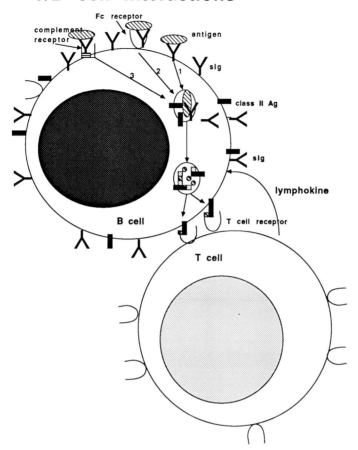

Figure 4 – 2 Schema for interaction of B cells and T cells in antigen presentation. Like the macrophage/T cell interaction, there are nonspecific mechanisms that allow for antigen entry (Fc receptor-mediated endocytosis (2), complement receptor-mediated endocytosis (3). However, in contrast to the nonspecific pathways, the B cell has the advantage of antigen-specific interactions through surface immunoglobulin (sIg) (1). Antigen can be avidly bound and internalized with processing, resulting in T-cell-specific epitopes. The T-cell receptor recognizes processed antigen bound to class II molecules and T cells become activated and secrete lymphokines (IL-2, γ-IFN, B-cell growth, and differentiation factors).

Since these cells are nonphagocytic and contain few lysosomes, antigen processing must be external to these cells either by cell surface proteolysis, or by requiring an additional accessory cell. Such a process has been suggested by Steinman and his coworkers, since dendritic cell-mediated events, in vitro, are dependent upon factors present in conditioned medium.[31] Therefore, although extremely efficient in function, dendritic cells are only a part of the accessory cell network.

Lastly, several groups have demonstrated that some epithelial and endothelial cells are capable of functioning as accessory cells since, under certain conditions, they can express class II Ag, phagocytose Ag, and secrete IL-1. Intestinal epithelial cells will be discussed in the final section of this chapter, but studies by Pober et al.[32] have documented the ability of Ia-bearing endothelial cells to stimulate allogeneic MLRs and present antigen to primed T cells in vitro. What is less clear is whether such cells function in this capacity in vivo. In certain disease states, such as Kawasaki's syndrome, a viral or autoimmune disease of endothelial cell lined blood vessels,[33] Ia-bearing endothelial cells may be the target of attack by self-reactive T cells, or alternatively, may be responsible for presenting auto- or neoantigens to T cells.[34] In either case, the aberrant expression of class II antigens in these cells is linked to the disease process. A similar hypothetical model has been proposed for autoimmune thyroid disease,[35] diabetes,[36] and psoriasis.[37] In these settings an initial triggering event results in inflammation and subsequent Ia expression on thyrocytes, islet cells, and basal keratinocytes, respectively. Since such areas are "privileged," i.e., not commonly exposed to foreign antigen, Ia molecules in these cells may present self antigens resulting in autoimmune tissue destruction. It is clear, however, that expression of class II antigens alone is not sufficient to induce an autoimmune response. Lo et al. inserted the class II gene, as a transgene, into mouse embryos along with an insulin promoter.[38] Although islet cells clearly expressed class II antigens in these transgenic mice, no diabetes or islet cell destruction (or even mononuclear cell infiltration) occurred in these animals. In summary, the expression of class II antigens may be necessary, but certainly not sufficient, for APC function and/or an autoimmune response.

ANTIGEN TRAFFICKING IN THE INTESTINE

In contrast to the peripheral immune system, the mucosal tissues require an adaptive mechanism to coexist with the external environment. Although there are several nonimmunologic mechanisms in place that reduce antigen access to the underlying mucosa (Table 4–1), specific pathways of antigen trafficking have been described in the intestine: the M cell or follicle-associated epithelium (the specialized epithelium overlying Peyer's patches), paracellular (through tight junctions), and transcellular (through the epithelium). What remains to be determined is which of these pathways predominates, and what consequences result from antigen uptake via each of these routes. There is evidence to suggest that, to some degree, each pathway is a viable mechanism for getting antigen into GALT, but perhaps the nature of the antigen or the desired resultant immune response dictates the route of entry.

M Cells

Well-defined lymphoid aggregates in mice and rats intimately associated with the overlying epithelium suggests an interactive role for lymphocytes and epithelial cells. Analysis of the surface epithelium overlying these lymphoid follicles (Peyer's patches) by electron microscopy (EM) has revealed the presence of specialized epithelial cells, characterized by elongated cytoplasm, reduction of microvilli, and maintenance of tight junctions with adjacent enterocytes (Fig. 4–3).[39] These follicle-associated epithelium (FAE) or M cells have been proposed as the major cell type responsible for antigen sampling in the gut.[40] Indeed, several studies have

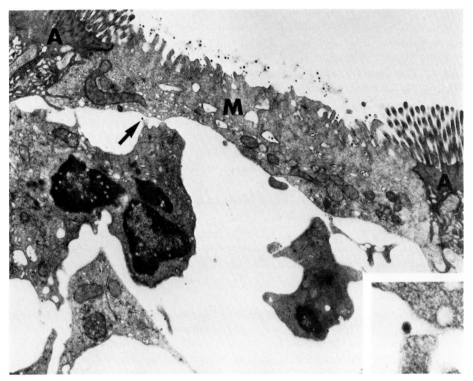

Figure 4–3 Electromicrograph of ileum overlying Peyer's patch (×11,500), 1 hour after inoculation with reovirus type 1 from a 10-day-old C3H/HeJ mouse. Virions are seen in the lumen, within vesicles in the M cell (M) (small arrow), and in the lamina propria adjacent to a macrophage (large arrow). Inset: Higher magnification of virion in lamina propria (×56,600). (Kindly provided by Dr. J. Wolf. Brigham and Woman's Hospital, Boston MA, and reproduced with permission.)

clearly documented the transport of particulate antigens (horseradish peroxidase),[41] reovirus,[42] cholera toxin,[43] bacteria,[44] and India ink[45] across the M cells. However, the M cell appears to be unique in its antigen transport mechanism in that processing of antigen within the M cell is not evident. Rather, the M cell appears to be acting as a conduit to transport antigen to lymphocytes and macrophages in the subepithelial space, and into the patch itself.[40] Lysosomes, as assessed by the presence of acid phosphatase-containing organelles, are not demonstrable in M cells[40] as opposed to adjacent enterocytes, where processing can occur (see below). Since M cells are thought to be derived from enterocytes, this loss of lysosomes may be part of the maturational process, although the true origin of M cells has not been clearly defined. In a series of elegant morphometric studies, Owen and his colleagues have clearly demonstrated Ag transport through the M cells associated with a concomitant influx of macrophages and lymphocytes, which would then be available to phagocytose Ag, transport Ag to the patch, and initiate a local immune response.[40] The inability of several investigators to reproducibly identify class II antigens on M cells provides further evidence for the lack of an Ag-presenting role by these cells.[46]

Still, there are several unique features of this system suggesting that M cells play a major role in antigen sampling in the normal gut. First, by scanning EM, M cells appear to be localized in "pits."[47] Particulate antigens can "fall" into those pits, resulting in greater antigen density overlying the M cell. Although the majority of such antigens are transported nonspecifically across the M cell, there is some evidence for the presence of specific antigen receptors (i.e., for reovirus 3) on these cells.[42] The selective advantage for having these specific receptors has not been elucidated to date, but it has been suggested that the immune response to specific antigens may be altered by the portal of entry into the GI tract (see below).

M cells have been described throughout the GI tract, being more abundant in the terminal ileum, and less notable in the colon[41] (consistent with areas of increased protein uptake).

The lack of efficient accessory cell function by the M cell dictates that antigen processing must occur elsewhere within the tissue itself. As previously mentioned, macrophages appear to "capture" antigen from the M cell and transport it to the underlying Peyer's patch. Ag-primed T and B cells are readily identified within the patch, but not in the surrounding lamina propria, supporting such a directed transport mechanism.[48] Within the patch itself, there are three putative antigen-presenting cells: dendritic cells, macrophages, and B cells, which function in a fashion similar to their counterparts in peripheral lymphoid tissues. However, within the patch, B cells become committed predominantly to IgA secretion.[49] Such isotype restriction is the result of regulatory influences of isotype-restricted T cells,[50] yet a novel role for dendritic cells in this system has been proposed. Spalding et al. have isolated Peyer's patch dendritic cells and demonstrated their ability to promote polyclonal B-cell IgA responses in vitro with either splenic or Peyer's patch T-cell help.[51] Such a concept would suggest remarkable tissue specificity for what have been previously considered nonspecific regulators of T-cell activation, and would require a rethinking of conventional antigen-presenting cells.

The unique homing of B cells (and, less well characterized, of T cells) from Peyer's patches to mesenteric nodes, thoracic duct, systemic circulation, and back to the lamina propria of mucosal structures (i.e., gut, lung, urinary tract, mammary gland) brings antigen-primed cells back to areas where they can mediate effector functions.[52] The role of tissue macrophages and dendritic cells in these areas (lamina propria) are still unknown and have not been easily addressed due to problems of technique and isolation. At this time, one can only hypothesize that these cells are active in non-M-cell antigen transport, activating primed cells in the lamina propria.

Paracellular Transport

In the intact intestine, the bowel maintains its integrity by virtue of a series of desmosomes and tight junctions between epithelial cells. Although ion transport is conceivable, macromolecules fail to negotiate this space. Only in areas of active inflammation or trauma will a breach of this barrier occur. This allows for direct interaction between the luminal contents and the lamina propria cells themselves.

The lack of an adequate model system has hampered the careful analysis of the importance and magnitude of this route of antigen entry. A recently described system, utilizing the malignant colonic carcinoma cell line T84 in monolayer cultures oriented on a basement membrane, has suggested that some toxins (i.e.,

Clostridium difficile toxin A) may disrupt desmosomes, allowing for transport of macromolecules through the intercellular spaces.[53] Interestingly, no intracellular trafficking was detectable in this system.

In diseases in which active inflammation is present, such as inflammatory bowel disease, antigen access through large mucosal breaks is probable, and may add to the continuous ongoing inflammatory process in these diseases.

Epithelial Cells

The role of the epithelial cell in protein transport from lumen to submucosa has been described by intestinal physiologists for several decades.[54,55] The enterocyte has also been defined as playing a key role in mucosal immunity, producing secretory component, and transporting IgA from the lamina propria into the lumen.[56] More recently, several groups have suggested a more novel role for epithelial cells: that of antigen-presenting cell. In order to achieve this status, the enterocyte would have to manifest all the requirements for antigen processing and presentation described in the beginning of this chapter: expression of class II molecules and ability to phagocytose and process (digest) a protein with subsequent re-expression of peptide-class II Ag complexes on the cell surface. Certainly the numbers of enterocytes far outnumber M cells, making an enterocyte-T cell interaction a more efficient process.

EXPRESSION OF CLASS II Ag ON ENTEROCYTES

As described earlier, several laboratories have recently described the presence of class II antigen (Ia molecules) on nonmononuclear cells.[57-60] The presence of Ia on intestinal enterocytes was initially described in a graft-versus-host disease model in the rat[59] in which cells of both the submucosa and the gut epithelium displayed heightened expression of class II Ag. These findings were extended into normal and inflamed tissues with the description of class II molecules on normal small bowel in rats[57] and in humans[58] by light and electron microscopy.[61] The distribution of class II Ag on enterocytes is predominantly on the luminal side of the cell, although one can detect them at lower density on the basolateral aspects of the cell as well. It is thought that the luminal expression on the enterocyte merely relates to the overlapping membranes of the microvilli on the luminal surface. The presence of class II antigens on normal colonocytes is more controversial, although when more sensitive techniques that amplify the antigen expressed are used,[58] there appears to be some basal expression of class II antigen on these cells as well. Such a finding makes inherent sense since the underlying lamina propria is comprised of inflammatory cells, capable of secreting inflammatory mediators such as gamma-interferon (γ-IFN), which are potent inducers of class II antigen expression.

One interesting observation is the pattern of class II antigen expression on epithelial cells in humans. While messenger RNA (mRNA) transcripts are detectable for all three surface HLA-D region molecules (DR, DP, DQ),[62] DQ is poorly expressed if at all. Although an exact functional role for each HLA-D subregion has not been completely characterized, it is possible that some antigeneic peptides are capable of binding only to DQ (or I-A in mouse),[13] and the lack of DQ leaves the host with a "hole in the repertoire,"[13] at least at the level of the mucosa.

As with several other cell types "aberrantly" expressing class II, attention has turned toward defining a disease or functional significance for its expression. In the case of thyrocytes, islet cells in the pancreas, the basal keratinocytes, class II Ag expression has been postulated to mediate presentation of autoantigens, resulting in autoimmunity. In the intestine this concept is less likely, since expression of class II antigen is present even in the normal state. Thus Ia molecules on entero-cytes can serve, as on monocytes, as a glycoprotein, which, when complexed to processed antigen, is able to activate primed T cells in the intraepithelial and subepithelial spaces. Alternately, it has been suggested that the class II antigen, abundantly expressed on the microvilli and hence on the luminal border of the enterocyte, serves as an antigen receptor by itself. Since many proteins may be catabolized within the lumen by acid and peptidases, externally "processed" pep-tides may bind and be transported across the enterocyte. In this scenario, the enterocyte would fulfill its "absorptive" and transport functions through the Ia molecules.

FUNCTIONAL ROLE FOR Ia+ ENTEROCYTES IN VITRO

The presence of class II antigens on the cell surface is necessary but not sufficient for a cell to function as an antigen-processing cell.[63] For example, Ia + B cells from patients with chronic lymphocytic leukemia are incapable of stimulating a primary mixed lymphocyte reaction.[63] These data suggest the requirement for additional factors (? IL-1) to mediate a stimulatory signal. Enterocytes are capable of stimu-lating a primary allogeneic mixed lymphocyte response,[58] although less vigorously than adherent cell populations containing dendritic cells, demonstrating that class II antigens on enterocytes are expressed in a form that is recognized, at least, by alloreactive cells. Furthermore, two groups have been able to demonstrate, in rats[57] and humans,[58] that enterocytes can process antigen, OVA, and tetanus toxoid respectively, and can activate primed T cells. Thus the enterocyte is functional as an antigen-processing cell in vitro, fulfilling all the requirements for such cells. The intriguing finding in both of these studies was the observation that there was selective activation of CD8 + suppressor T cells in cultures in which the enterocyte served as the antigen-presenting cell. This was of particular interest in light of the fact that several groups have reported that >98% of intraepithelial lymphocytes are CD8+.[64]

Since T-cell activation in the studies described above could be inhibited by antibodies to class II antigens, the dogma that CD4 + T cells are class II-restricted and CD8 + T cells are class I-restricted is challenged. Although the mechanism of CD8 + T-cell induction is as yet undetermined, there is evidence to support the presence of an additional CD8 ligand on the enterocyte.[65] Antibodies to CD8 but not CD4 inhibit the T-cell response to enterocytes, and isolated purified CD8 + T cells are capable of responding to epithelial cell stimulation. Such data negate the requirement for a CD4-CD8 + T cell interaction in this system.

Whether these functional properties can be translated into an in vivo phenome-non remains to be determined. The location of the class II Ag on the enterocyte raises questions as to whether there can be physiologic interactions with T cells.

Still, finding CD8 + T cells in the intraepithelial spaces, as well as the well-documented phenomenon of oral tolerance, which is mediated by induction of suppressor T cells (see Chapter 9), suggests that epithelial cells may truly function in an accessory cell capacity in vivo.

These experimental observations in two systems add support to the concept of a role for the enterocyte in normal antigen processing and presentation to local T-cell populations. The suppressor cell induction, although not antigen-specific, may help explain some unusual aspects of normal mucosal immunity: the highly regulated chronic inflammation seen in the lamina propria of normal individuals, and the suppression of systemic immune responses when one initially primes with an orally administered antigen. The mechanism of generating oral tolerance (by induction of antigen-specific suppressor cells) may be in part explained by enterocyte-mediated suppressor T-cell induction. This may result from the specific generation of tolerogenic peptides by the enterocyte. Such peptides have been isolated in the serum of tolerized mice[66] without clear knowledge of their origin. Processing of antigen by enterocytes appears to be less efficient than their monocyte counterparts,[65] with slower internalization and less rapid breakdown of protein (presumably due to a lower number of acid phosphatase-containing granules and a limited number of endopeptidases). With such a difference in processing ability, it is certainly conceivable that tolerogenic peptides may be the result of altered protein degradation and subsequent stimulation of suppressor cells recognizing such peptides.

CONCLUSIONS

In summary, the pathways of antigen handling by the gut are still being defined. There are unequivocal data supporting each of the mechanisms outlined in this chapter. The real question remains as to which mechanism(s) is predominant in a physiologic system. The most likely scenario is that specific antigens (particulate versus soluble) are handled differently and that, depending upon the mode of entry, the immune response generated will be different. Figure 4 – 4 outlines these possible scenarios:

1. The conventional hypothesis of antigen access through the M cell directs antigen into the Peyer's patch, which can result in the induction of an IgA-specific response and homing of antigen-specific B cells to other mucosal sites. Such a response is T-helper-dependent, class II-restricted, and may be associated with generation of poor immunologic memory.

2. A paracellular route of entry allows for local immune responses, mediated by lamina propria macrophages and dendritic cells without systemic priming. Conceivably this type of response may be responsible for the IgG responses seen in the GI tract.

3. The third pathway is via the epithelial cell and requires antigen processing of internalized peptides and presentation to either intraepithelial lymphocytes or local lamina propria T cells. The data to date suggest that this route results in the induction of a suppressed immune response and may be in part responsible for the induction of oral tolerance (generating "tolerogenic" peptides?).

Possible mechanisms for antigen entry in the intestine

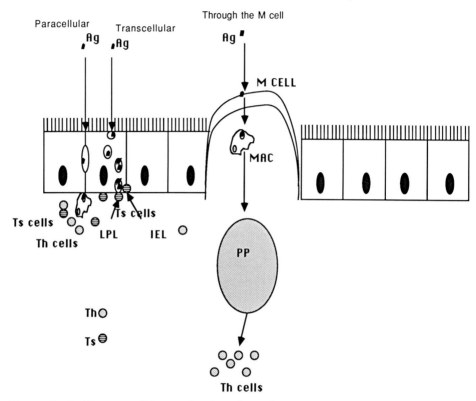

Figure 4–4 Three possible mechanisms for antigen entry into the GI tract and their possible immunologic outcomes. **1:** Through the M cell. Antigen may pass through the M cell without processing and be taken up by macrophages in the lamina propria (see also Fig. 4–3). Macrophages (MAC) travel to the underlying Peyer's patch (PP) where antigen (Ag) priming occurs. This type of event would result in the induction of a predominantly helper T cell (Th) response. **2:** Transcellular. Antigen is taken up actively by the enterocyte via pinocytosis, and protein degradation occurs by activation of proteolytic enzymes. Processed antigen binds to class II molecules and is re-expressed on the basolateral cell surface, where the complex can activate either intraepithelial lymphocytes (IEL) or lamina propria lymphocytes (LPL). Such a process would selectively activate suppressor T cells (Ts) and dampen an immune response or possibly result in a tolerant state. **3:** Paracellular. Antigen travels in between cells despite tight junctions (or in certain disease states, damaged tight junctions). No processing occurs until the intact antigen reaches the lamina propria, where tissue macrophages can take up the antigen and process and present it to LPLs. This type of event would most likely result in Th cell proliferation, although Th/Ts interactions may occur.

Since the nature of immunity in the intestine is one of nonresponsiveness, one might speculate that this last pathway plays a major role in mucosal immune responses. The validity of such an argument remains to be determined.

REFERENCES

1. Wolf JL, Bye WA: The membranous epithelial (M) cell and the mucosal immune system. *Annu Rev Med* 35:95–112, 1984.
2. Husband AJ, Gowans JL: The origin and antigen-dependent distribution of IgA-containing cells in the intestine. *J Exp Med* 148(5):1146–1160, 1978.
3. Joel DD, Laissur JA, LeFevre ME: Distribution and fate of ingested carbon particles in mice. *J Reticuloendothel Soc* 24:477–487, 1978.
4. Bienenstock J: Gut and bronchus associated lymphoid tissue: an overview. Adv Exp Med and Biol 149:471–497, 1982.
5. Katz DH, Hamaoka T, Benacerraf B: Cell interactions between histoincompatible T and B lymphocytes. II. Failure of physiologic cooperative interactions between T and B lymphocytes from allogeneic donor strains in humoral response to hapten-protein conjugates. *J Exp Med* 137:1405–1418, 1973.
6. Howard M, Farrar J, Hilfiker M, et al: Identification of a T cell-derived 6 cell growth factor distinct from interleukin 2. *J Exp Med* 155:914–923, 1982.
7. Mayer L, Fu SM, Kunkel HG: Human T cell hybridomas secreting factors for IgA-specific help, polyclonal B cell activation, and B cell proliferation. *J Exp Med* 156(6):1860–1865, 1982.
8. Meltzer MS, Oppenheim JJ: Bidirectional amplification of macrophage-lymphocyte interactions: enhanced lymphocyte activation factor production by activated adherent mouse peritoneal cells. *J Immunol* 118:77–82, 1977.
9. Krönke M, Scheurich P, Pfizenmaier K, et al: T-T cell interactions during in vitro cytotoxic T cell responses. VI. The role of T cell-derived colony-stimulating factor in helper T cell activation. *Eur J Immunol* 14(2):176–180, 1984.
10. Howard M, Paul WE: Regulation of B-cell growth and differentiation by soluble factors. *Annu Rev Immunol* 1:307–333, 1983.
11. Babbitt BP, Allen PM, Matsueda G, et al: Binding of immunogenic peptides to Ia histocompatibility molecules. *Nature* 317:359–361, 1985.
12. Björkman PJ, Saper MA, Samraoui B, et al: The foreign antigen binding site and T cell recognition regions of class I histocompatibility antigens. *Nature* 329:506–518, 1987.
13. Guillet JG, Lai MZ, Briner TJ, et al: Interaction of peptide antigens and class II major histocompatibility complex antigens. *Nature* 324:260–262, 1986.
14. Ziegler K, Unanue ER: Identification of a macrophage antigen-processing event required for I-region-restricted antigen presentation to T lymphocytes. *J Immunol* 127:1869–1875, 1981.
15. Ziegler HK, Unanue ER: Decrease in macrophage antigen catabolism caused by ammonia and chloroquine is associated with inhibition of antigen presentation to T cells. *Proc Natl Acad Sci USA* 79:175, 1982.
16. Lipsky PE, Ellner JJ, Rosenthal AS: Phytohemagglutinin-induced proliferation of guinea pig thymus-derived lymphocytes. *J Immunol* 116(3):868–875, 1976.
17. Rosenstreich DC, Farrar JJ, Dougherty S: Absolute macrophage dependency of T lymphocyte activation by mitogens. *J Immunol* 116(1):131–139, 1976.
18. Krogstad DJ, Schlesinger PH: Acid-vesicle function, intracellular pathogens, and the

action of chloroquine against plasmodium falciparum. *N Engl J Med* 317(a):542–549, 1987.

19. Samuelson LE, Schwartz RH: The use of antisera and monoclonal antibodies to identify the antigen-specific T cell receptor from pigeon cytochrome *c*-specific T cell hybrids. *Immunol Rev* 76:59–78, 1983.

20. Kouttab NM, Mehta S, Morgan J et al: Lymphokines and monokines as regulators of human lymphoproliferation. *Clin Chem* 30:1539–1545, 1984.

21. Kappler J, White J, Wegmann D, et al: Antigen presentation by Ia + B cell hybridomas to H-2 restricted T cell hybridomas. *Proc Natl Acad Sci USA* 79:3604–3607, 1982.

22. Chesnut RW, Colon S, Grey HM: Antigen presentation by normal B cells, B cell tumors, and macrophages: functional and biochemical comparison. *J Immunol* 128:1764–1768, 1982.

23. Rock KL, Benacerraf B, Abbas AK: Antigen presentation by hapten-specific B lymphocytes. I. Role of surface immunoglobin receptors. *J Exp Med* 160(4):1102–1113, 1984.

24. Kishimoto T: Factors affecting B-cell growth and differentiation. *Annu Rev Immunol* 3:133–157, 1985.

25. Scala G, Kuang YD, Hall RE, et al: Accessory cell function of human B cells. I. Production of both interleukin 1-like activity and an interleukin 1 inhibitory factor by an EBV-transformed human B cell line. *J Exp Med* 159:1637, 1984.

26. Steinman RM, Cohn ZA: Identification of a novel cell type in peripheral lymphoid organs of mice. I. Morphology, quantitation, tissue distribution. *J Exp Med* 137:1142, 1973.

27. Nussenzweig MC, Steinman RM: Contribution of dendritic cells to stimulation of the murine syngeneic mixed leukocyte reaction. *J Exp Med* 151:1196–1212, 1980.

28. Spalding DM, Williamson SI, Kropman WJ, et al: Preferential induction of polyclonal IgA secretion by murine Peyer's patch dendritch cell-T cell mixtures. *J Exp Med* 160:940, 1984.

29. Stingl K, Katz S, Clement L, et al: Immunologic functions of Ia-bearing epidermal langerhans cells. *J Immunol* 121(5):2005–2013, 1978.

30. Steinman RM, Kaplan G, Witmer MD, et al: Ultrastructure of mononuclear phagocytes developing in liquid bone marrow cultures. *J Exp Med* 149(1):1–16, 1979.

31. Witmer-Pack MD, Olivier W, Valinsky J, et al: Quantitation of surface antigens on cultured murine epidermal Langerhans cells: rapid and selective increase in the level of surface MHC products. *J Exp Med* 166(5):1484–1498, 1987.

32. Pober JS, Collins T, Gimbrone MA Jr, et al: Lymphocytes recognize human vascular endothelial and dermal fibroblast Ia antigens induced by recombinant immune interferon. *Nature* 305:726–729, 1983.

33. Leung DYM, Geha RS, Newburger JW, et al: Two monokines interleukin 1 and tumor necrosis factor, render cultured vascular endothelial cells suseptible to lysis by antibodies circulating during Kawaski syndrome. *J Exp Med* 164(6):1958–1972, 1986.

34. Pober JS, Gimbrone MA Jr, Collins T, et al: Interactions of T lymphocytes with human vascular endothelial cells: role of endothelial cells surface antigens. *Immunobiology* 168:483–494, 1984.

35. Bottazzo GF, Pujol-Burrell R, Hanafusa T, et al: Role of aberrant HLA-DR expression and antigen presentation in induction of endocrine autoimmunity. *Lancet* 2:1115–1119, 1983.

36. Bottazzo GF, Todd I, Mirakian R, et al: Organ-specific autoimmunity: a 1986 overview. *Immunol Rev* 94:137–169, 1986.

37. Gottlieb AB, Lifshitz B, Fu SM, et al: Marked increase in the frequency of psoriatic

arthritis in psoriasis patients with HLA-DR+ keratinocytes. *J Exp Med* 164(4):1013–1028, 1986.

38. Lo D, Burkly LC, Widera G, et al: Diabetes and tolerance in transgenic mice expressing class II MHC molecules in pancreatic beta cells. *Cell* 53(1):159–168, 1988.

39. Shimzu Y, Andrew W: Studies on the rabbit appendix. I. Lymphocyte-epithelial relations and the transport of bacteria from lumen to lymphoid nodule. *J Morphol* 123:231–249, 1967.

40. Owen RL, Apple RT, Bhalla DK: Morphometric and cytochemical analysis of lysosomes in rat Peyer's patch follicle epithelium: their reduction in volume fraction and acid phosphatase content in M cells compared to adjacent enterocytes. *Anat Rec* 216(4):521–527, 1986.

41. Owen RL: Sequential uptake of horseradish peroxidase by lymphoid follicle epithelium of Peyer's patches in the normal unobstructed mouse intestine: an ultrastructural study. *Gastroenterology* 72(3):440–451, 1977.

42. Wolf JL, Rubin DH, Finberg R, et al: Intestinal M cells: a pathway for entry of reovirus into the host. *Science* 212(449):471–472, 1981.

43. Shakhlamov VA, Gaider YA, Baranov VN: Electron-cytochemical investigation of cholera toxin absorption by epithelium of Peyer's patches in guinea pigs. *Bull Exp Biol Med* 90:1159–1161, 1981.

44. Owen RL, Pierce NF, Apple RT, et al: M cell transport of Vibrio cholerae from the intestinal lumen into Peyer's patches: A mechanism for antigen sampling and for microbal transepithelial migration. *J Infect Dis* 153(6):1108–1118, 1986.

45. Bockman DE, Cooper MD: Pinocytosis by epithelium associated with lymphoid follicles in the bursa of Fabricius, appendix and Peyer's patches. An electron microscopic study. *Am J Anat* 136:455–477, 1973.

46. Bjerke K, Brandtzaeg P: Lack of relation between expression of HLA-DR and secretory component (SC) in follicle-associated epithelium of human Peyer's patches. *Clin Exp Immunol* 71(3):502–507, 1988.

47. Owen RL, Jones AL: Epithelial cell specialization within human Peyer's patches: an ultrastructural study of intestinal lymphoid follicles. *Gastroenterology* 66:189–203, 1974.

48. Michalek SM, McGhee KR, Kiyono H, et al: The IgA response: inductive aspects, regulatory cells, and effector functions. *Ann NY Acad Sci* 409:48–71, 1983.

49. Craig SW, Cebra JJ: Peyer's patches: an enriched source of precursors for IgA-producing immunocytes in the rabbit. *J Exp Med* 134:188–200, 1971.

50. Elson CO, Heck JA, Strober W: T-cell regulation of murine IgA synthesis. *J Exp Med* 149(3):632–643, 1979.

51. Spalding DM, Griffin JA: Different pathways of differentiation of pre-B cell lines are induced by dendritic cells and T cells from different lymphoid tissues. *Cell* 44(3):507–515, 1986.

52. Lamm ME: Cellular aspects of immunoglobulin A. *Adv Immunol* 22:223–290, 1976.

53. Hecht G, Pothoulakis C, LaMont JT, et al: *Clostridium difficile* toxin A perturbs cytoskeletal structure and tight junction permeability of cultured human intestinal epithelial monolayers. *J Clin Invest* 82(5):1516–1524, 1988.

54. Walker WA, Isselbacher KJ: Uptake and transport of macromolecules by the intestine. Possible role in clinical disorders. *Gastroenterology* 67:531–550, 1974.

55. Bloch KJ, Wright JA, Bishara SM, et al: Uptake of polypeptide fragments of proteins by rat intestine in vitro and in vivo. *Gastroenterology* 95(5):1272–1278, 1988.

56. Mostov KE, Kraehnbuhl JP, Blobel G: Receptor-mediated transcellular transport of

immunoglobulin: synthesis of secretory component as multiple and larger transmembrane forms. *Proc Natl Acad Sci USA* 77(12):7257–7261, 1980.

57. Bland PW, Warren LG: Antigen presentation by epithelial cells of the rat small intestine. II. Selective induction of suppressor T cells. *Immunology* 58(1):9–14, 1986.

58. Mayer L, Shlien R: Evidence for function of Ia molecules on gut epithelial cells in man. *J Exp Med* 166(5):1471–1483, 1987.

59. Mason DW, Dallman M, Barclay AN: Graft-versus-host disease induces expression of Ia antigen in rat epidermal cells and gut epithelium. *Nature* 293(5828):150–151, 1981.

60. Selby WS, Janossy G, Masson DY, et al: Intestinal lymphocyte subpopulations in inflammatory bowel disease: an analysis by immunohistological and cell isolation techniques. *Clin Exp Immunol* 53(3):614–618, 1983.

61. Hirata I, Austin LL, Blackwell WH, et al: Immunoelectron microscopic localization of HLA-DR antigen in control small intestine and colon and in inflammatory bowel disease. *Dig Dis Sci* 31(12):1317–1330, 1986.

62. Mayer L, Eisenhardt D, Salomon P, et al: Submitted.

63. Halper JP, Fu SM, Gottlieb AB, et al: Poor mixed lymphocyte reaction stimulatory capacity of leukemic B cells of chronic lymphocytic leukemia patients despite the presence of Ia antigens. *J Clin Invest* 64(5):1141–1156, 1979.

64. Selby WS, Janossy G, Bofill M, et al: Lymphocyte subpopulations in the human small intestine. The findings in normal mucosa and in the mucosa of patients with adult coeliac disease. *Clin Exp Immunol* 52:219–228, 1973.

65. Mayer L, Eisenhardt D: Lack of induction of suppressor T cells by gut epithelial cells from patients with inflammatory bowel disease. The primary defect? *Gastroenterology* 92(5):1524 (abstract), 1987.

66. Ferguson A, Bruce MG, Strobel S: 'Processing' of antigen by the gut. *Monogr Allergy* 24:253–255, 1988.

CHAPTER 5

Migration of Lymphocytes Within the Mucosal Immune System

C. A. OTTAWAY

INTRODUCTION

Lymphocytes have two essential properties: they are the cellular substrate of anti-gen-specific immune responses, and they are highly motile cells that are able to cross endothelial barriers to travel from blood into tissues and from tissues into the lymph. The combination of these properties is the basis of lymphocyte migration and gives it its physiologic importance. The migration of lymphocytes and their progeny throughout the body facilitates the initiation and propagation of immune responses by permitting the continuous redistribution of the affector cell repertoire and the dissemination of responding effector cells to locations remote from their initial site of antigen presentation.

There are three major reasons why lymphoid cell migration to mucosal immune system, such as that of the intestine, are important. First, immunologic processes at these mucosal surfaces are at the front-lines of host defense. Second, the migration of lymphoid cells at the mucosae is extensive and highly specialized. Finally, alterations in mucosal lymphoid cell accumulation, and perhaps alterations in the regulation of this migration, are an integral feature of a variety of chronic immuno-inflammatory disease processes.

The purposes of this chapter are to focus attention on the physiologic basis of mucosal lymphocyte migration and to highlight our current concepts of how it is regulated.

LYMPHOCYTES IN THE INTESTINE

Lymphocytes are found in large numbers in the intestinal mucosa within three major distinguishable compartments (Table 5–1). The lymphoid cell constituents

49

Table 5–1 LYMPHOCYTE COMPARTMENTS OF THE INTESTINE

Compartment	Input	Constituents	Output
Peyer's patch	Lymphocytes Antigen	Affector cells $\cong$ 80% B $\cong$ 20% T CD4+ $\gg$ CD8+	Effectors Precursors
Lamina propria	Lymphocytes Antigen	Effector and affector cells $\cong$ 40% B $\cong$ 60% T	Ig responses T responses
Intraepithelial layer	Effectors Antigen	Effector cells $\cong$ 85% CD8+	T responses Other responses?

of these compartments differ substantially in fuction, phenotype, and fate. Although histologic sections suggest a stable distribution of cells in these compartments, the lymphoid constituents of these compartments are by no means static.

For example, lymphoid cells in the intraepithelial compartment (IEL) are predominantly CD8+ T cells in mice,[1] rats,[2] and humans.[3,4] This compartment consists almost entirely of effector cells,[1] and there is little evidence for local proliferation of lymphoid cells within this environment once the cells have moved to the epithelial side of the epithelial basement membrane.[5] Their life span, therefore, is probably limited by the life span of the epithelium itself. In the mouse, the T cells in this compartment use a T-cell receptor that is different from that found on the majority of T cells in the rest of the body. Whereas the majority of peripheral T cells (CD4+ or CD8+) have a T-cell receptor that consists of dimers of alpha and beta chains and is associated with the CD3 antigen, T cells of the IEL have a receptor made up of gamma and delta chain dimers.[6-8] These receptors are also associated with CD3, but, although the majority of IEL T cells express the CD8+ antigen, less than one-half of them also express Thy-1.[1,6,7] The situation in other species is not yet clear,[9,10] but the cells in this compartment probably represent a novel lineage of T cells specialized for antigen interactions at the epithelial surface.

Large numbers of lymphocytes exist within the lamina propria. The lymphocytes of this compartment are a mixed population of affector and effector cells. A sizeable proportion of these cells are B cells, many of which are terminally differentiated plasma cells producing exportable IgA and IgM, or IgG. The local production of secretory IgA within the mucosa is now recognized as a major mechanism for the interception of antigen from the intestinal lumen.[11,12] The life span of plasma cells, however, is also limited. For example, IgA plasma cells in the murine lamina propria have been estimated to have a turnover time on the order of only a few days.[13]

The principal immunologic affector organs of the intestinal mucosa are the aggregated gut-associated lymphoid tissues (GALT), such as Peyer's patches, tonsils and the appendix. Peyer's patches, for example, act as antigen detectors and processors. Their overlying epithelium consists of specialized microfold-containing cells that can actively sample the contents of the intestinal lumen; beneath this epithelium macrophages and dendritic cells are found that permit antigen presentation to lymphocytes.[14] Large numbers of B cells are found in the follicles of these structures, which are distributed around the T-cell and vascular corridors of the patches. It is now clear that Peyer's patches and their related GALT structures are the major sites at which the activation and programming of IgA-producing B cells and mucosally directed T-effector cells is initiated, and that the immune reactions that occur in these compartments generate the precursors of the effector populations that populate the other compartments of the intestinal mucosa.[15-18]

These considerations illustrate two central features of the mucosal immune system. First, effector lymphoid cell populations in the lamina propria and the epithelium are both topographically and temporally restricted. Second, these effector cells are the products of affector cell encounters with antigen that occur predominantly within a distinct affector compartment. It should come as no surprise, therefore, that communication between these compartments occurs and that the continued maintenance of immunologic effector competence depends upon the migration of cells between compartments. Furthermore, because of the major differences that are apparent in the constituents of these compartments, at least some aspects of the migration processes involved must be specialized and/or selective for particular cells at particular sites.

IMMUNOPHYSIOLOGY OF MUCOSAL LYMPHOID CELL MIGRATION

The extent to which lymphocytes migrate through the intestine is remarkable. It has been estimated that in mice approximately 2×10^8 lymphocytes per day are exchanged between the blood and intestinal lymph.[19] In rats, similar estimates suggest an intestinal exchange of approximately 10^9 lymphocytes per day,[20] while in the sheep, an animal that in size and cardiovascular capacity more closely resembles humans, the total throughput of lymphocytes for the intestine is of the order of 10^{10} cells per day.[21]

This prodigious traffic of lymphocytes involves both the organized lymphoid tissue such as Peyer's patches and the nonlymphoid lamina propria. In the cat[22] and the rat,[23] the density of lymphocytes exiting from the intestine is approximately tenfold higher in lymphatics draining Peyer's patch-containing regions than in those draining "nonlymphoid" intestine. Other experiments have demonstrated that the rate at which lymphocytes will enter Peyer's patches from the blood is an order of magnitude higher than the rate at which they will enter the nonlymphoid regions of the small intestine of rats and mice.[24,25] Thus the flux of lymphocytes through Peyer's patches is greater than that through the nonlymphoid intestine and reflects the higher efficiency with which lymphocytes enter the Peyer's patches. The portion of the intestine that contains macroscopically recognizable lymphoid tissue, however, is a small fraction of the total organ mass, and calculations of the relative distribution of lymphocyte migration between lymphoid and nonlymphoid regions of the intestine of rodents suggest that the total quantity of lymphocytes that migrate through these two regions is of similar total magnitude.[19,20]

For a lymphoid cell to migrate through intestinal tissue, it must: 1) be available in the blood; 2) be delivered to the intestinal vaculature; 3) attach to the endothelial surface of a postcapillary venule; 4) insinuate itself between endothelial cells; 5) transit the basement membrane of the endothelium; 6) locomote through the tissue stroma; and 7) find an appropriate exit through the fine lymphatic vessels and depart from the tissue.

A great variety of factors have been implicated as contributors to the process of lymphoid cell migration (Table 5–2). In applying these concepts to mucosal lymphoid cell migration, it is important to distinguish between different stages of lymphocyte activation and different sites of migration. The migratory properties of small lymphocytes and activated lymphoblasts differ in important ways. Moreover, there are differences in the interaction of each of these lymphoid cell types with lymphoid tissues such as Peyer's patches or lymph nodes, as opposed to their interaction with the nonlymphoid absorptive lamina propria of the intestine. Many of the general factors that influence migration to the mucosa have been reviewed elsewhere,[20,26] and further discussion will focus on specific factors as much as possible.

Migration Experiments In Vivo

In vivo studies of the physiology of lymphoid cell migration usually depend upon examining the distribution of lymphoid cell populations that have been labeled (isotopes, fluorescent dyes, chromosome markers) and transferred to the intravenous space of a suitable recipient (usually syngeneic). The distribution of the cells

Table 5–2   FACTORS THAT AFFECT LYMPHOID CELL MIGRATION TO THE MUCOSA

General Factors

Physiological factors
  Blood flow
  Density of cells in the blood
  Nutritional status of animal
Pathologic processes
  Inflammatory events
  Granuloma formation
  Drugs (ACTH, corticosteroids, cyclosporine A)

Specific factors

Lymphocyte phenotype
  B vs. T; CD4 vs. CD8
  State of activation (i.e., activated lymphoblast vs. "resting" lymphocyte)
  Tissue origin of lymphoblasts in all animals studied.
  Tissue origin of lymphocytes in some species (e.g., sheep).
  Lymphocyte surface determinants for Peyer's patches, lymph nodes, granuloma, other sites
  VIP receptors
  LFA-1
Endothelial phenotype
  HEV vs. other endothelia
  Carbohydrate determinants
  Specific surface proteins (e.g., addressins)
  Innervation
Mucosal stromal signals?

at some time is evaluated by examining labeled cells (amount, proportion, or density of the transferred cells) in a particular tissue or in blood or lymph of the recipient. In such experiments, small lymphocytes regularly will be found in large numbers in tissues such as Peyer's patches and mesenteric and other lymph nodes of the recipients, but few cells will accumulate within the mucosa of the intestine. The lack of accumulation of the lymphocytes in the intestine reflects a lower efficiency of uptake of the cells, and a lower probability that they will be retained in the lamina propria compared with the nodes or Peyer's patches.[20,26] This pattern of distribution of lymphocytes was first demonstrated by Gowans and his co-workers,[27] but it has been regularly affirmed by numerous investigators since.

In contrast, if actively dividing lymphoblasts that have been stimulated in vivo are selectively labeled (e.g., in vitro labeling with nucleotide precursors) and subjected to the same experimental protocol, lymphoblast populations obtained from either the thoracic duct lymph or mesenteric lymph nodes will accumulate readily in the intestinal mucosa, but will not accumulate in the Peyer's patches or mesenteric nodes to the same extent as small lymphocytes do.[28-33] Analyses of the time course of these types of experiments have shown that the efficiency with which mesenteric node lymphoblasts, for example, enter the intestine is not greater than that found for small lymphocytes, but that their retention by the tissues is greater.[24,26] In parallel, their ability to enter lymphoid tissues such as Peyer's patches and the mesenteric nodes is also not very different from that found for the small lymphocyte populations, but in these tissues, lymphoblasts are less likely to be retained than are the small lymphocytes.[24,26]

B and T Cells

A central concept that has emerged from migration studies is that small lymphocytes migrate extensively from the blood into secondary lymphoid tissues and other organs, and subsequently into the lymph draining those organs to return to the blood. The majority of the lymphocytes in the lymph draining the intestine are participating in this recirculation. Both B and T cells recirculate, and may do so differently in some tissues, but the migratory abilities of B and T cells appears to be similar in gut tissues of a variety of species.

For example, in sheep, the tempo with which lymphocytes obtained from the intestinal lymph will reappear in the mesenteric lymph after labeling and autologous transfusion is the same for B and T cells,[21] and studies in rodents suggest that both the admission and accumulation events for B and T cells in gut lymphoid tissue is quite similar. Lymphocytes in the thoracic duct (TD) of normal rats consist of approximately 70% T cells, but in athymic rats about 90% of the TD lymphocytes are Ig-bearing B cells.[34] If these lymphocyte populations are labeled and transfused to normal or athymic recipients, the lymphocytes from normal donors accumulate more readily in peripheral lymph nodes than do lymphocytes from athymic donors, but the lymphocytes from either donor will accumulate to an equivalent extent in the Peyer's patches of either type of recipient.[34,35] Furthermore, if rat TD lymphocytes are enriched for T cells and infused into normal recipients, these lymphocytes will accumulate to a greater extent in peripheral and mesenteric lymph nodes than they will in Peyer's patches.[36] Similarly, in mice, the relative localization of B and T cells of mixed lymphocyte populations is equivalent in Peyer's patches, but T cells will sustain a higher degree of localization in peripheral or mesenteric lymph nodes.[37] Kinetic assessment of the rate at which labeled lymphocyte populations are cleared from the blood into Peyer's patches demonstrates a similar clearance rate for populations that contain different proportions of B and T cells, but the rate at which these cells are cleared by mesenteric lymph nodes is higher when more T cells are present in the innoculum.[26]

Together, these studies suggest that, on average and unlike lymph nodes, there are no major differences in the ways in which B and T lymphocytes gain entry to the gut and Peyer's patches. The same is not true, however, when T cells are further discriminated with respect to their subsets. For example, Kraal and coworkers[38] examined the relative localization of CD8+ and CD8−T cells in mice at early times after cell transfer and observed differences in the distribution of these cells in different tissues. Specifically, they concluded that there was an enhanced ability of CD8−T cells to localize in Peyer's patches compared with subcutaneous lymph nodes. We have investigated the time course of accumulation of CD4-enriched and CD8-enriched T cell populations, and found both Peyer's patches and lymph nodes (inguinal and mesenteric) to have a consistent ability to clear CD4+ cells from the blood at a rate more than twofold greater than the rate found for CD8+ cells.[39] The retention of these lymphocytes in the tissues varied, however, both with T-cell phenotype and the organ concerned.[39]

Intestinal Migration Pools

A key question is the extent to which the intestinal compartments (Fig. 5–1) are a preferred route of migration for particular lymphocytes. In sheep, consistent evi-

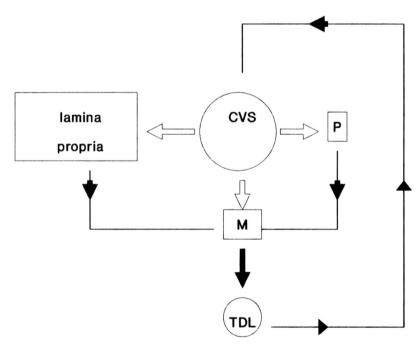

Figure 5–1 A schematic flow diagram for the migration of lymphocytes in different intestinal compartments. CVS, cardiovascular system; P, Peyer's patch; M, mesenteric lymph node; TDL, thoracic duct lymph.

dence has been found[40-43] that small lymphocytes emigrating from the gut in the intestinal lymph show a preferential, but by no means exclusive, ability to recirculate through the intestine rather than a tissue such as a subcutaneous lymph node after they are reinfused into the blood. Lymphocytes obtained from the lymph draining a subcutaneous lymph node show a complementary enhanced ability to remigrate through that nodal tissue rather than the intestine.[41,42] It has been shown that this bias in the migration potential of cells obtained from lymph compartments is also present when the cells are enriched for T cells[41] and is not a consequence of the presence of blast cells in the lymphoid cell preparation.[42] These observations are the basis for the view that there are at least two distinguishable pools of recirculating lymphocytes in this animal, one migrating preferentially through peripheral lymph nodes and one migrating through the gut.

The applicability of this concept to other species is currently unclear. Detailed studies of the in vivo migration of T and B small lymphocyte populations in rodents have failed to reveal any evidence that the migratory destination of the lymphocytes is primarily determined by their tissue of origin.[37,38,44,45] We will see below that distinguishable recognition mechanisms that affect the ability of lymphocytes to exit from the blood either in mucosal lymphoid tissue or subcutaneous lymph nodes are now clearly established in both rats and mice, but, so far, the evidence is consistent with the view that most normal lymphocytes express both sets of tissue determinants. In contrast to the situation with small lymphocytes, preferential migration of lymphoblasts in different nonlymphoid tissues is a consistent feature in all experimental species in which lymphoblast migration has been studied. The lymphoid tissue from which lymphoblast populations originate markedly restricts the range of tissues in which they will accumulate after transfer. For example, lymphoblasts that arise in subcutaneous lymph nodes will readily accumulate in inflamed skin or in the peritoneal cavity but are very limited in their ability to accumulate in the intestine.[31] Lymphoblasts from the thoracic duct, the mesenteric lymph node, or the intestinal lymph, however, will accumulate readily in the intestinal mucosa (Fig. 5-2), but do not accumulate in either normal or inflamed skin.[28-33]

Lymphoblasts originating in a particular mucosa can also have more than one mucosal destination. For example, gut-derived lymphoblasts can contribute to the IgA plasma cell population of the bronchial tree, the genitourinary tract, and the lactating breast,[46-49] and IgA-expressing lymphoblasts from the bronchus-associated lymphoid tissue can contribute to the plasma cell population of the intestine.[48] These observations have led to the idea that there is a common mucosal immune system, such that the activation of lymphoblasts in a particular mucosal site can result in the deployment of appropriate effector cells throughout that mucosa as well as other mucosal surfaces.[50]

With respect to the intestine, however, a large proportion of the activated blast cells found in the thoracic duct will have arisen in the gut-associated lymphoid tissues, and a large proportion of these will selectively take up residence in the intestinal mucosa. Furthermore, lymphoblasts in the thoracic duct have the ability to colonize the intestinal mucosa with intraintestinal selectivity depending upon their level of origin in the intestine. Pierce and Cray[51] studied the ability of thoracic duct populations obtained from intestinally immunized rats to result in antigen-specific plasma cells within the mucosa of syngeneic recipients after intravenous transfer. When donor rats were immunized with cholera toxin via the colon, the

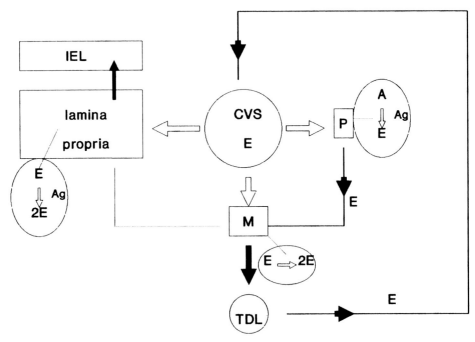

Figure 5 – 2 A schematic flow diagram for the migration of gut-originating lymphoblasts. A, affector cells; E, effector cells; potential sites of origin and expansion of
effector cells are indicated in ellipses; IEL, intraepithelial cells. Other abbreviations as
in Figure 1.

thoracic duct transfers resulted in specific antitoxin antibody-containing cells
throughout the intestine, but their density was approximately fivefold higher in the
colon than it was in the duodenum. In contrast, when donor immunization occurred via the duodenum, the density of the specific antibody-containing cells in
the duodenum of the recipients was 10 times higher than that found in the colonic
mucosa.[51]

Taken together, these observations suggest that following activation the way in
which lymphoid cells interact with tissues during migration changes substantially.
Furthermore, during activation and/or maturation, lymphoblasts must somehow
encode properties of their local environment that influence their ability to occupy
different mucosal tissues in a very precise manner.

The Issue of "Homing"

The preferential migration or selective tissue accumulation of particular lymphoid
cell populations is often referred to as "homing." Morris[52] has emphasized that this
anthropomorphic term is fraught with inferences that can interfere with our understanding of the proesses involved if we take the term too literally. For example,
without denying that certain lymphoid cell populations have the ability to migrate
to and/or accumulate in particular tissues in preferred ways, it would be incorrect
to infer that blood-borne lymphoid cells somehow have the ability to navigate to
predefined tissue destinations, or that lymphocytes have a fixed commitment to a

particular "home" throughout their life span. The specific factors that influence the selective or preferential migratory abilities of lymphocyte populations are still incompletely understood, but many processes are involved in lymphocyte migration. Selectivity in these processes can arise in at least two ways: selection as cells are admitted to a tissue, and selection after their arrival at that tissue.

MOLECULAR AND CELLULAR BIOLOGY OF LYMPHOID CELL MIGRATION

Under normal circumstances, blood-borne lymphocytes exit the blood stream by negotiating the endothelium of the postcapillary venules. To enter intestinal tissues, lymphocytes must reach the postcapillary venules in Peyer's patches, other lymphoid aggregates, or the mucosa, and must adhere to the endothelium to begin their migration. It is now clear that the marked efficiency with which lymphocytes gain entry to the lymphoid aggregates of the intestine is due to selective and specific interactions between surface determinants of lymphocytes and the endothelial cells of the postcapillary vessels of the lymphoid tissues. In lymphoid tissues such as Peyer's patches and lymph nodes, the endothelial cells lining these venules are specialized. In some species, the endothelial cells in the collecting venules have a cuboidal or columnar morphology and are referred to as high endothelial venules (HEV).[53] The "height" of the cells varies, however, and in some species, for example the sheep, the morphology of these cells is indistinguishable from that of other endothelia but still permits the efficient collection of lymphocytes.[54]

The concept that there is a specific interaction between lymphocytes and the specialized endothelial cells of the HEV arose originally from microscopic observations.[27,55-58] Detailed exploration of the molecular and cellular mechanisms involved, however, has come mainly from studies in which lymphocyte adhesion to the HEV endothelium is studied in vitro in parallel with in vivo studies. The pivotal development here was the introduction of in vitro methods for assessing the ability of lymphocytes to bind to HEV in histologic sections of lymphoid tissue such as Peyer's patches, lymph nodes, appendix, or tonsils.

Lymphocyte-Endothelial Binding

Stamper and Woodruff[59] first demonstrated that lymphocytes that recirculate in vivo can adhere to the endothelial cells of HEV in frozen sections of mucosal lymphoid tissues or lymph nodes when the lymphocytes are incubated on lymphoid tissue sections. This adherence shows a number of important features. First, although the lymphocytes need to be viable to attach themselves to the section, the section can be frozen and/or fixed with aldehyde reagents.[59-62] Second, recirculating lymphocytes demonstrate a high degree of binding to such sections, but preparations of lymphocytes obtained directly from the thymus or the bone marrow, which show little ability to recirculate, bind at least an order of magnitude less well to the sections. Furthermore, the binding of lymphocytes, which have good migratory abilities, is restricted to the HEV. Other vessels of the tissues do not support the adherence of lymphocytes in this assay.[59-62]

In various forms, this in vitro assay of the interaction of lymphocytes with the HEV of lymphoid tissues has been used in many investigations to define a number of determinants that control lymphocyte-endothelial cell interactions. What has emerged from these studies is the concept that the surface determinants that permit these interactions are found on both the lymphocytes and the endothelial cells, and that the determinants involved in mucosal tissues clearly differ from those involved in peripheral lymph nodes.

One of the first indications of an organ-specific bias in the interaction of lymphocytes with HEV came from studies of the ability of mouse lymphoma cell lines to bind to HEV in vitro.[63] It was found that, whereas some cell lines would bind to both Peyer's patch HEV and peripheral lymph node HEV, and others would bind to neither, there were some cell lines that demonstrated almost exclusive ability to bind to the HEV of one tissue but not the other.[63,64] Gallatin and his coworkers[65] exploited the ability of a particular cell line to bind to the HEV of subcutaneous lymph nodes, but not to Peyer's patch HEV by immunizing animals with that cell line. They produced monoclonal antibodies to the cell line and selected for antibodies that could affect the in vitro adherence of normal lymphocytes to lymph node HEV.[65] One selected antibody, designated MEL-14, has the ability to decrease the binding of normal murine lymphocytes and normal circulating human lymphocytes to either murine or human lymph node sections in vitro (Table 5–3). Furthermore, if normal murine lymphocytes are incubated with MEL-14 antibody prior to intravenous transfer to syngeneic recipients, the ability of the treated cells to accumulate at early times after cell transfer in the subcutaneous lymph nodes of the animals is impaired without any measurable difference in their ability to accumulate either in Peyer's patches or other tissues.[66] It has since been shown that the antigenic determinant with which MEL-14 reacts on the lymphocyte surface is an unusual ubiquinated glycoprotein of approximately 85–95 kD relative mass.[67]

There are two noteworthy features to these observations. First, the binding of this antibody to the lymphocyte surface affects the ability of the lymphocytes to adhere to the HEV in vitro, *and* to accumulated in vivo within particularly subcomponents of the lymphoid system. Second, although lymphocytes to which MEL-14 was bound were impaired in their ability to accumulate in peripheral lymph nodes of recipients, they were not impaired in their ability to enter Peyer's patches, and, in fact, lymphocytes with MEL-14 bound to their surface were recoverable from the Peyer's patches of the recipients.[65] These observations are most consistent with the idea that the determinant recognized by MEL-14 is involved in the attachment to the endothelial cells of the nodal HEV, and that most normal murine lymphocytes simultaneously express at least one other determinant that is involved with attachment and tissue entry via the endothelium of the gut-associated tissues.

A similar concept has emerged from studies in the rat, although this is based upon a difference in approach and a different set of determinants. Woodruff and her colleagues found that soluble protein factors, which could be isolated from the thoracic duct lymph of rats, had the ability to inhibit either the ability of thoracic duct lymphocytes (TDL) to adhere in vitro either to the HEV of cervical lymph node sections or the HEV of Peyer's patches.[53] These factors have been described as HEV binding factors for these specific targets (i.e., $HEBF_{LN}$ and $HEBF_{PP}$).[68] Heterologous antibodies to these factors were generated and shown to be directed against surface components of the TD lymphocytes. It has since been demonstrated that the same binding factors can be recovered from cultures of rat TDL cells,[69-71] and thus the factors that are isolatable from normal thoracic duct lymph

Table 5-3 PROPERTIES OF SOME MONOCLONAL ANTIBODIES TO LYMPHOCYTE SURFACE DETERMINANTS INVOLVED IN LYMPHOCYTE ENDOTHELIAL CELL INTERACTIONS*

MAb	Ref.	Produced in	Antigen used	Antigen recognized	Effect on lymphocyte-endothelial interaction
MEL-14	65	Mouse (IgG2)	Murine B lymphoma (C3H/eb)	Mouse: Ubiquinated glycoprotein, 85–95 kD Human: MEL-14 reacts with HERMES-1 of PBL	Mouse: ↓ Binding to LN ↓ Localization to LN Human: ↓ Binding of PBL to human LN
1B2	73	Mouse (IgG1)	Soluble HEV binding factor blocking PP	Rat: 80 kD protein	Rat: ↓ Binding to PP ↓ Localization to PP
A.11	72	Mouse (IgG1)	Soluble HEV binding factor blocking LN	Rat: 135 kD, 60 kD, and 40 kD proteins	Rat: ↓ Binding to LN ↓ Localization to LN
	53			Human: Reacts with PBL	Human: No effect on binding
3.A.7	53	Mouse	Soluble HEV binding factor from human serum	Human: Stains 85% PBL	Human: ↓ binding of PBL to rat cervical LN, no effect on binding to mesenteric LN
HERMES-1	74	Rat (IgG2a)	Human tonsil lymphocytes	Human: 90 kD protein	No direct effect on PBL binding in vitro
HERMES-3	76	Mouse (IgG2a)	HERMES-1 Ag from (KCA) B line that binds to appendix	Human: 85–95 kD protein stains 95% PBL	Human: ↓ Binding to appendix, no effect on LN binding

LN, lymph node; PP, Peyer's patch; PBL, human circulating lymphocytes.

* An MAb to an antigen designated LPAM-1 has now been identified which inhibits the adhesion of normal murine lymphocytes and some lymphoma cell lines to PP HEV in vitro. This antibody recognizes an epitope of a dimeric protein that is homologous to the human integrin receptor VLA-4. The effects of treatment with this antibody on migration in vivo have not been reported. (See Holzmann B, McIntyre B, Weissman LL, Identification of a murine Peyer's patch-specific lymphocyte homing receptor as an integrin molecule with an alpha chain homologous to human VLA-4alpha, *Cell* 56:37–46, 1989.)

are believed to be a shed product of circulating lymphocytes in vivo. The heterologous antibodies to these factors showed the ability to selectively interfere with the ability of rat TDL to bind to the HEV of either cervical lymph nodes or Peyer's patches, respectively.[53] Woodruff and Chin have since generated specific monoclonal antibodies to these binding factors (Table 5–3), which are able to affect both the in vitro adherence and the in vivo localization of transferred labeled lymphocytes in recipients.[72–73]

In both the rat and the mouse, therefore, there are separately recognizable lymphocyte determinants that appear to define the ability of lymphocytes to interact with the specialized endothelium of lymph nodes as opposed to the Peyer's patches. The determinants involved, however, appear to be different in these rodents. In particular, the determinant that is recognized on mouse lymphocytes by MEL-14 appears to be quite different from those recognized by A.11 on rat lymphocytes (Table 5–3),[53,65,72] even though the functional features that are perturbable by these antibodies are quite comparable. A very interesting feature, however, is that both the reagents developed in the rat and those developed in the mouse appear to have cross-reactivity with surface components of human lymphocytes (Table 5–3).

The extension of the ideas that have emerged from these studies to human lymphocytes has been a natural and important one, and has already suggested that the concept of multideterminants selective for particular lymphoid sites is warranted in humans. Woodruff and her colleagues have generated a monoclonal antibody (3.A.7, see Table 5–3) against soluble binding factor obtained from cultures of human circulating lymphocytes.[53] This antibody immunostains a large proportion of human lymphocytes and recognizes a surface determinant that participates in their ability to bind to rat cervical lymph node HEV in vitro.[53] It is pertinent to note that the ability of lymphocytes to adhere to HEV in vitro on tissue sections is not restricted by species barriers to any great extent, although allogeneic lymphocytes will not migrate or localize normally. Human lymphocytes, therefore, have the ability to bind to HEV in rat lymphoid tissues, and antibody 3A7 interferes with the ability of the human cells to attach to rat cervical, but not to mesenteric, lymph node sections in vitro.[53]

Jalkanen and her colleagues used a strategy of allogeneic lymphocyte immunization to generate antibodies to human lymphocyte determinants involved in HEV recognition.[74,75] These investigators immunized rats with human tonsil lymphocytes, generated hybridomas, and selected antibodies by their ability to immunostain human lymphocytes.[74] They generated an antibody, designated HERMES-1 (Table 5–3), which has not been implicated in HEV binding abilities but has some interesting properties. This antibody is directed at a glycoprotein that is also recognized by MEL-14, but appears to be directed at an epitope that is not used during the binding of cells to lymph node HEV. Thus the presence of the antibody does not affect the ability of either murine or human lymphocytes to bind to HEV in vitro, but the ability of different human cell lines to bind to HEV of the human appendix in vitro is paralleled by the degree to which they are immunostainable with the HERMES-1 antibody.[74,75]

This same group of workers[76] has used this reagent in an elegant way to further facilitate their search for specific human determinants. They used a particular human cell line that has the ability to adhere in vitro to sections of human appendix and partially purified the antigen to which HERMES-1 is directed from these cells.

This antigen, from the human cell line, was then used to immunize mice for hybridoma production, and antibodies were selected by their ability both to stain human lymphocytes and interfere with their ability to bind to the human appendix.[76] They selected an antibody designated HERMES-3, which cross reacts with both HERMES-1 and MEL-14, and in vitro decreases the ability of human cells to bind to the appendix, but has no effect on the ability of the cells to bind to the HEV of lymph node sections.[76]

The effects of antibodies 3A7 and HERMES-3 are provocative circumstantial evidence that human lymphocytes use a set of determinants that are similar in principal to those identified in the rodents, and that there are at least two distinguishable surface determinants involved in the ability of human cells to attach selectively to either the endothelium of lymph nodes or the endothelium of gut-associated lymphoid tissues such as the appendix and Peyer's patches (Table 5–3). It is important to recognize, however, that effects of these antibodies on the in vivo behavior of lymphocytes have not yet been tested. Furthermore, it needs to be recognized that strategies in which the selection of reagents through assays based upon HEV binding in vitro will, of necessity, select for effects that are maximally expressed under the conditions of that assay.

This bears upon our interpretation of the data for the following reasons. Although it would be simplest, and in many ways most attractive, to understand the process of selective migration in terms of single determinants that permit selective attachment processes at the endothelium, this aspect of the process is only one step in the migration process. Furthermore, although the molecular evidence so far has tended to emphasize the contribution of single determinants that have been amenable to present investigative approaches, even the attachment process is likely to be more complex than it at first seems. For example, there is evidence from parallel lines of investigation that other determinants of the lymphocyte can play a permissive role in selection during the early stages of migration.

One such factor is the leukocyte function associated antigen LFA-1, a lymphocyte surface determinant that has been implicated in other attachment events in vitro.[77] Investigations with both murine and human lymphocytes[78,79] indicates that the expression of LFA-1 affects the ability of lymphocytes to attach to HEV in vitro[78,79] and the ability of murine lymphocytes to localize in lymphoid tissues at early times after cell transfer.[78]

Other work has implicated the ability of lymphocytes to recognize and respond to neural signals that may be of particular importance in the intestine. For example, the neuropeptide vasoactive intestinal peptide (VIP) can influence the emigration of lymphocytes from lymph nodes in sheep,[80,81] and the entry of T cells from the blood into Peyer's patches and mesenteric lymph nodes in mice.[82,83] In mice, T cells have specific high-affinity receptors for VIP,[84] and the HEV of Peyer's patches and mesenteric nodes are innervated by VIP-immunostainable nerve fibers.[85] Interference with the ability of murine T cells to recognize this neuropeptide through perturbation of their VIP receptor expression affects the rate at which transferred T cells migrate into Peyer's patches and mesenteric nodes in vivo in a tissue-selective manner.[82,83] The concept that emerges from these studies is that selective patterns of innervation in the HEV, and selective expression of receptors by lymphocytes, may facilitate the interaction of the lymphocytes with the endothelium to modulate migration in both a tissue- and cell-specific fashion.

Studies of the dynamics of the interaction of blood-borne lymphocytes with the

HEV of Peyer's patches in vivo show that the attachment process is very rapid and of substantial strength.[86] Furthermore, the surface attachment between these cells in the intact animal achieves the strength required for the attached cell to withstand the flow of the blood in the vessel within a time period that is measured in milliseconds.[86] Thus it would not be surprising if a variety of concomitant molecular mechanisms were invoked during the attachment phase to facilitate this pivotal event. It seems likely that multifactorial contributions will be identified, perhaps with a key set of determinants operating to trigger a cascade of surface interactions that may be required to hold the cell at the endothelial surface while it begins its transit across the endothelial barrier.

Furthermore, it must be recognized that there is a substantial discontinuity between the efficiency with which lymphocytes can interact with endothelial cells in vitro as opposed to in vivo. For example, observations on the total numbers of lymphocytes that will adhere to the HEV on tissue sections in vitro indicate that the overall efficiency of the process is on the order of 10^{-4}–10^{-5}.[60,87] The attachment of lymphocytes directly to specialized endothelial cells derived from lymph nodes in culture is more efficient,[88] but still only yields an overall efficiency for attachment that is on the order of 10^{-2}–10^{-3}.[88] In vivo, however, the attachment and extraction of lymphocytes at these boundaries is extremely efficient and has regularly been found to be on the order of 10^{-1}–1.[26,86,89] Thus we must be cautious in extrapolating from the adherence assays to the in vivo situation without direct confirmation in the intact animal, because the dependency of the process on events that are affected at low efficiency may or may not be decisive when the system operates under physiologic conditions.

Another interesting apparent discrepancy in our present understanding is the selective interaction of lymphocytes with particular lymphoid tissues as it may occur for rodents, and perhaps for human lymphocytes, as opposed to the observations that have been made in sheep. It is clear that lymphocytes obtained from the gut lymph compartments of the sheep will display a bias in their ability to remigrate through the gut as opposed to peripheral locations such as a subcutaneous lymph node and vice versa.[40-43] The evidence in rodents and humans, however, is most consistent with the idea that the vast majority of circulating lymphocytes in these species simultaneously express determinants for both comparable destinations in their hosts. For example, approximately 90% of normal human circulating lymphocytes bear the determinants that are recognized both by the monoclonal antibodies 3.A.7 and HERMES-3.[53,76] Moreover, there is no direct evidence in rodents that the tissue of origin of cells, other than for blast cells, affects their migratory destination.

The reasons for this apparent discrepancy are not yet clear. One possibility is that there are species-specific differences in the molecular strategies that have been elaborated to promote migratory integrity. Another possibility is that the observations in the sheep depend upon the immunologic experience of the animal, and that memory cells may differ from virgin cells in the way in which, or the degree to which, they express tissue-specific determinants. For example, it is known that lymphocyte migration occurs extensively even in utero in the fetal sheep,[90] but that at this time there is no tissue-specific bias in the way in which cells collected from different lymph compartments will migrate. The asymmetric migration of lymphocytes in the sheep, therefore, is acquired postnatally, and it is possible that the cells that are contributing to this behavior may be cells that have had previous experience in one tissue or another. This scenario suggests that although hitherto unstimulated lymphocytes (virgin cells?) might express determinants for a variety of destinations, cells that have returned to the resting state after antigenic stimulation might be more restricted in the attachment determinants than they will express.

Endothelial Factors

Although most attention has been directed to the contributions of the lymphocyte to lymphocyte-endothelial interactions, the endothelial cells are not passive partners in the process. A variety of investigations have been aimed at determining the properties that the endothelial cell contributes to attachment and migration. Carbohydrate components on the surface of the endothelium at HEV have been implicated in the ability of these cells to participate in the selective attachment of lymphocytes. In particular, mannose-like determinants appear to play a role.[91-93] Furthermore, there are differences between different tissue sites. For example, enzyme treatment to remove the sialic acid residues on the endothelial cells of lymphoid tissue sections will disrupt the attachment of normal lymphocytes to lymph node sections, but does not affect the ability of lymphocytes to attach to Peyer's patch tissue sections.[94]

A number of monoclonal antibodies to the specialized endothelial cells of HEV have been generated (Table 5–4) that reveal some important properties. Duijvestijn and coworkers immunized rats with a stromal cell preparation of murine lymph nodes (subcutaneous and mesenteric) and after hybridization selected monoclonal antibodies that would stain endothelial cells in a variety of tissues.[95] They generated a number of monoclonals [termed mouse endothelial cell antibodies (MECA)] that reacted with endothelial cell components in a species-specific manner.[95] Some antibodies reacted with the endothelia of a wide variety of tissues, but one (MECA-325) appears to be selective in its ability to stain the endothelial cells of the HEV of both lymph nodes and Peyer's patches.[95] Although this antibody has no demonstrable ability to affect the adherence of lymphocytes to lymphoid tissue sections, it shows the interesting property of staining endothelial cells in experimental skin granulomas that formed in response to the injection of sheep red cells in the presence of Freund's complete adjuvant.[95] Furthermore, although it does not

Table 5–4 PROPERTIES OF SOME ENDOTHELIAL CELL MONOCLONAL ANTIBODIES

		Recognizes HEV in:					
Designation	Ref.	PLN	MLN	PP	Experi-mental granuloma	Antigen	Affects lymphocyte binding
Meca-325	95	Yes	Yes	Yes	Yes	ND	No
Meca-89	99	No	Yes	Yes	No	58–66 Kd protein	No
Meca-367	99	No	Yes	Yes	No	58–66 Kd protein	Yes

PLN, peripheral lymph nodes; MLN, mesenteric lymph nodes; PP, Peyer's patches; ND, not determined.

stain vessels in a variety of nonlymphoid tissues, it has been found to stain endo-thelial vessels in the postcapillary venules of the absorptive intestinal mucosa.[96] The vessels in these regions do not bear "high endothelial" morphology, but appear to be the sites through which both small lymphocytes[96] and lymphoblasts gain entry to the mucosa from the blood stream.[97,98]

Two other endothelial cell antibodies have been reported by Streeter and his coworkers[99] (Table 5–4). Antibodies MECA-89 and MECA-367 appear to recog-nize different epitopes of an endothelial cell protein that has a molecular weight of approximately 60,000 and is expressed by the HEV endothelial cells of Peyer's patches and mesenteric lymph nodes, but not by the HEV of subcutaneous lymph nodes, nor by the reacting endothelium in experimental granuloma of the skin.[99] Both MECA-89 and MECA-367 can also stain venules scattered throughout the absorptive lamina propria of the gut, although less densely than they stain the HEV of Peyer's patches.[99]

MECA-89 and MECA-367 have divergent effects on lymphocyte interactions with HEV endothelium in vitro and in vivo. MECA-367, but not MECA-89, treat-ment of lymphoid tissue sections inhibits the ability of mesenteric node lympho-cytes to bind to lymphoid tissue sections in a site-specific manner. Adhesion to the HEV of Peyer's patches is blocked by about one order of magnitude; adhesion to mesenteric node HEV is blocked by about 50%, but adhesion to peripheral lymph node sections is not affected by MECA-367 treatment.[99] In vivo, the early locali-zation of transferred mesenteric lymph node lymphocytes is perturbed by MECA-367, but not by MECA-89, pretreatment of syngeneic recipients. When animals received MECA-367 antibody intravenously prior to the transfer of labeled lymphocytes, the accumulation of cells in Peyer's patches was markedly decreased, mesenteric node accumulation was decreased by about 40%, and peripheral lymph node accumulation of the transferred cells was not measurably affected.[99]

Together, these observations suggest that the endothelial cell antigen recog-nized by MECA-367 participates in the adhesion of lymphocytes to HEV in a site-specific way. Whether this antigen is the complementary ligand, or a unique ligand, for the Peyer's patch-specific determinants at the surface of the lympho-cytes is not yet defined, but an important and new set of concepts has emerged. Streeter and his colleagues refer to the antigen recognized by MECA-367 as an "addressin," a vascular determinant involved in lymphocyte migration that is tissue-specific, signals positional information to circulating lymphocytes, and pro-motes topographically restricted cell-cell interactions.[99] The expectation is that a larger family of determinants that serve comparable functions in different tissue sites, and perhaps at different stages of endothelial cell differentiation, will be defined in the future.

CONCLUSIONS

The migration of lymphocytes and lymphoblasts in various intestinal compart-ments is an extensive, complex, and highly regulated set of processes. Much has been learned about the physiologic, cellular, and molecular bases of migration, but our knowledge is still incomplete. Further understanding of the factors that regu-late the selection of particular phenotypes of cells at the vascular endothelium, and those that promote the assembly of migrating populations of different lymphoid cells within the mucosa is essential if we are to bring basic understanding to the pathogenesis and pathophysiology of diseases of the intestine. Currently, the cellular and molecular factors that control the disposition of cells after they arrive within the tissues is largely undefined. For B lymphoblasts, it is clear that antigen can promote the retention and expansion of specific Ig-producing cells that reach the mucosa,[97] but the role of other signals is mostly unexplored. The fine detail that is emerging from the studies of the molecular determinants that influence lymphocyte-endothelial interactions suggest that other specific cell-cell and cell-surface interactions probably contribute during the residency of lymphoid cells within the intestinal stroma.

REFERENCES

1. Ernst PB, Befus AD, Bienenstock J: Leukocytes in the intestinal epitheliium: an unusual immunological compartment. *Immunol Today* 2:50–56, 1985.
2. Cerf-Bensussan N, Guy-Grand D, Lisouska-Grospierre B, et al: A monoclonal antibody specific for rat intestinal lymphocytes. *J Immunol* 136:76–82, 1986.
3. Selby WS, Janossy G, Bofill M, et al: Lymphocyte subpopulations in the human small intestine. The findings in normal mucosa and in the mucosa of patients with adult celiac disease. *Clin Exp Immunol* 52:219–224, 1983.
4. Spencer J, Dillon SB, Isaacson PG, et al: T cell subclasses in fetal human ileum. *Clin Exp Immunol* 65:553–558, 1986.
5. Marsh MN: Studies of intestinal lymphoid tissue. In Polak JM, Bloom SR, Wright NA, et al: *Basic Science in Gastroenterology: Structure of the Gut,* Ware, UK, Glaxo Group Research Ltd., 1982, p 87.
6. Goodman T, Lefrancois L: Expression of the gamma-delta T cell receptor in intestinal CD8+ intraepithelial lymphocytes. *Nature* 333:855–858, 1988.
7. Bonneville M, Janeway CA, Ito K, et al: Intestinal intraepithelial lymphocytes are a distinct set of gamma-delta T cells. *Nature* 336:479–481, 1988.
8. Janeway CA: Frontiers of the immune system. *Nature* 333:804–806, 1988.
9. Spencer J, Isaacson PG: Human T cell receptor expression (Letter). *Nature* 337:416, 1989.
10. Janeway CA: Human T cell receptor expression (Letter). *Nature* 337:416, 1989.
11. Owen RL, Jones AL: Epithelial cell specialization within Peyer's patches: an ultrastructural study of intestinal lymphoid follicles. *Gastroenterology* 66:189–203, 1974.
12. Parrott DMV: Structure and organization of lymphoid tissue in the gut. In Brostoff J, Challacombe S: *Food Allergy and Intolerance,* London, Baltiere Tindall, 1987, pp 3–26.
13. Mattioli CA, Tomasi TB: The life-span of IgA plasma cells in the mouse intestine. *J Exp Med* 138:452–459, 1973.
14. Ermack TH, Owen RL: Differential distribution of lymphocytes and accessory cells in mouse Peyer's patches. *Anat Rec* 215:144–152, 1986.
15. Keren DF, Holt PS, Collins H, et al: The role of Peyer's patches in the local immune response of rabbit ileum to live bacteria. *J Immunol* 120:1892–1896, 1978.
16. Kawanishi H, Saltzman L, Strober W: Mechanisms regulating IgA class-specific immunoglobulin production in murine gut associated lymphoid tissue. *J Exp Med* 157:433–450, 1983.
17. Kiyono H, Cooper MD, Kearney J, et al: Isotype specificity of helper T cell clones. Peyer's patch Th cells preferentially collaborate with mature IgA B cells for IgA responses. *J Exp Med* 159:798–811, 1984.

18. Kiyono H, Mosteller-Barnum L, Potts A, et al: Isotype specific immunoregulation. *J Exp Med* 161:731–747, 1985.

19. Ottaway CA: Neuropeptides, neurons and mucosal lymphoid cell migration. *Monogr Allergy* 24:157–166, 1988.

20. Ottaway CA: Lymphoid cell migration to the intestine in health and disease. In Losowsky MS, Heatley RV: *Gut Defenses in Clinical Practice.* Edinburgh, Churchill Livingstone, 1986, pp 48–66.

21. Reynolds J: Lymphocyte traffic associated with the gut: a review of studies in the sheep. In Husband AJ: *Migration and Homing of Lymphoid Cells II.* Boca Raton, CRC Press, 1988, pp 113–179.

22. Baker RD: The cellular content of chyle in relation to lymphoid tissue and fat transportation. *Anat Rec* 55:207–221, 1933.

23. Steer HW: An analysis of the lymphocyte content of rat lacteals. *J Immunol* 125:1845–1848, 1980.

24. Ottaway CA, Parrott DMV: A method for the quantitative analysis of lymphoid cell migration experiments. *Immunol Lett* 2:283–290, 1981.

25. Ottaway CA: The efficiency of entry of lymphoid cells into lymphoid and nonlymphoid tissues. *Adv Exp Med Biol* 149:219–224, 1982.

26. Ottaway CA: Dynamic aspects of lymphoid cell migration. In Husband AJ: *Migration and Homing of Lymphoid Cells I.* Boca Raton, CRC Press, 1988, pp 167–194.

27. Gowans J, Knight EJ: The route of recirculation of lymphocytes in the rat. *Proc R Soc (B)* 59:257–282, 1964.

28. Hall JG, Parry D, Smith M: The distribution and differentiation of lymph-borne immunoblasts after intravenous transfer into syngeneic recipients. *Cell Tissue Kinet* 5:269–276, 1972.

29. Hall JG, Scollay R, Smith M: Recirculation of lymphocytes through peripheral lymph nodes and other tissues. *Eur J Immunol* 6:117–128, 1976.

30. Guy-Grand D, Griscelli C, Vassalli P: The gut associated lymphoid system: nature and properties of the large dividing cells. *Eur J Immunol* 4:435–441, 1974.

31. Rose M, Parrott DMV, Bruce R: Migration of lymphoblasts to the small intestine. I. Effect of *Trichinella spiralis* infection on the migration of mesenteric lymphoblasts in syngeneic mice. *Immunology* 31:723–730, 1976.

32. Rose M, Parrott DMV, Bruce R: Migration of lymphoblasts to the small intestine. II. Divergent migration of mesenteric and peripheral immunoblasts to sites of inflammation in the mouse. *Cell Immunol* 27:36–45, 1976.

33. Smith M, Martin A, Ford WL: Migration of lymphoblasts in the rat. *Monogr Allergy* 16:203–231, 1980.

34. Fossum S, Smith M, Ford WL: The migration of lymphocytes across specialized vascular endothelium VII. The migration of T and B lymphocytes from the blood of the athymic rat. *Scand J Immunol* 17:539–549, 1983.

35. Fossum S, Smith M, Ford WL: The recirculation of T and B lymphocytes in the athymic rat. *Scand J Immunol* 17:551–557, 1983.

36. Smith M, Ford WL: The recirculating lymphocyte pool of the rat: a systematic description of the migratory behaviour of recirculating lymphocytes. *Immunology* 49:83–92, 1983.

37. Stevens SK, Weissman I, Butcher EC: Differences in the migration of B and T lymphocytes: organ-selective localization in vivo and the role of lymphocyte-endothelial recognition. *J Immunol* 128:844–850, 1982.

38. Kraal G, Weissman I, Butcher EC: Differences in in vivo distribution and homing of T cell subsets to mucosal vs. nonmucosal lymphoid organs. *J Immunol* 130:1097–2001, 1983.

39. Fisher L, Ottaway CA: The kinetics of migration of CD4 and CD8 lymphocytes in vivo. manuscript submitted.
40. Scollay R, Hopkins J, Hall J: Possible role of surface Ig in non-random migration of small lymphocytes. *Nature* 260:528–534, 1976.
41. Cahill RNP, Poskitt D, Frost H, et al: Two distinct pools of recirculating T lymphocytes: migratory characteristics of nodal and intestinal T lymphocytes. *J Exp Med* 145:420–426, 1977.
42. Chin W, Hay JB: A comparison of lymphocyte migration through intestinal lymph nodes, subcutaneous lymph nodes and chronic inflammatory sites of sheep. *Gastroenterology* 79:1231–1239, 1980.
43. Reynolds J, Heron I, Dudler L, et al: T cell recirculation in the sheep: migratory properties of cells from lymph nodes. *Immunology* 47:415–423, 1982.
44. Freitas A, Rose M, Parrott D: Murine mesenteric and peripheral lymph nodes: a common pool of small T cells. *Nature* 270:731–734, 1977.
45. Freitas A, Rose M, Rocha B: Random recirculation of small T lymphocytes from the thoracic duct lymph in mice. *Cell Immunol* 56:29–36, 1980.
46. Roux ME, McWilliams M, Phillips-Quagliata J, et al: Origin of IgA secreting cells in the mammary gland. *J Exp Med* 146:1311–1316, 1977.
47. Weisz-Carrington P, Roux M, McWilliams M, et al: Hormonal induction of the secretory immune system in the mammary gland. *Proc Natl Acad Sci USA* 75:2928–2933, 1978.
48. McDermott M, Bienenstock J: Evidence for a common mucosal immunological system I. Migration of B immunoblasts into intestinal, respiratory and genital tissues. *J Immunol* 122:1892–1897, 1979.
49. McDermott M, Clark D, Bienenstock J: Evidence for a common mucosal immunological system II. Influence of the estrous cycle on B immunoblast migration into genital and intestinal mucosa. *J Immunol* 124:2536–2541, 1980.
50. Scicchitano R, Stanisz A, Ernst P, et al: A common mucosal immune system revisited. In Husband AJ: *Migration and Homing of Lymphoid Cells II.* Boca Raton, CRC Press, 1988, pp 1–34.
51. Pierce N, Cray S: Determinants of localization, magnitude and duration of a specific mucosal IgA plasma cell response in enterically immunized rats. *J Immunol* 128:1311–1316, 1982.
52. Morris B: The homing of lymphocytes. *Blood Cells* 6:3–7, 1980.
53. Woodruff JJ, Clarke LM, Chin YH: Specific cell-adhesion mechanisms determining migration pathways of recirculating lymphocytes. *Annu Rev Immunol* 5:201–222, 1987.
54. Trevella W, Morris B: Reassortment of cell populations within the lymphoid apparatus of the sheep. In: *Blood Cells and Vessel Walls.* Ciba Foundation Symposium 71, 1980, pp 127–139.
55. Schoefl GI: The migration of lymphocytes across the vascular endothelium in lymphoid tissues: a reexamination. *J Exp Med* 136:568–579, 1972.
56. vanEwijk W, Borns N, Rozing J: Scanning electron microscopy of homing and recirculating lymphocyte populations. *Cell Immunol* 19:245–253, 1975.
57. Anderson A, Anderson N: Lymphocyte emigration from high endothelial venules in rat lymph nodes. *Immunology* 31:731–739, 1970.
58. Cleaesson M, Jorgenson O, Ropke C: Light and electron microscopic studies of the paracortical postcapillary high endothelial venules. *Z Zellforsch Mikrosk Anat* 119:195–206, 1971.
59. Stamper HB, Woodruff JJ: Lymphocyte homing into lymph nodes: In vitro demonstration of the selective affinity of recirculating lymphocytes for high endothelial venules. *J Exp Med* 144:828–931, 1976.

60. Stamper HB, Woodruff JJ: An in vitro model of lymphocyte homing. I. Characterization of the interaction between thoracic duct lymphocytes and specialized high endothelial venules of lymph nodes. *J Immunol* 119:772–779, 1977.

61. Woodruff JJ, Rasmussen RA: In vitro adherence of lymphocytes to unfixed and fixed high endothelial cells of lymph nodes. *J Immunol* 123:2369–2376, 1979.

62. Butcher EC, Scollay R, Weissman I: Lymphocyte adherence to high endothelial venules: characterization of a modified in vitro assay and examination of the binding of syngeneic and allogeneic lymphocytes. *J Immunol* 123:1996–1999, 1979.

63. Butcher EC, Scollay R, Weissman I: Organ specificity of lymphocyte interactions with organ specific determinants on high endothelial venules. *Eur J Immunol* 10:556–561, 1980.

64. Butcher EC: The regulation of lymphocyte traffic. *Curr Top Microbiol Immunol* 128:85–122, 1986.

65. Gallatin WM, Weissman I, Butcher EC: A cell surface molecule involved in organ-specific homing of lymphocytes. *Nature* 304:30–34, 1983.

66. Jalkanen S, Wu N, Bragatze R, et al: Human lymphocyte and lymphoma homing receptors. *Annu Rev Med* 38:467–476, 1987.

67. Siegleman M, Bond M, Galatin MW, et al: Cell surface molecule associated with lymphocyte homing is a ubiquinated branched-chain glycoprotein. *Science* 231:823–829, 1986.

68. Chin YH, Rasmussen RA, Cakiroglu A, et al: Lymphocyte recognition of lymph node high endothelium. VI. Evidence of distinct structures mediating binding to high endothelial cells of lymph nodes and Peyer's patches. *J Immunol* 133:2961–2968, 1984.

69. Chin YH, Carey G, Woodruff JJ: Lymphocyte recognition of lymph node high endothelium. I. Inhibition of in vitro binding by a component of thoracic duct lymph. *J Immunol* 125:1764–1769, 1980.

70. Chin YH, Carey G, Woodruff JJ: Lymphocyte recognition of lymph node high endothelium. II. Characterization of an in vitro inhibitory factor isolated by antibody affinity chromatography. *J Immunol* 125:1770–1778, 1980.

71. Chin YH, Carey G, Woodruff JJ: Lymphocyte recognition of lymph node high endothelium. V. Isolation of adhesion molecules from lysates of rat lymphocytes. *J Immunol* 131:1368–1375, 1983.

72. Rasmussen RA, Chin YH, Woodruff JJ, et al: Lymphocyte recognition of lymph node high endothelium VII. Cell surface proteins involved in adhesion defined by monoclonal anti-HEBF$_{LN}$ (A.11) antibody. *J Immunol* 135:19–27, 1985.

73. Chin YH, Rasmussen RA, Woodruff JJ, et al: A monoclonal anti-HEBF$_{PP}$ antibody with specificity for lymphocyte surface molecules mediating adhesion to Peyer's patch high endothelium of the rat. *J Immunol* 136:2556–2561, 1986.

74. Jalkanen S, Bargatze R, Herron L, et al: A lymphoid cell surface glycoprotein involved in endothelial cell recognition and lymphocyte homing in man. *Eur J Immunol* 16:1195–1202, 1986.

75. Jalkanen S, Reichart R, Gallatin MW, et al: Homing receptors and the control of lymphocyte migration. *Immunol Rev* 91:39–60, 1986.

76. Jalkanen S, Bragatze R, Toyos J, et al: Lymphocyte recognition of high endothelium: antibodies to distinct epitopes of an 85–95 kD glycoprotein antigen differentially inhibit lymphocyte binding to lymph nodes, mucosal or synovial endothelial cells. *J Cell Biol* 105:983–990, 1987.

77. Shaw S, Luce G: The lymphocyte function associated antigen (LFA-1) and CD2/LFA-3 pathways of antigen independent human T cell adhesion. *J Immunol* 139:1037–1045, 1987.

78. Hamann A, Jablonski-Westrich D, Duijvestijn A, et al: Evidence for an accessory role of

LFA-1 in lymphocyte-high endothelial interactions during homing. *J Immunol* 140:693–699, 1988.

79. Pals S, den Otter A, Miedema F, et al: Evidence that leukocyte function associated antigen-1 is involved in recirculation and homing of human lymphocytes via high endothelial venules. *J Immunol* 140:1851–1853, 1988.

80. Moore TC: Modification of lymphocyte traffic by vasoactive neurotransmitter substances. *Immunology* 52:511–517, 1984.

81. Moore TC, Spruck CH, Said SI: Depression of lymphocyte traffic in sheep by vasoactive intestinal peptide. *Immunology* 64:475–478, 1988.

82. Ottaway CA: In vitro alteration of receptors for vasoactive intestinal peptide changes in the in vivo localization of mouse T cells. *J Exp Med* 160:1054–1069, 1984.

83. Ottaway CA: Evidence for local neuromodulation of T cell migration in vivo. *Adv Exp Biol Med* 186:637–645, 1985.

84. Ottaway CA, Greenberg GR: Interaction of vasoactive intestinal peptide with mouse lymphocytes: specific binding and modulation of mitogen responses. *J Immunol* 132:417–423, 1984.

85. Ottaway CA, Lewis D, Asa S: Vasoactive intestinal peptide containing nerves in Peyer's patches. *Brain Behav Immun* 1:148–158, 1987.

86. Bjerknes M, Cheng H, Ottaway CA: Dynamics of lymphocyte endothelial interactions in vivo. *Science* 231:402–405, 1986.

87. Jalkanen S, Butcher EC: In vitro analysis of the homing properties of human lymphocytes: developmental regulation of functional receptors for high endothelial venules. *Blood* 66:577–582, 1985.

88. Ager A: Isolation and culture of high endothelial cells from rat lymph nodes. *J Cell Sci* 87:133–144, 1987.

89. Hay J, Hobbs B: The flow of blood to lymph nodes and its relation to lymphocyte traffic and immune responses. *J Exp Med* 145:31–37, 1977.

90. Cahill RNP, Heron I, Poskitt D, et al: Lymphocyte recirculation in the sheep fetus. In: *Blood Cells and Vessel Walls.* Ciba Foundation Symposium 71. 1980, pp 145–157.

91. Stoolman L, Rosen S: Possible role for cell-surface carbohydrate binding molecules in lymphocyte recirculation. *J Cell Biol* 96:722–727, 1983.

92. Stoolman L, Tenforde T, Rosen S: Phosphomannosyl receptors may participate in the adhesive interaction between lymphocytes and high endothelial venules. *J Cell Biol* 99:1535–1542, 1984.

93. Sprangrude G, Braaten B, Daynes R: Molecular mechanisms of lymphocyte extravasation. I. Studies of two selective inhibitors of lymphocyte recirculation. *J Immunol* 132:354–361, 1984.

94. Rosen S, Singer M, Yednock T, et al: Involvement of sialic acid on endothelial cells in organ-specific lymphocyte recirculation. *Science* 228:1005–1008, 1985.

95. Duijvestijn A, Kerkove M, Bargatze R, et al: Lymphoid tissue and inflammation-specific endothelial cell differentiation defined by monoclonal antibodies. *J Immunol* 138:713–719, 1987.

96. Jeurissen S, Duijvestijn A, Sontag Y, et al: Lymphocyte migration into lamina propria of the gut is mediated by specialized HEV-like blood vessels. *Immunology* 62:273–277, 1987.

97. Husband AJ: Kinetics of extravasation and redistribution of IgA-specific antibody containing cells in the intestine. *J Immunol* 128:1355–1359, 1982.

98. Bienenstock J, Befus A, McDermott M, et al: Regulation of lymphoblast traffic in mucosal tissue with emphasis of IgA. *Fed Proc* 42:3213–3216, 1983.

99. Streeter PR, Berg EL, Rouse B, et al: A tissue-specific endothelial cell molecule involved in lymphocyte homing. *Nature* 331:41–46, 1988.

PART **TWO**

THE EFFERENT LIMB OF THE MUCOSAL IMMUNE SYSTEM

CHAPTER 6

Humoral Immunity

WILLIAM R. BROWN

THOMAS M. KLOPPEL

INTRODUCTION

The secretion of secretory IgA (sIgA) into external body fluids, including those of the hepatobiliary and gastrointestinal tracts, is the hallmark of the mucosal immune system. Indeed, the magnitude of IgA's contribution to the immunologic material of the host is astonishing; in man, the combined synthesis of systemic and secretory IgA (about 66 mg/kg/day) makes IgA the major immunoglobulin,[1] and the intestine, in which IgA is clearly the predominant immunoglobulin, contains the largest accumulation of lymphoid tissues in the body.[2] Despite this predominance of IgA, it is important to keep in mind that all the other immunoglobulin isotypes (IgG, IgM, IgE, and IgD) are also present in tissues and fluids of the gastrointestinal tract, and they too contribute to mucosal immunologic reactions. In addition, it is important to emphasize, as will be elaborated in the next chapter, that cellular immune reactions in the digestive tract are of considerable importance and that immunologic defenses constitute only a portion of the total array of host defense mechanisms operative at mucosal surfaces.

In this chapter we shall first briefly review the nonimmunologic defense mechanisms of the gastrointestinal tract, then describe the mechanisms for the entry of immunoglobulins of the various isotypes into gastrointestinal and biliary secretions, and finally discuss the biologic roles of the secreted immunoglobulins.

This work was supported in part by the Veterans Administration.

NONIMMUNOLOGIC DEFENSE MECHANISMS AT MUCOSAL SURFACES

It is reasonable to consider the nonimmunologic defense mechanisms of the gut (listed in Table 6–1) when considering the humoral defense mechanisms, as the two components are often complementary or synergistic in their actions.

The normal bacterial flora of the intestinal tract appear to play a particularly useful role in regulating the growth of pathogenic bacteria in the gut. These organisms produce endogenous antibiotics (bacteriocins) and secrete toxic short-chain fatty acids that are directly harmful to particular pathogens.[3] The normal flora may also inhibit the adherence of bacteria to intestinal epithelial cells, inactivate bacterial toxins, and compete with pathogens for nutrients. In addition, the indigenous bacteria of the intestine stimulate the mucosal immune system, thereby preparing it to respond to pathogenic organisms.[4] An example of the salutary effects of the normal flora is that the deliberate feeding of nonpathogenic *Escherichia coli* to infants can prevent colonization or infection with gastrointestinal pathogens.[5] Peristaltic activity of the bowel is important to sweep away potential pathogens before they bind to and colonize the epithelial surface; such bowel activity may be performed synergistically with mucous secretion and antibodies, which cause the agglutination and/or immobilization of organisms. Mucins present in mucous secretions can bind to and coat various bacteria, viruses, and parasites, thus retarding their interactions with epithelial cells.[6] In certain circumstances, the presence of antibodies can enhance the activities of mucus: antibody-antigen complexes reportedly can stimulate the secretion of mucus from intestinal goblet cells,[7] and some antibodies can form physical bonds with mucus, so that bacteria with antibodies bound to their surfaces become more heavily coated with mucus.[8] The secretion of gastric acid inhibits the growth of bacteria in the stomach and upper intestinal tract, although gastric achlorhydria usually does not lead to overgrowth of intestinal bacteria unless there is an associated motility disorder or immunologic deficiency.[9] Lactoferrin, an iron-binding protein, can inhibit the growth of *E. coli* and other organisms by depriving them of iron; IgA antibodies can enhance this function by preventing organisms from releasing their own iron-binding factor.[10] Unconjugated bile acids can inhibit the growth of anaerobic bacteria in the upper small intestine. Lysozyme, an enzyme present in many foods, has lytic effects on many organisms, including *Streptococcus mutans* (an oral pathogen) and *Candida*

Table 6–1 NONIMMUNOLOGIC DEFENSES AT MUCOSAL SURFACES

Normal bacterial flora
Peristalsis
Secretion of mucus
Secretion of gastric acid
Antipathogenic substances in secretions
    Lactoferrin
    Bile salts
    Lysozyme
    Lactoperoxidase

albicans.[11] Lactoperoxidase has antimicrobial effects on *S. mutans* in the presence of hydrogen peroxide, an effect that also can be enhanced by the action of IgA antibodies.[12]

Numerous clinical examples illustrate the dependence of the host on both non-immunologic and immunologic factors in the defense of the gastrointestinal tract. Obstruction of the biliary ducts or the intestine can lead to severe infection or bacterial overgrowth even in the presence of an entirely intact immunologic apparatus. Conversely, immunologic deficiency states, such as AIDS and other immunologic deficiencies, can lead to serious and diverse gastrointestinal infections despite the presence of normally functioning nonimmunologic defenses.

MECHANISMS FOR ENTRY OF IMMUNOGLOBULINS INTO BILE AND INTESTINAL FLUIDS

The quantities of immunoglobulins present in secretions of the liver and digestive tract, and the sources and routes of entry of the immunoglobulins into the fluids, vary markedly among the various isotypes. It is impossible to state accurately the concentrations of immunoglobulins in the fluids because of several variables (mostly uncontrollable) that affect their quantification. These include the effects of differences in the sizes of immunoglobulin molecules or fragments in the fluids compared with the sizes of immunoglobulin standards used in various assays, nonspecific precipitin reactions between intestinal fluids and some antisera in immunodiffusion assays,[13] variable enzymatic degradation of the immunoglobulins,[14-16] and variable degrees of dilution of the immunoglobulins in vivo. Despite these problems, reasonable estimates of the concentrations of most of the immunoglobulins are available, and the clear-cut preponderance of IgA in the fluids has almost always been observed. Concentrations of IgA on the order of 0.3 g/l compared with concentrations of IgM and IgG of about 0.2 g/l and 0.1 g/l, respectively, in human intestinal fluids have been commonly reported,[17] but the variation among individuals is great, and we have generally observed higher ratios of IgA to the other two major immunoglobulin isotypes.[15-18] The concentrations of IgE and IgD are much lower than those of the other immunoglobulins, as discussed later. Concentrations of IgA in hepatic bile of postoperative patients in the range of 0.2 to 2.0 g/l were reported in two studies[19,20] and 1.4 to 8.8 g/l in another[21]; the concentrations of IgG and IgM in the bile are very much less. The proportions of plasma cells that populate the intestinal mucosa roughly reflect the relative concentrations of immunoglobulins in the intestinal fluids; in the healthy human small or large bowel, ratios on the order of about 10:1-0.5 for IgA, IgM, and IgG cells have generally been recorded.[17]

Depending on their isotype and molecular configuration, immunoglobulins can enter intestinal fluids and bile either by transudation from the plasma or interstitial fluids (monomeric IgA, IgG, IgE, and IgD) or by active, carrier-mediated transport across epithelia. The latter pathway is used extensively by dimers or larger polymers of IgA and by IgM; the majority of these two immunoglobulin isotypes that enter intestinal fluids is synthesized locally in plasma cells within the bowel wall.

IgA

In its classic 11S form, sIgA consists of two pairs of immunoglobulin heavy chains and light chains, one secretory component (SC), and one J (joining) chain. In the human, unlike several other species, the majority of circulating IgA is in the monomeric form. Another characteristic of human IgA is that there are two subclasses: IgA1 and IgA2. IgA1 dominates in serum by a margin of about 4:1, whereas approximately equal amounts of IgA1 and IgA2 are found in secretions.[1,22,23]

The delivery of IgA into external secretions involves a unique and complex series of inter- and intracellular events and the cooperation of at least two cell types (for reviews see references 24–32). In response to oral immunization, IgA-specific B cells, mostly in gut-associated lymphoid tissues, i.e., Peyer's patches, home to subepithelial layers of various mucosal tissues and differentiate into IgA-secreting plasma cells (32; see preceding chapters). In the plasma cells, precursor immunoglobulin heavy chains (alpha) and light chains (lambda or kappa) assemble to form monomeric IgA (mIgA) molecules; in the presence of an additional peptide, the J chain, the monomeric units join to create dimers and other polymeric forms of IgA (pIgA), which are secreted from the cell into the connective tissue milieu.[33–36] From there the pIgA may diffuse in two directions: toward the epithelium or toward the draining lymphatics. Either route allows for the initiation of the second phase of the IgA delivery system, i.e., the interaction of the Fc portion of the pIgA molecule with the polymeric immunoglobulin receptor, secretory component (membrane form of secretory component; mSC), which is present on the abluminal surface of epithelial cells and, in some species, on hepatocytes. As will be evident from the following discussion, many of the intracellular events in the synthesis of mSC and the transport of pIgA into secretions have been defined by studies on hepatocytes of the rat (Fig. 6–1).

Binding of pIgA to mSC

The first step in the transcytosis of pIgA is the binding of pIgA to mSC.[37] This binding, which was first studied in vitro with purified preparations of IgA and free or membrane-associated SC, is a saturable, reversible, and time-dependent process; the stoichiometry is one polymer of IgA for one molecule of SC. The affinity binding constant for pIgA and free SC is $\sim 10^8/M^{-1}$; for pIgA and mSC it is $\sim 10^9/M^{-1}$, suggesting that the interaction of pIgA with mSC is slightly stronger.[38,39] It is important to stress that only polymeric forms of IgA are capable of interacting with SC with high affinity.[39–43] The J chain, which links IgA monomers together[44,45] via disulfide bonds, is required for the binding of IgA to SC and subsequent transport of IgA,[46] although SC does not bind directly to the J chain. The NH_2-terminal first homologous domain of SC is necessary for pIgA binding,[47] and a tyrosine residue in the pIgA molecule may play a role in the binding of pIgA to SC, since binding and transcellular transport of IgA are often decreased after iodination IgA (48–50; our unpublished results).

IgA is thought to first interact with SC noncovalently[51]; later, disulfide interchange between a reactive sulfhydryl group on the IgA molecule and a disulfide bond on SC occurs, thereby forming a covalent disulfide bond between one IgA heavy chain and SC.[40,52–56] Interestingly, even though there is great species crossaffinity between IgA and SC,[43] the ability of IgA from one species to covalently bind to SC of different species is quite variable.[57]

BLOOD

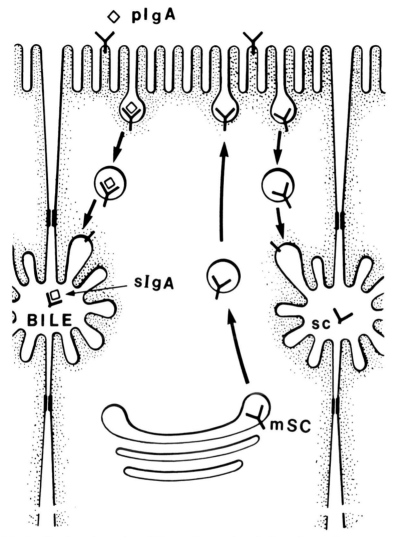

FIGURE 6 – 1 The transhepatocellular pathway for pIgA and secretory component. Secretory component is synthesized as a transmembrane glycoprotein (mSC) by epithelial cells, e.g., enterocytes, and (in some species) hepatocytes. In rat hepatocytes, SC is expressed on the sinusoidal surface of the hepatocyte, where it is available to bind polymeric IgA (pIgA) from the circulation. The pIgA-SC complex is internalized and transported by vesicles across the cell to the bile canalicular membrane of the hepatocyte. There, the transmembrane form of mSC is proteolytically processed to yield a smaller, soluble form of SC that remains complexed to pIgA. The pIgA-SC complex, now termed secretory IgA (sIgA), is released into the bile, and the membrane anchoring fragment is left behind. The synthesis of mSC, expression on the sinusoidal membrane, and secretion of free or uncomplexed SC into bile appear to be constituitive processes and proceed in the absence of pIgA. (From Brown WR, et al: The liver and IgA: immunological, cell biological and clinical implication. *Hepatology,* in press.)

Biosynthesis and Expression of mSC

mSC, like most integral plasma membrane proteins, is synthesized in the rough endoplasmic reticulum, processed in the Golgi, and transported to the plasma membrane. However, since SC is a soluble protein in secretions as well as a cell-surface receptor for pIgA, it follows an especially complicated intracellular biosynthetic pathway. Several studies have documented that mSC is the precursor of soluble SC: Mostov et al.,[58] using mRNA isolated from rabbit mammary gland, first showed in vitro that SC is synthesized as a molecule larger than that form secreted into milk. Kuhn and Kraehenbuhl[59] documented that the membrane forms of SC from rabbit mammary gland and liver were larger than comparable forms of SC present in milk and bile, respectively; importantly, those workers showed that the larger, membrane forms were structurally related to the secreted forms. Using HT29 cells (human colonic adenocarcinoma cell line), Mostov and Blobel[60] demonstrated, by means of biosynthetic pulse labeling/chase experiments, that the secreted form of SC (~ 77 kD) is derived from the NH_2 terminus of a larger transmembrane form of SC (~ 95 kD). Studies with rabbit mammary gland similarly suggested a precursor-product relationship between the membrane and secreted forms of SC.[24]

A more complete understanding of the structure of SC was attained when the gene for rabbit mSC was cloned and sequenced.[61] The deduced amino acid sequence indicated that the mSC molecule contains a leader sequence of 18 amino acids, an extracytosolic domain of 630 amino acids, a membrane-spanning domain of 23 amino acids and a cytosolic tail of 102 amino acids. The extracytosolic portion contains five 100–115-amino acid domains that are homologous to each other and to immunoglobulin kappa-chain variable regions.[61] Interestingly, rabbit SC, unlike human and rat SC, is heterogeneous, as a result of multiple alleles and mRNA processing; the latter produces deletions of certain intramolecular domains of the extracytosolic portion of SC.[62–64]

Recently, Larkin et al.[65] have shown that, in intact liver, the 120-kD plasma membrane form of mSC is phosphorylated at serine residue(s) located within the cytosolic tail of the molecule; consequently, the biliary form of SC is not phosphorylated. Musil and Baenziger[66] demonstrated in cultured primary rat hepatocytes that two species of mSC (105 and 109 kD), which were resistant to Endo H digestion, were phosphorylated; these experiments suggest that phosphorylation of SC does not require the presence of ligand (IgA). The possible role of phosphorylation or other posttranslational processing events in the intracellular sorting of SC remains to be clarified.

Endocytosis and Transcellular Routing of IgA-mSC Complexes

IgA binds to mSC that is diffusely localized along and in invaginations of the basolateral plasma membrane[67] that often appear to be coated.[68,69] In isolated hepatocytes, the binding of IgA induces clustering of mSC-IgA complexes; the clustering is sensitive to agents like cytochalasin B, which disrupt microfilaments.[69] After pIgA binds mSC on the basolateral surface of the cell, the IgA-mSC complexes are internalized into coated endocytic vesicles.[67,68,70] Soon after endocytosis, the IgA-mSC complexes are localized in a vesicular-tubular network.[68] In this network, the sorting of IgA from other endocytosed ligands presumably occurs. The sorted, IgA-mSC-containing vesicles then migrate across the cell, avoiding interaction with lysosomes, and fuse with the apical plasma membrane.[67,71,72] The transcellular migration appears to involve discrete vesicles, as opposed to a continuous intracellular tubule,[72] and depends upon functioning microtubules, as treatment with colchicine abolishes the transport of IgA.[57,73,74] The IgA transport vesicles from rat liver have been partially isolated and are characterized as approximately 140 nm in diameter, with a density of 1.07–1.08 g/ml.[75] Detailed biochemical characterization of the IgA transport vesicle is still needed.

Intracellular Sorting of mSC

One of the most remarkable aspects of the IgA delivery pathway is that SC does not require the presence of IgA for its biosynthesis, intracellular transport, or secretion. Both in liver perfusion studies[75,77] and in experiments with cultured cells,[58,66,78–81] SC follows its usual intracellular route: synthesis of the larger membrane form of SC, expression of the mSC at the basolateral cell surface, internalization and transcytosis of the mSC to the apical pole, and exocytosis of a smaller, soluble SC. That SC can be properly routed within the cell, even in the absence of IgA, strongly suggests that determinants of the complex intracellular sorting mechanisms that guide mSC first to the basolateral domain of the cell and then to the apical domain inherently reside within the mSC molecule. Indeed, eloquent studies by Mostov and colleagues, using expression of a normal or mutated mSC gene in cultured, polarized epithelial cells (Madrin Darby canine kidney cells; MDCK), have shown that mSC could be synthesized from the transfected normal gene expressed on the basolateral surface of the MDCK cells; the mSC was capable of binding and transporting IgA across the cell to the apical domain, where the IgA-SC complex was secreted.[82] Subsequent studies showed that the deletion of the cytoplasmic domain of mSC prevented its localization to the basolateral surface and thereby subsequent endocytosis of IgA,[83] whereas deletion of the membrane-anchor and cytosolic tail produced a soluble SC protein that was primarily routed to the apical pole of the cell and secreted into the apical medium.[84] These experiments suggest that the cytoplasmic portion of mSC is responsible for the initial targeting of mSC to the basolateral domain of the cell, whereas the extracytosolic portion of mSC (or SC) contains the appropriate signals for rerouting mSC to the apical domain of the cell. However, the mechanisms that operate to utilize these sorting domains remain to be determined.

Exocytosis of IgA-SC Complexes

The culmination of the IgA delivery pathway involves the proteolytic solubilization of the IgA-mSC complex at the apical pole of the cell. At this step, mSC is proteolytically processed to yield two proteins: a soluble form of SC, which is released into the external milieu still in complex with IgA, and a transmembrane anchoring fragment that contains the cytoplasmic tail of mSC, which remains with the membrane. The exact mechanism and location of this proteolytic event (in the transport vesicle or at the luminal membrane) remain obscure. Through the use of monoclonal antibodies specific for the cytoplasmic tail of mSC, it has been shown that the cytosolic tail (or slightly degraded fragments) can be released into the bile.[85]

Musil and Baenziger[86] recently demonstrated, in cultures of primary rat hepatocytes, that the cleavage of the membrane form of SC to the secreted form occurs at the cell surface and is a direct result of the action of a leupeptin- and antipain-inhibitable thiol protease. However, since their studies utilized nonpolar cells, the specific location of the proteolysis of mSC is unknown, although it is likely to be at the canalicular membrane. Interestingly, in the small intestine, we[87] have shown that SC in the enterocyte undergoes two proteolytic processing events: the first solubilizes SC; the second reduces the size of soluble SC by 10 kD. This latter processing is accomplished by a brush border metalloendoprotease that appears to have high specificity for SC.

Transport of IgA into Bile

The role of SC in the hepatobiliary transport of IgA in the rat was conclusively establshed through the results of several studies: 1) pIgA was effectively transported, whereas there was minimal or no detectable transport of sIgA (prepared from breast fluids or bile),[88,89] preformed complexes of pIgA with SC, or mIgA,[67,88] which, in contrast to pIgA, bind to SC poorly or not at all; 2) polymeric Fc fragments of an IgA myeloma protein, obtained by protease digestion, which were capable of binding in vitro to SC, were actively transferred in vivo into bile, whereas the corresponding Fab fragments, which did not bind to SC, were not transported[89]; 3) IgA polymers recovered from rat bile were entirely or mostly complexed with SC[88,90]; 4) heterologous IgG antibodies to rat SC injected into the circulation of rats were transported into bile, whereas control, nonimmune IgG was not,[88,89] and the transport of the anti-SC antibodies was diminished by competition from simultaneously injected purified rat SC or human pIgA[89]; and 5) pIgA immune complexes were transported into bile, and the transport could be inhibited by preincubation of the complexes with SC.[91]

The ability of cultured rat hepatocytes to synthesize and secrete SC was demonstrated initially by Socken et al.[92] and Zevenbergen et al.[93] At about the same time, Mullock et al.[94] showed in whole rats that biosynthetically labeled, immunorecognizable SC appeared sequentially in the Golgi, plasma membrane, and then in the bile. Sztul et al.[95] first showed that rat liver Golgi contained membrane forms of SC that were larger than biliary forms of SC. We[96] also identified forms of SC in rat liver membranes that were larger (~115 and 105 kD) than the immunologically related biliary form of SC (~85 kD), and found evidence for proteolytic processing of membrane SC to the soluble form. In pulse-labeling and subcellular fractionation experiments in rat liver, Sztul et al.[97,98] demonstrated that mSC was synthesized first as a 105-kD Endo H-sensitive form in the rough endoplasmic reticulum and then processed to 116 kD and eventually to a 120-kD Endo H-resistant form in the Golgi; both the 116-kD and 120-kD forms were transported to the sinusoidal plasma membrane; some conversion from 116 to 120 kD presumably occurred at the plasma membrane. Radioactivity initially observed in large membrane forms of SC was subsequently found in biliary SC (~80 kD).[95] Solari et al.,[89,99] using subcellular fractionation and immunoblotting in the rat liver, obtained similar results: an Endo H-sensitive 105-kD SC band in the rough endoplasmic reticulum and an Endo H-resistant 115-kD SC band in the Golgi. In the rat, most of the circulating pIgA is cleared by hepatocytes and delivered into the bile. This clearance probably reflects two attributes of the IgA: 1) an ability to bind mSC; and 2) an appropriate size to penetrate the fenestrae that are present in the endothelium of the hepatic sinusoids. For example, it is reported that smaller polymers of IgA and Fc (alpha) are cleared from the plasma more quickly than larger polymers.[100] Additionally, pentameric IgM and large IgA immune complexes (described below) are generally transported less efficiently into bile than IgA dimers.[88,91] Consequently, if the IgA polymer is of the appropriate size and capable of interacting with SC, the IgA should be cleared rapidly from the blood and delivered quantitatively into bile. Indeed, recent results (unpublished) from our laboratories documented that all of a biosynthetically labeled, rat hybridoma pIgA was cleared from the plasma within 5 min of injection, and all of the injected material was recovered in bile within 60–90 min.

Clearance and Biliary Secretion of IgA-Antigen Complexes

The discovery that IgA-antigen complexes could be removed from the circulation and delivered into bile suggested an additional role for the SC-mediated hepatic transport of IgA. The availability of a myeloma pIgA (MOPC 315) with antibody specificity for proteins haptenated with DNP or TNP allowed many investigators to examine the transhepatocellular transport of IgA-antigen complexes.[91,101,102–109] These studies showed that IgA-antigen complexes as well as other immune complexes may be cleared by a variety of receptors on many different cells in the liver. However, it appears that only clearance of pIgA-immune complexes by mSC on the sinusoidal surface of the hepatocyte promotes efficient transcytosis of the IgA-antigen-mSC complexes and their secretion into bile. The physiologic role of other hepatic receptors for IgA and other immunoglobulin immune complexes requires more study.

Influence of Hormones, Aging, Bile Flow, and Other Factors on SC Expression and IgA Transport

The synthesis and expression of mSC appears to be regulated during the development of the organism and during cellular differentiation. In the rat intestine, immunorecognizable SC appears in enterocytes between 10 and 15 days after birth, a time corresponding to the appearance of IgA-producing plasma cells in the lamina propria,[110] and reaches levels of adult expression by 40 days.[111] In contrast, in the human, SC is expressed in fetal tissues prior to the appearance of IgA or IgA plasma cells.[112] In the intestine, SC expression is dominant in the cells from the lower two-thirds of the crypt and is diminished in the more differentiated cells at the villus tip.[111,113] Interestingly, the expression of SC is often diminished in carcinomas, and the level of its expression often correlates with the degree of malignancy.[114–116] Schmucker et al.[117] have shown in the rat that the transport of IgA into bile decreases with age; the decrease in transport is a direct result of an age-related decrease in the expression of SC.[118]

The regulation of the expression of mSC and, consequently, the delivery of pIgA into external secretions, as well as the induction of the secretory immune response in general, may depend on hormonal and other chemical influences and may be tissue-specific.[119–121,122] For example, the amount of SC synthesized by uterine or lacrimal cells may be influenced by sex steroids, whereas in hepatocytes, glucocorticoids perform a regulating function[123]; the increase in the expression of SC apparently resides at both the levels of transcription and of translation.[123–125] Additionally, the synthesis and secretion of SC by HT-29 cells can be increased by treatment with gamma-interferon,[126,127] tumor necrosis factor-alpha,[128] or by growing the cells in glucose-free, galactose-substituted medium.[129] The physiologic consequences of these increases in SC expression and the related effect on the delivery of IgA into secretions remain to be explored.

The transport of IgA into bile is also affected by agents that affect bile flow. Even cannulation of the bile duct can affect the delivery pathway. For example, Hinton et al.[130] reported that the concentration of IgA in bile decreased to about 75% of the initial concentration within 3 hr after bile duct cannulation; this decrease was not due to interruption of enterohepatic circulation of IgA, since no such pathway normally exists. Similar results were obtained by Seo et al.,[131] who reported that IgA levels fell to 25% of normal after 4.5 hr of bile duct cannulation. Perhaps in relation to cannulation, Rank and Wilson[132] showed that chronic retardation of bile flow reduced the biliary concentration of IgA while not affecting other biliary proteins. We[133] demonstrated that transient bile duct ligation (2 hr) dramatically decreased the ability of the liver to transport IgA in the period subsequent to ligation, while not affecting the biliary secretion of other proteins, including SC. In the rat, it has also been shown that pharmacologic doses of estradiol, an agent which retards bile flow, decreases the plasma clearance and biliary secretion of IgA.[134] The mechanisms that link IgA transport to bile flow are unknown, but perhaps when they are understood, they will aid our understanding of the transhepatocellular delivery of IgA from blood to bile.

Species Differences in the Hepatobiliary Processing of IgA

The early reports on the hepatic transport of IgA in the rat were followed by similar studies conducted on several other species, with remarkable differences recorded. It soon became clear that although the rabbit, like the rat, could transport much pIgA from plasma into bile,[90,135,136] the guinea pig,[137-139] dog,[136] and sheep[137-139] could not transfer the immunoglobulin nearly as efficiently. Humans fell into the category of inefficient hepatic transporters of IgA.[19,140-142] The species differences in hepatic transport of pIgA are clearly related to differences in the locations of SC in hepatobiliary tissues. In those species in which transport of pIgA is moderate or high (rat, rabbit, mouse) SC, when searched for immunohistochemically, is found on hepatocytes. In contrast, those that transport IgA poorly (man, dog, guinea pig) do not express SC on hepatocytes; rather, it is located on intrahepatic and extrahepatic biliary epithelium.[29,33,126,136,141,142,143-145] No logical explanation for the species differences in hepatocellular locations of SC has been put forth. There does not seem to be a correlation between the amount of pIgA entering the circulation from sites of synthesis in the intestinal mucosa and the locations of SC. For example, the concentrations of IgA in mesenteric or thoracic duct lymph are reportedly several times higher than in the serum of rats,[146,147] mice,[147] guinea pigs,[146] and dogs,[147] even though only the rat and mouse have the hepatobiliary mechanism for effectively transferring the excess IgA into bile. We[148] and others[149] have found that human thoracic duct lymph is not enriched for pIgA compared with plasma, nor is much pIgA contributed to the systemic circulation by portal vein blood.[148,150]

The proportions of biliary IgA that are derived from clearance of plasma pIgA versus synthesis within the hepatobiliary tissues vary among species. For example, whereas around 90% of biliary pIgA in the rat and mouse is derived from the plasma,[151] the corresponding figure in man is about 50%.[19,141] The source of the remaining pIgA in human hepatic bile has not been directly identified. Normally, not many IgA-containing lymphoid cells are present in the human liver.[142,152] However, we[153] have found large numbers of plasma cells containing IgA, SC, and J chain surrounding the accessory glands in the extrahepatic bile ducts and just beneath the luminal surface epithelium of the ducts. At the ultrastructural level, IgA and SC in the epithelial cells had the characteristic features of SC-mediated endocytic transport of IgA. We suspect, then, that the biliary duct mucosa is the source of much of the IgA that is secreted into human hepatic bile. Recently, Carter et al.[154,155] demonstrated in the rat that oral administration of an antigen induced antigen-specific IgA-secreting plasma cells to home to the liver. Whether humans respond in a similar manner remains to be determined.

The net result of differences in the hepatic transport and synthesis of IgA is a marked difference in the amounts of IgA entering the intestinal lumen via bile, compared with direct secretion across the intestinal mucosa. Whereas the biliary excretion of pIgA is about 35 mg/kg/day in rats and rabbits, it is only on the order of 1 mg/kg/day in the human, guinea pig, and dog.[156] On the other hand, the relative amount of IgA entering the human intestinal lumen via direct secretion by the bowel mucosa is much higher.[157] The contrasting patterns of the expression of SC in hepatobiliary tissues and the transport of IgA by the liver and intestine in rat and man are illustrated in Figure 6–2.

IgM

IgM in secretions has many of the physical and functional characteristics of IgA. IgM is able to combine with SC in vitro with the same affinity as IgA binds[40] and is present in certain secretions in association with SC.[15,158] Immunocytochemical studies have demonstrated that IgM, like IgA, is present in the identical cellular and ultrastructural sites in human intestinal mucosa as SC.[158,159] Together, these observations support the concept that IgM shares with pIgA the SC-mediated pathway to the exterior. However, we[15] found that IgM in human intestinal fluids is infrequently complexed with SC and is largely in the form of fragments of the intact molecule. We also found, in experiments with preformed complexes of IgM and SC, that SC was readily dissociated from IgM when incubated in whole intestinal fluids, and the IgM moiety was largely fragmented. The striking difference between SC-IgM and sIgA in resistance to digestive proteases probably reflects the fact that SC is firmly bound to dimeric IgA by disulfide bonds and noncovalent forces, whereas IgM is bound to SC "loosely" and noncovalently.[40] Although we could not exclude the possibility that some or most of the IgM that enters the intestinal fluids does not travel the SC-mediated route, the evidence overall favors SC-mediated secretion of IgM, followed by degradation of sIgM by proteases present in luminal fluids.

IgG

The IgG in external secretions originates either from the local glandular mucosa, where it can be synthesized, or from the serum; its delivery into the external environment is thought to occur by passive diffusion across the epithelium.[160] A specific transporting system for IgG has not been identified, nor has SC been found associated with IgG in external secretions.[161] IgG plasma cells have been identified by means of immunohistochemical techniques in glandular mucosae. However, the number of IgG-producing plasma cells in the lamina propria of the human jejunum

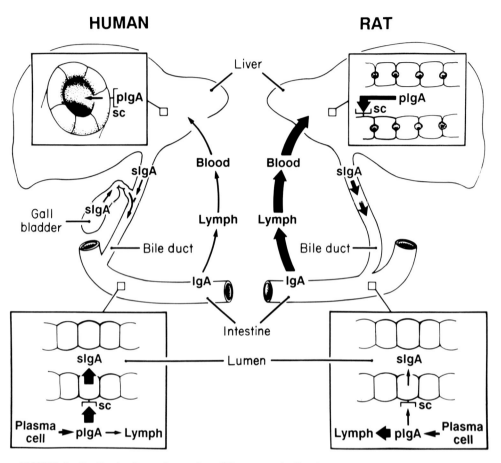

FIGURE 6–2 Illustration of species differences in the transport of IgA into the intestinal lumen. In the rat, only a small proportion of the pIgA that is synthesized by plasma cells in the intestinal mucosa enters the intestinal lumen directly, by way of the SC-mediated transport pathway across intestinal epithelial cells; the majority of pIgA enters the mesenteric lymph and then the blood circulation, and is cleared by transport into bile, by way of SC-mediated transport across hepatocytes. About 90% of the total IgA that enters the intestine of rats is derived from the hepatic clearance of plasma pIgA. In man, large amounts of pIgA synthesized in the intestinal mucosa enter the intestine directly via the SC-mediated transport across intestinal epithelial cells. A minority of the pIgA enters the mesenteric lymph and the blood circulation; this pIgA is probably cleared via a pathway across periductular capillaries and then the epithelium of biliary ductules in the liver. In addition, pIgA synthesized in the mucosa of the extrahepatic biliary ducts and the gall bladder is secreted across the epithelium of those structures and enters the bile. The result of these transport pathways in man is that most of the pIgA that enters the intestine is secreted directly across the intestinal wall; a minority comes from bile, and probably most of that fraction is derived from local synthesis in the biliary ducts and gall bladder mucosa, rather than by clearance of plasma pIgA. (From Brown WR, et al: The liver and IgA: Immunological, cell biological and clinical implication. *Hepatology,* in press.)

is five to tenfold less than the number of IgM-producing cells and 20- to 50-fold less than the number of IgA-producing plasma cells.[162] In the ileum, the numbers of IgG and IgM-producing cells are similar but still fourfold less than the number of IgA cells[163]; similar ratios have been obtained in the colon.[164] These numbers correspond with the ratios of the concentrations of immunoglobulins found in secretions. Interestingly, in many diseases of the gut, the number of IgG plasma cells increases substantially and often surpasses the number of IgA-producing cells,[165] and the amount of IgG recovered in secretions also increases, presumably due to leaky epithelium.[166] IgG, being very sensitive to peptic and tryptic digestion, is often present in fragmented forms in intestinal fluids.

IgE

IgE is present in such low concentrations in human intestinal fluids that it must be measured by radioimmunoassay or similarly sensitive methods, but we[167] found detectable IgE in small intestinal fluids from 92% of healthy persons or patients with various gastrointestinal diseases. We also observed that the immunologically reactive IgE was present largely in a relatively low molecular weight fraction (about 40,000 daltons) and, on the basis of the observed degradation products of an IgE myeloma protein, is probably an e_1 determinant-containing fragment of the amino terminus of the Fc region.[16] Thus, like IgM and IgG, much of the IgE that enters intestinal fluids is evidently rapidly lysed to smaller fragments. IgE in external secretions is not linked to SC, and there is no evidence for an active transport pathway for IgE to the exterior.[168]

Whether IgE plasma cells are present at all in the intestinal mucosa had been the subject of debate. Although Tada and Ishizaka[169] reported the presence of these cells in the intestine as well as other mucosae and we[167] found IgE cells to be on the order of about 2% of all immunoglobulin-containing cells in the gut, others[170] reported that the putative IgE plasma cells were actually mast cells with cytophilic IgE attached. That IgE plasma cells are truly present in the intestine was verified by documenting the morphology of the IgE-positive cells by immunoelectron microscopy,[171] although the cells have not been enumerated by that method. This last observation accords with reports that most of the IgE present in secretions is synthesized locally, not derived from transudation of serum IgE,[168] and that synthesis of IgE by mucosal specimens in vitro has been observed.[172] There had also been suspicion that IgE-containing cells in the intestinal mucosa are not of intestinal origin because of a paucity of IgE-bearing cells in gut-associated aggregated lymphoid tissues. However, Durkin et al.[173] have reported that 20% of Peyer's patch lymphoid cells in germ-free rats are IgE-bearing cells. Those authors speculate that IgE B cells do indeed have their genesis in Peyer's patches but often are not found there because antigen exposure causes maturation and rapid exit of the cells from the patches.

IgD

IgD does not appear to be a secretory immunoglobulin. Its concentrations in secretions are not elevated above those in serum, and there is no special transport pathway for IgD into secretions.

BIOLOGIC ACTIVITIES OF ANTIBODIES IN THE ALIMENTARY TRACT

In considering the activities of antibodies in the alimentary tract, it is important to appreciate some of the unique attributes of the mucosal immune system. This system must respond vigorously to mucosal pathogens while at the same time remaining unresponsive to the myriad antigens present in gut commensals and foods; it must help to exclude exogenous antigens from entering the internal milieu of the body, while still allowing the uptake and processing of nutrients; it must regulate the response of the systemic immune system to common environmental materials that might otherwise engage the system in autoimmune reactions or other counterproductive responses. In addition, the biologic actions of antibodies in the digestive tract sometimes have to be carried out in a harsh environment of potent proteolytic enzymes and the detergent action of bile acids.

IgA

Properties of sIgA

In certain respects, sIgA is well suited to meet the demands placed on antibodies in the digestive tract. It is highly resistant to digestion by pancreatic proteases. We[174] found that 11S IgA in colostrum and duodenal fluid, and IgA diphtheria antitoxins in nasal secretions, were much more resistant to degradation by trypsin and human duodenal fluid than was IgG. This resistance is the result of the association of polymeric IgA with SC, as demonstrated by experiments using in vitro combination of the two molecules.[175] Another feature of sIgA that has been touted as advantageous is its relationship to the complement system. Throughout the years, although there were reports of activation of both the classical[176-178] and the alternative[179,180] complement pathways by IgA, they could be challenged on grounds that aggregated or very large molecules of IgA were involved. Moreover, studies that compared the bactericidal properties of IgG, IgM, and IgA detected little or no bactericidal activity associated with IgA,[181-183] and in a study that used blood group antigens, IgA did not activate complement.[184] The validity of reports that sIgA can interact with lysozyme and complement to effect augmented bactericidal activity[185,186] has also been questioned.[17] Although recent reports have more convincingly demonstrated activation of complement by IgA — sIgA as well as serum IgA[187-190] — the biologic significance of this complement activation still has to be questioned: despite IgA's ability to deposit C3, IgA can apparently block complement-mediated bacteriolysis by IgG and IgM.[187,191,192] Thus the presence of IgA might reduce the possibility of complement-mediated reactions involving other immunoglobulin classes from occurring on mucosal surfaces; this could be particularly advantageous in the environment of the intestinal lumen, where the antigenic challenge facing the mucosal immune system is enormous. The relative lack of complement components in intestinal secretions[193] also weighs against a major role of IgA-complement reactions in the gut.

IgA also has a complex role with respect to phagocytosis. This role has been at least partially clarified since the discovery of surface receptors for IgA on effector cells such as granulocytes and monocytes.[194-197] It appears that IgA can inhibit phagocytosis on a nonspecific basis but enhance phagocytosis as well as killing on a specific basis. For example, heat-aggregated IgA decreased neutrophil binding and phagocytosis of *Candida* organisms coated with specific IgG anti-*Candida* antibodies and complement.[198] On the other hand, specific IgA antibodies have facilitated phagocytosis of *Neisseria gonorrhoeae* or *Pseudomonas aeruginosa*[199,200] and the lysis of *Neisseria meningitidis* by macrophages.[191] With particular relevance to the intestine, IgA antibodies from intestinal fluids specifically enhanced the natural antibacterial activity of murine intestinal leukocytes to a *Shigella* strain in an in vitro assay[201]; whether such IgA-mediated cellular cytotoxicity reactions are an important first line of defense against infectious agents in the alimentary tract deserves clarification.

A peculiarity of IgA, the biologic significance of which is still not completely clear, is the susceptibility of IgA1 to proteases produced by certain bacteria. Such enzymes, produced by *Streptococcus sanguis, Streptococcus pneumoniae, N. meningitidis, N. gonorrhoeae* and *Hemophilus influenzae* can cleave molecules of the IgA1 subclass at sites within the hinge region of the heavy chains.[202-207] Most of the IgA proteases are specific for human IgA1; IgA proteins from several animal species, other isotypes of human immunoglobulins, and human IgA2 are not susceptible. The association of IgA molecules with SC does not make them resistant to the bacterial IgA proteases, but sIgA may be at somewhat of an advantage in this regard because of its relatively high proportion of IgA2.[22,23] It has been proposed that the cleavage of IgA1 antibodies by the proteases might result in loss of antibody activity, e.g., aggregation of particulate antigens, or interference with Fc-mediated functions.[208] In the intestinal tract, however, bacteria producing the proteases are present without causing untoward effects.[207]

The Antigen Exclusion Role of IgA

One of the most frequently touted roles of sIgA is inhibition of uptake of nonviable antigens at mucosal surfaces. While this proposed activity is supported by some experimental evidence, its biologic significance remains unestablished. Frequently cited support for the immune exclusion role of mucosal antibodies comes from the work of Walker and colleagues,[209,210] who found that oral or intense parenteral immunization with horseradish peroxidase or bovine albumin inhibited, in an antigen-specific manner, absorption of those antigens by everted gut sacs in vitro. The mechanism responsible for this inhibition appeared to be increased adsorption of antigen, in the form of complexes with specific antibodies, to the mucous coat of the intestinal surface, followed by degradation of the antigen by pancreatic proteases. Treatment of intestinal loops from immunized animals with dithiothreitol to remove the mucous layer eliminated the inhibition of antigen uptake, and ligation of the pancreatic ducts prevented the enhanced degradation of antigen-antibody complexes[211,212]; subsequent in vivo experiments supported these findings.[212] It is important to note, though, that the inhibition of antigen uptake in the rat was attributed to IgG1 antibodies, not IgA. Direct evidence for the role of IgA in this activity is still lacking. IgA-deficient persons have been found to have increased amounts of certain ingested food antigens in their circulation and increased titers of precipitating antibodies to milk proteins and the presence of circulating IgA immune complexes.[213,214] While these observations support the concept of sIgA being a barrier to antigenic penetration of the intestinal surface, they do not prove it; other defects in the mucosa of IgA-deficient persons might lead to increased absorption of intact antigens, and such persons may have impaired mechanisms for the removal of antigens from the circulation, once absorbed, or have defective systemic immunologic tolerance to foreign protein antigens.

The immune exclusion role of sIgA, even if it is operative, is probably not a major mechanism by which systemic reactions to dietary antigens are avoided; even in immune animals, the reduction in absorption of antigens is only on the order of 50%, which seems unlikely to substantially reduce the possibility of an immune response. Nevertheless, at times of possible disruption of the integrity of the intestinal mucosa, as perhaps in infection or allergy, sIgA in the secretions or on the epithelial surface might be critical in preventing absorption of harmful antigens.

Even though sIgA may not be able to abolish the absorption of unwanted antigens, the role of IgA in disposing of the antigens, once absorbed, should not be discounted. As we have discussed, the liver of some species can quite efficiently clear IgA-antigen complexes via the SC-mediated transport pathway and discard the complexes into the bile.[91,101,102-109] Even though the human liver does not have this effective clearance mechanism, its hepatocytes, through their binding of IgA1 proteins to the asialoglycoprotein receptor or other receptors,[215] might be able to take up antigens complexed with IgA1 and degrade them intracellularly. In addition, immunoelectron micrographic studies have demonstrated the presence of IgA2 on the surfaces and within endocytic-like vesicles of Kupffer cells in the human liver[216]; perhaps these phagocytic cells can also dispose of antigens associated with IgA. The role of the liver in handling IgA or IgA immune complexes may be highly relevant in disease states in which IgA is prominently deposited along the sinusoids of the liver (especially in alcoholic liver disease)[217] or in the skin or kidneys (IgA nephropathy).

Inhibition of Adherence

A logical extension of the concept of immune exclusion of soluble antigens is that, by a similar mechanism, IgA might interfere with the attachment of bacteria to the intestinal surface; the data supporting this possibility are fairly persuasive. Years ago, Williams and Gibbons[218] reported that purified IgA could inhibit the adhesion in vitro of oral streptococci to buccal epithelial cells. Local IgA has also been shown to inhibit the adhesion of *E. coli* to urinary tract epithelium[219,220] and of streptococci to dental enamel.[221] In the intestine, a similar mechanism has been demonstrated in experimental *Vibrio cholera* infection[222]; intestinal loops prepared in orally immunized mice were partially protected from the effects of live cholera organisms, and the protection appeared to be due to the action of specific antibodies excluding the organisms from attaching to the gut wall. The mechanisms in the inhibition of bacterial attachment are not fully defined, but antibody binding to specific adhesion determinants on the microorganisms is one possibility. Similar observations have been made in studies on the enteroadherent *E. coli* rabbit model of diarrhea (RDEC), in which specific IgA antibodies in milk have passively protected recipient animals,[223] and some evidence suggests that IgA antibodies in intestinal fluids can be similarly protective.[224,225] In the case of *Salmonella*, sIgA antibodies attached to organisms may prevent their adherence by causing a decrease in hydrophobicity and in negative charge of the organisms.[226,227]

A highly interesting observation made in mice and humans is that the indigenous bacteria of the intestine were coated with IgA but potentially pathogenic microorganisms were not.[4,228] The authors of that work have suggested that a large antigenic load, such as that of the indigenous flora, is required in order to stimulate a mucosal IgA response. Their observation that bacteria flourishing in the bowel lumen are coated with IgA is also persuasive evidence of the limited role of IgA antibodies in phagocytosis and killing of bacteria.

Other Antimicrobial Functions of IgA

Among the most convincing data on the antimicrobial effects of mucosal IgA is the work of Ogra et al.[229] of about 20 years ago, showing that oral immunization with live or killed poliovirus produced a mucosal IgA antibody response, but immunization with killed (Salk) virus did not. The mucosal response was associated with a striking resistance to reinfection of mucosal areas, a phenomenon not observed after parenteral immunization (although the latter route of immunization is effective in preventing paralytic disease, probably because of the production of serum IgG antibodies). sIgA antibodies can neutralize cholera toxin,[230] probably by preventing binding of the toxin to epithelial cells. Purified cholera toxin is a potent immunogen that, when administered properly to animals, can prevent disease.[231] In attempts to immunize against cholera in man, various modifications of cholera toxin have been used as immunogens; one of the most promising has been a combination of the B subunit of the cholera toxin molecule with formalin- or heat-inactivated classical or El Tor cholera vibrios.[232] We[233] and others[234] have found that IgA-cholera toxin antibodies secreted into the bile of rats that have been immunized via the intestinal tract can protect against the secretory effects of cholera toxin in the intestine; this is evidence that the sIgA antibodies can retain antitoxin activity in the powerful detergent milieu of bile.

The actions of sIgA in protecting against intestinal parasites is not well defined, although it is suspected that the antibodies interfere with the attachment of the organisms to the epithelial surface or inhibit motility of the organisms by binding to flagellae. Experimental giardiasis is one of the best-studied models of the role of antibodies in an intestinal parasitic infection. The results of studies on immunoglobulin-deficient mice[235] and nude mice (which because of their lack of helper/inducer T cells could not produce anti-*Giardia muris* antibodies)[236,237] indicate that antibodies (perhaps both IgA and IgG) in intestinal fluids are important in eradication of the parasites. The exact mechanism of this eradication is not known, but an antibody-mediated cellular cytotoxicity has been suggested.[238] The emphasis ascribed to antibodies in these animal studies accords with the very high frequency of giardiasis in immunoglobulin-deficient persons, especially those with the common variable hypogammaglobulinemia.[239]

sIgA Antibodies in Bile

sIgA antibodies to several intestinal microorganisms have been demonstrated under "natural" conditions or after experimental immunization (for a complete list see reference 240). The relevance of these antibodies in protecting the biliary ducts or the intestine remains to be established. Since, in man, the intestinal mucosa contributes most of the IgA present in the intestinal fluid,[157] the biliary antibodies are probably not crucial to protection of the intestine.

Overall, the status of IgA in the immunologic protection of mucous membranes is still incompletely defined. Doubtless, though, the role of IgA is highly complex and intertwined with the roles of other immunoglobulins and nonimmunologic defenses. IgA may be less important in protection against infectious agents than was believed when it was initially touted as the "first line of defense," even though it probably possesses more biologic activities than was envisioned when the idea was first proposed. Doubt about the overall significance of sIgA is supported by the well-known observation that persons selectively deficient in IgA are usually not bothered by exceedingly frequent gastrointestinal or other mucosal infections and do not have excessive numbers of bacteria in their small intestinal fluids.[18] It is possible that in those persons the mucosal antibody-mediated protective role of IgA is taken over by IgM, since they respond to intranasal polio immunization with local IgG and IgM responses[241] and possess increased numbers of IgM plasma cells in the intestinal lamina propria.[242,243] Nevertheless, the importance of sIgA in the overall balance of mucosal immune responses should not be discounted. It might be that through its role as an inhibitory molecule, preventing the activation of potent immunologic reactions, e.g., those involving neutrophils and the complement cascade, or in preventing misrecognition of self-antigens, sIgA has its greatest utility. In this connection, it is noteworthy that autoimmune diseases seem to occur with increased frequency in patients who are selectively IgA-deficient.[18]

IgM

There is little direct evidence for the participation of IgM in the defense of the intestine. Although IgM possesses opsonizing ability through complement activation, the role of complement in intestinal secretions, as already mentioned, is probably limited. Direct evidence for the efficacy of IgM, as well as IgG, in the intestine has been provided by studies in which the in vivo and vitro antibacterial activities of IgG, IgM, and IgA antibodies to *V. cholerae* were compared[244]; IgM and IgG showed pronounced antibacterial activity, both through complement-mediated killing and opsonization. According to one report,[245] IgM is the major secretory immunoglobulin in the intestinal tract of children. Thus, during the time when the IgA system is developing, IgM antibodies might be especially important. Another occasion when IgM antibodies might be very useful is when IgA is absent, as in IgA deficiency states (see above), in which IgM might "substitute" for IgA.

One reason to question the effectiveness of secreted IgM in intestinal fluids is its susceptibility to proteolysis,[15] as we have mentioned. A major function of IgM antibodies, i.e., the agglutination of bacteria, would be expected to be impaired by degradation of the molecule. This speculation is supported by the observation that IgA antibodies retained agglutinating activity in intestinal secretions better than did IgM antibodies.[246]

IgG

The role of IgG antibodies in mucosal defenses of the intestine has not been nearly as extensively studied as that of IgA, and IgG has generally been considered less important than IgA. This opinion derives in part from the fact that the concentration of IgG is much less than that of IgA in human intestinal fluids [although in the rat[247] and ruminant,[248,249] IgG is a major secretory immunoglobulin]. Other evidence suggesting a lesser role for IgG is that IgG has no specific transport pathway to the exterior and is highly sensitive to proteolysis by peptic and tryptic enzymes present in digestive tract fluids.[174] The significance of this latter "defect" of IgG may have been exaggerated, however, because the Fab fragments of IgG that are produced by tryptic digestion may still be capable of performing important functions, e.g., neutralizing toxins or inhibiting the adherence of microorganisms.[250] On the other hand, one can speculate that the cleavage of the Fc region of IgG might accomplish the useful function of preventing the intact IgG molecule from binding to various effector cells, and thereby reducing its ability to mediate inflammatory reactions at the mucosal surface. Some hints of the possible hazards of having IgG antibodies present in the mucosa come from the observations that serum antibodies, while inhibiting the passage of specific antigen through the mucosa, actually enhanced the penetration of bystander antigens,[251,152] perhaps because the formation of IgG immune complexes produced a cellular inflammatory response, resulting in increased leakiness of the mucosa. In the respiratory tract, evidence suggests that serum IgG antibodies, in the absence of local antibody responses, may be damaging to lung tissues,[253] presumably through the formation of locally deposited immune complexes.

IgG antibodies are reportedly capable of performing functions ascribed to IgA, e.g., exclusion of antigens,[247] prevention of adhesion of bacteria to the intestinal wall,[254] and neutralization of viruses.[240,255] We have mentioned the evidence that IgG in animal models can be protective against *Giardia* organisms.[236,237] Another potentially important role of IgG in the intestine is the stimulation of the secretion of mucus. In rats, IgG immune complexes on the mucosal surface have triggered the release of mucus from goblet cells.[7] The possibility that such a mechanism is also present in man has been raised by our recent finding of a specific binding site for the Fc region of IgG, which appears most associated with goblet cells, in the human small intestine and colon.[256]

The generally accepted principal role for IgG in the mucosa is that of a "second line of defense." This action presumably occurs largely within the mucosa, where IgG cells are relatively numerous (taking into account the rather low concentration of IgG in the intestinal fluids), and considerable IgG is present in the interstices of the cellular elements.[159,160,257,258] At times of penetration of potentially pathogenic antigens into the mucosa, the action of IgG antibodies to contain the infection might be crucial. The potential for IgG to induce unwanted inflammatory responses in the bowel wall has already been discussed. The relationship of this potential to the prominent increase in mucosal IgG-containing cells observed in inflammatory bowel disease[164] deserves further study. IgG plasma cells in the bowel mucosa might also be a major contributor to the IgG content of serum, especially of antibodies to microorganisms encountered in the gut, but this possibility has not been systematically examined.

A persuasive bit of evidence in favor of a critical role for IgG, as well as of IgM antibodies, in gut defenses is the high frequency of intestinal infections in patients with generalized immunoglobulin deficiencies, e.g., those with the common variable hypogammaglobulinemia.[239,259] As many as two-thirds of such patients who have diarrhea may have infection with *Giardia lamblia*,[239,259] and they may also have an increased frequency of shigellosis, salmonellosis, and campylobacteriosis.[259-261] Additional support for the role of IgG and IgM antibodies (as well as IgA antibodies) in intestinal defenses may be forthcoming from more extensive probing of the immunologic defects leading to intestinal infections in AIDS patients, in whom some workers[262] emphasize the role of defective humoral antibody responses as a consequence of the T-helper deficiencies that characterize the disease.

IgE

On the basis of the low concentrations of IgE in intestinal fluids and the few IgE cells in the intestinal mucosa, it would seem that IgE is only a minor player in the immunologic activities of the digestive tract. However, IgE appears to play an important role both in the mediation of intestinal allergic reactions (true food allergies) and defense against certain intestinal parasites. An IgE reaction is invariably a part of the immune response to infection with helminth parasites, and raised serum levels of IgE in parasitized persons are characteristic, although the mechanism by which IgE antibodies help protect against these infections has not been extensively studied. The best characterized mechanism is that in which degranulation of mast cells occurs as a result of cross-linking of surface IgE by antigen, releasing vasoactive amines that render the epithelium more permeable to serum immunoglobulins, which can enter the bowel lumen and attack the parasite. A protease that is specifically released from mucosal mast cells during anaphylaxis and that can attack the collagenous matrix of the intestinal mucosa, thereby altering water and electrolyte transport, has been identified.[263] Experimentally, rats immunized passively with serum antibody against *Nippostrongylus brasiliensis* and subsequently given intestinal anaphylaxis expel the worms faster than allergic rats lacking serum antibodies to the worm.[264] It appears that IgE is not essential for the expulsion but has a potentiating effect on the immune serum.[265] In addition to this effect of IgE, mast cell products themselves may have activity against parasites[266,267] and IgE antibodies complexed to antigen within the intestinal lumen may trigger the release of mucus from goblet cells,[268] thereby aiding expulsion of the worms.

Although IgE has been reported capable of several activities usually ascribed only to other immunoglobulin isotypes (opsonization, cytotoxicity, blocking of bacterial adherence),[269] we suspect that because of the low concentrations of IgE in intestinal fluids and the extensive fragmentation of whatever IgE is present,[16] these activities are not of much biologic importance. On the other hand, we (Brown and Lee) have speculated that the proteolysis of IgE in the intestine could be important in preventing allergic reactions because the amino-terminal part of Fc fragments of IgE are incapable of mediating passive cutaneous anaphylaxis.[270] The subject of food allergy is discussed in detail in Chapter 23. We simply mention here that the majority of allergic reactions to food are believed to be due to IgE-mediated, mast cell-dependent immediate hypersensitivity reactions.[271] There are reports of increased amounts of IgE in the intestinal fluids[272,273] and of IgE cells in the intestinal lamina propria[274] of patients with this kind of food sensitivity, but the validity and significance of these results are in doubt because of the difficulties in enumerating the low numbers of IgE cells in the mucosa, the proteolysis of IgE in intestinal fluids, and the lack of specificity of the presumptive abnormal findings.

IgD

Although there may be some special role for the small amounts of IgD that seep into intestinal secretions, none has been defined. If IgD is an important component of mucosal defenses, it seems to act mostly at sites other than the gastrointestinal tract. Low but definite numbers of IgD B cells can be found normally in the tonsils, lacrimal-nasal glands, and salivary glands.[275] Furthermore, in IgA deficiency, normally occurring IgA plasma cells in those tissues are replaced by large numbers of

IgD plasma cells, whereas in the gastrointestinal mucosa they are replaced by IgM and IgG plasma cells.[275] The difference in the distribution of IgD plasma cells has prompted the suggestion that a mucosal minisystem exists, characterized by IgD precursor development in tonsils and selective homing of such precursors to respiratory mucosal glands.[276]

REFERENCES

1. Conley ME, Delacroix D: Intravascular and mucosal immunoglobulin A: two separate but related systems of immune defense. *Ann Intern Med* 106:892–899, 1987.
2. Brandtzaeg P: Role of J chain and secretory component in receptor-mediated glandular and hepatic transport of immunoglobulins in man. *Scand J Immunol* 22:111–46, 1985.
3. Mackowiak P: The normal microbial flora. *N Engl J Med* 307:83–93. 1982.
4. Van Saene HKF, van der Waaij D: A novel technique for detecting IgA coated potentially pathogenic microorganisms in the human intestine. *J Immunol Methods* 30:87–96, 1979.
5. Lodinova R, Korych B, Bartakova Z, et al: Prevention and treatment of gastrointestinal infections in infants by using immunobiological methods. *Ann NY Acad Sci* 409:841–844, 1983.
6. Gibbons RJ: Review and discussion of role of mucus in mucosal defense. In Strober W, Hanson LA, Sell KW: *Recent Advances in Mucosal Immunity.* New York, Raven, 1982, p 343.
7. Lake AM, Bloch KJ, Neutra MR, et al: Intestinal goblet cell mucus release. II. In vivo stimulation by antigen in the immunized rat. *J Immunol* 122:834–837, 1979.
8. Clamp JR: The relationship between secretory immunoglobulin A and mucus. *Biochem Soc Trans* 5:1579–81, 1977.
9. Hermans PE, Diaz-Buxo JA, Stobo JD: Idiopathic late-onset immunoglobulin deficiency. Clinical observations in 50 patients. *Am J Med* 61:221–237, 1976.
10. Rogers HJ, Synge C: Bacteriostatic effect of human milk on *E. coli:* the role of IgA. *Immunology* 34:19–28, 1978.
11. Goodman H, Pollock JS, Katona LI, et al: Lysis of *Streptococcus mutans* by hen egg white lysozyme and inorganic sodium salts. *J Bacteriol* 146:764–774, 1981.
12. Moldoveanu Z, Tenovuo J, Pruitt KM, et al: Anti-bacterial properties of milk: IgA-peroxidase-lactoferrin interactions. *Ann NY Acad Sci* 409:848–850, 1983.
13. Brown WR: Nonimmunoglobulin precipitin lines between intestinal fluids and antisera in immunodiffusion studies: an explanation for their occurrence and how they can be avoided. *J Lab Clin Med* 77:326–334, 1971.
14. Brown WR, Newcomb RW, Ishizaka K: Proteolytic degradation of secretory and serum immunoglobulins and diphtheria antitoxin. *J Clin Invest* 49:1374–1380, 1987.
15. Richman LK, Brown WR: Immunochemical characterization of IgM in human intestinal fluids. *J Immunol* 119:1515–1519, 1977.
16. Brown WR, Lee EH: Studies on IgE in human intestinal fluids. *Int Arch Allergy Appl Immunol* 50:87–94, 1976.
17. Hanson LA, Brandtzaeg P: The mucosal defense system. In Stiehm ER, Fulginiti VA: *Immunologic Disorders in Infants and Children.* Philadelphia, Saunders, 1980, p 137.
18. Brown WR, Savage DD, Dubois RB, et al: The intestinal microflora of immunoglobulin-deficient and normal human subjects. *Gastroenterology* 62:1143–1152, 1972.

19. Delacroix DL, Hodgson HJF, McPherson A, et al: Selective transport of polymeric immunoglobulin A in bile. *J Clin Invest* 70:230–241, 1982.

20. Kutteh WH, Prince SJ, Phillips JO, et al: Properties of immunoglobulin A in serum of individuals with liver diseases and in hepatic bile. *Gastroenterology* 82:184–193, 1982.

21. Nagura H, Nakane PK, Smith PD, et al: IgA in human hepatic bile and liver. *J Immunol* 126:587–595, 1981.

22. Mestecky J, Russell MW: IgA subclasses. *Monogr Allergy* 19:27–301, 1986.

23. Delacroix DL, Dive C, Rambaud JC, et al: IgA subclasses in various secretions and in serum. *Immunology* 47:383–385, 1982.

24. Solari R, Kraehenbuhl JP: The biosynthesis of secretory component and its role in the transepithelial transport of IgA dimer. *Immunol Today* 56:17–20, 1985.

25. Ahnen DJ, Brown WR, Kloppel TM: Secretory component. The polymeric immuno globulin receptor. What's in it for the hepatologist and gastroenterologist. *Gastroenterology* 89:667–682, 1985.

26. Ahnen DJ, Brown WR, Kloppel TM: Secretory component. The polymeric immuno-globulin receptor. In Conn PM: *The Receptors,* Vol III. Orlando, FL, Academic Press, 1986, p 2.

27. Mestecky J, McGhee JR: Immunoglobulin A (IgA): molecular and cellular interactions involved in IgA biosynthesis and immune response. *Adv Immunol* 40:153–245, 1987.

28. Mestecky J, Russell MW, Jackson S, et al: The human IgA system: a reassessment. *Clin Immunol Immunopathol* 40:105–114, 1986.

29. Brandtzaeg P, Valnes K, Scott H, et al: The human gastrointestinal secretory immune system in health and disease. *Scand J Gastroenterol* 20:17–38. 1985.

30. Underdown BJ, Schiff JM: Immunoglobulin A: strategic defense initiative at the mu-cosal surface. *Ann Rev Immunol* 4:389–417, 1986.

31. Mestecky J, Schrohenholer RE, Kulhavy R, et al: Association of S-IgA subunits. *Adv Exp Med Biol* 45:99–109, 1974.

32. Bienenstock J: Gut and bronchus-associated lymphoid tissue: an overview. *Adv Exp Med Biol* 149:471–477, 1982.

33. Brandtzaeg P: Role of J chain and secretory component in receptor-mediated glandu-lar and hepatic transport of immunoglobulins in man. *Scand J Immunol* 22:111–146, 1985.

34. Mestecky J, Preud'homme JL, Crago SS, et al: Presence of J chain in human lymphoid cells. *Clin Exp Immunol* 39:371–385, 1980.

35. Nagura H, Nakane PK, Brown WR: Ultrastructural localization of J-chain in human intestinal mucosa. *J Immunol* 123:1044–1050, 1979.

36. Brandtzaeg P: Immunohistochemical characterization of intracellular J chain and binding site for secretory component (SC) in the human immunoglobulin (Ig)-produc-ing cells. *Mol Immunol* 20:941–966, 1983.

37. Brown WR, Isobe K, Nakane PK, et al: Studies on translocation of immunoglobulins across intestinal epithelium. IV. Evidence for binding of IgA and IgM to secretory component in intestinal epithelium. *Gastroenterology* 73:1333–1339, 1977.

38. Kuhn LC, Kraehenbuhl JP: Role of secretory component, a secreted glycoprotein, in the specific uptake of IgA dimer by epithelial cells. *J Biol Chem* 254:11072–11081, 1979.

39. Kuhn LC, Kraehenbuhl JP: Interaction of rabbit secretory component with rabbit IgA dimer. *J Biol Chem* 254:11066–11071, 1979.

40. Brandtzaeg P: Human secretory component. IV. Immunoglobulin binding properties. *Immunochemistry* 14:178–188, 1977.

41. Weicker J, Underdown BJ: A study of the association of human secretory component with IgA and IgM proteins. *J Immunol* 114:1337–1344, 1975.

42. Radl J, Klein F, van der Berg P: Binding of secretory piece to polymeric IgA and IgM paraproteins in vitro. *Immunology* 20:843–852, 1971.

43. Underdown BJ, Socken DJ: A comparison of secretory component-immunoglobulin interactions amongst different species. *Adv Exp Med Biol* 107:503–511, 1978.

44. Halpern MS, Koshland ME: Novel subunit in secretory IgA. *Nature* 228:1276–1278, 1970.

45. Garcia-Pardo A, Lamm ME, Plaut AG, et al: J chain is covalently bound to both monomer subunits in human secretory IgA. *J Biol Chem* 256:11734–11738, 1981.

46. Brandtzaeg P, Prydz H: Direct evidence for an integrated function of J chain and secretory component in epithelial transport. *Nature* 311:71–73, 1984.

47. Frutiger S, Hughes GJ, Fonck C, et al: High and low molecular weight rabbit secretory components. Evidence for the deletion of the second and third domains in the smaller peptide. *J Biol Chem* 262:1712–1715, 1987.

48. Schiff JM, Fisher MM, Underdown BJ: Receptor-mediated biliary transport of immunoglobulin A and asialoglycoprotein: sorting and missorting of ligands revealed by two radiolabeling methods. *J Cell Biol* 98:79–89, 1984.

49. Schiff JM, Fisher MM, Jones AL, et al: Human IgA as a heterovalent ligand: Switching from the asialoglycoprotein receptor to secretory component during transport across the rat hepatocyte. *J Cell Biol* 102:920–931, 1986.

50. Schiff JM, Fisher MM, Underdown BJ: Secretory component as the mucosal transport receptor: separation of physiochemically analogous human IgA fractions with different receptor-binding capacities. *Mol Immunol* 23:45–56, 1986.

51. Lindh E, Bjork I: Binding of secretory component to dimers of immunoglobulin A in vitro. *Eur J Biochem* 62:263–270, 1976.

52. Lindh E, Bjork I: Relative rates of the non-covalent and covalent binding of secretory component to an IgA dimer. *Acta Pathol Microbiol Scandc* 85:449–453, 1977.

53. Underdown BJ, De Rose J, Plaut A: Disulfide bonding of secretory component to a single monomer subunit in human secretory IgA. *J Immunol* 118:1816–1821, 1977.

54. Murkofsky NA, Lamm ME: Effect of a disulfide interchange enzyme on the assembly of human secretory immunoglobulin A from immunoglobulin A and free secretory component. *J Biol Chem* 254:12181–12184, 1979.

55. Garcia-Pardo A, Lamm ME, Plaut AG, et al: Secretory component is covalently bound to a single sub-unit in human secretory IgA. *Mol Immunol* 16:477–482, 1979.

56. Hanly CW, Chang CH, Schiffer M: A model for Secretory Component-IgA Interactisms. *Fed Proc Fed Am Soc Exp Biol* 44:1299, 1985 (abstr).

57. Socken DJ, Underdown BJ: Comparison of human, bovine and rabbit secretory component-immunoglobulin interactions. *Immunochemistry* 15:499–506, 1978.

58. Mostov KE, Kraehenbuhl JP, Blobel G: Receptor-mediated transcellular transport of immunoglobulin: synthesis of secretory component as multiple and larger transmembrane forms. *Proc Natl Acad Sci USA* 77:7257–7261, 1980.

59. Kuhn LC, Kraehenbuhl JP: The membrane receptor for polymeric immunoglobulin is structurally related to secretory component. Isolation and characterization of membrane secretory component from rabbit liver and mammary gland. *J Cell Biol* 256:12490–12495, 1981.

60. Mostov K, Blobel G: A transmembrane precursor of secretory component. *J Biol Chem* 257:11816–11821, 1982.

61. Mostov KE, Friedlander M, Blobel G: The receptor for transepithelial transport of IgA and IgM contains multiple immunoglobulin-like domains. *Nature* 308:37–43, 1984.

62. Knight KL, Rosenzweig M, Lichter EA, et al: Rabbit secretory IgA: identification and genetic control of two allotypes of secretory component. *J Immunol* 112:877–882, 1974.

63. Kuhn LC, Kocher HP, Hanly WC, et al: Structural and genetic heterogeneity of the receptor mediating translocation of immunoglobulin A dimer antibodies across epithelia in the rabbit. *J Biol Chem* 258:6653–6659, 1983.

64. Frutiger S, Hughes GJ, Hanly WC, et al: The amino-terminal domain of rabbit secretory component is responsible for noncovalent binding of immunoglobulin A dimers. *J Biol Chem* 261:16673–16681, 1986.

65. Larkin JM, Sztul ES, Palade GE: Phosphorylation of the rat hepatic polymeric IgA receptor. *Proc Natl Acad Sci USA* 83:4759–4763, 1986.

66. Musil LS, Baenziger JU: Intracellular transport and processing of secretory component in cultured rat hepatocytes. *Gastroenterology* 93:1194–1204, 1987.

67. Takahashi I, Nakane PK, Brown WR: Ultrastructural events in the translocation of polymeric IgA by rat hepatocytes. *J Immunol* 128:1181–1187, 1982.

68. Geuze HJ, Slot JW, Strous GJAM, et al: Intracellular receptor sorting during endocytosis: comparative immunoelectron microscopy of multiple receptors in rat liver. *Cell* 37:195–204, 1984.

69. Gebhardt R, Robenek H: Ligand-dependent redistribution of the IgA receptor on cultured rat hepatocytes and its disturbance by cytochalasin B. *J Histochem Cytochem* 35:301–309, 1987.

70. Limet JN, Quintart J, Schneider Y-J, et al: Receptor-mediated endocytosis of polymeric IgA and galactosylated serum albumin in rat liver. Evidence for intracellular ligand sorting and identification of distinct endosomal compartments. *Eur J Biochem* 146:539–548, 1985.

71. Courtoy PJ, Limet JN, Quintart J, et al: Transfer of IgA into rat bile: ultrastructure demonstration. *Ann NY Acad Sci* 409:799–802, 1983.

72. Hoppe CA, Connolly TP, Hubbard AL: Transcellular transport of polymeric IgA in the rat hepatocyte: biochemical and morphological characterization of the transport pathway. *J Cell Biol* 101:2113–2123, 1985.

73. Nagura H, Nakane PK, Brown WR: Translocation of dimeric IgA through neoplastic colon cells in vitro. *J Immunol* 123:2359–2368, 1979.

74. Goldman IS, Jones AL, Hradek GT, et al: Hepatocyte handling of immunoglobulin A in the rat: the role of microtubules. *Gastroenterology* 85:130–140, 1983.

75. Mullock BM, Luzio JP, Hinton RH: Preparation of a low-density species of endocytic vesicle containing immunoglobulin A. *Biochem J* 214:823–827, 1983.

76. Mullock BM, Jones RS, Hinton RH: Movement of endocytic shuttle vesicles from the sinusoidal to the bile canalicular face of hepatocytes does not depend on the occupation of receptor sites. *FEBS Lett* 113:201–205, 1980.

77. Kloppel TM, Brown WR, Reichen J: Mechanisms of secretion of proteins into bile. Studies in the perfused rat liver. *Hepatology* 6:587–594, 1986.

78. Limet JN, Schneider YL, Vaerman JP, et al: Binding, uptake and intracellular processing of polymeric rat immunoglobulin A by cultured rat hepatocytes. *Eur J Biochem* 125:437–443, 1982.

79. Gebhardt R: Primary cultures of rat hepatocytes as a model of canalicular development, biliary secretion, and intrahepatic cholestasis. III. Properties of the biliary transport of immunoglobulin A as revealed by immunofluorescence. *Gastroenterology* 84:1462–1470, 1983.

80. Jones AL, Huling S, Hradek GT, et al: Uptake and intracellular disposition of IgA by rat hepatocytes in monolayer culture. *Hepatology* 2:769–776, 1982.

81. Deitcher DL, Neutra MR, Mostov KE: Functional expression of the polymeric immunoglobulin receptor from cloned cDNA in fibroblasts. *J Cell Biol* 102:911–919, 1986.

82. Mostov KE, Deitcher DL: Polymeric immunoglobulin receptor expressed in MDCK cells transcytoses IgA. *Cell* 46:613–621, 1986.

83. Mostov KE, Kops AD, Deitcher DL: Deletion of the cytoplasmic domain of the polymeric immunoglobulin receptor prevents basolateral localization and endocytosis. *Cell* 47:359–364, 1986.

84. Mostov KE, Breitfeld P, Harris JM: An anchor-minus form of the polymeric immunoglobulin receptor is secreted predominantly apically in Madrin-Darby canine kidney cells. *J Cell Biol* 105:2031–2036, 1987.

85. Solari R, Racine L, Tallichet C, et al: Distribution and processing of the polymeric immunoglobulin receptor in the rat hepatocyte: morphological and biochemical characterization of subcellular fractions. *J Histochem Cytochem* 34:17–23, 1986.

86. Musil LS, Baenziger JU: Cleavage of membrane secretory component of soluble secretory component occurs on the cell surface of rat hepatocyte monolayers. *J Cell Biol* 104:1725–1733, 1987.

87. Ahnen DJ, Singleton JR, Hoops TC, et al: Posttranslational processing of secretory component in the rat jejunum by a brush border metalloprotease. *J Clin Invest* 77:1841–1848, 1986.

88. Fisher MM, Nagy B, Bazin H, et al: Biliary transport of IgA. Role of secretory component. *Proc Natl Acad Sci USA* 76:2008–2012, 1979.

89. Lemaitre-Coelho I, Altamirano GA, Barranco-Acosta C, et al: In vivo experiments involving secretory component in the rat hepatic transfer of polymeric IgA from blood into bile. *Immunology* 43:261–270, 1981.

90. Jackson GDF, Lemaitre-Coelho I, Vaerman JP, et al: Rapid disappearance from serum of intravenously injected rat myeloma IgA and its secretion into bile. *Eur J Immunol* 8:123–126, 1978.

91. Socken DJ, Simms ES, Nagy BR, et al: Secretory component-dependent hepatic transport of IgA antibody-antigen complexes. *J Immunol* 127:316–319, 1981.

92. Socken DJ, Jeejeebhoy KN, Bazin H, et al: Identification of secretory component as an IgA receptor on rat hepatocytes. *J Exp Med* 150:1538–1548, 1979.

93. Zevenbergen JL, May C, Wanson JC, et al: Synthesis of secretory component by rat hepatocytes in culture. *Scand J Immunol* 11:93–97, 1980.

94. Mullock BM, Hinton RH, Peppard J, et al: Distribution of secretory component in hepatocytes and its model of transfer into bile. *Biochem J* 190:819–826, 1980.

95. Sztul ES, Howell KE, Palade GE: Intracellular and transcellular transport of secretory component and albumin in rat hepatocytes. *J Cell Biol* 97:1582–1591, 1983.

96. Kloppel TM, Brown WR: Rat liver membrane secretory component is larger than free secretory component in bile. Evidence of proteolytic conversion of the membrane form to the free form. *J Cell Biochem* 24:307–318, 1984.

97. Sztul ES, Howell KE, Palade GE: Biogenesis of the polymeric IgA receptor in rat hepatocytes. I. Kinetic studies of its intracellular forms. *J Cell Biol* 100:1248–1254, 1985.

98. Sztul ES, Howell KE, Palade GE: Biogenesis of the polymeric IgA receptor in rat hepatocytes. II. Localization of its intracellular forms by cell fractionation studies. *J Cell Biol* 100:1255–1261, 1985.

99. Solari R, Kraehenbuhl JP: Biosynthesis of the IgA antibody receptor: a model for the transepithelial sorting of a membrane glycoprotein. *Cell* 36:61–71, 1984.

100. Schiff JM, Endo Y, Kells DIC, et al: Kinetic differences in hepatic transport of IgA polymers reflect molecular size. *Fed Proc* 42:1341, 1983 (abstr).

101. Russell MW, Brown TA, Mestecky J: Role of serum IgA. Hepatobiliary transport of circulating antigen. *J Exp Med* 153:968–976, 1981.

102. Stokes CR, Swarbrick ET, Soothill JF: Immune elimination and enhanced antibody responses: functions of circulating IgA. *Immunology* 40:455–458, 1980.

103. Peppard J, Orlans E, Payne AW, et al: The elimination of circulating complexes containing polymeric IgA by excretion in the bile. *Immunology* 42:83–89, 1981.

104. Socken DJ, Simms ES, Nagy B, et al: Transport of IgA antibody-antigen complexes by the rat liver. *Mol Immunol* 18:345–348, 1981.

105. Peppard JV, Orlans E, Andrew E, et al: Elimination into bile of circulating antigen by endogenous IgA antibody in rats. *Immunology* 45:467–472, 1982.

106. Brown TA, Russell MW, Mestecky J: Hepatobiliary transport of IgA immune complexes: molecular and cellular aspects. *J Immunol* 128:2183–2186, 1982.

107. Harmatz PR, Kleinman RE, Bunnell BW, et al: Hepatobiliary clearance of IgA immune complexes formed in the circulation. *Hepatology* 2:328–333, 1982.

108. Brown TA, Russell MW, Kulhavy R, et al: IgA-mediated elimination of antigens by the hepatobiliary route. *Fed Proc* 42:3218–3221, 1983.

109. Skogh T, Edebo L, Stendahl O: Gastrointestinal uptake and blood clearance of antigen in the presence of IgA antibodies. *Immunology* 50:175–180, 1983.

110. Nagura H, Nakane PK, Brown WR: Breast milk IgA binds to jejunal epithelium in suckling pets. *J Immunol* 120:1333–1337, 1978.

111. Buts JP, Delacroix D: Oncogenic changes in secretory component expression by villous and crypt cells of rat small intestine. *Immunology* 54:181–187, 1985.

112. Ogra SS, Ogra PL, Lippes J, et al: Immunohistologic localization of immunoglobulins, secretory component, and lactoferrin in the developing human fetus. *Proc Soc Exp Biol Med* 139:570–574, 1972.

113. Brown WR, Isobe Y, Nakane PK: Studies on translocation of immunoglobulins across intestinal epithelium. II. Immunoelectron microscopic localization of immunoglobulins and secretory component in human intestinal mucosa. *Gastroenterology* 71:985–995, 1976.

114. Ahnen DJ, Nakane PK, Brown WR: Ultrastructural localization of carcinoembryonic antigen in normal intestine and colon cancer. Abnormal distribution of CEA on the surfaces of colon cancer cells. *Cancer* 49:2077–2090, 1982.

115. Poger ME, Hirsch BR, Lamm ME: Synthesis of secretory component by colonic neoplasms. *Am J Pathol* 82:327–339, 1976.

116. Rognum T, Brandtzaeg P, Orjasaeter H, et al: Immunohistochemical study of secretory component, secretory IgA and carcinoembryonic antigen in large bowel carcinomas. *Pathol Res Pract* 170:126–145, 1980.

117. Schmucker DL, Gilbert R, Jones AL, et al: Effect of aging on the hepatobiliary transport of dimeric immunoglobulin A in the male Fischer rat. *Gastroenterology* 88:436–443, 1985.

118. Daniels CK, Schmucker DL, Jones AL: Age-dependent loss of dimeric immunoglobulin A receptors in the liver of the Fischer 344 rat. *J Immunol* 134:3855–3858, 1985.

119. Wira CR, Sandoe CP: Sex steroid hormone regulation of IgA and IgG in rat uterine secretions. *Nature* 268:534–536, 1977.

120. Weisz-Carrington P, Roux ME, McWilliams M, et al: Hormonal induction of the secretory immune system in the mammary gland. *Proc Natl Acad Sci USA* 75:2928–2932, 1978.

121. McDermott MR, Clark DA, Bienenstock J: Influence of the estrous cycle on B immunoblast migration into genital and intestinal tissues. *J Immunol* 124:2536–2539, 1980.

122. Sullivan DA, Wira CR: Variations in the levels of free secretory component in rat mucosal secretions. *J Immunol* 130:1330–1335, 1983.

123. Wira CR, Colby E: Regulation of secretory component by glucocorticoids in primary cultures of rat hepatocytes. *J Immunol* 134:1744–1748, 1985.

124. Sullivan DA, Underdown BJ, Wira CR: Steroid hormone regulation of free secretory component in the rat uterus. *Immunology* 49:379–386, 1983.

125. Wira CR, Stern J, Colby E: Estradiol regulation of secretory component in the uterus of the rat: evidence for involvement of RNA synthesis. *J Immunol* 133:2624–2628, 1984.

126. Tomana M, Kulhavy R, Mestecky J: Receptor-mediated binding and uptake of immunoglobulin A by human liver. *Gastroenterology* 94:762–770, 1988.

127. Sollid DM, Kvale D, Brandtzaeg P, et al: Synthesis of cytoplasmic and functional membrane SC induced by gamma interferon. *Adv Exp Med Biol* 216:1109–1116, 1987.

128. Kvale D, Lovhaug D, Sollid LM, et al: Tumor necrosis factor-alpha up-regulates expression of secretory component, the epithelial receptor for polymeric Ig. *J Immunol* 140:3086–3089, 1988.

129. Rao CK, Kaetzel CS, Lamm ME: Induction of secretory component synthesis in colonic epithelial cells. *Adv Exp Med Biol* 216:1071–1077, 1987.

130. Hinton RH, Ah-Sing E, Jones RS, et al: Enterohepatic circulation of IgA does not occur in rats. *Biosci Rep* 1:575–580, 1981.

131. Seo JK, Grant KE, Sullivan DA, et al: Biliary IgA content following common duct cannulation in the rat. *Adv Exp Med Biol* 216:1133–1138, 1987.

132. Rank J, Wilson ID: Changes in IgA following varying degrees of biliary obstruction in the rat. *Hepatology* 3:241–247, 1983.

133. Kloppel TM, Hoops TC, Gaskin C, et al: Uncoupling of the biliary secretory pathways for IgA and its receptor, secretory component, by brief periods of cholestasis. *Am J Physiol* 253:G232–G240, 1987.

134. Goldsmith MA, Jones AL, Underdown BJ, et al: Alterations in protein transport events in rat liver after estrogen treatment. *Am J Physiol* 253:G195–G200, 1987.

135. Delacroix DL, Denef AM, Acosta GA, et al: Immunoglobulins in rabbit hepatic bile: selective secretion of IgA and IgM and active plasma-to-bile transfer of polymeric IgA. *Scand J Immunol* 16:343–350, 1982.

136. Delacroix DL, Furtado-Barreira G, de Hemptinne B, et al: The liver in the IgA secretory immune system. Dogs, but not rats and rabbits, are suitable models for human studies. *Hepatology* 3:980–988, 1983.

137. Hall JG, Gyure LA, Payne AWR: Comparative aspects of the transport of immunoglobulin A from blood to bile. *Immunology* 41:899–902, 1980.

138. Orlans E, Peppard JV, Payne AWR, et al: Comparative aspects of the hepatobiliary transport of IgA. *Ann NY Acad Sci* 409:411–427, 1983.

139. Vaerman JP, Lemaitre-Coelho I, Limet J, et al: Hepatic transfer of polymeric IgA from plasma to bile in rats and other mammals. A survey. In Strober W, Hanson LA, Sell KW: *Recent Advances in Mucosal Immunity*. New York, Raven, 1982, p 233.

140. Dooley JS, Potter BJ, Thomas HC, et al: A comparative study of the biliary secretion of human dimeric and monomeric IgA in the rat and in man. *Hepatology* 2:323–327, 1982.

141. Delacroix DL, Vaerman JP: Function of the human liver in IgA homeostasis in plasma. *Ann NY Acad Sci* 409:383–401, 1983.

142. Nagura H, Smith PD, Nakane PK, et al: IgA in human bile and liver. *J Immunol* 126:587–595, 1981.

143. Fukuda Y, Nagura H, Asai J, et al: Possible mechanisms of elevation of serum secretory immunoglobulin A in liver diseases. *Am J Gastroenterol* 81:315–324, 1986.

144. Kater L, Jobsis AC, de la Faille-Kuyper EH, et al: Alcoholic hepatic disease. Specificity of IgA deposits in liver. *Am J Clin Pathol* 71:51–57, 1979.

145. Delacroix DL, Courtoy PJ, Rahier J, et al: Localization and serum concentration of secretory component during massive necrosis of human liver. *Gastroenterology* 86:521–531, 1984.

146. Vaerman J-P, Andre C, Bazin H, et al: Mesenteric lymph as a major source of serum IgA in guinea pigs and rats. *Eur J Immunol* 3:580–584, 1973.

147. Kaartinen J, Imir R, Klokars M, et al: IgA in blood and thoracic duct lymph: concentration and degree of polymerization. *Scand J Immunol* 7:229–232, 1978.

148. Brown WR, Smith PD, Lee E, et al: A search for an enriched source of polymeric IgA in human thoracic duct lymph, portal vein blood and aortic blood. *Clin Exp Immunol* 48:85–90, 1982.

149. Cruchard A, Lapperrouza C, Megevand R: Agammaglobulinemia in monozygous twins: therapeutical prospects. *Birth Defects* 4:315–327, 1968.

150. Challacombe SJ, Greenall C, Stoker TAM: A comparison of IgA in portal and peripheral venous blood. *Immunology* 60:111–116, 1987.

151. Delacroix DL, Malburny GN, Vaerman JP: Hepatobiliary transport of plasma IgA in the mouse: contribution to clearance of intravascular IgA. *Eur J Immunol* 15:893–899, 1985.

152. Hadziyannis S, Feizi T, Scheuer PJ, et al: Immunoglobulin-containing cells in the liver. *Clin Exp Immunol* 5:499–514, 1969.

153. Nagura H, Tsutsumi Y, Hasegawa H, et al: IgA plasma cells in biliary mucosa. A likely source of locally synthesized IgA in human bile. *Clin Exp Immunol* 54:671–680, 1983.

154. Carter L, Jackson GDF: Antibody synthesis in the rat liver: a source of biliary IgM, IgA and IgG following injection of horse erythrocytes into the intestine or Peyer's patches. *Adv Exp Med Biol* 216b:1147–1156, 1987.

155. Carter L, Barrington PJ, Cooper GN, et al: Antibody synthesis in the rat liver: an association between antibody-forming cells in the liver and biliary antibodies following intravenous injection of horse erythrocytes. *Int Arch Allergy Appl Immunol* 82:153–158, 1987.

156. Delacroix DL, Vaerman JP: Function of the human liver in IgA homeostasis in plasma. *Ann NY Acad Sci* 409:383–401, 1983.

157. Jonard PP, Rambaud JC, Dive C, et al: Secretion of immunoglobulins and plasma proteins from the jejunal mucosa. *J Clin Invest* 74:525–535, 1984.

158. Brandtzaeg P: Human secretory immunoglobulin M: an immunochemical and immunohistochemical study. *Immunology* 29:559–570, 1975.

159. Brown WR, Isobe Y, Nakane PK: Studies on translocation of immunoglobulins across intestinal epithelium. II. Immunoelectron microscopic localization of immunoglobulins and secretory component in human intestinal mucosa. *Gastroenterology* 71:985–995, 1976.

160. Brandtzaeg P: Human secretory immunoglobulins. *Clin Exp Immunol* 8:69–85, 1971.

161. Tomasi TB, Grey HM: Structure and function of immunoglobulin A. *Prog Allergy* 16:81–213, 1972.

162. Baklien K, Fausa O, Thune PO, et al: Immunoglobulins in jejunal mucosa and serum from patients with dermatitis herpetiformis. *Scand J Gastroenterol* 12:126–168, 1977.

163. Baklien K, Brandtzaeg P: Immunohistochemical characterization of local immunoglobulin formation in Crohn's disease of the ileum. *Scand J Gastroenterol* 11:447–457, 1976.

164. Brandtzaeg P, Baklien K, Fausa O, et al: Immunohistochemical characterization of local immunoglobulin formation in ulcerative colitis. *Gastroenterology* 66:1123–1136, 1974.

165. Baklien K: Immunopathology of the gut: a Study of the Immunoglobulin Systems of the Human Intestine. Oslo, University Hospital, 1977.

166. Brandtzaeg P, Baklien K: Intestinal secretion of IgA and IgM: a hypothetical model. In: *Immunology of the Gut.* Ciba Foundation Symposium 46 (New Series). Amsterdam, Elsevier, 1977, p 77.

167. Brown WR, Borthistle BK, Chen ST: Immunoglobulin E (IgE) and IgE-containing cells in human gastrointestinal fluids and tissues. *Clin Exp Immunol* 20:227–237, 1975.

168. Newcomb RW, Ishizaka K: Physicochemical and antigenic studies on human E in respiratory fluid. *J Immunol* 105:85–89, 1970.

169. Tada T, Ishizaka K: Distribution of E-forming cells in lymphoid tissues of the human and monkey. *J Immunol* 104:377–387, 1970.

170. Mayrhofer G, Bazin M, Gowans JL: Nature of cells binding anti-IgE in rats immunized with *Nippostrongylus brasiliensis:* IgE synthesis in regional nodes and concentration in mucosal mast cells. *Eur J Immunol* 6:537–545, 1976.

171. Patterson S, Roebuck P, Platts-Mills TAE, et al: IgE plasma cells in human jejunum demonstrated by immune electron microscopy. *Clin Exp Immunol* 46:301–304, 1981.

172. Platts-Mills TA: Local production of IgG, IgA, and IgE antibodies in grass pollen hay fever. *J Immunol* 122:2218–2225, 1979.

173. Durkin HG, Bazin H, Waksman BH: Origin and fate of IgE-bearing lymphocytes. I. Peyer's patches as differentiation site of cells simultaneously bearing IgA and IgE. *J Exp Med* 154:640–648, 1981.

174. Brown WR, Newcomb RW, Ishizaka K: Proteolytic degradation of exocrine and serum immunoglobulins. *J Clin Invest* 49:1374–1380, 1970.

175. Lind E, Bjork I: Binding of secretory component to dimers of immunoglobulin A in vitro. Mechanisms of the covalent bond formation. *Eur J Biochem* 62:263–270, 1976.

176. Burritt MF, Calvancio NJ, Mehta S, et al: Activation of the classical complement pathway by Fc fragment of human IgA. *J Immunol* 118:723–725, 1977.

177. Iida K, Fujita T, Inai S, et al: Complement fixing abilities of IgA myeloma proteins and their fragments. The activation of complement through the classical pathway. *Immunochemistry* 13:747–752, 1976.

178. Williams BD, Slaney JM, Price JF, et al: Classical pathway activation of complement system by IgA anti-C3 antibody. *Nature* 259:52–53, 1976.

179. Colten HR, Bienenstock J: Lack of C3 activation through classical or alternative pathways by human secretory IgA anti-blood group A antibody. *Adv Exp Med Biol* 45:305–314, 1974.

180. Robertson J, Caldwell JR, Castle JR, et al: Evidence for the presence of components of the alternative (properdin) pathway of complement activation in respiratory secretions. *J Immunol* 117:900–903, 1976.

181. Eddie DS, Shulkin MC, Robbins JB: The isolation and biologic activities of purified secretory IgA and IgG anti-*Salmonella typhimurium* O antibodies from rabbit intestinal fluid and colostrum. *J Immunol* 106:181–190, 1971.

182. Reed WP, Albright EL: Serum factors responsible for killing of *Shigella. Immunology* 26:205–215, 1974.

183. Heddle RJ, Knop J, Steele EJ, et al: The effect of lysozyme on the complement dependent bactericidal action of different antibody classes. *Immunology* 28:1061–1066, 1975.

184. Colten HR, Bienenstock J: Lack of C3 activation through classical or alternate pathways by human secretory secretory IgA anti blood group A antibody. *Adv Exp Med Biol* 45:305–308, 1974.

185. Adinolfi M, Glynn AA, Lindsay M, et al: Serological properties of A antibodies to *Escherichia coli* present in human colostrum. *Immunology* 10:517–526, 1966.

186. Hill IR, Porter P: Studies of bactericidal activity to *Escherichia coli* of porcine serum and colostral immunoglobulins and the role of lysozyme with secretory IgA. *Immunology* 26:1239–1250, 1974.

187. Griffis JMcL, Jarris GA: Interaction of serum IgA with complement components: the molecular basis of IgA blockade. *Adv Exp Med Biol* 216B:1303–1309, 1987.

188. Rits M, Bazin H, Vaerman J-P: Partial activation of rat complement through the alternative pathway by rat insoluble IgA immune complex. *Adv Exp Med Biol* 216B:1311–1316, 1987.

189. Pfaffenbach G, Lamm ME, Gigli I: Activation of guinea pig alternative complement pathway by mouse IgA immune complexes. *J Exp Med* 155:231–247, 1982.

190. Hiemstra PS, Biewanga J, Gorter A, et al: Activation of complement by human serum IgA, secretory IgA and IgA1 fragments. *Mol Immunol* 25:527–533, 1988.

191. Lowell GH, Smith LF, Griffiss JM, et al: Antibody-dependent mononuclear cell-mediated antimeningococcal activity. Comparison of the effects of convalescent and post-immunization IgG, IgM, and IgA. *J Clin Invest* 66:260–267, 1980.

192. Griffiss JM: Bactericidal activity of meningococcal antisera. Blocking by IgA of lytic antibody in human convalescent sera. *J Immunol* 114:1779–1784, 1975.

193. Reynolds HY, Thompson RE: Pulmonary host defences. I. Analysis of protein and lipids in bronchial secretions and antibody responses after vaccination with *Pseudomonas aeruginosa*. *J Immunol* 111:358–368, 1973.

194. Fanger MW, Pugh J, Bernier GM: The specificity of receptors for IgA on human polymorphonuclear cells and monocytes. *Cell Immunol* 60:324–334, 1981.

195. Fanger MW, Goldstine SN, Shen L: Cytofluorographic analysis of receptors for IgA on human polymorphonuclear cells and monocytes and the correlations of receptor expression with phagocytosis. *Mol Immunol* 20:1019–1027, 1983.

196. Gauldie J, Richards C, Lamontagne L: Fc receptors for IgA and other immunoglobulins on resident and activated alveolar macrophages. *Mol Immunol* 20:1029–1037, 1983.

197. Strober W, Hague NE, Lum LG, et al: IgA-Fc receptors on mouse lymphoid cells. *J Immunol* 121:2440–2445, 1978.

198. Wilton JM: Suppression by IgA of IgG-mediated phagocytosis by human polymorphonuclear leucocytes. *Clin Exp Immunol* 34:423–428, 978.

199. Bisno AL, Ofek I, Beachey EH, et al: Human immunity to *Neisseria gonorrhoeae:* acquired serum opsonic antibodies. *J Lab Clin Med* 86:221–229, 1975.

200. Reynolds HY, Kazmierowski JA, Newball HH: Specificity of opsonic antibodies to entrance phagocytosis of *Pseudomonas aeruginosa* by human alveolar macrophages. *J Clin Invest* 56:376–385, 1975.

201. Tagliabue A, Nencioni L, Villa L, et al: Antibody-dependent cell-mediated antibacterial activity of intestinal lymphocytes with secretory IgA. *Nature* 306:184–186, 1983.

202. Bricker J, Mulks MH, Plaut AG, et al: IgA1 proteases of *Haemophilus influenza:* Cloning and characterization in *Escherichia coli* K-12. *Proc Natl Acad Sci USA* 80:2681–2685, 1983.

203. Kilian M, Mestecky J, Kulnavy R, et al: IgA1 proteases from *Haemophilus influenzae, Streptococcus pneumoniae,* and *Streptococcus sanguis:* comparative immunochemical studies. *J Immunol* 124:2596–2600, 1980.

204. Male CJ: Immunoglobulin A1 protease production by *Haemophilus influenzae and Streptococcus pneumoniae. Infect Immun* 26:254–261, 1979.

205. Mestecky J, McGhee JR, Crago SS, et al: Molecular-cellular interactions in the secretory IgA response. *J Reticuloendothel Soc* 28:45S–60S, 1980.

206. Mulks MH, Plaut AG: IgA protease production as a characteristic distinguishing pathogenic from harmless *Neisseriaceae. N Engl J Med* 299:973–976, 1978.

207. Mehta SK, Plaut AG, Calvanico NJ, et al: Human immunoglobulin A: production of an Fc fragment by an enteric microbial proteolytic enzyme. *J Immunol* 111:1274–1276, 1973.

208. Mestecky J, McGhee RJ, Crago SS, et al: Molecular-cellular interactions in the secretory IgA response. *J Reticuloendothel Soc* 28:45S–60S, 1980.

209. Walker WA, Isselbacher KJ, Bloch KJ: Intestinal uptake of macromolecules: effect of oral immunization. *Science* 177:608–610, 1972.

210. Walker WA, Isselbacher KJ, Bloch KJ: Intestinal uptake of macromolecules. II. Effect of parenteral immunization. *J Immunol* 111:221–226, 1973.

211. Walker WA, Wu M, Isselbacher KJ, et al: Uptake of macromolecules. IV. The effect of pancreatic duct ligation on breakdown of antigen and antigen-antibody complexes on the intestinal surface. *Gastroenterology* 69:1223–1229, 1975.

212. Pang KY, Walker WA, Bloch KJ: Intestinal uptake of macromolecules. Differences in distribution of protein antigen in control and immunized rats. *Gut* 22:1018–1024, 1981.

213. Cunningham-Rundles C, Brandeis WE, Good RA, et al: Milk precipitins, circulating immune complexes and IgA deficiency. *Proc Natl Acad Sci USA* 75:3387–3389, 1978.

214. Cunningham-Rundles C, Brandeis WE, Good RA, et al: Bovine antigens and the formation of circulating immune complexes in selective immunoglobulin A deficiency. *J Clin Invest* 64:272–279, 1979.

215. Tomana M, Kulhavy R, Mestecky J: Receptor-mediated binding and uptake of immunoglobulin A by human liver. *Gastroenterology* 94:762–770, 1988.

216. Amano K, Tsukuda K, Takeuchi T, et al: IgA depositions in alcoholic liver disease. An immunoelectron microscopic study. *Am J Clin Pathol* 89:22–28, 1988.

217. Van de Wiel A, Schurman HJ, van Riessen D, et al: Characteristics of IgA deposits in liver and skin of patients with liver disease. *Am J Clin Pathol* 86:724–730, 1986.

218. Williams RC, Gibbons RJ: Inhibition of bacterial adherence by sIgA—a mechanism of antigen disposal. *Science* 177:697–699, 1972.

219. Sohl-Akerlund A, Ahlstedt S, Hanson LA, et al: Antibody responses in urine and serum against *Escherichia coli* O antigen in childhood urinary tract infection. *Acta Pathol Microbiol Scandc* 87:29–36, 1979.

220. Svanborg-Eden C, Svennerholm AM: SIgA and IgG antibodies prevent adhesion of *Escherichia coli* to human urinary tract epithelial cells. *Infect Immun* 22:790–797, 1978.

221. Kilian M, Roland K, Mestecky J: Interference of sIgA with sorption of oral bacteria to hydroxyapetite. *Infect Immun* 31:942–951, 1981.

222. Fubara ES, Freter R: Protection against enteric bacterial infection by secretory IgA antibodies. *J Immunol* 111:395–403, 1973.

223. Boedeker EC, Cheney CP, Cantey JR: Inhibition of enteropathogenic *Escherichia coli* (strain RDEC-1) adherence to rabbit intestinal brush borders by milk immune secretory immunoglobulin A. *Adv Exp Med Biol* 216B:919–930, 1987.

224. McQueen C, Hooven-Lewis C, Dinari G, et al: Mucosal specific IgG production is sustained relative to IgA during an *E. coli* infection as measured by organ culture of rectal biopsies. *Clin Res* 33:411A, 1987.

225. McQueen C, Shoham H, Boedeker E: Intragastric inoculation with an *E. coli* pilus attachment factor (AF/R1) protects against subsequent colonization by an enteropathogen (*E. coli* strain RDEC-1). *Adv Exp Med Biol* 216:911–918, 1987.

226. Magnusson KE, Stendhal O, Stjernstrom I, Edebo L: Reduction of phagocytosis surface hydrophobicity and change of *Salmonella typhimurium* 395 MR10 by reaction with sIgA. *Immunology* 36:439–447, 1979.

227. Magnusson KE, Stjernstrom I: Mucosal barrier mechanisms. Interplay between secre-

tory IgA (sIgA), IgG and mucins on the surface properties and association of *Salmonellae* with intestine and granulocytes. *Immunology* 45:239–248, 1982.

228. van der Waaij D, Heidt PJ: Food and Immunology. Uppsala, Almquist and Wiksell, 1977, p 133.

229. Ogra PL, Karzon DT, Righthand F, et al: Immunoglobulin response in serum and secretions after immunization with live and inactivated polio vaccine and natural infection. *N Engl J Med* 279:893–900, 1968.

230. Svennerholm AM: Nature of protective cholera immunity. In Ouchterlony J, Holmgran J: *Cholera and Related Diarrheas.* Basel, Karger, 1980, p 171.

231. Pierce NF, Cray WC Jr, Sacci JB Jr, et al: Oral immunization against experimental cholera: the role of antigen form and antigen combination in evoking protection. *Ann NY Acad Sci* 409:724–733, 1983.

232. Holmgren J, Svennerholm AM, Clemens J, et al: An oral B sorbent-whole cell murine against cholera: from concept to successful field trial. *Adv Exp Med Biol* 216:1649–1660, 1987.

233. Tamaru T, Brown WR: IgA antibodies in rat bile inhibit cholera toxin-induced secretions in ileal loops in situ. *Immunology* 55:579–583, 1985.

234. Vaerman JP, Derijck-Langendries A, Rits M, et al: Neutralization of cholera toxin by rat bile secretory IgA antibodies. *Immunology* 54:601–603, 1985.

235. Snider DP, Gordon J, McDermott MR, et al: Chronic *Giardia muris* infection in anti-IgM-treated mice. I. Analysis of immunoglobulin and parasite-specific antibody in normal and immunoglobulin-deficient animals. *J Immunol* 134:4153–4162, 1985.

236. Heyworth MF: Antibody response to *Giardia muris* trophozoites in mouse intestine. *Infect Immun* 52:568–571, 1986.

237. Heyworth MF, Carlson JR, Ermak TH: Clearnace of *Giardia muris* infection requires helper/inducer T lymphocytes. *J Exp Med* 165:1743–1748, 1987.

238. Kaplan BS, Uni S, Aikawa M, et al: Effector mechanism of host resistance in murine giardiasis: specific IgG and IgA cell-mediated toxicity. *J Immunol* 134:1975–1981, 1985.

239. Brown WR, Butterfield D, Savage D, et al: Clinical, microbiological and immunological studies in patients with immunoglobulin deficiencies and gastrointestinal disorders. *Gut* 13:441–449, 1972.

240. Brown WR, Kloppel TM: The liver and IgA: immunological, cell biological and clinical implication. *Hepatology,* in press.

241. Ogra PL, Coppola PR, MacGillivray MH, et al: Mechanisms of mucosal immunity to viral infections in IgA deficiency syndromes. *Proc Soc Exp Biol Med* 145:811–816, 1974.

242. Eidelman S, Davis SD: Immunoglobulin content of intestinal mucosal plasma cells in ataxia telangiectasia. *Lancet* 1:884–886, 1968.

243. Crabbe PA, Heremans JF: Lack of IgA in serum of patients with steatorrhea. *Gut* 7:119–127, 1966.

244. Steele EJ, Chaicumpa W, Rowley D: Isolation and biological properties of three classes of rabbit antibody to *Vibrio cholera. J Infect Dis* 130:93–103, 1974.

245. Savilahti E: Immunoglobulin containing cells in the intestinal mucosa and immunoglobulins in the intestinal juice in children. *Clin Exp Immunol* 11:415–25, 1972.

246. Haneberg B: Human fecal agglutinins to rabbit erythrocytes. *Scand J Immunol* 3:71–76, 1974.

247. Walker WA, Isselbacher KJ, Bloch KJ: Intestinal uptake of macromolecules: effect of oral immunization. *Science* 177:608–610, 1972.

248. Newby TJ, Bourne FJ: The nature of the local immune system of the bovine mammary gland. *J Immunol* 118:461–465, 1977.

249. Mach J-P, Pahud J-J: Secretory IgA-a major immunoglobulin in most bovine external secretions. *J Immunol* 106:552–563, 1971.

250. Rowley D: Specific immune antibacterial mechanisms in the intestines of mice. *Am J Clin Nutr* 27:1417–1423, 1974.

251. Tolo K, Brandtzaeg P, Jonsen J: Mucosal penetration of antigen in the presence or absence of serum derived antibody. *Immunology* 33:733–743, 1977.

252. Bloch KJ, Walker WA: Effect of locally induced intestinal anaphylaxis on uptake of a bystanding antigen. *J Allergy Clin Immunol USA* 67:312–316, 1981.

253. Roska AK, Garancis JC, More VL, Abramoff P: Immune complex disease in guinea pig lungs. I. Elicitation by aerosol challenge, suppression with cobra venom factor, and passive transfer with serum. *Clin Immunol Immunopathol* 8:213–224, 1977.

254. Jones GW, Rutter JM: Contribution of the K88 antigen of *Escherichia coli* to enteropathogenicity; protection against disease by neutralizing the adhesive properties of K88 antigen. *Am J Clin Nutr* 27:1441–1449, 1974.

255. Wells PW, Snodgrass DR, Herring JA, Dawson AMcL: Antibody titers to lamb rotavirus in colostrum and milk of vaccinated ewes. *Vet Rec* 103:46–48, 1978.

256. Kobayashi K, Blaser MJ, Brown WR: Identification and partial characterization of an Fcγ binding site in human intestinal epithelium. *Gastroenterology* 94:A231, 1988.

257. Brandtzaeg P: Structure synthesis and external transfer of mucosal immunoglobulins. *Ann Immunol* 124C:417–438, 1973.

258. Brandtzaeg P: Mucosal and glandular distribution of immunoglobulin components. *Immunology* 26:1101–1114, 1974.

259. Ament ME, Ochs HD, Davis SD: Structure and function of the gastrointestinal tract in primary immunodeficiency syndromes: a study of 39 patients. *Medicine* 52:227–248, 1973.

260. Ahnen DJ, Brown WR: *Campylobacter enteritis* in immune-deficient patients. *Ann Intern Med* 96:187, 1982.

261. Hermans PE, Diaz-Buxo JA, Stobo JD: Idiopathic late-onset immunoglobulin deficiency. *Am J Med* 61:221–237, 1976.

262. Heyworth MF, Owen RL: Gastrointestinal aspects of acquired immunodeficiency syndrome. *Surv Dig Dis* 3:197–209, 1985.

263. Patrick MK, Dunn IJ, Buret A, et al: Mast cell protease release and mucosal ultrastructure during intestinal anaphylaxis in the rat. *Gastroenterology* 93:1–9, 1988.

264. Barth EE, Jarrett WF, Urquhart GM: Studies on the mechanism of the self cure reaction in rats infected with *Nippostrongylus brasiliensis*. *Immunology* 10:459–464, 1966.

265. Musoke AJ, Williams J, Leid WR: Immunological response of the rat to infection with *Taenia taeniae formis*. VI. The role of immediate hypersensitivity in resistance to reinfection. *Immunology* 34:565–570, 1978.

266. Briggs NT: Hypersensitivity in murine trichinosis. *Ann NY Acad Sci* 113:456–466, 1963.

267. Rothwell TLW, Prichard RK, Love RJ: Studies on the role of histamine and 5-HT in immunity against the nematode *Trichostrongylus colubriformis*. *Int Arch Allergy Appl Immunol* 46:1–13, 1974.

268. Lake AM, Bloch KJ, Sinclair KJ, Walker WA: Anaphylactic release of intestinal goblet cell mucus. *Immunology* 39:173–178, 1980.

269. Tlaskalova-Hogenova H, Simeckova J, Vetvicka V, et al: Opsonic, cytotoxic, precipitating, blocking of bacterial adherence, and other activities of monoclonal IgE antibody compared with IgA and IgM. *Immunology* 52:427–433, 1984.

270. Ishizaka K, Ishizaka T, Lee EH: Biologic function of the Fc fragments of E myeloma protein. *Immunochemistry* 7:687–702, 1970.

271. Metcalfe DD: Food hypersensitivity. *J Allergy Clin Immunol* 73:749–766, 1984.

272. Belut D, Moneret-Vautrin DA, Nicolas JP, et al: IgE levels in intestinal juice. *Dig Dis Sci* 25:323–331, 1980.

273. Freier S, Lebenthal E, Freier M, et al: IgE and IgD antibodies to cow milk and soy protein in duodenal fluid: effects of pancreozymin and secretin. *Immunology* 4971:69–75, 1983.

274. Shiner M, Ballard J, Smith ME: The small-intestinal mucosa in cow's milk allergy. *Lancet* 1:136–139, 1975.

275. Brandtzaeg P, Gjeruldsen ST, Korsrud F, et al: The human secretory immune system shows striking heterogeneity with regard to involvement of J chain-positive IgD immunocytes. *J Immunol* 122:503–510, 1979.

276. Brandtzaeg P: The secretory immune system of lactating human mammary glands compared with other exocrine organs. *Ann NY Acad Sci* 49:353–382, 1983.

CHAPTER 7

Mucosal Cellular Immunity

CLAUDIO FIOCCHI

INTRODUCTION

The traditional view that humoral immunity is the predominant form of defense mechanism in the gastrointestinal tract can be ascribed to two basic observations. The first is the well-recognized abundance of mature plasma cell in the normal intestinal mucosa. The second is the production of secretory IgA, a unique type of immunoglobulin with the peculiar capacity of performing a highly effective role in local immune defense, without triggering potentially harmful and tissue-damaging effects. This simplistic view is challenged by the fact that the composition of lymphoid tissue in the gastrointestinal tract is not restricted to elements and products of the B-cell system, and that a vast array of other immunocytes are also present, such as T lymphocytes, macrophages, mast cells, and other leukocytes (Fig. 7–1). Obviously, all of them exert their functions locally and therefore must be considered in the global assessment of local defense mechanisms, since mucosal immunity, like any other immune defense system, results from the integration of several diverse cellular types and activities.[1]

The normal human intestinal mucosa is rich in T cells, which are second in number only to plasma cells. While these are located exclusively in the lamina propria, T lymphocytes are distributed more widely, being found not only in the lamina propria but also in the epithelial layer. T cells are detected early in ontogeny.[2,3] Intraepithelial lymphocytes (IEL) are present in the human fetal intestine; they express the CD3 (pan T cell) phenotype and already exhibit a predominance of CD8 positive (suppressor/cytotoxic phenotype) over CD4 positive (helper/inducer phenotype) cells.[3] This peculiar differential distribution persists and becomes even more accentuated in postnatal life. CD3 positive cells are also noticed in the fetal lamina propria clustered in small aggregates. Considering that the intestine is free

E   Epithelium

LP   Lamina propria

SE   Subepithelial space

④   CD4 T cell

⑧   CD8 T cell

     Macrophage

     Dendritic cell

     Mast cell

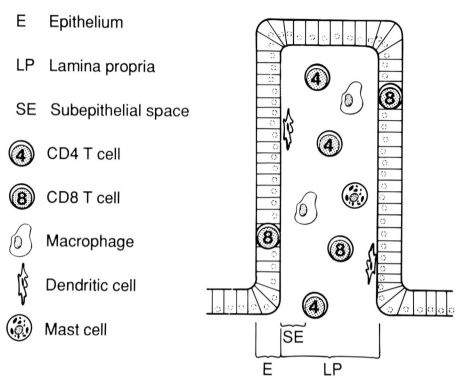

FIGURE 7–1 Schematic representation and spatial distribution of the main cell types mediating cellular immunity in the epithelium and the lamina propria of the villous intestinal mucosa.

of bacterial and dietary products until birth, this early and selective accumulation of T cells is intriguing, suggesting that the distribution of elements mediating cellular immunity follows specific migratory or homing patterns, and is not strictly an antigen-dependent phenomenon. Furthermore, the preferential but broad distribution of gut mucosal T-cell subsets, which persists throughout adult life, strongly indicates that cellular immunity is aimed at a wide range of activities in several different compartments, resulting in interactions with many other immune and nonimmune cells. This is especially true for T cells, which have a central regulatory role even on secretory IgA synthesis by controlling IgA B-cell isotype differentiation,[4] as will be discussed elsewhere in this book. The focus of this chapter will be on mucosal T lymphocytes and classical mechanisms of cell-mediated immunity, such as proliferative responses, immunoregulatory activity, and cytotoxicity. In addition, other cell types and functions that participate directly or indirectly in cell-mediated phenomena will be examined. Finally, how cellular immunity may be implicated in the pathogenesis of human intestinal diseases will be briefly discussed. Human studies will be emphasized, with reference to animal models whenever appropriate.

INTRAEPITHELIAL LYMPHOCYTES

The inclusion of IEL as part of intestinal mucosal cell-mediated immunity is well justified by two fundamental characteristics of this unique population of immuno-cytes. The first is their predominant thymic origin, and the second is their strategic location among the epithelial cells that separate the antigen-rich intestinal lumen from the subepithelial lymphoid tissue of the lamina propria. These observations strongly suggest that IEL play a key role in local immune homeostasis.

IEL are located within the epithelium, usually between villous epithelial cells, and above the basal lamina.[5] In the normal bowel, their number varies according to the segment examined, being progressively less common from the small to the large bowel.[6] Intraepithelial lymphocytes constitute up to 39% of the epithelial cells of the normal human jejunum,[7] whereas in the colon only up to 3%.[8] Although the reason for this difference is not known, it may be related to the quantity and type of antigenic material at different sites along the gastrointestinal tract. Most IEL (up to 60%) are granulated, but the number, size, and content of the cytoplasmatic granules vary considerably among different species.[9] As IEL have been seen cross-ing the basal lamina,[10] they are almost certainly not a static population, but whether they travel to or from the lamina propria, or in both directions is un-known.[11] Recent evidence suggests that IEL are derived from activated lamina propria T cells.[12] Since this discussion is restricted to the role of IEL in cell-mediated immunity, the reader interested in a comprehensive review of these cells is referred to other reports.[5,9,11,13]

The number of IEL is relatively small in the human gut, and methods for isolation and recovery are still unsatisfactory. For these reasons, the present un-derstanding of IEL is based primarily on animal studies, rodents in particular. In addition, there appear to be considerable differences in many morphologic, pheno-typic, and functional aspects of these cells among various species.[9,13] Thus, because many aspects of IEL can not be generalized, it will be useful to consider human and animal studies separately.

Animal Intraepithelial Lymphocytes

Morphologic and Phenotypic Characteristics

In mice approximately 50% of IEL are of thymic origin. Their precursors probably derive from Peyer's patches, where they are activated by local stimuli and then leave, migrating to the mesenteric lymph nodes, thoracic duct, and home back to the intestinal mucosa.[14] The true nature of murine IEL has been a matter of controversy, as some investigators have claimed that IEL represent a "novel type" of T cell that acts as a precursor of mast cells.[15] Unlike typical mast cells, fresh granulated IEL do not contain histamine and lack high-affinity receptors for IgE.[16] When cultured with interleukin-2 (IL-2), granulated IEL develop into cells with enhanced cytotoxicity for YAC-1 and P815 target cells and display T-cell markers (Thy1+, Lyt1, Lyt2+). In contrast, if cultivated in the presence of interleukin-3 (IL-3), the derived cells stain metachromatically, contain large amounts of hista-mine, and express high-affinity receptors for IgE.[17] Thus it appears that mast cell precursors do exist in the epithelium, they are distinct from T lymphocytes, and their development into mature mast cells depends on local factors including soluble products of mucosal T cells.[18]

In view of evidence for considerable heterogeneity within the IEL population, the use of morphologic characteristics alone is certainly not an optimal way to classify and distinguish its various subsets. A multitude of studies reported detailed analyses of surface markers on murine IEL and generally agreed that about one-half of them express pan T-cell markers (Thy1). The majority of Thy1+ IEL also express the Lyt2 (suppressor/cytotoxic, CD8 phenotype) marker. In mice, extensive investigation of the coexpression of Thy1+ and Thy1− cells with additional markers has created a highly complex picture, with several subsets, some fairly well defined in function and number, and others whose function and proportion are yet to be firmly established (Table 7–1). In other species, T cells with a suppressor/cytotoxic phenotype also tend to be predominant among IEL.[19-22]

The use of newer antibodies recognizing unique surface antigens unrelated to T- and non-T-cell lineage recently allowed a novel approach to the phenotypical characterization of IEL. In rats, the monoclonal antibody RGL-1 identifies the majority of lymphocytes in the intestinal lamina propria and the epithelium, but only less than 2% of cells in other lymphoid organs.[23] RGL-1 also recognizes 95% of granular IEL, but less than 0.1% of blood large granular lymphocytes. A similar monoclonal antibody, M290, detects almost exclusively Lyt2+, L3T4+ lymphocytes residing in or immediately adjacent to mice gut epithelium.[24] An additional mean of distinguishing IEL and their subsets may be through assessment of their T-cell receptor (TCR). Recent studies have demonstrated that murine and avian IEL express preferentially the TCR1 phenotype (γ-δ TCR homologue) in association with the CD8 phenotype, as opposed to the vastly more common TCR2 phenotype (α-β TCR homologue), which is found on the majority of cells in the peripheral blood and lymphoid organs in association with the CD4 phenotype.[25,26] The exact significance of these unique antigens and receptors on IEL is not clear, but they probably reflect specific tissue homing patterns and perhaps distinctive physiologic roles.

Functional Characteristics
The most attractive aspect in the study of IEL resides in the investigation of their functional properties, since these may provide clues to their biologic significance in vivo. Most of the attention has been focused on cytotoxic activities. The presence, among IEL, of cell subsets containing granular lymphocytes has stimulated much interest in their potential for mediating spontaneous cytotoxicity, in light of their similarity to large granular lymphocytes (LGL), which are responsible for most of the natural killer (NK) cell activity in the peripheral circulation. Tagliabue and associates demonstrated that murine IEL possess strong NK activity against YAC-1 cells.[27] This function is mediated by a subset of granular lymphocytes that

Table 7–1 SURFACE PHENOTYPE AND FUNCTIONAL ACTIVITY OF MURINE INTRAEPITHELIAL LYMPHOCYTES

Phenotype	Function	Proportion (%)
Thy1+ (Lyt1+,Lyt2+?)	CTL	30–40
Thy1+,Lyt1+,Lyt2+	CTL precursor	
Thy1+,Lyt1−,Lyt2−AsGm1−,NK1−	NK	<10
Thy1−	Splenic NK suppressor	?
?	NC	?
Thy1−,Lyt2−	Mast cell precursor NK	<10
Thy1−,Lyt1−,Lyt2+,Lyt3−	?	40–50

CTL, cytotoxic T lymphocyte; NK, natural killer cell; NC, natural cytotoxic cell. [Adapted from Ernst et al. (9), with permission.]

display a Thy1.2+, Lyt1.1−, Lyt2.1− phenotype, different from that of splenic NK cells.[28] Additional studies have confirmed that clear differences exist between epithelial LGL and morphologically similar cells from other compartments.[29] Actually, in the whole population of murine IEL, the proportion displaying spontaneous cytotoxicity is relatively small, not exceding 15% of all cells.[9] Some of them may even be restricted to specific types of cytotoxic functions, as demonstrated by the existence of a unique IEL subset (asialo-GM1+, Thy1−, Lyt1−, Lyt2−) effective against enteric murine coronavirus.[30] Natural killer cell activity mediated by IEL has also been reported in rats, guinea pigs, and chickens.[31−33]

T cells that specifically recognize and are cytolytic for allogenic tumor cells to which animals have been sensitized can be found in the gut epithelium of mice,[34] indicating the presence of classical cytotoxic T lymphocytes (CTL) and CTL precursors.[35] During the process of generating antigen-specific CTL, activation of additional nonspecific spontaneous cytotoxic cells can occur.[36] Mitogen-induced cytotoxicity, another nonspecific killer function also mediated by T cells, has been reported using guinea pigs IEL.[32] Additional cytolytic functions of murine IEL include natural cytotoxicity against tumor targets,[37] spontaneous antibacterial activity,[38] and antibody-dependent cellular cytotoxicity, which can be mediated by secretory IgA against bacteria.[39]

Limited information is available on other, noncytotoxic functions of murine IEL, but they are probably no less important, and some are likely to be directly involved in local cell-mediated immunity. IEL can exert an NK suppressor function,[40] modulate expression of Ia on intestinal epithelial cells,[41] and participate in the inflammatory response leading to development of crypt cell hyperplasia during small intestinal graft-versus-host disease (GVHD).[42]

Human Intraepithelial Lymphocytes

Morphologic and Phenotypic Characteristics

Like their murine counterparts, human IEL are also of thymic origin, containing and an even higher proportion of cells displaying mature T-cell markers. Early studies utilizing relatively crude anti-T-cell antisera recognized the predominantly T-cell nature of IEL in fixed sections of human small and large bowel.[43,44] These findings were followed by a series of investigations using immunofluorescence or immunoperoxidase techniques and highly specific monoclonal antibodies able to recognize cell surface antigens associated with various types of lymphocytes. Selby and collaborators were the first to report that over 95% of stomach and proximal small bowel IEL were T lymphocytes (Hle-1+, HuTLA+), whereas in the colon their proportion varied between 85% and 95%. In neither location did IEL express Ia-like (HLA-DR) antigens [class II antigens of the major histocompatibility complex (MHC)] and surface or cytoplasmatic immunoglobulin.[45] The same group of investigators also reported that the majority (67–90%) of intraepithelial T cells (HuTLA+) reacted with the OKT8 monoclonal antibody, indicating that they belonged to the suppressor/cytotoxic (CD8) subset. Interestingly, the lamina propria contained a substantially lower proportion of OKT8+ cells (27–56%).[46] The different distribution of T-cell subsets between the intraepithelial and lamina propria compartments in normal adult human intestinal mucosa was confirmed by showing that only 16% of intraepithelial T cells were OKT4+ (CD4 phenotype), as opposed to 69% of lamina propria T cells. Intraepithelial lymphocytes failed to express the Tac (anti-IL-2 receptor) activation antigen and C3b receptor (C3RTO5−).[47,48] It was also observed that most OKT8+ IEL were negative for Leu1, an antigen expressed on most peripheral blood T cells, suggesting the existence of different subsets of CD8 cells within the intestinal mucosa.[47] As noted in rodents, some human IEL have cytoplasmic granules and ultrastructural features comparable to those of peripheral blood LGL. However, in spite of these similarities, small bowel IEL are not stained by the Leu7 (anti-HNK-1) or Leu11 (anti-CD16) monoclonal antibodies, which recognize essentially all LGL responsible for the bulk of NK activity in the circulation.[49,50] Intraepithelial lymphocytes are also not stained by the H366 monoclonal antibody, which identifies the subset of cytotoxic T cells within the CD8 population.[51] Most of the above immunohistochemical studies have been confirmed by immunoelectronmicroscopy.[52]

The strategic location of IEL strongly suggests that these cells may be actively involved in local antigen processing. Therefore, it would be expected that most of them exhibit some evidence of cell activation. Surprisingly, this is not the case, at least as detected by the lack of sporadic expression of HLA-DR antigens, Tac antigen, T9 antigen (transferrin receptor found on dividing cells), or recognition by OKT10 (for "activated" lymphocytes) and Ki67 (for proliferating nuclei) monoclonal antibodies.[50,51,53] Only a small proportion (11%) of normal jejunal IEL express the T2 "T blast" antigen (CD7), and most of them are CD8 cells.[50]

As previously mentioned, the differential distribution of CD4 and CD8 cells between IEL and lamina propria mononuclear cells (LMPC) occurs in intrauterine life.[3] However, other factors, such as anatomic location and antigenic exposure, probably contribute to the final distribution of T-cell subsets in adult life. For instance, the T-cell population is quite different in the epithelium covering Peyer's patches as opposed to that of the villous epithelium. In the follicle-associated epithelium the number of IEL is significantly higher, and 40% of them are CD4 cells, in marked contrast to 6% detected in distant sites.[54] In the colon the number of IEL is 50–80% lower than in the jejunum, and the ratio of CD4 to CD8 cells can be much higher than in the small bowel.[51] The exact reason for these differences is not apparent, but they are likely to reflect a functional adaptation of IEL to various microenvironments.

The search for more specific characteristics for human IEL has led to isolation of a novel membrane molecule on these cells.[55] The same group of investigators that described a monoclonal antibody (RGL-1) directed to rat IEL[23] has recently reported the development of a comparable antibody (HML-1) for human IEL. In tissues and isolated cells, HML-1 stains all subsets of IEL, including >99% of granular IEL, 40% of lamina propria T cells, and 30% of mesenteric lymphoblasts, but only rare cells in other lymphoid compartments. Because of these results and association with RGL-1, it appears the HML-1 may define a differentiation antigen expressed on mucosa-associated T cells. The functional properties of this antigen remain undefined, but they may be involved in traffic and homing of cells, or local immune defense mechanisms.[56] As far as the type of T-cell receptor on human IEL goes, a few preliminary experiments indicate that most cells exhibit the α-β homologue (TCR1), and not the rare γ-δ homologue (TCR2) found in murine IEL.[55]

Functional Characteristics

In comparison with the detailed data on morphologic and phenotypic characteristics of human IEL, studies of their function have been extremely few. Nevertheless, the limited amount of reported data tends to indicate that they possess unusual functional properties. Intraepithelial lymphocytes have a low rate of spontaneous proliferation and do not respond to the lectins phytohemagglutinin, concanavalin A, and pokeweed mitogen, even after addition of autologous macrophages or IL-2.[57,58] They are capable, however, of modulating immunoglobulin production by peripheral blood and autologous LPMC.[57,59] In spite of their morphologic resemblance to peripheral blood LGL, isolated human IEL do not mediate NK activity, as shown by their failure to kill K562 target cells, alone or after stimulation with interferon (IFN)-α, phytohemagglutinin, or using indomethacin or cimetidine during their isolation.[58] The intriguingly low proliferative capacity of human IEL was explored by Ebert and collaborators.[60] These investigators showed that the low proliferative response was partially due to the predominance of CD8 cells among IEL, and that stimulation actually occurred in the absence of proliferation, as detected by production of IL-2. The most interesting finding was that IEL could be triggered to proliferate to a high level by the addition of sheep red blood cells, suggesting that these cells may be activated by alternate pathways.

What can we conclude, from presently available information, about the role of IEL in the mucosal immune system? It is well known that the number of IEL increases significantly in a number of diseases, such as gluten-sensitive enteropathy, tropical sprue, dermatitis herpetiformis with bowel involvement, giardiasis, cow's milk protein intolerance, and microscopic and collagenous colitis,[61–66] but usually not in Crohn's disease, ulcerative colitis, and Whipple's disease.[13] We do not know, however, what these changes, or lack of them, really reflect. Considering their predominant CD8, Leu7−, Leu11−, H366− phenotype associated with a lack of spontaneous or inducible cytotoxic activity, ability to modulate immunoglobulin synthesis, and low proliferative capacity, these characteristics taken together suggest that human IEL represent long-lived immunoregulatory cells, possibly suppressing response to antigens passing through the villous epithelium. The selective decrease in the number of CD8 cells, with a concomitant increase of CD4 cells only in epithelia covering areas actively involved in antigen absorption and processing, such as Peyer's patches,[54] is in agreement with the above hypothesis. To confirm this, IEL must become available in much greater numbers, perhaps through cloning techniques, to permit pursuing additional studies of their immunomodulatory capacity.

LAMINA PROPRIA MONONUCLEAR CELLS

The bulk of lymphoid tissue within the wall of the human gastrointestinal tract is found within the lamina propria. The local immunocyte population probably varies in number and composition depending on the quantity and quality of the lumenal content, but generally decreases from the small toward the large bowel.[67] This population is much more heterogeneous than that present in the epithelium, being composed of mature plasma cells, T cells, various cells of the monocytic-macrophage lineage, mast cells, and other less frequent elements such as eosinophils, basophils, and neutrophils. These quantitative and qualitative differences between IEL and LPMC suggest that both compartments have different, although probably integrated roles in local cell-mediated immune responses. In fact, LPMC cover a substantially wider and more complex range of activities than IEL. To properly address all relevant aspects, the various cellular components of the lamina propria will be discussed separately, with emphasis on T cell-mediated functions. Aspects dealing with humoral immunity have been discussed in the preceding chapter.

Morphologic and Phenotypic Characteristics

In Situ Cells

Information on the types of cells present in immunohistochemically stained tissue sections of the intestinal lamina propria was accrued in parallel with the study of IEL. While observing that IEL were almost exclusively T cells, the presence of large numbers of T cells was also noted within the lamina propria.[43,44] It became apparent that the distribution of T-cell subsets was different between the two compartments, as the proportion of CD8 cells was smaller (39%) in the lamina propria than in the epithelium (70%) of both the small and large bowel.[46] About one-fourth to one-third of all lamina propria cells are CD3, CD2 lymphocytes, as shown by staining with the anti-T3, anti-Leu1, and anti-T11 monoclonal antibodies.[49,68] CD4 (OKT4+, Leu3+, T4+) lymphocytes are the predominant subset, their proportion varying from 68% to 71%, whereas CD8 (OKT8+, Leu2+, T8+) lymphocytes constitute 28–32% of all T cells.[47,48,68] There is some indication that T cells are more common in the small bowel than in the colon,[6] and that the ratio of CD4 to CD8 cells changes according to the segment of the digestive tract, averaging 3:2 in the jejunal and 5:2 in the colonic mucosa.[51] In addition, cells expressing helper/inducer or suppressor/cytotoxic phenotypes in the absence of the CD3 phenotype have been reported among LPMC.[49]

Antibodies that stain NK cells, such as Leu7 (anti-HNK-1), Leu11 (anti-CD16), Leu19 (anti-NKH-1), NKTa, and NKTb, identify no or very few (up to 1.8%) cells within the lamina propria.[6,47,49,68,69] Similarly to IEL, there is limited evidence for in situ activation of LPMC, as few of these are recognized by the Tac, IL-2R1, I2 (anti-HLA-DR), T10, T2, 4F2, T9, Ki67, and Ta1-RD1 antibodies.[6,46–51,53,68,69] In agreement with this observation, only rare lymphoblasts positive for [³H]thymidine are shown by autoradiography.[70] Approximately 40% of lamina propria T cells bear a mucosa-associated antigen identified by the HML-1 antibody.[55]

Isolated Cells

More information on the types of mucosal T and other immune cells in humans has been obtained through the study of purified preparation of isolated LPMC. This has provided important complementary data, which allow a more detailed evaluation of phenotypically defined T-cell subsets and their functional properties. When compared with peripheral blood mononuclear cells, mucosal cells obtained by mechanical or enzymatic techniques are usually fairly heterogenous in size and nucleocytoplasmatic ratio, the majority being composed of small mature lymphocytes with few blast cells.[71–74] Molecular genetic analysis of immunoglobulin and T-cell antigen receptors shows that LPMC have a polyclonal nature.[75] Several studies investigated the relative frequency of lymphoid cell subsets in LPMC isolates, based on morphology, sheep red blood cell rosetting, IgG-coated sheep erythrocyte rosetting, surface immunoglobulin, staining for nonspecific esterase, and identification by monoclonal antibodies.[8,69,71–74,76–81] Based on these criteria, T cells represent 50–60% of LPMC, B cells 20–25%, Fc receptor-bearing cells and NK less than 5%, and macrophages about 10%, in addition to a variable proportion (0–27%) of "null" cells depending on the methods used to define each cell subset.[82]

Phenotypic studies of murine LPMC have been limited. In one report, approximately 25% were Thy1+, 12% Lyt1+, 15% Lyt2+, and 40% expressed surface immunoglobulin.[40]

Detailed analyses of intestinal mucosal T-cell subsets using double-label flow cytometry have been reported by James and coworkers. In humans, these investigators found that, when compared with peripheral blood mononuclear cells, T lymphocytes contained a significantly higher percentage of Leu3+,Leu8− and Leu3+,2H4− cells (helper-inducer phenotype), and a corresponding decrease in Leu3+,Leu8+ and Leu3+,2H4+ cells (suppressor-inducer phenotype). In addition, they contained fewer Leu2+,Leu15+ cells (suppressor-effector pheontype), but similar proportions of Leu1+,9.3+ cells (cytotoxic phenotype).[83] Similar findings were observed in nonhuman primates, except that percentages of Leu2+,Leu15+ and Leu1+,9.3+ cells were approximately equal to those found in the blood and spleen.[84] As an extension of these observations, Kanof and coworkers investigated the expression of the Leu8 antigens on lamina propria CD4 T cells.[85] This antigen subdivides helper cells into two distinct subsets with strong (CD4,Leu8−) and weak (CD4,Leu8+) capacity to provide help for immunoglobulin synthesis. These investigators found that while the majority (64%) of peripheral blood CD4 cells coexpressed Leu8, only a small number (9.5%) of mucosal CD4 did so, both in isolated cells and tissue sections. Thus it appars that helper/inducer and cytolytic cells constitute the bulk of T cells within the intestinal lamina propria. This phenotypic expression has a matching functional counterpart, as will be discussed in the following sections.

Some evidence of cellular activation is found among isolated LPMC, as demonstrated by the formation of stable E-rosette by T cells.[76,78] However, considering the extremely rich antigenic and mitogenic milieu surrounding these cells in vivo, the expression of early activation markers is relatively infrequent, in agreement with the in situ immunohistochemical studies. Freshly isolated, unstimulated LPMC expressing the Tac antigen are 1–5%, while the T9 and 4F2 antibodies recognize about 5% and 13% of LPMC, respectively.[69,86] A different situation may exist in other animals, as LPMC from nonhuman primates have a significantly increased proportion of IL-2R+ (CD25) and HLA-DR+ T cells compared with peripheral blood, mesenteric lymph nodes, and spleen.[87]

Functional Characteristics

State of Activation and Proliferative Activity

According to several studies discussed in the preceding section, LPMC represent an "activated" population, as shown by some morphologic and phenotypic characteristics displayed by in situ and isolated cells. In agreement with this observation, the functional assessment in vitro also reflects an enhanced state of activation. The rate of spontaneous proliferation of LPMC, measured by uptake of [³H]thymidine, is substantially higher than that of peripheral blood mononuclear cells,[71,78,88,89] except in one study that employed a mechanical method for cell isolation.[72] The number of T cells forming stable E-rosettes (at 37°C) increases with time in culture.[78] The examination of the proliferative response of LPMC to the lectin mitogens phytohemagglutinin, concanavalin A, and pokeweed mitogen has given variable results. Some studies found that LPMC respond somewhat less than peripheral blood cells,[71,76,88] whereas one study found generally comparable responses.[78] Depending on the part of the intestinal mucosa (small or large bowel) from which LPMC are extracted, noticeable differences can be observed in the degree of proliferation to the same mitogens.[78] As far as the kinetics of the proliferative response go, this is generally comparable to that of peripheral lymphocytes, including the appearance of cells displaying early activation markers recognized by the 4F2, T9, and anti-Tac monoclonal antibodies.[78,86]

LPMC also proliferate when exposed to bacterial antigens, including several bacteroides, *Staphylococcus aureus,* lipolysaccharide from two different *Escherichia coli,* enterobacterial common antigen, and cell-wall-defective *Pseudomonas-*like bacteria, but not lipid A.[78,90] However, in a recent study of an infectious model of lymphogranuloma venereum proctitis in monkeys, LPMC from involved and uninvolved bowel did not proliferate in response to antigen-specific stimulation in vitro, in contrast to the vigorous response of lymphocytes from peripheral circulation, draining lymph nodes, and spleen.[91] Whether or not this phenomenon occurs in humans is not known. Lamina propria mononuclear cells are able to recognize and proliferate in response to alloantigens, functioning as both inducers and responders in a mixed lymphocyte culture.[73,92]

Recent studies of the proliferative response of LPMC to IL-2 and the accompanying intracellular events and products have been of great help in the understanding of the state of activation of LPMC. After incubation with IL-2, human LPMC show a strong proliferative activity, with a remarkable increase (from 3.7% to 63.6%) in the number of Tac+ cells and less of HLA-DR+ cells.[69] The same phenomenon is observed with LPMC from nonhuman primates, which respond to IL-2 more vigorously than cells from any other lymphoid organ.[87] As demonstrated by Northern blotting with a specific cDNA probe, these monkeys' fresh LPMC contain mRNA for the IL-2 receptor, in contrast to mononuclear cells from peripheral blood and mesenteric lymph nodes, which only show detectable levels of IL-2R mRNA after culture with concanavalin A. None of the unstimulated cell populations produce IL-2, but after mitogen-induced activation LPMC produce significantly more IL-2 than cells from the blood, and express mRNA for IL-2, while circulating lymphocytes do not.

Recently, some reports have shown that interleukin-4 [IL-4, B-cell growth factor (BCGF)] has the capacity to stimulate LPMC in both humans and monkeys.[93,94] Preliminary experiments in our laboratory show that, as compared with IL-2, human recombinant IL-4 is a weak inducer of proliferation from freshly isolated LPMC. However, when these are incubated in vitro with phytohemagglutinin or IL-2, IL-4 induces a vigorous, dose-dependent proliferative response.[94] Thus it appears that LPMC have the capacity to respond to IL-4, but this depends on their state of activation.

Immunoregulatory Function

Preliminary evidence that human LPMC exert immunomodulatory activity was provided by studies showing generation of potent suppressor cells by mitogen stimulation. After incubation with either concanavalin A or phytohemagglutinin, LPMC significantly suppress mitogen- and alloantigen-induced proliferative responses of peripheral blood cells.[78,95,96] This suppressor function may have some specificity, as LPMC inhibit the response of mucosal lymphocytes to a significantly greater degree than that of peripheral blood cells.[97] In addition to inhibiting proliferation, LPMC also have the capacity to regulate immunoglobulin secretion by both intestinal mucosal and circulating B cells.[98-100] Using purified populations of mucosal T cells derived from normal and inflamed gut, and pokeweed mitogen-stimulated peripheral blood B cells in mixing experiments, lamina propria and peripheral blood T cells show comparable helper T cell function.[99,100] In one study this helper activity of LPMC was not isotype-restricted, being comparable for synthesis of IgM, IgA, and IgG,[100] while in another study IgA and IgM, but not IgG secretion was enhanced.[59] In regard to suppressor cell function, unstimulated intestinal T cells do not significantly suppress immunoglobulin synthesis. CD8-enriched LPMC display marginal suppression, while mucosal T cells do exhibit significant suppression after stimulation with concanavalin A. Thus it can be concluded that helper T-cell activity predominates in the human intestinal mucosa under normal and inflammatory conditions.[99,100] A parallel situation is found in the mucosa of nonhuman primates, also under physiologic and pathologic situations.[84,101] In these animals, the helper function of lamina propria T cells can be enhanced by IL-2.[102] In addition, antigen-specific helper activity of mucosal T cells for polyclonal immunoglobulin synthesis can be demonstrated in the absence of a proliferative response after in vitro stimulation by a specific antigen *(Chlamidia trachomatis).*[91]

Two recent studies have carefully assessed the immunoregulatory activity of the CD4 and CD8 subsets in human intestinal mucosa.[85,103] Based on the observation that lamina propria CD4 cells have a decreased expression of the Leu8 antigen compared with peripheral CD4 cells, differences in the regulation of immunoglobulin synthesis could be anticipated between these two compartments. In fact, the helper function of intestinal CD4 T cells is significantly stronger than that of peripheral blood cells: after incubation with anti-Leu8 antibody, peripheral CD4 T cells display suppressor function, while their intestinal counterparts do not.[85] No differences are observed in the helper function of CD4,Leu8− T cells and the suppressor function of CD4,Leu8+ T cells from both the intestine and the blood. Therefore it was concluded that the detected difference in helper function between gut and circulating CD4 T cels is due to quantitative differences of CD4,Leu8+ cells. In a second study, the same system of pokeweed mitogen-stimulated immunoglobulin secretion as the target of immunoregulatory activity was used, but CD8 T cells were evaluated as mediators of regulation.[103] Depending on the experimental conditions, lamina propria CD8 T cells exhibit either suppressor or helper activity. A dissociation between peripheral blood and mucosal CD8 cell suppressor function can be revealed by adding CD4 cells — lamina propria CD8 cells augment, while peripheral blood CD8 cells suppress immunoglobulin synthesis. The authors concluded that mucosal CD8 cells have a spectrum of immunomodulatory activity, with CD4 cells representing the target of CD8 cell activity.

In summary, regulatory cells and related events occuring in the intestinal lamina propria are complex and certainly deserve further investigation. However, from the presently available information, it is apparent that LPMC are constituted predominantly of T cells in a state of continuous activation, resulting in a shift of their predominant function toward a preferential helper activity mediated by CD4 cells.[104]

Cytokine Production
Cytokines are nonantibody-soluble products of immunologically activated cells, including lymphocytes (lymphokines) and macrophages (monokines). They act at

all levels of the immune response, and there is evidence to demonstrate that they play an important role also in mucosal immunity, under both physiologic and pathologic conditions.[105] Despite their enhanced state of activation, cultured LPMC do not spontaneously produce IL-2.[89] However, after stimulation with phorbol myristate acetate, phytohemagglutinin, concanavalin A, anti-CD3 monoclonal antibody, or combinations of these, substantial levels of IL-2 activity are detected in the culture supernatants.[87,89,106] Two observations are particularly relevant in regard to the response pattern observed in the above experimental systems. First, unlike peripheral blood lymphocytes, LPMC produce IL-2 after culture with phorbol myristate acetate alone,[89] and second, after mitogen stimulation, LPMC produce more IL-2 than lymphocytes from other lymphoid organs, providing additional evidence for preactivation of lamina propria cells.[87] CD4 T cells are responsible for most of the produced IL-2, whereas CD8 T cells contribute much less (unpublished observations). IL-2 produced in the intestinal mucosa probably regulates various immune functions, such as helper activity[102] and cytotoxicity.[106]

Intestinal LPMC exhibit several other cytokine activities. As observed with IL-2, LPMC do not spontaneously produce IFN-γ, but do so after stimulation by IL-2 or phytohemagglutinin.[107] This LPMC-derived endogenous IFN-γ can modulate HLA-DR expression.[108] IL-1 bioactivity is detected in fresh and cultured intestinal tissues as well as in their culture supernatants.[109,110] Essentially all intestinal mucosal IL-1 production derives from LPMC, which contain intracellular IL-1 and release it into the culture medium (unpublished observations). Finally, initial evidence has been reported for the spontaneous and mitogen-stimulated production of colony stimulating factors by LPMC.[111]

Intense research efforts are required to fully understand the exact role of these various cytokines in the regulatory and effector functions of intestinal immunity. However, it should be noted that the biological impact of these soluble mediators is probably not restricted to immune cells. Recent reports have demonstrated that recombinant IFN-γ and tumor necrosis factor-α (TNF-α) have the capacity to enhance the in vitro expression of secretory component by epithelial cell lines.[112,113] If similar phenomena occur in vivo, the role of mucosal cytokines will include not only cell-mediated immune events but also crucial lymphoepithelial interactions.[114]

Cytotoxic Activity

Among the various immune functions of human LPMC, none has received more attention than the investigation of their cytotoxic potential. This probably reflects an intense interest in searching for mechanisms that mediate cell death and can ultimately lead to the tissue damage encountered in some gastrointestinal diseases.[115] Several different cytotoxic systems exist, and essentially all have been investigated using intestinal mucosal cells (Table 7–2). For the sake of clarity, each will be discussed separately.

Antibody-Dependent Cellular Cytotoxicity

Antibody-dependent cellular cytotoxicity (ADCC) is mediated by a cell bearing an Fc receptor for IgG that binds to an antigen on the surface of the target cell. Reports on the existence of ADCC in the intestinal mucosa have been variable, in part because of methodologic differences in the extraction of intestinal LPMC,[74,116] but more likely because of the selection of target cells. Absent or insignificant ADCC

Table 7–2 CYTOTOXIC ACTIVITY OF ISOLATED HUMAN INTESTINAL LAMINA PROPRIA MONONUCLEAR CELLS

Type	Target	Effector cell	Level of activity	Reference
Antibody-dependent		LPMC	Insignificant	79
	PG33	LPMC	Insignificant	116, 118
	Chang	LPMC	Insignificant	117
	LPS-coated Chang	LPMC	Low-moderate	73, 88, 118,
	Chicken RBC	IEL + LPMC	Moderate	119
	Sheep RBC			120
Mitogen-induced	Chang	LPMC	Moderate-strong	88, 116
	P185	LPMC	Moderate-strong	121
	Chicken RBC	LPMC	Moderate-strong	116
	Human RBC	LPMC	Moderate-strong	118
	RPMI-4788	LPMC	Moderate-strong	122
Cell-mediated lympholysis	Alloantigens	LPMC	Absent	92
Natural killer	Chang	LPMC	Insignificant	88, 116, 118
	K562	LPMC	Insignificant	68, 88, 118, 121
	K562	LPMC	Moderate	80, 124
	K562	NKH1+	Strong	131
	K562	Single cell	Moderate	130
	MOLT4	Single cell	Moderate	130
	Raji	Single cells	Absent	130
	RPMI-4788	LPMC	Moderate-strong	128
	KATO III	IEL + LPMC	Strong	120
Induced IL-2	K562	LPMC	Strong	68,69,106
	K562	CD2+,CD3−, Leu7−,CD16−	Strong	123
	K562	CD2+,CD3−, CD8+,CD4−, CD16−,Leu19−	Strong	131
	Daudi	LPMC	Moderate	68, 69, 106
	MOLT 4	LPMC	Moderate	133
	HL60	LPMC	Moderate	133
	HT-29	LPMC	Moderate	133
	U937	LPMC	Moderate	133
	RPMI-SE	LPMC	Moderate	133
IFN-γ	K562	LPMC	Absent	68
IFN-α, β	K562	LPMC	Low-moderate	122, 123, 124

Table 7 – 2 *(continued)*

Type	Target	Effector cell	Level of activity	Reference
Anti-CD3	K562	CD2+,CD3+, CD8+CD4−, CD16−,Leu7−	Moderate-strong	137
Against intestinal targets	Fresh colonocytes	Single cell	Moderate	130
	Fresh colonocytes	LPMC	Moderate	136
	Fresh colonocytes	LPMC	Absent	134
	Fresh colon cancer	LPMC	Absent	133
	Gut fibroblasts	LPMC	Moderate	133
	ECAC	CD2+,CD3+, CD16−	Moderate	81

LPMC, lamina propria mononuclear cells; IEL, intraepithelial lymphocytes; RBC, red blood cells; IL-2, interleukin2; IFN, interferon; ECAC, epithelial cell-associated components.

has been found against lymphoblastoid, Chang, and lipolysaccharide-coated Chang cells,[79,116,117] whereas chicken red blood cells usually exhibit moderate-to-strong susceptibility to lamina propria effector cells.[73,88,118,119] Moderately low levels of ADCC for sheep erythrocytes have been observed in the only study reporting the use of a mixture of IEL and LPMC extracted from the gastric mucosa.[120]

Mitogen-Induced Cytotoxicity
Mitogen-induced cellular cytotoxicity (MICC) has been invariably found to be mediated by LPMC, after incubating these cells with lectins such as phytohemagglutinin or wheat germ agglutinin. High levels of killing are obtained against Chang and P815 cells as well as human and chicken erythrocytes.[88,116,118,121] Additionally, concanavalin A and pokeweed mitogen can enhance the level of cytotoxicity against the human colon cancer cell line RPMI-4788 well above background killing.[122]

Cell-Mediated Lympholysis
Killing of allogeneic targets after in vitro sensitization, as in cell-mediated lympholysis (CML), apparently is not mediated by LPMC, even though an appropriate proliferative response is measurable after reexposure to the foreign antigen.[92] Lack of effector cells or inhibition of their activity could be responsible for this unique finding.

Natural Killer Cell Activity
Spontaneous cell-mediated cytotoxicity (SCMC) (or NK activity) by LPMC has been the most widely investigated. Initially, there has been substantial controversy over whether or not the intestinal lamina propria contain NK cells, mostly due to considerable methodologic differences in the selection of effector cells, time of incubation (4, 18, or 24 hours ^{51}Cr release assays), and choice of target cells. Several investigators found insignificant or low level killing of K562 or Chang cells.[68,88,116,118,121,123] Some authors attributed the poor NK activity of LPMC to the

paucity of Leu7+ cells among them, and obtained moderate cytotoxicity against K562 by increasing the effector to target ratios to match the level of Leu7+ cells to that of the peripheral blood.[80,124] Other possible causes implicated in the low NK function were ascribed to inhibitory substances released during the ezymatic isolation process,[125,126] and the preferential compartmentalization of NK cells in the vascular bed as opposed to the mesenteric lymph nodes and gut mucosa.[127] However, the same intestinal LPMC that fail to kill K562 cells are effective in destroying the RPMI-4788 colon cancer cell line,[128] and unseparated mononuclear cells from human gastric mucosa are cytotoxic for the KATO-III stomach cancer cell line.[120] These two reports suggest that gut NK cells may be quite selective in their lytic capacity. Gut NK activity may also vary among species, as nonhuman primates consistently exhibit CD16-mediated spontaneous cytotoxicity, although at levels lower than those observed in the peripheral blood.[129] This NK activity persists unchanged under gut inflammatory conditions.[101]

Other approaches toward demonstrating NK activity by LPMC have included enrichment of NK by depletion of adherent cells, density gradients, or the use of indomethacin during the microcytotoxicity assay, but they all failed to enhance killing above baseline.[68,123] Using an alternate method that consists of a single cell assay in agar, spontaneous killing of MOLT4 but not Raji cells was demonstrable.[130] However, definitive evidence that intestinal LPMC can mediate NK activity was provided by Shanahan and coworkers.[131] These investigators showed that intestinal mucosal cells that do not kill K562 cells in a 4 hour assay become strongly cytolytic against the same targets after enrichment for NKH1+ cells, which constitute only 2–3% of the unseparated LPMC. Unlike their peripheral blood counterparts, mucosal NKH1+ cells were Leu11−.

Induced Cytotoxicity
In view of the relatively weak cytotoxic potential of human LPMC, several investigators have attemped to boost their activity using a variety of inducers. The most widely utilized has been IL-2, which invariably induces lymphokine-activated killer (LAK) cells from gut lamina propria cells. Such intestinal LAK cells show a broad spectrum of cytotoxicity against different types of targets, including the K562 (myelogenous leukemia), Daudi (Burkitt lymphoma), MOLT4 (T-cell leukemia), HL60 (promyelocytic leukemia), U937 (hysticocytic lymphoma), RPMI-SE (renal cell carcinoma), and HT-29 (colon cancer) cell lines, autologous blasted LPMC, hapten-modified autologous LPMC, and normal intestinal fibroblasts.[68,69,106,123,132–134] LAK cells can be induced from both human and monkey LPMC.[129] Defined phenotypes have been attributed to intestinal precursor/effector LAK cells, such as CD2+,CD3−,Leu7−,CD16−[123] and CD2+,CD3−,CD4−,CD8+,CD16,Leu19−.[131] Nevertheless, it is likely that they actually represent a heterogeneous population, since various subsets with different phenotypes can mediate IL-2-induced cytotoxcity.[69] Interferon has also been used to augment LPMC cytotoxic activity using different types and amounts of this lymphokine. Results have been variable, ranging from no effect with low doses of IFN-γ,[68] to a minimal or moderate increase with high doses of IFN-α or -β[122–124,132] IL-1 does not enhance LPMC cytotoxic activity, either alone or in combination with IL-2.[135] In contrast, preliminary experiments in our laboratory indicate that IL-4 can upgrade or downgrade the cytotoxicity of LPMC, and this modulatory action varies with the state of cell activation.[94]

Cytotoxicity Against Gut-Related Targets
Most of the forms of cytotoxicity discussed in the preceding sections provide information reflecting the overall ability of intestinal mucosal mononuclear cells to mediate nonspecific lytic phenomena. However, if these cells have a role in immune-mediated destruction of the gut associated with clinical manifestations, they must be able to destroy relevant tissues, i.e., cells of intestinal origin. Limited evidence exists to support the latter hypothesis. In additon to the ability to kill some long-term transformed gastrointestinal cell lines of gastrointestinal origin, there are few studies showing that LPMC can spontaneously kill fresh autologous human colonic epithelial cells in vitro.[129,136] These reports contrast with others denying that the same type of effector cells can destroy autologous or allogeneic fresh colonocytes or colon cancer cells, even after activation with high doses of IL-2.[133,134] Cytotoxicity against defined intestinal epithelial antigens [epithelial cell-associated components (ECAC)] has also been demonstrated in vitro using LPMC from inflammatory bowel disease, but not normal gut.[81] The effector cell in this system is not MHC-restricted and bears the CD2+,CD3+,CD16− phenotype. This is quite intriguing, as recent evidence shows that human intestinal mucosal mononuclear cells are excellent mediators of anti-CD3 T-cell cytotoxicity, which is mediated by CD2+,CD3+,CD8+,CD4−,CD16−,Leu7− cells.[123,131,137] This killer function is triggered by antibodies to the CD3 component of T cells, is non-major histocompatibility complex-restricted, and is believed to reflect in vivo primed CTL function. Thus the intestine may be an immunologic compartment enriched for such cytolytic T cells, which may become nonspecifically activated by stimuli from the mucosal microenvironment and perhaps mediate local tissue damage in certain pathologic situations.[137]

In summary, the various types of cytotoxic cells and mechanisms that may be operative in the gut are different and generally weaker than comparable elements present in the peripheral circulation. However, intestinal immunocytes can be induced to exhibit vigorous cytotoxic function after appropriate stimulation. It cannot be excluded that both the relative quiescence of killer activity and the need for inducers represent local mechanisms of mucosal homeostasis, perhaps aimed at preventing an excessive immune reactivity. There is still no definitive proof that immunologically mediated cytotoxicity is responsible for triggering or sustaining pathologic events in the gut, but data accumulated so far support this possibility. Of the several systems that might be involved, NK activity is the least likely to be of importance, whereas ADCC, cytokine-induced, and anit-CD3-induced cytotoxic activity may be of direct relevance.

ANTIGEN-PRESENTING CELLS

Morphologic and Phenotypic Characteristics of In Situ Cells

Antigen presentation is usually the initiating event in a chain of immune cell interactions, and is obviously of critical importance for the development of an appropriate immune response. Thus cells responsible for or involved in antigen uptake, processing, and presentation play a fundamental role in determining how and what types of helper, suppressor, or effector activities will result from the ensuing immune response. The term antigen-presenting cells is commonly used to describe various cell types that may be involved in antigen processing, such as monocytes, macrophages, dendritic cells, and veiled cells. Different morphologic, phenotypic, and functional characteristics distinguish these various types of cells. However, the exact relationship among them is not entirely clear in most tissues and organs, including the digestive system. Intestinal epithelial cells can function as antigen-presenting cells under some circumstances, and they are discussed elsewhere in this book.

Macrophages are easily identified by their morphologic characteristics in the mucosa of the gastrointestinal tract, where they are found mostly in the subepithelial areas of the lamina propria. This location was origianlly thought to have a functional significance in the local mechanisms of defense, and this macrophage-epithelial association was defined as a "subepithelial reticulohistiocytic complex".[138] Histologically, the frequency of macrophages is estimated to be approximately 300 cells/mm^2.[139] Essentially all macrophages strongly express class II (HLA-DR) antigens on their surface.[53] However, in spite of this common characteristic related to their function as antigen-presenting cells, it is becoming increasingly evident that intestinal macrophages represent an extremely heterogenous group of cells, with preferential distribution along the different segments of the gut, in both normal and pathologic conditions. In one study using histochemical and immunohistologic methods, 80–90% of small intestinal HLA-DR+ macrophages possessed stellate processes and exhibited strong membrane adenosine triphosphate activity but weak acid phosphatase and nonspecific esterase activity; in the colon, however, 60–70% of HLA-DR+ macrophages were large, round, and showed strong acid phosphatase and nonspecific esterase activity but no adenosine triphosphatase activity.[140] These morphologic and histochemical differences were interpreted as indicating different functional characteristics between small and large bowel macrophages: small intestinal macrophages could be involved in processing absorbed soluble antigens, while colonic macrophages could serve as phagocytis "scavenger" cells for particulate antigen. Another recent report using monoclonal antibodies defining specific subsets of antigen-presenting cells also supports the concept of heterogeneity. Allison and collaborators used the antibodies RFD1 to detect interdigitating (antigen-presenting) cells, RFD7 for mature macrophages, RFD9 for epithelioid and tingible body macrophages, and UCHM1 for monocytes.[141] In normal colonic mucosa, RFD1 detected the majority of macrophages located immediately beneath the epithelium, while RFD7 identified cells scattered throughout the lamina propria, with 87% of the cells exhibiting double staining. RFD9 positive cells were confined to lymphoid aggregates, while UCHM1 positive cells were rare. In both studies, a wide spectrum of phenotypic changes was observed during inflammatory conditions (ulcerative colitis and Crohn's disease), suggesting major shifts of macrophage subpopulations in response to an altered immunologic environment. The exact meaning of the heterogeneity of antigen-presenting cells in the normal and diseased intestine can not be understood simply by enumeration, no matter how detailed, of cell phenotypes in fixed tissue section. Only the combination of phenotypic assessment with the study of the functional properties of antigen-presenting cells can provide precise information of the role of these cells in health and disease.

Studies on Isolated Cells

Unfortunately, there is a scant amount of information on the functional characterization of antigen-presenting cells in the intestinal mucosal immune system. This situation is particularly true in humans, since available data are limited due to considerable technical difficulties in isolation, purification, and in vitro culture of the various types of antigen-presenting cells. In histologically normal small intestinal or colonic mucosa, macrophages constitute approximately 10% of isolated LPMC obtained by enzymatic digestion, with cell yields varying from 1.6 to 3.4 × 10^6 cells/g of wet tissue.[142,143] Isolated intestinal macrophages show typical morphology after surface adherance, most are HLA-DR+, and approximately one-half have Fc receptors.[142] Functional assessment has been extremely limited, essentially restricted to the demonstration of phagocytic ability for sheep red blood cells and bacteria, and secretion of the constitutive enzyme lysozyme.[142-145] Preliminary experiments in our laboratory demonstrate that intestinal macrophages synthesize and release substantial amounts of IL-1 in normal and pathologic conditions.[146]

Another type of intestinal antigen-presenting cell has been described using a technique of time-lapse cinematography in a series of studies by Wilders and collaborators.[147-149] These cells have been named "veiled cells" due to their display of moving cytoplasmatic extensions. They express class II antigens but no immunoglobulin or T-cell markers on their surface, as expected for cells of non-B, non-T-cell lineage. While veiled cells are easily detected in the lymphoid follicles and lamina propria of various animal species they are extremely rare in normal human colonic mucosa, their number increasing only during an active inflammatory process.[149]

None of the above studies actually addressed some of the most crucial functional aspects of macrophages and related cells, such as antigen processing and presentation, helper and suppressor activity for antigen- and mitogen-induced proliferation, induction of helper (CD4) cells, cytotoxic capacity, etc. Although the morphologic, phenotypic, and in vitro characteristics gathered so far strongly suggest that antigen-presenting cells in the gut exert functions similar to those of equivalent cells from other organs and systems, efforts must be expanded to test those functions in culture. In addition, potential peculiarities of behavior that may represent adaptation or response to the unique intestinal environment should be investigated and carefully characterized.

MAST CELLS

Types and Distribution

The study of mast cells has been classically associated with allergic phenomena mediated by immediate hypersensitivity reactions, usually involving reaginic IgE. Although this concept is still valid, the spectrum of actions of mast cells has been considerably broadened, and includes a substantial participation in cellular immunity.[150] This new wider view of mast cells is of particular relevance to mucosal immunity, because of their distribution, type, and function in the gastrointestinal tract, as well as participation in some gastrointestinal diseases.

Mast cells are easily recognized by the presence of large metachromatically staining granules containing a variety of biologically active substances. Mast cells tend to be more abundant in those parts of the body in direct contact with the external environment, such as the skin, the respiratory tract, and the digestive system.[151,152] In the latter, they are found all along its length, scattered in the epithelium, mucosa, submucosa, muscle, and serosa, although their number tends to decrease from the jejunum and ileum toward the colon and the rectum.[153] A more precise understanding of the distribution and types of intestinal mast cells was obtained after appreciation of two fundamental aspects. The first deals with the special staining characteristics of tissue mast cells, in both animals and humans. The number of detectable mast cells is crucially dependent on the method of fixation, as demonstrated by Strobel and collaborators in specimens of human jejunum.[154] The second is the realization that human mast cells, as their animal counterparts, are quite heterogeneous, but can be divided into two basic types: the "typical" or connective tissue mast cell, and the "atypical" or mucosal mast cell. Typical and atypical mast cells differ in regard to size, morphology, dye binding properties, histamine content, response to stimulatory and inhibitory signals, T-cell dependence, and types of proteoglycans produced (Table 7–3). Both types are present in the human intestine, where the mucosal mast cell can be found in the epithelium and lamina propria, whereas the connective tissue mast cell tends to be more restricted to the submucosa, muscularis mucosae, and serosa.[152,155,156] Using differential staining with formalin or basic lead acetate, additional differences can be demonstrated in reference to distribution along different segments of the intestine, mucosal mast cells being more abundant in all layers of the large bowel and also in the lamina propria and muscle of the small bowel.[157]

Functional Aspects

Because of their relatively small number and difficult isolation, information on human mucosal mast cells is limited. Therefore some relevant aspects of these cells are covered by studies performed in animals, mostly the mouse and rat. As previously discussed, considerable controversy existed until recently on the origin of mucosal mast cells and their relationship to intestinal T cells. Initially, it was proposed that the mouse granulated intraepithelial lymphocyte was a precursor of mucosal mast cells.[15] However, later studies tend to suggest that both cell types have different progenitors and a separate ontogeny.[158,159]

Table 7–3 COMPARATIVE PROPERTIES AND FUNCTIONS OF CONNECTIVE TISSUE AND MUCOSAL MAST CELLS IN THE RAT

Characteristic	Connective tissue (typical)	Mucosal (atypical)
Fixative	Formaldehyde	Basic lead acetate (Carnoy)
Life span	Long	Short (thymus-dependent)
Precursor cell	Local	Bone marrow
Size	Larger	Smaller
Number of granules	Larger	Smaller
Histamine content	Greater	Smaller
Serotonin content	Greater	Smaller
Serin protease	RMCP I	RMCP II
Fc receptors for IgE	More	Fewer
Innervation	–	+
Effect of membrane-stabilizing antiallergic substances	+	–
Effect of corticosteroids	–	Decreased RMCP degranulation

RMCP I, II, rat mast cell protease type I and type II.

[Adapted from Pabst (186), with permission.]

A common approach to the investigation of the function of intestinal mast cells has been the use of helminth-infected rats, which display intense mast cell hyperplasia, thus facilitating cell isolation, mediator measurement, and the study of differentiation, proliferation, and regulatory events.[160,161] Isolated rat intestinal mast cells have been shown to be morphologically, histochemically, and functionally different from peritoneal mast cells.[160] Similar studies have been extended to nonhuman primates, and showed that mucosal mast cells differ from those derived from the lungs.[162,163] Finally, two separate groups of investigators have recently described the isolation and preliminary functional characterization of human intestinal mucosal mast cells.[164,165] The achieved level of purification and enrichment (up to 8%) is suboptimal; nevertheless, it represents a starting point for the initial in vitro assessment of gut mucosal mast cell biologic composition and function. In the first report mucosal mast cells were indistinguishable from those extracted from human lung in their morphologic and functional aspects.[164] In the second report they were found to be composed of two histochemically distinct populations, one analogous to rat peritoneal and connective tissue mast cells, and another similar to rat intestinal mast cells.[165] Whether these diverse characteristics reflect different functions is still unknown, but this is obviously of great interest because of possible implications in normal and pathologic conditions of the gut.

A particularly intriguing and novel aspect relevant to mucosal mast cells is the increasingly large body of evidence indicating a close relationship among these cells, neuropeptides, the enteric nervous system, and intestinal immunity.[166] Substance P induces mucosal mast cell secretion,[167,168] nerve growth factor induces histamine release,[166] and an intimate physical contact has been described between mucosal mast cells and peptidergic nerve fibers.[169] Given the importance of neuroregulation for mucosal immunity, the above studies suggest that mucosal mast cells may serve as a link between the neuroendocrine and immune systems in the intestine.

Abundant data have also been accumulated to support the role of mast cells in various cell-mediated immune events, such as delayed-type hypersensitivity, cytotoxicity, immunoregulation, and inflammation.[150] However, the exact relationship between cellular immunity, mucosal mast cells, and disease is still unclear. In well-defined animal models of enteropathy, such as GVHD, typical pathologic changes putatively mediated by cellular immune responses still occur even after profound depletion of mucosal mast cells, suggesting that they may not have a significant pathogenic input.[170] Nevertheless, mast cell hyperplasia in the bowel wall has been well documented in several human diseases, as in gluten-sensitive enteropathy, Crohn's disease, and many parasitic infections.[171-173] In addition, initial evidence exists for active participation of mucosal mast cells in gut inflammation, as indicated recently by Fox and coworkers.[174] These authors showed that mast cells derived from intestine involved in inflammatory bowel disease release de novo greater amounts of histamine when compared with autologous mast cells from uninvolved intestine. Thus it is clear that knowledge of the function of mucosal mast cells is too limited, at present, to permit a full understanding of their function in intestinal immunity, and in particular their controversial role as inducers of or responders to intestinal diseases. The methodology for isolation of human gut mucosal mast cells is now at hand, and its application to a variety of in vitro systems should supply the means of answering some of these crucial questions.

ROLE OF CELLULAR IMMUNITY IN INTESTINAL DISEASES

In the preceding paragraphs considerable evidence has been presented to show the variety of cell types, products, and activities that are potentially involved in cell-mediated immune phenomena in the intestine. However, direct evidence that gut injury in humans and related clinical manifestations are the result of immunologic events occurring in the intestinal wall is still lacking at present. Nevertheless, there is compelling circumstantial evidence suggesting that T-cell-mediated immune responses play a significant role in the pathogenesis of some gastrointestinal diseases. Many clinical entities manifested by enteropathy and malabsorption are likely to be caused by local cellular reactions to food or enteric antigens, such as celiac disease, cow's milk protein intolerance, various food allergies (soya, rice, fish, chicken), giardiasis, helminthiases, tropical sprue, GVHD, etc.[175] These entities share not only some clinical manifestations, but, more importantly, also some common mucosal pathologic findings, represented by lymphocytic infiltration, increased number of intraepithelial lymphocytes, villous atrophy, and crypt cell hyperplasia. Therefore, if these changes can be shown to be the consequence of T-cell activation, lymphokine release, or cytotoxicity by T or NK cells in the microenvironment of the gut mucosa, this would provide direct evidence for a cause and effect reltionship between cellular immunity and pathogenesis.

Induction of immunologically mediated gut injury is obviously easier to demonstrate in animal models, and several have been explored with variable degree of success: GVHD, allograft rejection, contact sensitivity, *Nippostrongylus brasiliensis* infestation, and hypersensitivity to dietary antigens.[175] Among them, the most widely used experimental model and the one that has provided the most useful data is the induction of GVHD-associated enteropathy in mice.[176] This model can be conveniently modulated by changing some of the experimental parameters, such as the use or lack of irradiation, age and type of the animals, and timing of the phase of the rejection phenomenon. In an extensive series of reports, Mowat and co-workers have gathered substantial data to support the involvement of cell-mediated immunity in the development of gut pathologic abnormalities. Crypt cell hyperplasia and increased number of intraepithelial lymphocytes occur during the early response of intestinal GVHD.[177] This early response, called proliferative phase, is induced by helper T cells.[178] Elimination of NK cells induces a milder form of intestinal GVHD, indicating that these cells are also an important component of the local response.[179] In addition, mucosal T cells appear to influence epithelial cell renewal and differentiation in both normal and pathologic conditions.[180] Both soluble mediators and specific cytotoxic T lymphocytes are probably implicated in local effector mechanisms, but acting at different stages: the former are more likely to be involved in the early proliferative stage marked by nonspecific cytotoxicity, whereas the latter appear during a later destructive stage.[181,182] In reality, both stages merely represent a progressive form of a mucosal delayed-type hypersensitivity reaction. Evidence for the essential role of soluble products of activated immune cell in gut tissue injury has recently been provided by Piguet and collaborators.[183] In the acute phase of intestinal GVHD, these authors demonstrated that local release of TNF-α is associated with epithelial cell alterations and increases the inflammatory reaction, and both effects can be prevented by administration of antibodies specific for the cytokine.

The validity of the previous observations, and the possibility that activation of mucosal T cells is not restricted to experimental animal enteropathies, but actually plays an equally relevant role in the pathogenesis of intestinal lesions in humans, have been substantially strengthened by the elegant study by MacDonald and Spencer.[184] Using organ cultures of human fetal small intestine stimulated by pokeweed mitogen or anti-CD3 antibody, these investigators were able to show that in situ activation of mucosal T cells, demonstrated by the appearance of IL-2 receptors on cell surfaces and detection of IL-2 in the culture supernatants, was rapidly followed by profound morphologic changes manifested by crypt cell hyperplasia and villous atrophy. These effects were directly related to the number of T cells in the specimens and could be prevented by the addition of cyclosporin A, an inhibitor of T-cell activation. Essentially identical changes can be found in focal microscopic lesions in the jejunum of patients with Crohn's disease,[185] thus suggesting that they may be the result of local T-cell-mediated immune responses.

In conclusion, there is considerable indirect evidence, in both animals and humans, to support the hypothesis of an intimate association between an active intestinal mucosal cell-mediated immune response and the concomitant development of pathologic abnormalities. However, this is not sufficient yet to establish a direct cause and effect relationship, and definitive proof that cellular immune responses are actually responsible for human intestinal diseases will require further research to define all the implicated effector mechanisms and their respective targets.

REFERENCES

1. Bienenstock J, Ernst PB, Underdown BJ: The gastrointesinal tract as an immunologic organ-state of the art. *Ann Allergy* 59:17–20, 1987.
2. Orlic D, Lev R: An electron microscopic study of intraepithelial lymphocytes in human fetal small intestine. *Lab Invest* 37:554–561, 1977.
3. Spencer J, Dillon SB, Isaacson PG, et al: T cell subclasses in fetal human ileum. *Clin Exp Immunol* 65:553–558, 1986.
4. Strober W, Sneller MC: Cellular and molecular events accompanying IgA B cell differentiation. *Monogr Allergy* 24:181–190, 1988.
5. Otto HF: The interepithelial lymphocyte of the intestinum. Morphological observations and immunologic aspects of intestinal enteropathy. *Curr Top Pathol* 57:81–121, 1973.
6. Hirata I, Berrebi G, Austin LL, et al: Immunohistological characterization of intraepithelial and lamina propria lymphocytes in control ileum and colon and in inflammatory bowel disease. *Dig Dis Sci* 31:593–603, 1986.
7. Ferguson A: Celiac disease and gastrointestinal food allergy. In Ferguson A, MacSween RNM: *Immunological Aspects of the Liver and the Gastrointestinal Tract.* Lancaster, England, MTP Press Ltd, 1967, p 152.
8. Bartnik W, ReMine SC, Chiba M, et al: Isolation and characterization of colonic intraepithelial and lamina propria lymphocytes. *Gastroenterology* 78:976–985, 1980.
9. Ernst PB, Befus AD, Bienenstock J: Leukocytes in the intestinal epithelium: an unusual immunological compartment. *Immunol Today* 6:50–55, 1985.
10. Toner PG, Ferguson A: Intraepithelial cells in the human intestinal mucosa. *J Ultrastruc Res* 34:329–344, 1971.

11. Ferguson A: Intraepithelial lymphocytes of the small intestine. *Gut* 18:921–937, 1977.

12. MacDonald TT, Spencer JM, Monk TJ: Evidence that intraepithelial lymphocytes are derived from activated lamina propria T cells in human small intestine. *International Coeliac Symposium.* London, 1988, p 12 (Abstract).

13. Dobbins WO: Human intestinal intraepithelial lymphocytes. *Gut* 27:972–985, 1986.

14. Guy-Grand D, Griscelli C, Vassalli P: The gut associated lymphoid system: nature and properties of the large dividing cells. *Eur J Immunol* 4:435–443, 1974.

15. Guy-Grand D, Griscelli C, Vassalli P: The mouse gut lymphocyte, a novel type of T cell. Nature, origin and traffic in mice in normal and graft-versus-host conditions. *J Exp Med* 148:1661–1677, 1978.

16. Petit A, Ernst PB, Befus AD, et al: Murine intestinal intraepithelial lymphocytes I. Relationship of a novel Thy1−, Lyt1−, Lyt2+, granulated subpopulation to natural killer cells and mast cells. *Eur J Immunol* 15:211–215, 1985.

17. Ernst PB, Petit A, Befus AD, et al: Murine intestinal intraepithelial lymphocytes II. Comparison of freshly isolated and cultured intraepithelial lymphocytes. *Eur J Immunol* 15:216–221, 1985.

18. Guy-Grand D, Dy M, Luffau G, et al: Gut mucosal mast cells. Origin, traffic, and differentiation. *J Exp Med* 160:12–28, 1984.

19. Lyscom N, Brueton MJ: Intraepithelial, lamina propria and Peyer's patches lymphocytes of the rat small intestine: isolation and characterization in terms of immunoglobulin markers and receptors for monoclonal antibodies. *Immunology* 45:775–783, 1982.

20. Heijden FLVD: Mucosal lymphocytes in the rat small intestine: phenotypical characterization in situ. *Immunology* 59:397–399, 1986.

21. Arnaud-Battandier F, Nelson DL: Immunologic characteristics of intestinal lymphoid cells of the guinea pig. *Gastroenterology* 82:248–253, 1982.

22. Nagi AM, Babiuk LA: Bovine gut-associated lymphoid tissue — morphologic and functional studies. I. Isolation and characterization of leukocytes from the epithelium and the lamina propria of bovine small intestine. *J Immunol Methods* 105:23–37, 1987.

23. Cerf-Bensussan N, Guy-Grand D, Lisowska-Grospierre B, et al: A monoclonal antibody specific for rat intestinal lymphocytes. *J Immunol* 136:76–82, 1986.

24. Kilshaw PJ, Baker KC: A unique surface antigen on intraepithelial lymphocytes in the mouse. *Immunol Lett* 18:149–154, 1988.

25. Goodman T, Lefrançois L: Expression of the γ-δ T-cell receptor on intestinal CD8+ intraepithelial lymphocytes. *Nature* 333:855–858, 1988.

26. Bucy RP, Chen C-LH, Cihak J, et al: Avian T cells expressing γ-δ receptors localize in the splenic sinusoids and the intestinal epithelium. *J Immunol* 141:2200–2205, 1988.

27. Tagliabue A, Luini W, Soldateschi D, et al: Natural killer cell activity of gut mucosal lymphoid cells in mice. *Eur J Immunol* 11:919–922, 1981.

28. Tagliabue A, Befus AD, Clark DA, et al: Characteristics of natural killer cells in the murine intestinal epithelium and lamina propria. *J Exp Med* 155:1785–1796, 1982.

29. Alberti S, Colotta F, Spreafico F, et al: Large granular lymphocyte from murine blood and intestinal epithelium: comparison of surface antigens, natural killer activity, and morphology. *Clin Immunol Immunopathol* 36:227–238, 1985.

30. Carman PS, Ernst PB, Rosenthal KL, et al: Inraepithelial lymphocytes contain a unique subpopulation of NK-like cells active in the defense of gut epithelium to enteric murine coronavirus. *J Immunol* 136:1548–1553, 1986.

31. Flexman JP, Shellam GR, Mayrhofer G: Natural cytotoxicity, responsiveness to interferon and morphology of intra-epithelial lymphocytes from the small intestine of the rat. *Immunology* 48:733–741, 1983.

32. Arnaud-Battandier F, Bundy BM, O'Neil M, et al: Cytotoxic activities of gut mucosal lymphoid cells in guinea pigs. *J Immunol* 121:1059–1065, 1978.

33. Chai J-Y, Lillehoj HS: Isolation and functional characterization of chicken intestinal intra-epithelial lymphocytes showing natural killer cell activity against tumour target cells. *Immunology* 63:111–117, 1988.

34. Davies MDJ, Parrott DMV: Cytotoxic T cells in small intestine epithelial, lamina propria and lung lymphocytes. *Immunology* 44:367–371, 1981.

35. Ernst PB, Clark DA, Rosenthal KL, et al: Detection and characterization of cytotoxic T lymphocyte precursors in the murine intestinal intraepithelial leukocyte population. *J Immunol* 136:2121–2126, 1986.

36. Klein JR, Kagnoff MF: Nonspecific recruitment of cytotoxic effector cells in the intestinal mucosa of antigen-primed mice. *J Exp Med* 160:1931–1936, 1984.

37. Tagliabue A, Villa L, Scapigliati G, et al: Peyer's patches lymphocytes express natural cytotoxicity but not natural killer activity. *Nat Immun Cell Growth Regul* 3:95–101, 1983.

38. Nencioni L, Villa L, Boraschi D, et al: Natural and antibody-dependent cell-mediated activity against *Salmonella typhimurium* by peripheral and intestinal lymphoid cells in mice. *J Immunol* 130:903–907, 1983.

39. Tagliabue A, Nencioni L, Villa L, et al: Antibody-dependent cell-mediated antibacterial activity of intestinal lymphocytes with secretory IgA. *Nature* 306:184–186, 1983.

40. Parrott DMV, Tait C, MacKenzie S, et al: Analysis of the effector functions of different populations of mucosal lymphocytes. *Ann NY Acad Sci* 409:307–320, 1983.

41. Cerf-Bensussan N, Quaroni A, Kurnick JT, et al: Intraepithelial lymphocytes modulate Ia expression by intestinal epithelial cells. *J Immunol* 132:2244–2251, 1984.

42. Mowat AMcI, Ferguson A: Intraepithelial lymphocyte count and crypt hyperplasia measure the mucosal component of the graft-versus-host reaction in mouse small intestine. *Gastroenterology* 83:417–423, 1982.

43. Strickland RG, Husby G, Black WC, et al: Peripheral blood and intestinal lymphocyte sub-populations in Crohn's disease. *Gut* 16:847–853, 1975.

44. Meuwissen SGM, Feltkamp-Vroom TM, de la Riviere AB, et al: Analysis of the lympho-plasmacytic infiltrate in Crohn's disease with special reference to identification of lymphocyte-subpopulations. *Gut* 17:770–780, 1976.

45. Selby WS, Janossy G, Jewell DP: Immunohistological characterization of intraepithelial lymphocytes of the human gastrointestinal tract. *Gut* 22:169–176, 1981.

46. Selby WS, Janossy G, Goldstein G, et al: T lymphocyte subsets in human intestinal mucosa: the distribution and relationship to MHC-derived antigens. *Clin Exp Immunol* 44:453–458, 1981.

47. Selby WS, Janossy G, Bofill M, et al: Lymphocyte subpopulations in the human small intestine. The findings in normal mucosa and in the mucosa of patients with adult coeliac disease. *Clin Exp Immunol* 52:219–228, 1983.

48. Selby WS, Janossy G, Bofill M, et al: Intestinal lymphocyte subpopulations in inflammatory bowel disease: an analysis by immunohistological and cell isolation techniques. *Gut* 25:32–40, 1984.

49. Cerf-Bensussan N, Schneeberger EE, Bhan AK: Immunohistologic and immunoelectron microscopic characterization of the mucosal lymphocytes of human small intestine by the use of monoclonal antibodies. *J Immunol* 130:2615–2622, 1983.

50. Malizia G, Trejdosiewcz LK, Wood GM, et al: The microenvironment of coeliac disease: T cell phenotypes and expression of the "T blast" antigen by small bowel lymphocytes. *Clin Exp Immunol* 60:437–446, 1985.

51. Trejdosiewcz LK, Malizia G, Badr-el-Din S, et al: T cell and mononuclear phagocyte populations of the human small and large intestine. *Adv Exp Med Biol* 216A:465–473, 1987.

52. Vecchi M, Berti E, Primignani M, et al: In situ identification of immune competent cells in gastrointestinal mucosa: an evaluation by immunoelectromicroscopy. *Virchows Arch [Pathol Anat]* 406:407–415, 1985.

53. Hirata I, Austin LL, Blackwell WH, et al: Immunoelectron microscopic localization of HLA-DR antigen in control small intestine and colon and in inflammatory bowel disease. *Dig Dis Sci* 31:1317–1330, 1986.

54. Bjerke K, Brandtzaeg P, Fausa O: T cell distribution is different in follicle-associated epithelium of human Peyer's patches and villous epithelium. *Clin Exp Immunol* 74:270–275, 1988.

55. Cerf-Bensussan N, Jarry A, Brousse N, et al: A monoclonal antibody (HML-1) defining a novel membrane molecule present on human intestinal lymphocytes. *Eur J Immunol* 17:1279–1285, 1987.

56. Jarry A, Cerf-Bensussan N, Brousse N, et al: Same peculiar subset of HML1+ lymphoctes present within normal intestinal epithelium is associated with tumoral epithelium of gastrointestinal carcinomas. *Gut* 29:1632–1638, 1988.

57. Greenwood JH, Austin LL, Bobbins WO: In vitro characterization of human intestinal intraepithelial lymphocytes. *Gastroenterology* 85:1023–1035, 1983.

58. Cerf-Bensussan N, Guy-Grand D, Griscelli C: Intraepithelial lymphocytes of human gut: isolation, characterization and study of natural killer activity. *Gut* 26:81–88, 1985.

59. Danis VA, Heatley RV: Evidence for regulation of human colonic mucosal immunoglobulin secretion by intestinal lymphoid cells. *J Clin Lab Immunol* 22: 7–11, 1987.

60. Ebert EC, Roberts AI, Brolin RE, et al: Examination of the low proliferative capacity of human jejunal intraepithelial lymphocytes. *Clin Exp Immunol* 65:148–157, 1986.

61. Marsh MN: Functional and structural aspects of the epithelial lymphocyte, with implications for coeliac disease and tropical sprue. *Scand J Gastroenterol (Suppl)* 114:55–75, 1985.

62. Marsh MN, Mathan M, Mathan VI: Studies of intestinal lymphoid tissue. The secondary nature of lymphoid cell "activation" in the jejunal lesions of tropical sprue. *Am J Pathol* 112:302–312, 1983.

63. Corazza GR, Frazzoni M, Gasbarrini G: Jejunal intraepithelial lymphocytes in coeliac disease: are they increased or decreased? *Gut* 25:158–162, 1984.

64. Wright SG, Tomkins AM: Quantification of the lymphocytic infiltrate in jejunal epithelium in giardiasis. *Clin Exp Immunol* 29:408–412, 1977.

65. Phillips AD, Rice SJ, France NE, et al: Small intestinal intraepithelial lymphocyte levels in cow's milk protein intolerance. *Gut* 20:509–512, 1979.

66. Lazenley AJ, Yardley JH, Giardiello FM, et al: Lymphocytic ("microscopic") colitis: a comparative histopathologic study with particular reference to collagenous colitis. *Hum Pathol* 20:18–28, 1989.

67. Lloyd G: A study of mast cells and immunoglobulins in inflammatory bowel disease. M.Sc. Thesis. University of Manchester, England, 1975.

68. Fiocchi C, Tubbs RR, Youngman KR: Human intestinal mucosal mononuclear cells exhibit lymphokine-activated killer cell activity. *Gastroenterology* 88:625–637, 1985.

69. Fiocchi C, Youngman KR, Yen-Lieberman B, et al: Modulation of intestinal immune reactivity by interleukin 2. Phenotypic and functional analysis of lymphokine-activated killer cells from human intestinal mucosa. *Dig Dis Sci* 33:1305–1315, 1988.

70. Konttinen YT, Bergroth V, Nordstrom D, et al: Lymphocyte activation in vivo in the intestinal mucosa of patients with Crohn's disease. *J Clin Lab Immunol* 22:59–63, 1987.

71. Clancy R: Isolation and kinetic characteristics of mucosal lymphocytes in Crohn's disease. *Gastroenterology* 70:177–180, 1976.

72. Goodacre R, Davidson R, Singal D, et al: Morphologic and functional characteristics of human intestinal lymphoid cells isolated by a mechanical technique. *Gastroenterology* 76:300–308, 1979.

73. Fiocchi C, Battisto JR, Farmer RG: Gut mucosal lymphocytes in inflammatory bowel disease. Isolation and preliminary functional characterization. *Dig Dis Sci* 24:705–717, 1979.

74. Bland PW, Richens ER, Britton DC, et al: Isolation and purification of human large bowel mucosal lymphoid cells: effect of separation technique on functional characteristics. *Gut* 20:1037–1046, 1979.

75. Kaulfersch W, Fiocchi C, Waldmann TA: Polyclonal nature of the intestinal mucosal lymphocyte populations in inflammatory bowel disease. A molecular genetic evaluation of the immunoglobulin and T-cell antigen receptors. *Gastroenterology* 95:365–370, 1988.

76. Bull DM, Bookman MA: Isolation and functional characterization of human intestinal mucosal lymphoid cells. *J Clin Invest* 59:966–974, 1977.

77. Eade OE, St Andre-Ukena S, Moulton C, et al: Lymphocyte subpopulations of intestinal mucosa in inflammatory bowel disease. *Gut* 21:675–682, 1980.

78. Fiocchi C, Battisto JR, Farmer RG: Studies on isolated gut mucosal lymphocytes in inflammatory bowel disease. Detection of activated T cells and enhanced proliferation to *Staphylococcus aureus* and lipolysaccharides. *Dig Dis Sci* 26:728–736, 1981.

79. Bookman MA, Bull DM: Characteristics of isolated intestinal mucosal lymphoid cells in inflammatory bowel disease. *Gastroenterology* 77:503–510, 1979.

80. Gibson PR, Dow EL, Selby WS, et al: Natural killer cells and spontaneous cell-mediated cytotoxicity in the human intestine. *Clin Exp Immunol* 56:438–444, 1984.

81. Roche JK, Fiocchi C, Youngman K: Sensitization to epithelial antigens in chronic mucosal inflammatory disease. Characterization of human intestinal mucosa-derived mononuclear cells reactive with purified epithelial cell-associated components in vitro. *J Clin Invest* 75:522–530, 1985.

82. Fiocchi C: Intestinal mucosal lymphocytes: a new approach to the pathogenesis of inflammatory bowel disease. In Rachmilewitz D: *Inflammatory Bowel Disease 1986.* The Hague, Martinus Nijhoff Publishers, 1986, p 73.

83. James SP, Fiocchi C, Graeff AS, et al: Phenotypic analysis of lamina propria lymphocytes. Predominance of helper-inducer and cytolytic T-cell phenotype and deficiency of suppressor-inducer phenotypes in Crohn's disease and control patients. *Gastroenterology* 91:1483–1489, 1986.

84. James SP, Graeff AS, Zeitz M: Predominance of helper-inducer T cells in mesenteric lymph nodes and intestinal lamina propria of normal nonhuman primates. *Cell Immunol* 107:372–383, 1987.

85. Kanof ME, Strober W, Fiocchi C, et al: CD4 positive Leu-8 negative helper-inducer T cells predominate in the human intestinal lamina propria. *J Immunol* 141:3029–3036, 1988.

86. Pallone F, Fais S, Squarcia O, et al: Activation of peripheral blood and intestinal lamina propria lymphocytes in Crohn's disease. In vivo state of activation and in vitro response to stimulation as defined by the expression of early activation antigens. *Gut* 28:745–753, 1987.

87. Zeitz M, Greene WC, Peffer NJ, et al: Lymphocyte isolated from the intestinal lamina propria of normal nonhuman primates have increased expression of genes associated with T-cell activation. *Gastroenterology* 94:647–655, 1988.

88. Bland PW, Britton DC, Richens ER, et al: Peripheral, mucosal, and tumour-infiltrating components of cellular immunity in cancer of the large bowel. *Gut* 22:744–751, 1981.

89. Fiocchi C, Hilfiker ML, Youngman KR, et al: Interleukin 2 activity of human intestinal mucosa mononuclear cells. Decreased levels in inflammatory bowel disease. *Gastroenterology* 86:734–742, 1984.

90. Fiocchi C, Parent K, Mitchell P: Proliferative response of gut mucosal lymphocytes from Crohn's disease patients to enterobacterial common antigen, lipopolysaccharide and cell wall-defective bacteria. In Pena AS, Weterman IT, Booth CC, Strober W: *Recent Advances in Crohn's Disease.* The Hague, Martinus Nijhoff Publishers, 1981, p 433.

91. Zeitz M, Quinn TC, Graeff AS, et al: Mucosal T cells provide helper function but do not proliferate when stimulated by specific antigen in lymphogranuloma venereum proctitis in nonhuman primates. *Gastroenterology* 94:353–366, 1988.

92. MacDermott RP, Bragdon MJ, Jenkins KM, et al: Human intestinal mononuclear cells. II. Demonstration of naturally occurring subclasses of T cells which respond in the allogeneic mixed leukocyte reaction but do not effect cell-mediated lympholysis. *Gastroenterology* 80:748–757, 1981.

93. Kwan WC, Tierney SJ, James SP: Interleukin-4 (IL-4) is an autocrine T cell factor in the afferent limb of the mucosal immune system of nonhuman primates. *Gastroenterology* 94:245, 1988 (Abstract).

94. Fiocchi C, Levine AD, West GA, et al: Interleukin 4 (IL4) modulates proliferative and cytotoxic responses of human intestinal mucosal mononuclear cells. *Gastroenterology* 96:152, 1989 (Abstract).

95. Goodacre RL, Bienenstock J: Reduced suppressor cell activity in intestinal lymphocytes from patients with Crohn's disease. *Gastroenterology* 82:653–658, 1982.

96. Fiocchi C, Youngman KR, Farmer RG: Immunoregulatory function of human intestinal mucosa lymphoid cells: evidence for enhanced suppressor cell activity in inflammatory bowel disease. *Gut* 24:692–701, 1983.

97. Smith EB, Leapman SB, Filo RS, et al: Specificity of the suppressor cell activity of intestinal lymphocytes. *Am J Surg* 145:164–168, 1983.

98. Clancy R, Cripps A, Chipchase H: Regulation of human gut B lymphocytes by T lymphocytes. *Gut* 25:47–51, 1984.

99. James SP, Fiocchi C, Graeff AS, et al: Immunoregulatory function of lamina propria T cells in Crohn's disease. *Gastroenterology* 88:1143–1150, 1985.

100. Elson CO, Machelski E, Weiserbs DB: T cell-B cell regulation in the intestinal lamina propria in Crohn's disease. *Gastroenterology* 89:321–327, 1985.

101. James SP, Graeff AS, Zeitz M, et al: Cytotoxic and immunoregulatory function of intestinal lymphocytes in *Chlamydia trachomatis* proctitis of nonhuman primates. *Infect Immun* 55:1137–1143, 1987.

102. James SP, Graeff AS: Effect of IL-2 on immunoregulatory function of intestinal lamina propria T cells in normal non-human primates. *Clin Exp Immunol* 70:394–402, 1987.

103. Lee A, Sugerman H, Elson CO: Regulatory activity of the human CD8+ cell subset: a comparison of CD8+ cells from the intestinal lamina propria and blood. *Eur J Immunol* 18:21–27, 1988.

104. James SP, Zeitz M, Kanof ME, et al: Activation and regulatory function of lamina propria T cells: implications for inflammatory bowel disease. In Goebbell H, Peskar BM, Malchoh: *Inflammatory Bowel Diseases: Basic Research and Clinical Implications.* Lancaster, England, MTP Press Limited, 1988, p 95.

105. Fiocchi C: Lymphokines and the intestinal immune response. Role in inflammatory bowel diseases. *Immunol Invest* 18:91–102, 1989 (in press).

106. Kusugami K, Youngman KR, West GA, et al: Lymphokine-activated killer cell activity of human intestinal mucosal mononuclear cells. Induction by endogenous interleukin

2 distinguishes Crohn's disease, ulcerative colitis, and control cells. *Gastroenterology* 97:1–9, 1989.

107. Lieberman BY, Fiocchi C, Youngman KR, et al: Interferon γ production by human intestinal mucosal mononuclear cells. Decreased levels in inflammatory bowel disease. *Dig Dis Sci* 33:1297–1304, 1988.

108. Ouyang Q, El-Youssef M, Yen-Lieberman B, et al: Expression of HLA-DR antigens in inflammatory bowel disease mucosa: role of intestinal lamina propria mononuclear cell-derived interferon γ. *Dig Dis Sci* 33:1528–1536, 1988.

109. Ligumsky M, Simon PL, Karmeli F, et al: Interleukin-1 — possible mediator of the inflammatory response in ulcerative colitis (UC). *Gastroenterology* 94:263, 1988 (Abstract).

110. Sartor RB, Chapman EJ, Schwab JH: Increased interleukin-1 beta concentrations in resected inflammatory bowel disease (IBD) tissue. *Gastroenterology* 94:399, 1988 (Abstract).

111. Pullman W, Hapel AJ, Doe WF: Colony stimulating factor production by intestinal lamina propria cells is increased in inflammatory bowel disease. *Gastroenterology* 94:361, 1988 (Abstract).

112. Sollid LM, Kvale D, Brandtzaeg P, et al: Interferon-γ enhances expression of secretory component, the epithelial receptor for polymeric immunoglobulins. *J Immunol* 138:4303–4306, 1987.

113. Kvale D, Lovhaug D, Sollid LM, et al: Tumor necrosis factor-α upregulates expression of secretory component, the epithelial receptor for polymeric Ig. *J Immunol* 140:3086–3089, 1988.

114. Brandtzaeg P, Sollid LM, Thrane PS, et al: Lymphoepithelial interactions in the mucosal immune system. *Gut* 29:1116–1130, 1988.

115. James SP, Strober W: Cytotoxic lymphocytes and intestinal disease. *Gastroenterology* 90:235–240, 1986.

116. Chiba M, Bartnik W, ReMine SG, et al: Human colonic intraepithelial and lamina proprial lymphocytes: cytotoxicity in vitro and the potential effects of the isolation method on their functional properties. *Gut* 22:177–186, 1981.

117. Clancy R, PucciA: Absence of K cells in human gut mucosa. *Gut* 19:273–276, 1978.

118. MacDermott RP, Franklin GO, Jenkins KM, et al: Human intestinal mononuclear cells. I. Investigation of antibody-dependent, lectin-induced, and spontaneous cell-mediated cytotoxic capabilities. *Gastroenterology* 78:47–56, 1980.

119. Chiba M, Shorter RG, Thayer WR, et al: K-cell activity in lamina proprial lymphocytes from the human colon. *Dig Dis Sci* 24:817–822, 1979.

120. Sakai Y, Koizumi K: Cell-mediated cytotoxicity of mononuclear cells isolated from cancer and normal mucosa of the stomach. *Gastroenterology* 82:1374–1380, 1982.

121. Falchuk ZM, Barnhard E, Machado I. Human colonic mononuclear cells: studies of cytotoxic function. *Gut* 22:290–294, 1981.

122. MacDermott RP, Bragdon MJ, Kodner IJ, et al: Deficient cell-mediated cytotoxicity and hyporesponsiveness to interferon and mitogen lectin activation by inflammatory bowel disease peripheral blood and intestinal mononuclear cells. *Gastroenterology* 90:6–11, 1986.

123. Hogan PG, Hapel AJ, Doe WF: Lymphokine-activated and natural killer cell activity in human intestinal mucosa. *J Immunol* 135:1731–1738, 1985.

124. Gibson PR, Jewell DP: Local immune mechanisms in inflammatory bowel disease and colorectal carcinoma. *Gastroenterology* 90:12–19, 1986.

125. Gibson PR, Hermanowicz A, Jewell DP: Factors affecting the spontaneous cell-mediated cytotoxicity of intestinal mononuclear cells. *Immunology* 53:267–274, 1984.

126. Gibson PR, Hermanowicz A, Verhaar HJJ, et al: Isolation of intestinal mononuclear cells: factors released which affect lymphocyte viability and function. *Gut* 26:60–68, 1985.

127. Gibson PR, Verhaar HJJ, Selby WS, et al: The mononuclear cells of human mesenteric blood, intestinal mucosa and mesenteric lymph nodes: compartmentalization of NK cells. *Clin Exp Immunol* 56:445–452, 1984.

128. Beeken WL, Gundel RM, St. Andre-Ukena S, et al: In vitro cellular cytotoxicity for a human colon cancer cell line by mucosal mononuclear cells of patients with colon cancer and other disorders. *Cancer* 55:1024–1029, 1985.

129. James SP, Graeff AS: Spontaneous and lymphokine-induced cytotoxic activity of monkey intestinal mucosal lymphocytes. *Cell Immunol* 93:387–397, 1985.

130. Targan S, Britvan L, Kendal R, et al: Isolation of spontaneous and interferon inducible natural killer cells from human colonic mucosa: lysis of lymphoid and autologous epithelial target cells. *Clin Exp Immunol* 54:14–22, 1983.

131. Shanahan F, Brogan M, Targan S: Human mucosal cytotoxic effector cells. *Gastroenterology* 92:1951–1957, 1987.

132. Gibson PR, Jewell DP: The nature of the natural killer (NK) cell of human intestinal mucosa and mesenteric lymph node. *Clin Exp Immunol* 61:160–168, 1985.

133. Trudel JL, Youngman KR, West GA, et al: Lymphokine-activated killer (LAK) cells from human intestinal mucosa: cytotoxic activity against tumor cell lines and modified self but not autologous and allogeneic colon cancer cells. *J Surg Res* 44:445–454, 1988.

134. Gibson PR, Van de Pol E, Pullman W, et al: Lysis of colonic epithelial cells by allogeneic mononuclear and lymphokine activated killer cells derived from peripheral blood and intestinal mucosa: evidence against a pathogenic role in inflammatory bowel disease. *Gut* 29:1076–1084, 1988.

135. Fiocchi C: Induction, modulation and characterization of lymphokine-activated killer cells from human intestinal mucosa. In Strober W, Lamm ME, McGhee JR, James SP: *Mucosal Immunity and Infections at Mucosal Surfaces.* New York, Oxford University Press, 1988, p 248.

136. Shorter RG, McGill DB, Bahn RC: Cytotoxicity of mononuclear cells for autologous colonic epithelial cells in colonic diseases. *Gastroenterology* 86:13–22, 1984.

137. Shanahan F, Deem R, Nayersina R, et al: Human mucosal T-cell cytotoxicity. *Gastroenterology* 94:960–967, 1988.

138. Donnellan WL: The structure of the colonic mucosa. The epithelium and subepithelial reticulohistiocytic complex. *Gastroenterology* 49:496–514, 1965.

139. Yunis E, Sherman FE: Macrophages of rectal lamina propria in children. *Am J Clin Pathol* 53:580–591, 1970.

140. Selby WS, Poulter LW, Hobbs S, et al: Heterogeneity of HLA-DR positive histiocytes of human intestinal lamina propria: a combined histochemical and immunological analysis. *J Clin Pathol* 36:379–384, 1983.

141. Allison MC, Cornwall W, Poulter LW, et al: Macrophage heterogeneity in normal colonic mucosa and in inflammatory bowel disease. *Gut* 29:1531–1538, 1988.

142. Golder JP, Doe WF: Isolation and preliminary characterization of human intestinal macrophages. *Gastroenterology* 84:795–802, 1983.

143. Beeken W, Mieremet-Ooms M, Ginsel LA, et al. Enrichment of macrophages in cell suspensions of human intestinal mucosa by elutriation centrifugation. *J Immunol Methods* 73:189–201, 1984.

144. Winter HS, Sessions Cole F, Huffer LM, et al: Isolation and characterization of resident macrophages from guinea pig and human intestine. *Gastroenterology* 85:358–363, 1983.

145. Beeken W, Northwood I, Beliveau C, et al: Phagocytes in cell suspensions of human colonic mucosa. *Gut* 28:976–980, 1987.

146. Simon PL, West GA, Rachmilewitz D, et al: Investigation of interleukin 1 (IL1) activity in the intestinal mucosa of Crohn's disease (CD) and ulcerative colitis patients. *Gastroenterology* 96:473, 1989 (Abstract).

147. Wilders MM, Drexhage HA, Weltervreden EF, et al: Large mononuclear Ia-positive veiled cells in Peyer's patches. I. Isolation and characterization in rat, guinea pig and pig. *Immunology* 48:453–460, 1983.

148. Wilders MM, Sminia T, Plesch BEC, et al: Large mononuclear Ia-positive veiled cells in Peyer's patches. II. Localization in rat Peyer's patches. *Immunology* 48:461–467, 1983.

149. Wilders MM, Drexhage HA, Kokjé M, et al: Veiled cells in chronic idiopathic inflammatory bowel disease. *Clin Exp Immunol* 55:377–387, 1984.

150. Befus D, Fujimaki H, Lee TDG, et al: Mast cell polymorphism: present concepts, future directions. *Dig Dis Sci* (Suppl) 33:16–24, 1988.

151. Lemanske Jr RF, Atkins FM, Metcalfe DD: Gastrointestinal mast cells in health and disease. Part I. *J Pediatri* 103:177–184, 1983.

152. Barrett KE, Metcalfe DD: The mucosal mast cell and its role in gastrointestinal allergic disease. *Clin Rev Allergy* 2:39–53, 1984.

153. Norris HT, Zamcheck N, Gottlieb LS: The presence and distribution of mast cells in the human gastrointestinal tract at autopsy. *Gastroenterology* 44:448–455, 1963.

154. Strobel S, Miller HRP, Ferguson A: Human intestinal mucosal mast cells: evaluation of fixation and staining techniques. *J Clin Pathol* 34:851–858, 1981.

155. Bienenstock J, Befus AD, Pearce F, et al: Mast cell heterogeneity: derivation and function, with emphasis on the intestine. *J Allergy Clin Immunol* 70:407–412, 1982.

156. Barrett KE, Metcalfe DD: Mast cell heterogeneity: evidence and implications. *J Clin Immunol* 4:253–261, 1984.

157. Befus D, Goodacre R, Dyck N, et al: Mast cell heterogeneity in man. I. Histologic studies of the intestine. *Int Arch Allergy Appl Immunol* 76:232–236, 1985.

158. Schrader JW, Scollay R, Battye F: Intramucosal lymphocytes of the gut: Lyt-2 and Thy-1 phenotype of the granulated cells and evidence for the presence of both T cells and mast cell precursors. *J Immunol* 130:558–564, 1983.

159. Schrader JW, Lewis SJ, Clark-Lewis I, et al: The persisting (P) cell: histamine content, regulation by a T cell-derived factor, origin from a bone marrow precursor and relationship to mast cells. *Proc Natl Acad Sci USA* 78:323–327, 1981.

160. Befus AD, Pearce FL, Gauldie J, et al: Mucosal mast cells. I. Isolation and functional characteristics of rat intestinal mast cells. *J Immunol* 128:2475–2480, 1982.

161. Pearce FL, Befus AD, Gauldie J, et al: Mucosal mast cells. II. Effects of anti-allergic compounds on histamine secretion by isolated intestinal mast cells. *J Immunol* 128:2481–2486, 1982.

162. Barrett KE, Metcalfe DD: The histologic and functional characterization of enzymatically dispersed intestinal mast cells of nonhuman primates: effects of secretagogues and anti-allergic drugs on histamine secretion. *J Immunol* 135:2020–2026, 1985.

163. Barrett KE, Szucs EF, Metcalfe DD: Mast cell heterogeneity in higher animals: a comparison of the properties of autologous lung and intestinal mast cells from nonhuman primates. *J Immunol* 137:2001–2008, 1986.

164. Fox CC, Dvorak AM, Peters SP, et al: Isolation and characterization of human intestinal mucosal mast cells. *J Immunol* 135:483–491, 1985.

165. Befus AD, Dyck N, Goodacre R, et al: Mast cells from human intestinal lamina propria. Isolation, histochemical subtypes, and functional characterization. *J Immunol* 138:2604–2610, 1987.

166. Bienenstock J, Denburg J, Scicchitano R, et al: Role of neuropeptides, nerves and mast cells in intestinal immunity and physiology. *Monogr Allergy* 24:124–133, 1988.

167. Shanahan F, Lee TDG, Bienenstock J, et al: The influence of endorphins on peritoneal and mucosal mast cell secretion. *J Allergy Clin Immunol* 74:499–504, 1984.

168. Shanahan F, Denburg JA, Fox J, et al: Mast cell heterogeneity: effects of neuroenteric peptides on histamine release. *J Immunol* 135:1331–1337, 1985.

169. Stead RH, Tomioka M, Quinonez G, et al: Intestinal mucosal mast cells in normal and nematode-infected rat intestine are in intimate contact with peptodergic nerves. *Proc Natl Acad Sci USA* 84:2975–2979, 1987.

170. Ferguson A, Cummins AG, Munro GH, et al: Roles of mucosal mast cells in intestinal cell-mediated immunity. *Ann Allergy* 59:40–43, 1987.

171. Strobel S, Busuttil A, Ferguson A: Human intestinal mucosal mast cells: expanded population in untreated coeliac disease. *Gut* 24:222–227, 1983.

172. Dvorak AM, Monohan RA, Osage JE, et al: Crohn's disease: transmission electron microscopic studies. II. Immunologic inflammatory response: alterations of mast cells, basophils, eosiniphils and the microvasculature. *Hum Pathol* 11:606–619, 1980.

173. Gustowska LR, Ruitenberg RJ, Elgersma A, et al: Increase in mucosal mast cells in the jejunum of patients with *Trichinella spiralis*. *Int Arch Allergy Appl Immunol* 71:304–308, 1983.

174. Fox CC, Moore WC, Bayless TM, et al: Enhanced mast cell histamine release in idiopathic inflammatory bowel disease. In MacDermott RP: *Inflammatory Bowel Disease. Current Status and Future Approach.* Amsterdam, Excerpta Medica, 1988, p 355.

175. Kay RA, Ferguson A: Intestinal T cells, mucosal cell-mediated immunity and their relevance to food allergic disease. *Clin Rev Allergy* 2:55–68, 1984.

176. MacDonald TT, Ferguson A: Hypersensitivity reaction in the small intestine. III. The effects of allograft rejection and of graft-versus-host disease on epithelial cell kinetics. *Cell Tissue Kinet* 10:301–312, 1977.

177. Mowat AMcI, Ferguson A: Hypersensitivity reactions in the small intestine. VI. Pathogenesis of the graft-verses-host reaction in the small intestinal mucosa of the mouse. *Transplantation* 32:238–243, 1981.

178. Mowat AMcI, Borland A, Parrott DMV: Hypersensitivity reactions in the small intestine. VII. The intestinal phase of murine graft-versus-host reaction is induced by Lyt2- T cells activated by I-A alloantigens. *Transplantation* 41:192–198, 1986.

179. Mowat AMcI, Felstein MV: Experimental studies of immunologically mediated enteropathy. II. Role of natural killer cells in the intestinal phase of murine graft-versus-host reaction. *Immunology* 61:179–183, 1987.

180. Mowat AMcI, Felstein MV, Baca ME: Experimental studies of immunologically mediated enteropathy. III. Severe and progressive enteropathy during graft-versus-host reaction in athymic mice. *Immunology* 61:185–188, 1987.

181. Felstein MV, Mowat AMcI: Experimental studies of immunologically mediated enteropathy. IV. Correlation between immune effector mechanisms and type of enteropathy during a GvHR in neonatal mice of different ages. *Clin Exp Immunol* 72:108–112, 1988.

182. Mowat AMcI, Felstein MV, Borland A, et al: Experimental studies of immunologically mediated enteropathy. Development of cell mediated immunity and intestinal pathology during a graft-versus-host reaction in irradiated mice. *Gut* 29:949–956, 1988.

183. Piguet P-F, Grau GE, Allet B, et al: Tumor necrosis factor-cachectin is an effector of skin and gut lesions of the acute phase of the graft-vs-host disease. *J Exp Med* 166:1280–1289, 1987.

184. MacDonald TT, Spencer J: Evidence that activated mucosal T cells play a role in the pathogenesis of enteropathy in human small intestine. *J Exp Med* 167:1341–1349, 1988.

185. Entrican JH, Busuttil A, Ferguson A: Are the focal microscopic jejunal lesions in Crohn's disease produced by a T-cell-mediated immune response? *Scand J Gastroenterol* 22:1071–1075, 1987.

186. Pabst R: The anatomical basis for the immune function of the gut. *Anat Embryol* 176:135–144, 1987.

PART THREE

REGULATION

CHAPTER 8

IgA B-Cell Development

WARREN STROBER

GREGORY R. HARRIMAN

MICHAEL C. SNELLER

INTRODUCTION

One of the defining features of the mucosal immune system is its preferential utilization of the IgA immunoglobulin class for its B cell response to antigenic challenge. Over the years, this central aspect of mucosal immune function has led to a wide-ranging series of investigations directed at understanding the Ig class-specific cellular and molecular mechanisms that underlie IgA B cell differentiation. In this chapter we shall examine the results of these investigations and, in doing so, attempt to construct a coherent overview of the factors controlling the major component of the mucosal humoral response.

To set the discussion in a broad prospective, we will begin with a brief description of the anatomy of the mucosal immune system and thus the cellular microenvironment in which IgA B cells develop and mature. We will then proceed to a discussion of the molecular aspects of B cell differentiation so as to define the biochemical processes that govern B cell differentiation generally and IgA B cell differentiation particularly. Finally, we will go on to our main subject, an account of the factors involved in the emergence of IgA B cells and their subsequent regulation.

ANATOMY OF THE MUCOSAL IMMUNE SYSTEM

The mucosal immune system can be divided into two parts on the basis of its morphology and function.[1] The first of these is the so-called organized lymphoid tissues, which consist of the mucosal follicles present in the wall of the intestinal and respiratory tracts. These are known respectively as the gut-associated lymphoid tissue (GALT) and the bronchus-associated lymphoid tissue (BALT). The second is the diffuse lymphoid tissues that are widely distributed beneath the epithelial cells in the mucosal areas. The organized tissues are generative or "afferent" lymphoid areas where antigens (and mitogens) bring about initial cell activation and differentiation. Conversely, the diffuse lymphoid tissues are receiving or "efferent" lymphoid areas where antigens interact with cells to bring about terminal differentiation leading to antibody production or cytotoxic reactions. These two parts of the mucosal system are linked by a "homing" mechanism by which cells (particularly B cells) that have developed in the organized tissues leave the latter and migrate to the diffuse lymphoid tissues. Recent studies suggest that this homing mechanism is dependent on the presence of lymphocyte receptors that recognize organ- or tissue-specific endothelial cell "addressins" in the various mucosal organs, and that facilitate site-specific passage of lymphocytes through endothelial cells.[2,3]

The morphology of the mucosal follicles is distinguished from those in the systemic lymphoid system by the fact that antigens enter the former by way of specialized epithelial cells, known as M cells, which transport antigen from the gut lumen via pinocytosis to the cells in the follicle proper.[4] The area immediately subjacent to the M cells, the so-called dome area, is rich in cells potentially capable of antigen presentation, such as macrophages, dendritic cells, and B cells.[5] These cells are readily pulsed by antigens that have entered the system by the oral route.[6] The dome area is also rich in T cells, which, in most cases, bear the CD4 antigen.

Below the dome area is the follicular/germinal center area. In this region B cells are the predominant cell type, although scattered T cells are also found. The germinal centers are not unlike those in systemic lymphoid tissues in that they contain many relatively differentiated, membrane IgD− B cells.[7] However, B cells in this location differ from those in systemic germinal centers by the fact that a large fraction bear membrane IgA (mIgA).[7] Terminally differentiated B cells (plasma cells) are conspicuously absent from the mucosal follicles, presumably because B cells exit the follicle as they begin transformation into plasma cells.

As for the diffuse mucosal lymphoid tissues, these are made up of a complex assortment of cells, including T cells, B cells, macrophages, and several nonlymphoid cell types. Cells located above the epithelial basement membrane, among the epithelial cells, are called intraepithelial lymphocytes (IEL) and are composed of several types of T cells, but not B cells.[8] It has been shown in the mouse that a large fraction of the intraepithelial T cells bear the $\gamma\delta$ T-cell receptor, rather than the $\alpha\beta$ receptor.[9] Cells in the lamina propria (LPL) are composed of both T cells and B cells (as well as macrophages, granulocytes, and mast cells). The T cells consist, in part, of CD4+ cells that are distinguished from those in other tissues by the fact that they bear surface molecules indicative of cell activation (e.g., IL-2 receptors) and that they secrete a panoply of lymphokines that favor B-cell differentiation.[10] The B cells consist largely of IgA plasma cells secreting dimeric or polymeric IgA that is ultimately transferred to the mucosal surface by an IgA-specific transport mechanism.[1]

Restating the above information from the point of view of the IgA B cell, we can say that organized mucosal lymphoid tissues contains developing B cells that advance to the stage of mIgA expression, sIgA+ B cells. The latter then migrate to the mesenteric node and to the diffuse mucosal areas, where they undergo terminal differentiation and secrete IgA. As we shall see, these various steps in the IgA B cell differentiation cycle are governed by lymphokines and cytokines secreted by regulatory cells present in the various mucosal sites. A final point is that while most IgA B cell development takes place in mucosal tissues, it remains possible that some IgA B cells develop in other areas as well. In this regard, the bone marrow contains substantial numbers of B cells capable of producing IgA, and there is some evidence that many of these cells are generated locally rather than at mucosal sites.[11]

CELLULAR AND MOLECULAR EVENTS OCCURRING DURING B CELL DEVELOPMENT

The B Cell Lineage

During most of their life cycle, cells that ultimately become IgA B cells share a differentiation process with B cells of other isotypes. Thus we preface our discussion of IgA B cell development with a consideration of overall B cell development.

B cells have their origin in pluripotential stem cells present in fetal liver and adult bone marrow. The earliest cells of the B lineage are recognizable by the fact that they bear certain B-cell-specific surface markers detected by monoclonal antibodies.[12] These early B cells develop into "pre-B cells", that express cytoplasmic (but not surface) μ-heavy chains and then into "immature B cells" that express complete IgM molecules on the cell surface. Immature B cells, in turn, become "mature B cells" that co-express membrane IgM (mIgM) and IgD (mIgD). Finally, mature B cells undergo isotype switch differentiation into membrane IgG-, IgE-, IgA-expressing B cells and terminal differentiation into Ig-secreting plasma cells. B cell development prior to switch and terminal differentiation is initiated or regulated either by direct interactions with regulatory cells (such as stromal cells or T cells) or by exposure to various cytokines and lymphokines. In contrast, switch and terminal differentiation require B cells that have been activated by antigen (or *in vitro* by mitogen). An overview of B cell development is shown in Figure 8–1.

Molecular Genetics of B-Cell Development

The cellular transformations described above reflect a series of molecular events that involve the ordered rearrangement and deletion of DNA gene segments (genes) encoding the heavy and light chains of the Ig molecule. Prior to the onset of B cell development, the region of the genome dedicated to the Ig molecule consists of many structural genes separated by intervening DNA. Thus, the variable region of the heavy chain gene region consists of several hundred to more than a thousand variable (V) genes, 10 to 20 diversity (D) genes, and four joining (J) genes,[16] followed, in turn, by the various heavy chain constant (C_H) region genes. In the human the heavy chain gene complex is located on chromosome 14,[17] while in the mouse it is located on chromosome 12.[18] The light chain genes are organized in a similar manner except no D genes are present.[16] Two separate families of light chain genes, designated kappa (κ) and lambda (λ), are present, each lying on a different chromosome.[18-20] In the mouse, the κ locus consists of four functional Jκ segments located upstream from a single constant region κ gene (Cκ); in contrast, the murine λ gene locus consists of only two Vλ genes located upstream from two Jλ-Cλ genes.[21] An overview of the molecular events occurring during B cell development is shown in Fig. 8–2.

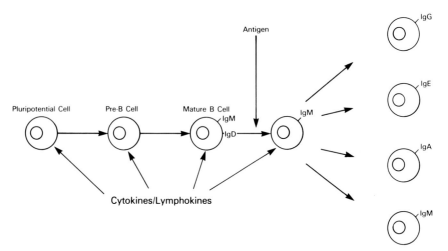

Figure 8 – 1   The B-cell developmental pathway. A pluripotential B cell located in the adult bone marrow is induced to differentiate into pro-B cells, first displaying B-cell-specific markers. The pro-B cells develop into pre-B cells that can synthesize μ heavy chains but not light chains; these cells lack surface Ig. The pre-B cells develop into mature, surface IgM/IgD-bearing and IgM-bearing B cells that can be activated by antigen and that undergo either isotype switch differentiation into IgG, IgA, and IgE B cells and/or terminal differential into IgM, IgG, IgA, and IgE-producing plasma cells. Each of these steps requires one or more cytokines or lymphokines; however, only the last two steps require antigen.

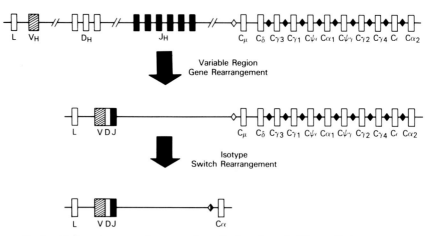

Figure 8 – 2   Molecular events occurring during B-cell differentiation heavy chain rearrangement. In the germline state the heavy chain gene complex is composed of many hundred variable (V) region genes, ~10 D region genes, and 6 J region genes. These undergo rearrangement as indicated in the text to form a recombined VDJ gene that encodes the variable region of the Ig molecule. The Ig gene in this state is found in sIgM-bearing B cells. During isotype switching a second rearrangement occurs depending on recombination between the $C\mu$ switch region and one of the downstream C_H switch regions. The resultant Ig gene is found in an sIgG-, sIgE- or sIgA-bearing B cell depending on which recombination occurs.

Variable Region Gene Assembly

The formation of a functional heavy chain variable region (V_H) is accomplished by the joining of individual V-D-J genes into a functional V_H gene. Such joining is accomplished by a series of site-specific interactions between DNA sequences flanking the structural genes that are followed by DNA loop formation and deletion.[16] The site-specific interactions involve sequences that are made up of a conserved 7 base pair (bp) sequence (heptamer) located immediately adjacent to the structural gene, as well as a conserved 9 bp sequence (nonamer) which is separated from the heptamer by a nonconserved spacer region that is either 12 or 23 bp in length. Recombination (joining of two gene segments) only occurs between a sequence whose heptamers and nonamers are separated by 12 bp and a segment whose heptamers and nonamers are separated by 23 bp.[22,23] D_H genes are always flanked by heptamer-nonamer sequences separated by 12 bp spacers and thus can join only to the 3′ end of the V_H genes and the 5′ end of all J_H genes since these genes are always flanked by heptamer-nonamer sequences separated by 23 bp spacers; conversely, V_H genes cannot join to J_H genes, since both are flanked by a heptamer-nonamer sequence separated by 23 bp spacers. Although V_H-D_H joining is permitted by the 12/23 joining rule, it is not observed; instead, D_H-J_H joining occurs first, followed by V_H-$D_H J_H$ joining.[24] Light chain V and J segments are also flanked by the appropriate recognition sequences and recombine in accordance with the 12/23 joining rule.[16]

The exact mechanism by which the above DNA rearrangements occur is not known, but based on the various joining patterns that have been observed, a multistep process has been proposed.[25] In the first step the genes to be joined are brought into alignment, and a double-stranded DNA cleavage occurs at the junction of the coding sequence and the flanking recognition sequences. Next, back-to-back fusion of the recognition sequences occurs, followed by deletion of the latter along with intervening DNA. Before the joining of the two coding sequences, modifications involving deletion and/or addition of bases to the coding sequences can occur (referred to as N-region insertion). Available evidence suggests that the enzyme terminal deoxynucleotidyl transferase (TdT) is involved in this modification process.[26]

The formation of the light chain variable region occurs via a mechanism similar to that governing the heavy chain variable region, with two important exceptions. First, deletion of bases before joining is more limited, and addition of bases (N-region insertion) is rarely seen.[27] Second, DNA sequences between the V and J light chain genes are not always deleted after rearrangement.[28-31] Several possible mechanisms have been proposed to explain this retention of intervening sequences, including sister chromatid exchange, reintegration of deleted sequences, and an inversion joining mechanism.

The rearrangement process, regardless of its exact mechanisms, is by its very nature imprecise. Thus, in order to produce a complete protein, the various Ig gene segments must be joined so that their coding sequences are in the same translational reading frame (which should occur in approximately one of three rearrangements), and the joined segments must be free of any in-phase translation termination codons. Rearrangements that do not exhibit these characterstics will fail to give rise to functional Ig proteins and are referred to as nonproductive rearrangements. If one of every three VDJ rearrangements is productive, one would predict that 40% of developing B cells will have nonproductive VDJ rearrangements on both chromosomes. Recent studies of Abelson virus transformed pre-B-cell lines (which are undergoing VDJ rearrangements) are in accord with this prediction.[24] B cells having nonproductive rearrangements on both chromosomes presumably represent dead-end cells that do not undergo further development.

From the above description of variable region gene assembly, the mechanisms underlying antibody diversity become clear. First, such diversity is the product of the random selection of different combinations of V-D-J genes on both the heavy and light chain. Second, it occurs as a result of somatic mutation occurring after V region assembly.[32] Third and finally, it occurs as a result of in-frame variability in the joining sites or insertion of bases (N-region insertions) at the joining sites. The molecular events involved in variable region gene assembly occur in the B cell during its pre-B-cell stage, prior to the time it displays an antigen receptor. Thus the generation of diversity is independent of antigen stimulation; nevertheless, the latter is ultimately involved in the selection and expansion of particular cell clones.

Regulation of Variable Region Assembly

The formation of a functional Ig variable region during B cell development is a tightly regulated process characterized by the fact that the variable region genes are assembled in a strict order and that only one heavy chain allele and one light chain allele are expressed in a given B cell (a phenomenon known as allelic exclusion). Regarding the variable region gene assembly order, studies employing a variety of transformed pre-B cell lines and normal pre-B cells indicate that heavy chain variable region assembly always precedes light chain variable region assembly and that the generation of a productive VDJ rearrangement terminates further heavy chain gene assembly and initiates light chain rearrangement.[33-38] Recent evidence suggests that it is the production of a complete μ-heavy chain protein that serves to regulate these two events.[39,40] As for light chain gene assembly, older studies of a number of B cell lines indicate that assembly of the κ gene precedes that of the λ gene.[41-44] The key event governing this order seems to be the production of a light chain protein that can pair with the pre-existing heavy chain to form a complete Ig molecule;[45] once this occurs, further light chain gene rearrangement ceases. Newer studies, however, indicate that this sequential model ($\kappa \rightarrow \lambda$) may need to be modified, in that small populations of murine B cells coexpress λ and λ light chains.[46]

Regarding allelic exclusion, present evidence suggests that it is the production of the μ-protein that signals the cessation of heavy chain rearrangement and the beginning of light chain rearrangement, whereas the production of a complete Ig molecule stops light chain rearrangement.[46,47]

Ig Gene Expression

Ig gene expression is under the control of a promotor region located upstream of the RNA polymerase start site of each V gene as well as an enhancer region located in the intron region separating the recombined VDJ genas and the first C_H gene.[48,49] In recent years it has become apparent that initiation of transcription involves the activity of DNA binding proteins, which bind to the promotor and enhancer regions and increase their accessibility to transcriptional machinery.[49] Thus, although all cells have the requisite promotor/enhancer regions associated with their Ig genes, only B cells have the necessary DNA binding proteins that allow these regions to become operational. In addition, the promotor region of the Ig gene in B cells may have an enhanced capacity to interact with DNA binding proteins because it has undergone a DNA rearrangement that brings the promotor region into physical proximity to the enhancer region.

The Ig promotor region contains a conserved octameric DNA sequence, ATTTGCAT, (OCTA site) which lies just upstream of the TATA box (the major RNA polymerase binding site).[50] It has been shown that lymphoid cells contain a specific DNA binding protein, NF-A2, which is inducible by lypopolysaccharide (LPS) and which binds to the OCTA site.[50,51] It is postulated that such binding leads to or enhances the accessibility of the promotor region to RNA polymerase and/or other necessary transcriptional factors and is thus a key step (if not *the* key step) in Ig gene activation.

The Ig enhancer region, on the other hand, contains a number of sites that interact with DNA binding proteins.[51] These include so-called E sites ($E_1 - E_4$ in the C_H gene and $E_1 - E_3$ in the $C\kappa$ gene) having a consensus sequence of CAGGTGGC, a B site in the $C\kappa$ gene having the sequence GGACTTTCC, and an OCTA site in the C_H gene that is identical to the OCTA sequence associated with the Ig promotor already mentioned. The E sites bind several different proteins that are widely distributed in different cell types. Nevertheless such binding in vivo occurs only in B cells, suggesting that specific chromatin conformation or other factors determine actual binding. On the other hand, a DNA binding factor that binds to the B site, NF-κB, does seem to have some B-cell specificity, since the level of this binding factor correlates with κ gene expression and is dependent on the presence of B-cell activators (such as LPS).[49,52] Interestingly, evidence has been presented that NF-κB is present in many cells but in an inactive form that is maintained by the presence of other proteins; thus control of NF-κB activity may relate to its state of activation.[52] Finally, the OCTA site present in both the promotor and enhancer regions also interacts with a lymphoid cell-specific factor, which, as mentioned above, is known as NF-A2.[49] However, while the OCTA site is necessary for promotor activity, it is not necessary for enhancer activity (at least in the systems so far studied). This illustrates the fact that there is some redundancy in the control system for Ig gene expression.

The synthesis or activity of the nuclear binding proteins that control Ig gene transcription are in turn controlled by poorly understood mechanisms related to level of cell differentiation and activation. In this regard, it is important to mention here a possibility that we will return to later, namely that cytokines and lymphokines may influence the rate of synthesis or the state of activation of nuclear binding factors.

Ig Heavy Chain Class Switching

Following heavy chain V region assembly the heavy chain Ig gene is composed of a rearranged VDJ segment juxtaposed to the IgM constant region (Cμ). Similarly, the rearranged light chain gene is composed of either a Vκ-Jκ or Vλ-Jλ segment juxtaposed to either the Cκ or Cλ genes respectively. At this point the immature B cell is expressing membrane IgM (mIgM). At a somewhat later stage of development the B cell begins to coexpress mIgD and mIgM. This is accomplished by the production of a long primary mRNA transcript that includes the VDJ sequences along with the Cμ and Cδ sequences. This transcript is then alternatively spliced to give rise to $C\mu$ and $C\delta$ mRNA transcripts that each contain the same VDJ variable region genes.[53]

The next stage of B-cell development involves a process known as isotype switch differentiation, whereby a given mIgM-bearing B cell is able to give rise to cells that express the same variable region as the parent IgM B cell in association with one or another of the various C_H regions. In the mouse there are eight genetically and structurally defined Ig heavy chain classes and/or subclasses: IgM, IgD, IgG3, IgG1, IgG2b, IgG2a, IgE, and IgA. In the human, this basic arrangement seems to have undergone duplication in that the $C\mu$ and $C\delta$ genes are followed by two tandem segments each containing $C\gamma$, $C\epsilon$, and $C\alpha$ genes.[54] These distinct Ig isotypes are capable of mediating a variety of specialized effector functions. Thus, the membrane bound form of IgM serves as the B cell antigen receptor responsible for triggering most primary B cell responses, whereas the secretory form of IgM is the first class of antibody produced in the humoral immune response and is efficient at fixing complement and at agglutinating antigens. In contrast, IgG, because of its capacity to bind to cells via the Fc receptor, is an essential component in the opsonization of bacteria and other organisms. IgA, because of its secretion onto mucosal surfaces, plays an important role in defense against pathogens that might gain entry via the oral and respiratory tracts. Thus, by associating a given variable region with different heavy chain isotypes, the immune system is able to use the same antibody receptor to mediate a variety of effector functions.

The precise mechanisms involved in isotype switching are, in principle, similar to those responsible for variable region gene assembly reviewed above. In the one most generally accepted (the "looping out" model), DNA sequences (switch sites) located 5' to the $C\mu$ and 5' to a downstream C_H gene are brought together, and the intervening DNA in the loop thus formed is deleted.[55] In a second mechanism, one that probably occurs only under special circumstances if it occurs at all (the sister chromatid exchange model), switching results from "crossing over" between sister chromatids, which takes place after chromosome replication and before cell division.[56] Such crossing over could produce a reverse in the order of the C_H genes, such as that observed in certain plasmacytoma cell lines.[56] The structure of the switch sites, i.e., the locus of recombination in either model, has been determined by comparing the DNA sequences in the regions 5' to C_H genes in cells in which Ig genes are not expressed (e.g., liver cells) with the 5' DNA sequences in cells expressing one or another isotype (e.g., plasma cells). In this way it has been shown that the switch sites are DNA regions containing tandem repeats sharing dispersed TGACC and TGGG sequences.[55]

Further details concerning the events occurring during switch recombination are gradually becoming known. An important recent finding is that transcription of a downstream C_H gene can occur prior to its recombination with the VDJ genes.[57] This suggests that the same DNA binding proteins that bind to particular regions of DNA and increase their accessibility to RNA polymerases may also increase their accessibility to recombinases. In addition, such DNA binding factors may have a direct role in the formation of the "loops" that occur during switch recombination or serve as points of attachment for switch recombinases, which secondarily form the loops.

That downstream C_H genes are transcribed prior to recombination fits with recent studies establishing that B cells pass through a stage in which they express sIgM in association with another, more downstream isotype and that in such double isotype-expressing cells the downstream C_H gene is not rearranged, i.e., is in a germline configuration.[58-60] The mechanism underlying such double C_H gene expression may involve the synthesis of a long primary mRNA transcript encoding both the $C\mu$ gene followed by the downstream C_H gene followed by the processing of the long transcript to yield message for the individual immunoglobulins that are expressed on the cell surface. Alternatively, it is possible that $C\mu$ and downstream C_H gene message are produced separately, and the latter is subsequently "trans-spliced" to VDJ message or else is expressed as protein that does not contain variable region (VDJ) determinants. Additional studies of clonal cells lines capable of undergoing switch recombination will be necessary to decide between these possibilities.

IgA B-CELL SWITCH DIFFERENTIATION

Having discussed the general cellular and molecular mechanisms governing the differentiation of all B cells, we are now in a position to turn our attention to a process occurring during the development of one kind of B cell, the IgA B cell. Here, we must consider first the isotype switch differentiation step that results in the differentiation of sIgM-expressing B cells into sIgA-expressing B cells, since this is necessarily the step that establishes the B cell as an IgA B cell.

Antigen-Driven, Random IgA B-Cell Differentiation

An initial concept of IgA B cell isotype switch, one put forward by Cebra et al., was that such switching was a B cell centered process unaffected by regulatory signals emanating from other cells.[61-63] These investigators started with the assumptions that: 1) switch differentiation occurs in a more or less random fashion and involves progressively more downstream C_H genes; and 2) switch differentiation is facilitated by cell activation or division. They then postulated that the pattern of isotype expression of a B cell population was related mainly to the level of antigenic exposure to which the population had been subjected and thus in the case of B cells that have undergone a number of rounds of antigen-driven activation/proliferation, one necessarily sees a large number of cells expressing relatively downstream C_H genes. Finally, they postulated that the occurrence of IgA B cells in the mucosal area follows from the fact that mucosal B cells are more exposed to antigenic/mitogenic stimuli than B cells in other lymphoid areas and that in the mouse the $C\alpha$ gene is the most downstream of the Ig genes. A problem that arises in applying this reasoning to human systems is that in humans the Ig gene region is composed of two blocks of C_H genes with a $C\alpha1$ gene at the end of one block and a $C\alpha2$ gene at the end of another (see discussion above). In this case, therefore, the theory would have to be modified so as to include the possibility that random switching events have an intermediate $C\alpha$ gene stop point in addition to the obligate stop point at the end of the entire Ig gene set.

In support of this "B cell centered" theory of IgA switch differentiation, Cebra et al. marshalled evidence that the expression of the IgA isotype in the mucosal B cell population was critically dependent on the level of antigenic stimulation to which the cell population had been exposed.[61-63] Thus, using the Klinman splenic focus assay in which the clonal progeny of individual B cells seeded into spleens of irradiated mice are examined, these authors showed that many more "IgA-only" clones were found in mice exposed to a full panoply of mucosal antigens/mitogens (conventional animals) as compared with mice exposed to a limited number of such antigens/mitogens (germ-free animals). In addition, they demonstrated that antigen challenge of mice by the oral route led to the appearance of increased numbers of IgA-only clones or clones secreting IgA as well as other isotypes.

While these data are undoubtably valid, they nevertheless fall considerably short of proving any particular theory of IgA B cell differentiation. The difficulty lies in the fact that the systems studied were complex and, in fact, the B cells ultimately assayed developed in a milieu containing T cells and other cells. Thus one can also use the data presented to argue that the main effect of increased antigenic-mitogenic challenge on IgA B cell development was not on B cells directly, but rather on T cells or other cells and the release of factors by the latter that direct the course of B cell differentiation. As a matter of fact, Mongini and Paul in later work using the same splenic focus assay as that used by Cebra et al. showed that clonal B cell populations derived from athymic animals manifest poor IgA responses and that the latter are augmented when T cells are added to the system.[64] In addition, they showed that clonal B cell populations secreting IgA do not cosecrete any of the IgG subclasses; thus IgA B cells appear to originate independently of IgG B cells.[65] The Mongini data, therefore, quite clearly pointed to a more complex concept of IgA B cell isotype differentiation, one in which the path of B cell differentiation is regulated by "outside" factors.

Another kind of evidence in favor of random B cell switching, one that applies to B cells generally, not just IgA B cells, comes from recent molecular studies of isotype switching in human B cell neoplasms.[66,67] Here it was found that (regardless of the specific tumor type) the Ig gene on the allellically excluded, inactive chromosome was not usually switched to the same C_H gene as the C_H gene on the active chromosome. Since a directed switch would, theoretically at least, have led to the same C_H deletions on both chromosomes, these data argue that switching is random. However, these data are at odds with data obtained in murine systems wherein it was found that B cell hybridomas usually manifested correlated switches on both chromosomes.[68] Thus it is possible that the human data, in that it relies on neoplastic B cells, does not reflect physiologic switching events.

Directed, Cytokine/Lymphokine-Dependent IgA B-Cell Differentiation

In opposition of a B cell-centered concept of IgA switch differentiation is the concept that such differentiation is a directed process involving signals that address cells in a Ig class-specific fashion and emanating from cells other than B cells. The initial support for this view was the observation that the ability of the whole animal to synthesize IgA depends on the integrity of the T cell system. Thus it was shown in early studies that thymectomized animals have decreased IgA antibody responses and that nude (congenitally athymic) mice have low serum IgA levels.[69,70] Similarly, it was found that in humans with severe thymic abnormalities, such as those with ataxia-telangiectasia, one observes IgA deficiency.[71] These in vivo observations were ultimately complemented by several in vitro studies. Thus, in the early 1980s, Elson et al. showed that concanavalin A (con A)-stimulated T cells added to cultures of LPS-activated B cells had a profound effect on isotype expression, depending on the T cell source: con A-activated Peyer's patch T cells suppressed both IgM and IgG production and enhanced IgA production, whereas con A-activated splenic T cells suppressed production of all Ig classes, including IgA.[72] These effects could be obtained regardless of the B cell source, indicating that they were T cell-specific rather than B cell-specific. Altogether, these studies pointed quite clearly to the possibility that T cells regulate IgA responses in a class-specific manner. As such, they presaged the studies of Mongini et al., mentioned above, in which it was shown that T cells are probably involved in IgA B cell expression.

Subsequent studies of the role of regulatory cells in IgA B cell development began to address the question of whether the regulatory effect could be exerted at the level of IgA switch differentiation. In initial studies of this kind, Kawanishi and his colleagues studied the capacity of clonal Thy 1+ cells derived from Peyer's patches or spleen to induce sIgM+ B cells to differentiate into sIgA+ B cells.[73,74] In these studies purified populations of sIgM+ B cells obtained from Peyer's patches were cultured *in vitro* with or without cloned Thy 1+ cells (putative T cells) from Peyer's patches or spleen, in the presence of the B cell stimulant LPS. It was found that the sIgM+ B cells cultured with LPS alone or in the presence of cloned Thy 1+ cells from spleen gave rise to sIgM+ and sIgG+ B cells as well as IgM- and IgG-producing plasma cells after 5 days of culture, but very few IgA+ B cells or IgA-producing plasma cells. In contrast, the same B cells cultured with Peyer's patch clonal Thy 1+ cells led to the appearance of large numbers of sIgA+ B cells and decreased numbers as sIgG+ B cells. To address the question of whether such sIgA+ B cells derived from the preferential expansion of a small, previously inapparent, subpopulation of sIgA+ B cells still present in the purified sIgM+ B cell population, the cloned Thy 1+ cells were cocultured with preselected sIgA+ B cells to determine if the latter would proliferate faster than sIgM+ B cells in similar cocultures. It was found that sIgA+ and sIgM+ B cells have similar proliferation rates, and it was thus concluded that the sIgA+ B cells had not arisen from a hidden sIgA+ B cell subpopulation. Finally, it was determined that the sIgA+ B cells appearing in such cultures were able to secrete IgA if they were subsequently exposed to T cell-derived factors that enhance terminal B cell differentiation.[74] In summary then, the Peyer's patch-derived Thy 1+ T cells appeared to be capable of inducing sIgM+ B cells to undergo isotype switch to functional sIgA+ B cells and that, as a corollary, IgA switch differentiation is a directed IgA-specific process governed by factors outside of the B cell.

On the basis of its Thy 1-positivity, Kawanishi et al. believed that the switch cell necessary for IgA B cell isotype differentiation was a T cell; however, this cell also expressed major histocompatibility complex (MHC) class II surface antigen, an antigen not found on murine T cells. Thus, in retrospect, the possibility must be considered that the cell responsible for bringing about isotype switching was another type of cell. Of particular relevance here are recent studies showing that when highly purified sIgM+ (sIgA−) Peyer's patch B cells are incubated with Peyer's patch stromal cells (in the presence of LPS), large numbers of B cells that express membrane IgA make their appearance, which, under appropriate conditions, can be made to secrete significant amounts of IgA (Harriman and Strober, unpublished data). These studies suggest that stromal cells can induce IgA-specific isotype switch and, by extension, that the switch cells studied by Kawanishi et al. were cells with stromal cell characteristics.

Further studies relevant to cells that might regulate IgA switch differentiation were those conducted by Spalding et al. in which pre-B cells, obtained by culture of bone marrow cells with IL-3, were used as the regulatable B cell population.[75] In this case, the pre-B cells were cultured with cellular aggregates containing both dendritic cells and T cells obtained from either the spleen or the Peyer's patch. In the former instance, the pre-B cells underwent differentiation and synthesized large amounts of IgM, but only small amounts of IgG/IgA, whereas in the latter instance, the pre-B cells underwent differentiation and synthesized large amounts of IgA and only modest amounts of IgM/IgG. The ability of the dendritic-T cell aggregates to enhance IgA secretion in these studies correlated with the source of the dendritic cells rather than T cells: the dendritic cells derived from Peyer's patches but not from the spleen manifested the IgA-enhancing effect, and the source of the T cells was immaterial. These studies, in utilizing a B cell population that is not likely to contain preswitched IgA B cells that can be selectively expanded by regulatory cells (rather than switched) validated the concept of directed IgA-specific isotype switching. In addition, they support the concept that such switching is at least partly due to a non-T cell present in the Peyer's patch.

Finally, studies conducted by Mayer et al. of the human immunodeficiency state known as the hyper-IgM syndrome also provided evidence of directed isotype switching.[76] The hyper-IgM syndrome is characterized by the presence of increased amounts of serum IgM and the absence of serum IgG or IgA. This abnormality is represented on the cellular level by B cells that express sIgM, but not sIgG or sIgA and that produce only IgM when cultured with mitogen (pokeweed mitogen) in the presence of either patient or normal T cells. However, if B cells from hyper-IgM patients are cultured with T cells from a particular T cell neoplasm (a patient with a certain form of T cell leukemia) they were able to undergo isotype switch and produce IgG alone or in combination with IgA. These studies show quite clearly, therefore, that T cells are indeed part of the switch differentiation process, perhaps in association with the non-T cell regulatory elements discussed above.

Taken together, the above cellular studies of IgA B cell development provide persuasive evidence that IgA switch differentiation is indeed a directed rather than random process. Nevertheless, certain important questions remain. The first relates to the fact that the findings so far obtained, despite considerable effort, do not completely rule out the possibility that the various regulatory cells (stromal cell, dendritic cell, or T cell) are acting to expand selectively hidden B cell subpopulations that are already committed to IgA differentiation, rather than causing de novo IgA switch differentiation. Definitive evidence that this is not the case would involve the use of potentially differentiable clonal B cell populations that have been determined to be B cells not committed to IgA differentiation using molecular techniques. Such a B cell population does not yet exist, but may become available in the future with the application of newly discovered lymphokines (e.g., IL-7) to in vitro B cell culture. A second question relates to the actually switching signals emitted by isotype switching cells. Here we have to turn to studies of the role of cytokines and lymphokines in B cell isotype differentiation, as discussed below.

Role of Cytokines/Lymphokines in IgA Switch Differentiation

As just mentioned, additional insights into B cell isotype switching may be derived from studies of the effects of various defined cellular factors (cytokines and lymphokines) on the B cell differentiation process. In initial studies of this type,

Vitetta and her colleagues showed that a lymphokine called BCDFγ and later identified as IL-4, induced LPS-stimulated B cells to produce IgG1 rather than IgG3.[77] Subsequently, Snapper and Paul showed that IL-4 added to LPS-stimulated B cell cultures led to a cell population containing a high proportion of sIgG1+ (40–50%) and sIgE+ (10%) B cells, some of which go on to secrete one or the other of these immunoglobulins.[78] Importantly, these IL-4 effects on IgG1 (and IgE) expression occurred at the expense of IgM and IgG3 expression and can be achieved by pretreating resting cells with the lymphokine.[79] These facts strongly suggest that the IL-4 does, in fact, bring about switch differentiation. Finally, Snapper and Paul have shown that a second lymphokine, IFN-γ, inhibits the IL-4 effect on IgG1 secretion and has an independent enhancing effect on IgG2a secretion.[80] This latter fact introduces the possibility that Ig class and subclass expression is under the general control of one or another specific lymphokine.

The aforementioned findings concerning IL-4 effects on IgG1 (and IgE) expression raise the immediate question of whether IL-4 also plays a role in IgA B cell differentiation. To address this question the capacity of IL-4 to influence IgA expression of normal B cells or B cell lines were recently studied by the present authors. In studies of normal B cells, purified sIgM+ B cells obtained from Peyer's patches and stimulated with LPS were cultured with and without IL-4. It was found that IL-4 brought about little if any IgA expression either in the form of membrane IgA or secreted IgA. Thus IL-4 does not act on normal B cells to induce IgA expression in the same way it does to induce IgG1 expression.

A different picture was obtained, however, in studies of a B cell line known at CH12.LX.[81] This B cell line is one composed of IgM expressing B cells (98% of the whole) that spontaneously differentiate into IgA-expressing cells at a low rate so that at any given time a cloned CH12.LX B cell contains a small proportion of IgA-expressing cells (2% of the whole). Presumably, therefore, the CH12.LX B cell population has some inherent committment to the expression of IgA, and indeed it can be shown that CH12.LX B cells contain germline (sterile) Cα transcripts, indicative of the presence of a significant proportion of cells with activated Cα genes. When IL-4 was added to cultures of CH12.LX cells containing presorted sIgM+ cells (in the absence of LPS), the number of cells expressing surface IgA was markedly increased. In addition, when IL-5 as well as IL-4 was added to the culture, IgA secretion was greatly increased. These findings suggest that IL-4 does, in fact, have an effect on the level of IgA expression, but only on cells that are already committed to such expression.

The studies on the effect of IL-4 on IgA B cell differentiation create some doubt as to whether IL-4 acts as a true switch lymphokine with regard to IgG1 (and IgE) B cell differentiation. In this regard, it remains possible that even if the effects of IL-4 are seen are on sIgM+ B cells, the latter may have already undergone subtle isotype-specific changes at the level of the C_H genes, and the effect of IL-4 may be to preferentially expand cells that have undergone an initial isotype switch step. Arguing against this possibility, however, are recent studies by Stavnezer et al. and Alt et al. showing that the treatment of normal B cells with LPS and IL-4 leads to downstream C_H gene activation, i.e., expression of germline γ1 and ε mRNA transcripts.[82,83] In addition, Alt et al. have shown that IL-4 inhibits γ2b sterile transcript expression that normally occurs in LPS-activated normal B cells and in Ableson virus-transformed B cells.[84] These data suggest that IL-4 does act as a switch factor in some forms of B cell switch differentiation, even if it does not do so in the case of IgA B cell switch differentiation.

A Theory of IgA B-Cell Switch Differentiation

While the information concerning IgA B cell differentiation, as discussed above, is still incomplete, it is nevertheless possible to draw a reasonably complete picture of the overall process (Fig. 8–3). The first step of the differentiation process appears to involve an interaction between cells of the mucosal follicular reticulum (stromal cells or dendritic cells) and sIgM+ B cells, which causes the latter to undergo IgA switch differentiation.[73-76] This interaction can consist of a direct cell-cell event or, alternatively, of a cytokine-mediated event. In the next step, T cells become involved, probably by providing accessory signals that confirm and establish the initial committment to IgA. As yet, the lymphokine involved in such T cell signalling has not been clearly defined, but IL-4 is the major candidate.

It appears likely that the signals that cause IgA switch differentiation operate by inducing DNA-binding factors that bind to $C\alpha$ switch regions. Initially, such binding is followed by transcription of the $C\alpha$ gene, while the latter is still in a germline configuration, and the production of sterile $C\alpha$ transcripts; in this manner, the B cell becomes an "ambiguous" cell that synthesizes both μ mRNA and α mRNA. Such a cell may develop into a B cell that is synthesizing both full-length μ mRNA and α mRNA, the latter via alternative splicing of a long primary mRNA transcript or via transplicing of VDJ mRNA and downstream $C\alpha$ mRNA. Alternatively, the ambiguous B cell may undergo a deletional rearrangement during which the $C\mu$ gene and the $C\gamma$ genes are deleted and the $C\alpha$ gene is brought into position near the VDJ gene. At this point the cell becomes a committed IgA B cell that is subject to a host of postswitch differentiation events, as discussed below.

POSTSWITCH IgA B-CELL DIFFERENTIATION

Cells developing in the Peyer's patches and definitely committed to IgA expression come under the influence of several postswitch regulatory factors that allow the cell to develop into terminally differentiated IgA-producing plasma cells. However,

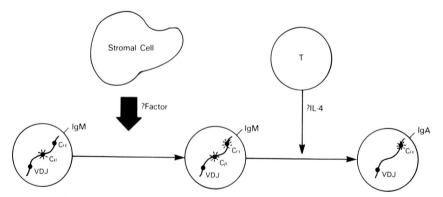

Figure 8–3 IgA B-cell switch differentiation. IgA B cell isotype switch differentiation probably depends on cell-cell interactions with or factors secreted by a stromal cell. In this step the $C\alpha$ gene is activated, and commitment to IgA B-cell differentiation is made. As indicated in the text, it is possible that T-cell factors (?IL-4) are also necessary for the terminal phase of this differentiation step.

very few IgA-producing plasma cells are actually found in the Peyer's patches, and it is likely that such postswitch differentiation either does not occur or is not completed at this site. On the other hand, there is emerging evidence that T cells in the mesenteric nodes and lamina propria differ from those in the mucosal follicles in their capacity to produce the lymphokines necessary for terminal B cell differentiation.[10] It is in these efferent sites, therefore, that one would expect to see the postswitch differentiation events.

Regulation of Postswitch IgA B-Cell Differentiation by Cells Bearing IgA-Fc Receptors

The first IgA-specific postswitch regulatory influences to be discovered were those involving T cells bearing IgA-Fc receptors (Tα cells). To put these studies into prospective, however, we must first discuss the extensive findings of Ishizaka and his colleagues relating to effects of T cells bearing IgE-Fc receptors (Tϵ) on IgE B cell development.[85,86] Ishisaka and his colleagues showed first that Tϵ cells can be induced by IgE (or by IgE-antigen complexes) to produce two types of IgE binding factors, which differ in their pattern of glycosylation: a factor that exhibits N-glycosylation and that potentiates IgE responses, and a factor that exhibits only O-glycosylation and that suppresses IgE responses. Second, they showed, using relevant hybridoma T cells, that T cells can be induced to produce either type of binding factor depending on whether they are stimulated in the presence of a regulatory molecule known as glycosylation-enhancing factor (GEF) or, alternatively, in the presence of a regulatory molecule known as glycosylation-inhibiting factor (GIF); GEF results in IgE binding factors that enhance IgE synthesis, whereas GIF results in IgE binding factors that inhibit IgE synthesis. Finally, these authors showed that IgE binding factors are antigenically related to IgE-Fc receptors and may therefore represent either secreted receptors or shed receptors (or a component thereof). On the basis of these findings, Ishisaka et al. proposed that T cells producing IgE binding factors interact with B cells bearing membrane IgE (i.e., postswitch IgE B cells) and have class-specific positive and negative regulatory effects. This potentially important conclusion, however, must be tempered by the knowledge that the regulatory effects observed were relatively small, (two to fourfold), and thus it remains to be clearly established that the regulatory effects of IgE binding factors are not merely adjunctive to other regulatory influences on IgE B cells. In the latter regard, we have already mentioned the fact that IL-4 may act as a switch factor that induces IgE switch differentiation and thus may influence IgE B cell differentiation in a more fundamental manner.[78]

Studies parallel to those just described on the regulatory role of Tα cells began with the discovery of Strober et al. and Lum et al. that a small but definite proportion of T cells in various lymphoid tissues of mice and humans do in fact bear IgA-Fc receptors.[87,88] These authors, as well as subsequent investigators, were best able to demonstrate such receptors using IgA-coated sheep red blood cells (SRBCs) in rosetting assays, rather than with the use of soluble IgA. This suggested early on that IgA-Fc receptors on T cells have a relatively low affinity for IgA and thus require multivalent IgA ligands to achieve high levels of receptor occupancy.

In subsequent studies of the functional capacities of Tα cells, the latter were found to have both positive and negative effects of the IgA response, just as in the case of the Tϵ cells already discussed. Turning to the positive effects first, it was shown by Kiyono et al. that cloned T cells derived from the mucosal follicles of animals immunized orally with various antigens (SRBCs) fell into two broad categories, those enhancing IgM and IgA and those enhancing responses to all Ig classes.[89] The T cell clones of interest, i.e., the ones preferentially supporting IgA (and IgM) responses were antigen-specific and MHC-restricted; in addition, they contained cells that bore IgA-Fc receptors. Finally, the form of help provided for the IgA response by these T cells was postswitch in character, since they exerted effects on B cells bearing sIgA and not on those lacking sIgA.[90]

In subsequent studies, the same authors showed that T cell hybridomas derived from the above T cell clones (by fusion with a T cell lymphoma cell) also provided help for IgM and IgA, but only if the hybridoma T cell bore IgA-Fc receptors.[91] These hybridoma T cells differed from the T cell clones in being capable of enhancing IgA responses of B cells having a specificity that differed from that of the T cells from which the clones were derived, although antigen still needed to be present in the culture medium (presumably as a B cell activator) for an enhanced IgA response to occur. The fact that the T cell clones were antigen-specific and the T cell hybridomas were not may be explained by assuming that the T cell clones could interact less efficiently than the T cell hybridomas with B cells and thus required an antigen bridge. As discussed below, this may relate, in turn, to the avidity of IgA-Fc receptors on the two cell types. An important additional point concerning these findings was that the help provided by one or more factors present in the supernatant of the T cell cultures could be absorbed out by solid-phase IgA (but not by solid-phase IgG or IgM) and thus consisted of one or more IgA binding factors. However, on further study such binding factors were found to provide both help and suppression: the factor(s) augmented IgA synthesis (about threefold) at moderate dilution and mildly suppressed IgA synthesis at low dilution.

The significance of these findings is not yet clear. One possibility is that Tα cells constitute an important component of postswitch IgA B cell differentiation and that they exert their effects on IgA B cells via release of IgA binding factors. In this view the IgA binding factors, as in the IgE system, interact with membrane-bound IgA on the B cell and thus induce terminal differentiation in an IgA class-specific fashion. However, as already mentioned, it is probable that IgA-Fc receptors have a low affinity for IgA and require multivalency to achieve significant binding. On this basis, released IgA binding factors would be expected to have low affinity for IgA and to lack physiologic significance. Another possibility is that Tα cells have a special effect on IgA response because of their capacity to manifest enhanced cell-cell interaction with IgA B cells (i.e., enhanced capacity to adhere to IgA B cells). This follows from the argument already advanced that binding of IgA to IgA-Fc receptors is more likely if multiple receptor-ligand interactions are initiated at the same time, as would be the case in a cell-cell interaction. As a corollary, the enhanced activity of the T cell hybridomas bearing IgA-Fc receptors (as compared with their clonal T cell parents) may relate to the fact that such cells have been selected for IgA enhancing activity and thus bear higher affinity IgA-Fc receptors than do the unselected T cell clones. The enhanced capacity of either the T cell clones or hybridomas to engage in cell-cell interactions would then provide for more efficient delivery of lymphokines to the IgA B cell, which, as discussed below, is also known to play a role in postswitch IgA B cell differentiation. In addition, it is possible that Tα cells are also influenced by putative cell-cell interaction and become more activated to produce differentiation factors following engagement of their IgA-Fc receptors by membrane-bound multivalent IgA.

Turning now to the negative regulatory effects observed with Tα cells, one should mention first the series of observations by Lynch et al. showing that mice carrying IgA plasmacytomas have, in their spleens, high numbers of Tα cells (as mice bearing IgG and IgM plasmacytomas have high numbers of Tγ and Tμ spleen cells, respectively).[92] Similarly, circulating T cell populations in humans bearing myelomas contain increased numbers of cells bearing Fc receptors for the immunoglobulin type of the myeloma.[92] These findings suggest that the number of T cells bearing Fc receptors for a particular immunoglobulin is to some extent regulated by the concentration of that immunoglobulin. In further studies by Lynch et al. it was shown that the Tα cells present in mice having high IgA levels were generally CD8-positive T cells that manifested IgA class-specific suppressor function.[93,94] This was illustrated by the facts that: 1) orally immunized mice manifested reduced IgA responses but unchanged IgG and IgM responses when such mice were preinfused with large numbers of T cells from mice bearing IgA plasmacytomas; and 2) T cell populations containing a high percentage of cells bearing IgA-Fc receptors inhibited in vitro growth and secretion of IgA plasmacytoma B cells (MOPC-315).

In additional studies related to such Tα cell-mediated suppressor function conducted by Yodoi et al., it was shown that normal human T cells as well as hybridoma T cells bearing IgA-Fc receptors are capable of producing IgA binding factors that cause significant suppression of pokeweed mitogen-induced IgA synthesis (but not IgG or IgM synthesis) by cultured peripheral blood cells.[95,96] The IgA-binding factor was a glycosylated protein having a molecular weight of ~56,000. Similarly, Sarfati et al. showed that human T cells incubated with IgA produced a factor that suppressed mitogen-induced IgA synthesis (but not IgM or IgG synthesis) by cultured peripheral blood cells.[97]

Taken together, the above studies point to the existence of a negative feedback circuit for IgA responses. In the presence of normal IgA levels or low IgA levels, the number of T cells bearing IgA-Fc receptors and the density of IgA-Fc receptor on such T cells may be low. However, as IgA levels increase, particularly IgA in multivalent form (IgA present on cell surfaces or complexed to antigen) IgA-Fc receptors on T cells are up-regulated, and one sees the appearance of T cells capable of suppressing the IgA response. As in the case of the positive effects of Tα cells discussed above, it is possible that the negative effects of Tα cells are mediated by cell-cell interaction or by the release of IgA-Fc binding factors. Both possibilities have some experimental support in that Williams and Lynch have shown that T cells bearing high levels of IgA-Fc receptors form clusters with B cells bearing IgA, and Roman et al. have shown, using MOPC-315 plasmacytoma cells as an indicator cell, that IgA binding factors bind to sIgA-bearing B cells and then suppress the latter's proliferation as well as their production of α heavy chain and λ light chain.[98,99] In view of the discussion above concerning the low affinity of IgA-Fc receptors, it seems likely that, in the end, direct cell-cell interaction will prove to be more important than released IgA binding factors in bringing about IgA-specific suppression under physiologic conditions. In addition, in this case the possibility must also be considered that locally formed IgA complexes give rise to multivalent IgA ligands that can interact with IgA-Fc receptors on T cells and thereby stimulate the latter to release Ig class-nonspecific suppressor factors.

Regulation of Postswitch IgA B-Cell Differentiation by Cytokines and Lymphokines

A second and perhaps dominant form of postswitch IgA B cell regulation is that mediated by cytokines and lymphokines. In point of fact, a host of cytokines/lymphokines have been shown to have regulatory effects on B cells, including IL-1, IL-2, IL-4, IL-5, IL-6, and IFN-γ in murine systems and several other less well characterized materials in human systems.[100] For the most part, the activity of these cytokines/lymphokines in postswitch B cell differentiation has been assumed to be isotype-nonspecific, i.e., they affect B cell differentiation of B cells of various isotypes. However, this has not been studied rigorously using isolated cell populations of a given isotype; hence the possibility remains that certain cytokines/lymphokine or cytokine/lymphokine combinations may affect B cells of one isotype more than another. In this regard, evidence has recently come forward that IL-5 acting alone or in combination with other lymphokines may have special effects on IgA B cell development, and it is to this lymphokine that we shall now turn our attention.

IL-5 is a lymphokine initially identified by Takatsu and his coworkers as T cell replacing factor (TRF-1, B151-K12 TRF) and by Swain and her colleagues as BCGF-II.[101] Functional studies of this molecule have shown that it acts on activated B cells either as a proliferation factor or as a differentiation factor. In addition, biochemical/molecular studies of this substance have established that it is a glycosylated protein consisting of two or more polypeptide chains of 112–113 amino acids that usually occur as a 45–60 kD dimer. Of interest, IL-5 also has potent eosinophil colony-stimulating activity, and there is emerging evidence that substances that antagonize IL-5 activity prevent eosinophil formation.[102]

Early on Takatsu et al. found that IL-5 enhanced both IgM and IgG antibody synthesis (IgA responses were not studied).[103] Later Kagnoff et al. showed that IL-5 containing T cell supernatants or purified IL-5 enhanced both IgM and IgA anti-polysaccharide responses (anti-α 1,3-dextran).[104] Up to this point, therefore, IL-5 did not seem to have an isotype-specific effect. Recently, however, it has been shown that when B cells are stimulated by LPS, IL-5 has relatively greater effects on IgA synthesis than on the synthesis of IgM or on any of the IgG subclasses.[105] Thus, in a polyclonal B cell activation system, IL-5 does appear to be a key lymphokine for IgA. This may have considerable significance to in vivo IgA responses in view of the fact that in the bacteria-rich environment of the mucosa, LPS (along with IL-5) may play an important role in maintaining IgA responses at a certain threshold level.

Recent studies of IL-5 using recombinant material have established that, in LPS-activated cell systems, IL-5 acts on sIgA+ cells, rather than sIgA− cells and is thus a postswitch differentiation factor.[106,107] In addition, it was shown that IL-5 increases IgA synthesis by enhancing B cell differentiation rather than proliferation. On the other hand, little is known about the molecular mechanisms underlying the activation of IL-5 on IgA B cell differentiation (or indeed on IgM/IgG B cell differentiation) other than the fact that IL-5 promotes synthesis of the secretory forms of μ, γ1 and α mRNA.[108]

As indicated above, other lymphokines besides IL-5 act on B cells to promote their terminal differentiation. In this regard, additive or synergistic effects of IL-5, IFN-γ, and IL-2 were reported by Kagnoff et al. and by Harriman et al.[109,110] In addition, in very recent studies, Kunimoto has shown, using B cells from Peyer's patches that were activated in vivo (presumably by environmental antigens), that IL-6 synergizes with IL-5 in promoting IgA responses.[111] This is in contrast to IgM/IgG responses wherein IL-1 and IL-6 appeared to be a more potent cytokine/lymphokine combination. Thus IL-5 and IL-6 may be a particularly important lymphokine combination for postswitch IgA B cell differentiation.

If certain lymphokines are key elements in postswitch IgA B cell differentiation, do there exist certain classes of T cells that preferentially secrete such lymphokines? An early answer to this question was provided by the studies of Elson and Strober mentioned earlier in which it was shown that con-A-activated T cells from Peyer's patches enhanced IgA responses and suppressed IgG and IgM responses, whereas similarly activated T cells from spleen suppressed Ig responses of all classes.[72] In the light of more recent knowledge concerning lymphokines, these data are best explained by assuming that Peyer's patch T cells (as well as mesenteric lymph node cells) are composed of cells that are better able to elaborate lymphokines that enhance IgA synthesis such as IL-5 than spleen T cells. Also relevant to this discussion is the recent discovery that T cells from all lymphoid sources can be grouped into those producing IL-4 and IL-5 on the one hand (TH_2 cells) and IL-2 and IFN-γ on the other (TH_1 cells).[112] On this basis it is attractive to postulate that TH_2 cells are particular prevalent in Peyer's patches and other mucosal tissues.

Having considered the role of cytokines/lymphokines on postswitch B cell differentiation it is important to return to the question of how cytokine/lymphokine effects relate to those mediated by Tα cells (Fig. 8–4). At this point, it is probably best to consider these two modes of IgA class-specific postswitch helper function as two sides of the same coin: on the one hand, Tα cells are IgA-specific helper cells by virtue of their capacity to interact with IgA B cells (via the IgA-Fc receptors); on the other hand, the actual help rendered is mediated by Ig class-nonspecific lymphokines. Stated differently, the ability of Tα cells to act as IgA-specific helper cells is based on the fact that such cells are best able to focus lymphokines on IgA B cells.

Ig CLASS-NONSPECIFIC FORMS OF IgA B-CELL REGULATION

Oral Tolerance

The regulation of IgA B cells is also brought about by general processes governing B cell responses in the mucosal system. One such process (or set of processes) is that involved in the phenomenon of oral tolerance, i.e., the marked tendency of an orally administered protein antigen to induce mucosal and systemic unresponsiveness to that antigen, even when the antigen is subsequently administered by a parenteral route.[113,114] It is widely believed that such tolerance is a necessary feature of an antigenic environment that is replete with "trivial" antigenic materials that would otherwise overwhelm mucosal immune responses needed for host defense.

A number of cellular mechanisms have been shown to account for oral tolerance. The first and most important involves the fact that the mucosal immune system usually responds to antigen with elaboration of antigen-specific suppressor T cells. Thus it can be shown in adoptive transfer experiments that an animal that has

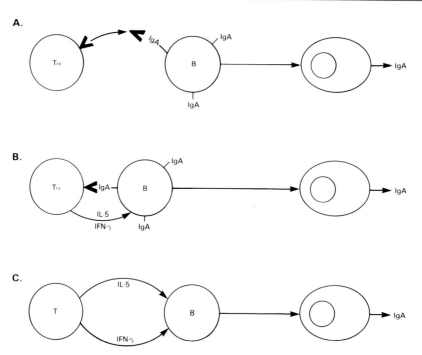

Figure 8–4 Postswitch IgA B-cell differentiation. IgA B-cell postswitch differentiation can potentially occur by several mechanisms: as indicated in **(A)**, a Tα cell can release an IgA binding factor (a form of the IgA-Fc receptor?) that binds to the IgA B cell and induces terminal differentiation; alternatively, as indicated in **(B)**, the same cell can enter into a cell-cell interaction with the IgA B cell and deliver non-isotype-specific lymphokine signals in an efficient fashion. Finally, as indicated in **(C)**, T cells not bearing IgA-Fc receptors may deliver lymphokine signals from a relatively long range.

undergone oral antigen challenge is the source of suppressor T cells that can transfer unresponsiveness to a second animal, even when the latter is challenged by a parenteral route.[115] The suppressor T cells transferable in this manner are found initially in the mucosal system and later in other lymphoid tissues; thus suppressor T cells initially induced at mucosal sites have the capacity to migrate widely. Another possible mode of suppressor T cell development following oral challenge, one not involving the mucosal immune system per se, is that antigen fragments formed in the gastrointestinal tract enter the circulation and induce suppressor T cells in systemic lymphoid tissues.[116]

The cellular interactions that give rise to suppressor T cells in mucosal tissues are probably similar to those in systemic lymphoid tissues. This being said, it is by no means clear why such suppressor T cells are more readily induced in the mucosa than elsewhere. One possibility is that mucosal follicles contain antigen-presenting cells that are particularly capable of initiating suppressor T cell cascades.[117] Another possibility is that antigen fragments formed in the mucosal immune environment are more tolerogenic than the antigens that initiate responses in the systemic immune environment.

A second mechanism of oral tolerance involves the induction of antigen-nonspecific T cells. Evidence for this mechanism is inherent in the observation that mice unresponsive to LPS (C3H/HeJ mice) manifest increased responses to orally administered antigens, as compared with LPS-responsive mice (C3H/H3N mice).[118,119] In addition, such mice have reduced suppressor T cell responses following oral antigen challenge and therefore do not display the phenomenon of oral tolerance (at least with respect to certain antigens). One explanation of the decreased oral tolerance in such mice is that the latter have an increased antigen-nonspecific contrasuppressor T cell activity that down-regulates mucosal suppressor T cells elaborated as a result of oral antigen challenge. Data in support of such increased contrasuppressor T cell activity in LPS-unresponsive mice will be discussed below. Another explanation is that LPS and other B cell mitogens that are present in the mucosal environment normally cause a certain level of B cell activation, and the activated B cells that result subsequently interact with so-called autoreactive T cells, which then develop into antigen-nonspecific suppressor T cells. In either case, one obtains decreased mucosal suppressor T cell activity that is antigen-nonspecific.

Yet a third mechanism of oral tolerance relates to the fact that antigens entering the mucosal immune system may induce clonal inhibition or clonal anergy of B cells and T cells present in the mucosal follicles. This possibility is supported by the fact that (at least in the case of sheep) Peyer's patches are the sites of massive cell turnover and cell death, just as is the thymus.[120]

While oral tolerance may generally involve B cell responses involving all Ig isotypes, it may in some instances spare IgA responses. Thus, in studies by Richman et al., it was shown that oral antigen challenge with a protein antigen led to profound suppression of antigen-specific IgG antibody responses, but preserved or even enhanced antigen-specific IgA antibody responses.[121] In explanation of this finding, one can invoke several of the mechanisms already discussed above, as well as one that relies on contrasuppressor T cells that specifically effects IgA responses (see data in support of this possibility below). Alternatively, one can postulate an Ig class-specific regulatory environment in which IgA class-specific helper T cells are stimulated pari passu with Ig class-nonspecific suppressor T cells to obtain net suppression of IgG and IgM responses along with net help for IgA responses. In any case, the selective preservation of IgA responses may have an important survival advantage to the organism, allowing positive IgA responses that are necessary for host defense function at mucosal surfaces, and disallowing potentially harmful systemic responses to antigens that gain entry to the internal system.

Mucosal Contrasuppressor T Cells

Contrasuppressor T cells are regulatory T cells that are defined by their capacity to reverse T cell-mediated suppression by rendering helper T cells resistant to suppressor T cell signals.[122] First described by Gershon et al., they are thought to be the cellular end product of a complex contrasuppressor T cell circuit that includes inducer, transducer, and effector T cells.[122] Evidence for the occurrence of contrasuppressor T cells in the mucosal immune system was obtained by Green et al., who showed that treatment of Peyer's patch T cell populations with antibodies that remove contrasuppressor-inducer cells or contrasuppressor-effector cells unmasks the presence of suppressor T cells in an in vitro detection system.[123] On this basis

Green et al. postulated that not only do contrasuppressor T cells occur in the mucosal system, but that such cells perform the vital function of allowing positive B cell responses in a lymphoid site where suppressor T cells ordinarily dominate (see discussion of oral tolerance above).

Data relevant to mucosal contrasuppressor T cells was subsequently accumulated by McGhee and his colleagues, who showed first that the reduced suppressor T cell activity following oral antigen challenge to LPS-unresponsive mice (C3H/HeJ mice) was accompanied by the presence in both Peyer's patch and spleen of a T cell population that could reverse oral tolerance in normal mice (LPS-responsive, C3H/HeN mice) both in vitro and in vivo.[124] At low antigen doses the relevant T cell was a cell that lacked markers commonly associated with helper T cells (L3T4), whereas at higher doses the relevant T cell, at least in the spleen, did bear this marker; in both cases, the relevant cell was able to adhere to the lectin *Vicia villosa*, which had previously been shown to specifically bind to contrasuppressor T cells.[125] On this basis, the oral tolerance reversing cell was termed a contrasuppressor T cell. While contrasuppressor T cells are increased in LPS-unresponsive mice, they are by no means absent in normal mice.

Of interest to the present discussion of IgA B cells, McGhee et al. have obtained evidence that the contrasuppressor T cells are isotype-specific: spleen cells with the contrasuppressor phenotype obtained from orally primed mice mediated contrasuppression for all Ig classes, whereas spleen contrasuppressor cells obtained from systemically primed mice exhibited contrasuppressor activity for IgM and IgG classes, but not IgA.[125] In addition, Peyer's patch contrasuppressor T cells exhibited more contrasuppression for IgA than IgM and IgG responses, and the IgA-specific contrasuppressor activity could be removed from cell populations by absorption of the cells to glutaldehyde-fixed IgA-specific helper T cell clones (such as those described above).[124]

These studies appeared to establish a phenotypically and functionally unique subset of cells that regulate IgA responses by reversing IgA-specific suppression. However, at this point in our knowledge, these cells must be redefined in terms of their capacity to produce various types of lymphokines, so as to determine if their effects are entirely on suppressor T cells (as would be the case of true contrasuppressor T cells) or on B cells (as would be the case if the contrasuppressor cell was really a form of helper T cell). In this regard, it has recently been shown that at least some cells that have characteristics of contrasuppressor T cells are able to produce IL-5 (Kagnoff MF, personal communication). In the last analysis, then, to prove the existence of "true" contrasuppressor T cells one must be able to show that there are T cells that act to turn off T cells producing "suppressor" lymphokines.

CONCLUSIONS

The picture of the IgA B cell development that emerges from the above discussion is that such development is a multistate process controlled by both positive and negative factors (Fig. 8–5). The key initial step involves isotype-switch differentiation, and very persuasive evidence has been presented that this is an induced event resulting from cellular interactions specific to the mucosal environment. Such interactions most likely involve a mucosal stromal or dendritic cell and a mucosal T cell that act through direct cellular contact with developing B cells or

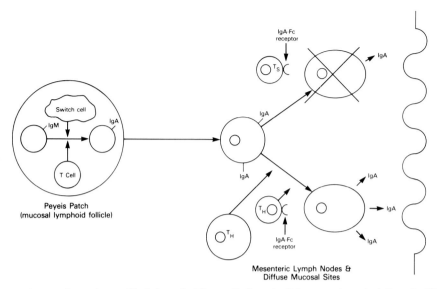

Figure 8 – 5 Overview of IgA B-cell differentiation. In this overview, IgA B-cell differentiation is considered a two-step process consisting of a switch step and a postswitch step. The former occurs in the mucosal follicles (Peyer's patches), whereas the latter occurs in the mesenteric nodes or in the diffuse mucosal lymphoid areas (lamina proprias). The postswitch steps, as shown, can involve enhancing and suppressing interactions, both on a IgA class-specific and -nonspecific basis.

through the release of specific cytokines or lymphokines that have not yet been completely defined. It is likely that the latter influence IgA-specific switch differentiation by inducing DNA-binding proteins that bind to and thereby make accessible key DNA switch sites located 5′ to the $C\alpha$ gene, thus allowing $C\alpha$ gene transcription and rearrangement. Recent evidence indicates that whereas IL-4 may be important to IgG subclass switch differentiation, it does not play a primary role in IgA switch differentiation. Nevertheless, it may act at a later stage in the switch process after the B cell has made an initial commitment to IgA differentiation.

Following IgA isotype switch differentiation, the IgA B cell is acted on by a number of forces that are both IgA class-specific and IgA class-nonspecific. Within the IgA-specific realm are the mechanisms involving T cells bearing IgA-Fc receptors. The thesis has been presented that these cells are either positive or negative regulators that have an increased capacity to interact with IgA B cells by virtue of their IgA-Fc receptors. This allows them to deliver differentiation signals via the secretion of various lymphokines so that what is essentially a IgA class-nonspecific mechanism of B cell help becomes IgA class-specific. Among the important lymphokines and cytokines secreted by such IgA-Fc receptor-bearing T cells as well as by other regulatory T cells acting on postswitch IgA B cells is the lymphokine known as IL-5. Evidence has been brought forward that the latter may be particularly important to IgA B cell differentiation, although clearly this lymphokine also has effects on the differentiation of cells committed to other isotypes. To bring about optimal IgA responses, IL-5 probably acts in conjunction with a number of other lymphokines.

Also affecting IgA B cell differentiation are the mechanisms underlying oral tolerance. For the most part, these involve both antigen-specific and antigen-non-specific suppressor T cells, which affect responses of all classes; however, such regulatory responses may not always apply to IgA responses. Thus oral antigen administration may result in positive IgA response in the face of negative IgG and IgM responses. In a related context, there is some evidence that suppressor T cell responses may be contrasuppressed in an IgA-specific fashion, but this requires additional study at the level of lymphokine production.

Overall, the complexity of IgA B cell differentiation as described here offers a number of challenging possibilities for the control and manipulation of IgA responses for therapeutic purposes. In this regard, it may soon be possible to design specific ways of magnifying IgA responses in an effort to combat pathogens that enter the body via the mucosal surfaces or to control untoward responses to antigens that enter through the mucosa and induce anti-self (autoimmune) responses.

REFERENCES

1. Strober W, Brown WR: The mucosal immune system. In Samter M: *Immunological Diseases,* ed 4. Boston, Little, Brown, 1988, pp 79–139.
2. Jalkanen S, Wu N, Bargatze RF, et al: Human lymphocyte and lymphoma homing receptors. *Annu Rev Med* 38:467–476, 1987.
3. Streeter PR, Berg EL, Rouse BTN, et al: A tissue-specific endothelial cell molecule involved in lymphocyte homing. *Nature* 331:41–46, 1988.
4. Sneller MC, Strober W: M cells and host defense. *J Infect Dis* 154:737–740, 1986.
5. Ermak TH, Owen RL: Differential distribution of lymphocytes and assessory cells in mouse Peyer's patches. *Anat Rec* 215:144–152, 1986.
6. Richman LK, Graeff AS, Strober W: Antigen presentation by macrophage-enriched cells from the mouse Peyer's patch. *Cell Immunol* 62:110–118, 1981.
7. Butcher EC, Rouse RV, Coffman RL, et al: Surface phenotype of Peyer's patch germinal center cells: implication for the role of germinal centers in B cell differentiation. *J Immunol* 129:2698–2707, 1982.
8. Ernst PB, Befus AD, Bienenstock J: Leukocytes in the intestinal epithelium: an unusual immunological compartment. *Immunol Today* 6:50–54, 1985.
9. Goodman T, LeFrancois L: Expression of the gamma-delta T cell receptor on intestinal CD8+ intraepithelial lymphocytes. *Nature* 333:855–858, 1988.
10. Zeitz M, Green WC, Peffer NJ, et al: Lymphocytes isolated from the intestinal lamina propria of normal non-human primates have increased expression of genes associated with T cell activation. *Gastroenterology* 94:647–655, 1988.
11. Kaiserlian D, Delaeroix D, Bach JF: The wasted mutant mouse. I. An animal model of secretory IgA deficiency with normal serum IgA. *J Immunol* 135:1126–1131, 1985.
12. Kincade PW, Lee G, Watanabe T, et al: Antigens displayed on murine B lymphocyte precursors. *J Immunol* 127:2262–2268, 1981.
13. Cooper MD: Pre-B cells: normal and abnormal development. *J Clin Immunol* 1:81–89, 1981.
14. Vittetta ES, Uhr JW: Immunoglobulin receptors revisited. *Science* 189:964–968, 1975.
15. Abney ER, Cooper MD, Kearney JF, et al: Sequential expression of immunoglobulins on developing mouse B lymphocytes: a systematic survey that suggests a model for the generation of immunoglobulin isotype diversity. *J Immunol* 120:2041–2049, 1978.
16. Tonegawa S: Somatic generation of antibody diversity. *Nature* 302:575–581, 1983.

17. Flanagan JG, Rabbitts TH: Arrangement of human immunoglobulin heavy chain constant region genes implies evolutionary duplication of a segment containing gamma, epsilon and alpha genes. *Nature* 300:709–713, 1982.

18. Hengartner H, Meo T, Muller E: Assignment of gene for Ig κ and H chains to chromosomes 6 and 12 in mouse. *Proc Natl Acad Sci USA* 75:4494–4498, 1978.

19. Swan D, D'Eustachio P, Leinwand L, et al: Chromosomal assignment of the mouse κ light chain gene. *Proc Natl Acad Sci USA* 76:2736–2739, 1979.

20. D'Eustachio P, Pravcheva D, Marcu K, et al: Chromosomal location of structural genes encoding murine Ig light chains. *J Exp Med* 151:1545–1550, 1980.

21. Eisen HN, Reilly EB: Lambda chains and genes in inbred mice. *Annu Rev Immunol* 3:337–365, 1985.

22. Early P, Huang H, Davis M, et al: An immunoglobulin heavy chain variable region gene is generated from three segments of DNA: V_H, D and J_H. *Cell* 19:981–992, 1980.

23. Sakano H, Maki R, Kurosawa Y, et al: Two types of somatic recombination are necessary for the generation of complete immunoglobulin heavy chain genes. *Nature* 286:676–683, 1980.

24. Alt FW, Yancopoulos GD, Blackwell TK, et al: Ordered rearrangement of immunoglobulin heavy chain variable region segments. *EMBO J* 3:1209–1219, 1984.

25. Alt FW, Baltimore D: Joining of immunoglobulin heavy chain gene segments: implication from a chromosome with evidence of three D-J_H fusions. *Proc Natl Acad Sci USA* 79:4118–4122, 1982.

26. Desiderio SV, Yancopoulos GD, Paskind M, et al: Insertion of N regions into heavy chain genes in correlated with expression of terminal deoxytransferase in B cells. *Nature* 311:752–755, 1984.

27. Yancopoulos G, Alt FW: Regulation of the assembly and expression of variable region genes. *Annu Rev Immunol* 4:339–368, 1986.

28. Steinmetz M, Altenburger W, Zauchau HG: A rearranged DNA sequence possibly related to the translocation of Ig gene segments. *Nucleic Acids Res* 8:1709–1720, 1980.

29. Hochtl J, Muller CR, Zachau HG: Recombined flanks of the variable and joining segment of Ig genes. *Proc Natl Acad Sci USA* 79:1383–1387, 1982.

30. Hochtl J, Zachau HG: A novel type of aberrant recombination in Ig genes and its implications for V-J joining mechanism. *Nature* 302:260–263, 1983.

31. Fedderson RM, Van Ness BG: Double recombination of a single Ig κ-chain allele: implications for the mechanism of rearrangement. *Proc Natl Acad Sci USA* 82:4793–4797, 1985.

32. Golub ES: Somatic mutation: diversity and regulation of the immune repertoire. *Cell* 48:723–724, 1987.

33. Levitt D, Cooper MD: Mouse pre-B cells synthesize and secrete μ heavy chains but not light chains. *Cell* 19:617–625, 1980.

34. Siden E, Alt FW, Shinefeld L, et al: Synthesis of immunoglobulin μ chain gene products precedes synthesis of light chains during B lymphocyte development. *Proc Natl Acad Sci USA* 78:1823–1827, 1981.

35. Coffman R, Weissman I: Gene rearrangement in pre-B cells. *J Mol Cell Immunol* 1:33–38, 1983.

36. Burrows P, LeJeune M, Kearney JF: Evidence that murine pre-B cells synthesise μ heavy chains but not light chains. *Nature* 280:838–840, 1979.

37. Maki R, Kearney JD, Paige C, et al: Immunoglobulin gene rearrangements in immature B cells. *Science* 209:1366–1369, 1980.

38. Perry RP, Kelley DE, Coleclough C, et al: Organization and expression of immunoglobulin genes in fetal liver hybridomas. *Proc Natl Acad Sci USA* 78:247–251, 1981.

39. Weaver D, Constantini F, Imanishi-Kavi T, et al: A transgenic immunoglobulin mu gene prevents rearrangement of endogenous genes. *Cell* 42:117–127, 1985.

40. Rusconi S, Kohler G: Transmission and expression of a specific pair of rearranged immunoglobulin μ and κ genes in a transgenic mouse line. *Nature* 314:330–334, 1985.

41. Hieter PA, Korsmeyer SJ, Waldman T, et al: Human immunoglobulin κ light chain genes are deleted or rearranged in λ-producing B cells. *Nature* 290:368–372, 1981.

42. Coleclough C, Perry R, Karjalainen K, et al: Aberrant rearrangements contribute significantly to the allelic exclusion of immunoglobulin gene expression. *Nature* 290:372–378, 1981.

43. Durdik J, Moore MW, Selsing E: Novel κ light chain gene rearrangement in mouse λ light chain-producing B lymphocytes. *Nature* 307:749–752, 1984.

44. Siminovitch KA, Bakhshi A, Goldman P, et al: A uniform deleting element mediates the loss of κ genes in human B cells. *Nature* 316:260–262, 1985.

45. Alt FW, Enea V, Bothwell ALM, et al: Activity of multiple light chain genes in murine myeloma lines expressing a single functional light chain. *Cell* 21:1–12, 1980.

46. Persiani DM, Durdik J, Selsing E: Active λ and κ antibody gene rearrangement in Abelson murine leukemia virus-transformed pre-B cell lines. *J Exp Med* 165:1655–1674, 1987.

47. Gollahon KA, Hagman J, Brenster RL, et al: Ig λ-producing B cells do not show feedback inhibition of gene rearrangement: *J Immunol* 141:2771–2780, 1988.

48. Wall R, Kuehl M: Biosynthesis and regulation of immunoglobulins. *Annu Rev Immunol* 1:393–422, 1983.

49. Grosschedl R, Baltimore D: Cell-type specificity of immunoglobulin gene expression is regulated by at least three DNA sequence elements. *Cell* 41:885–897, 1985.

50. Singh H, Sen R, Baltimore D, et al: A nuclear factor that binds to a conserved sequence motif in transcriptional control elements of immunoglobulin genes. *Nature* 319:154–158, 1986.

51. Lenardo M, Pierce JW, Baltimore D: Protein-binding sites in Ig gene enhancers determine transcriptional activity and inducibility. *Science* 236:1573–1577, 1987.

52. Sen R, Baltimore D: Inducibility of κ immunoglobulin enhancer-binding protein NF-κB by a posttranslational mechanism. *Cell* 47:921–928, 1986.

53. Moore KW, Rogers J, Hunkapiller T, et al: Expression of IgD may use both DNA rearrangement and RNA splicing mechanisms. *Proc Natl Acad Sci USA* 78:1800–1804, 1982.

54. Flanagan JG, Robbitts TH: Arrangement of human immunoglobulin heavy-chain constant region genes implies evolutionary duplication of a segment containing γ, ϵ, and α genes. *Nature* 300:709–713, 1982.

55. Shimizu A, Honjo T: Ig class switching. *Cell* 36:801–803, 1984.

56. Obata M, Kataoka T, Nakai S, et al: Structure of a rearranged $\gamma 1$ chain gene and its implication to immunoglobulin class-switch mechanism. *Proc Natl Acad Sci USA* 78:2437–2441, 1982.

57. Stavnezer J, Radcliffe G, Lin Y-C, et al: Immunoglobulin heavy-chain switching may be directed by prior induction to transcripts from constant-region genes. *Proc Natl Acad Sci USA* 85:7704–7708, 1988.

58. Yoita Y, Kumagai Y, Okumura K, et al: Expression of lymphocyte surface IgE does not require switch recombination. *Nature* 297:697–699, 1982.

59. Perlmutter AP, Gilbert W: Antibodies of the secondary response can be expressed without switch recombination in normal mouse B cells. *Proc Natl Acad Sci USA* 81:7189–7193, 1984.

60. Chen Y-W, Word C, Dev V, et al: Double isotype production of a neoplastic B cell line: II. Allelically excluded production of μ and γ1 heavy chains without C_H gene rearrangement. *J Exp Med* 164:562–579, 1986.

61. Gearhart PJ, Cebra JJ: Differentiated B lymphocytes. Potential to express particular antibody variable and constant regions depends on site of lymphoid tissue and antigen load. *J Exp Med* 149:216–227, 1979.

62. Fuhrman JA, Cebra JJ: Special features of the primary process for a secretory IgA response. B cell priming with cholera toxin. *J Exp Med* 153:537–544, 1981.

63. Cebra JJ, Fuhrman JA, Gearhart PJ, et al: B lymphocyte differentiation leading to a commitment of IgA expression may depend on cell division and may occur during antigen-stimulated clonal expansion. In Strober W, Hanson LA, Sell KW: *Recent Advances in Mucosal Immunity.* New York, Raven Press, 1982, pp 155–171.

64. Mongini PKA, Stein KE, Paul WE: T cell regulation of IgG subclass antibody production in response to T-independent antigens. *J. Exp. Med.* 153:1–12, 1981.

65. Mongini PKA, Paul WE, Metcalf ES: IgG subclass, IgE and IgA antitrinitrophenyl antibody production within trinitrophenyl-ficoll-responsive B cell clones. *J Exp Med* 157:69–85, 1983.

66. Barzillo GV, Cooper MD, Kubagawa H, et al: Isotype switching in human B lymphocte malignancies occurs by DNA deletion: evidence for nonspecific switch recombination. *J Immunol* 139:1326–1335, 1987.

67. Borzillo GV, Cooper MD, Bertolè LF, et al: Lineage and stage specificity of isotype switching in humans. *J Immunol* 141:3625–3633, 1988.

68. Hummel M, Berry JK, Dunnick W: Switch region content of hybridomas: the two spleen cell IgH loci tend to rearrange to the same isotype. *J Immunol* 138:3539–3548, 1987.

69. Clough JD, Mims LH, Strober W: Deficient IgA antibody responses to arsonilic acid bovine serum albumin (BSA) in neonatally thymectomized rabbits. *J Immunol* 106:1624–1629, 1971.

70. Pritchard H, Riddaway J, Micklem HS: Immune responses in congenitally thymusless mice. II. Quantitative studies of serum immunoglobulin, the antibody response to sheep erthrocytes, and the effect of thymus allografting. *Clin Exp Immunol* 13:135–138, 1973.

71. McFarlin DE, Strober W, Waldmann TA: Ataxia-telangiectasia. *Medicine* 51:281–314, 1972.

72. Elson CC, Heck JA, Strober W: T Cell regulation of murine IgA synthesis. *J Exp Med* 149:632–643, 1979

73. Kawanishi H, Saltzman L, Strober W: Mechanisms regulating IgA class-specific immunoglobulin production in murine gut-associated lymphoid tissues. I. T cells derived from Peyer's patches that switch sIgM B cells to sIgA B cells *in vitro. J Exp Med* 157:437–450, 1983.

74. Kawanishi H, Saltman L, Strober W: Mechanisms regulating IgA class-specific immunoglobulin production in murine gut-associated lymphoid tussies. II. Terminal differentiation of postswitch sIgA-bearing Peyer's patch B cells. *J Exp Med* 158:649–669, 1983.

75. Spalding DM, Griffin JA: Different pathways of differentiation of pre-B cell lines are induced by dentritic cells and T cells from different lymphoid tissues. *Cell* 44:507–515, 1986.

76. Mayer L, Kwan SP, Thompson C, et al: Evidence for a defect in "switch" T cells in patients with immunodeficiency and hyperimmunoglobulinemia M. *N Engl J Med* 314:409–413, 1986.

77. Isakson PC, Pure E, Vitetta ES, et al: T cell derived B cell differentiation factor(s). Effect on the isotype switch of murine B cells. *J Exp Med* 155:734–748, 1982.

78. Snapper CM, Finkelman FD, Stefang D, et al: IL-4 induces co-expression of intrinsic membrane IgG1 and IgE by murine B cells stimulated with lipopolysaccharide. *J Immunol* 141:489–498, 1988.

79. Snapper CM, Paul WE: B cell stimulating factor-1 (interleukin-4) prepares resting murine B cells to secrete IgG1 upon subsequent stimulation with bacterial lipopolysaccharide. *J Immunol* 139:10–17, 1987.

80. Snapper CM, Paul WE: Interferon-γ and B cell stimulatory factor-1 reciprocally regulate Ig isotype production. *Science* 236:944–947, 1987.

81. Kunimoto DY, Harriman GR, Strober W: Regulation of IgA differentiation in CH12LX B cells by lymphokines, IL-4 induces membrane IgM-positive CH12LX cells to express membrane IgA and IL-5 induced membrane IgA-positive CH12LX cells to secrete IgA. *J Immunol* 141:713–720, 1988.

82. Stavnezer J, Radcliffe G, Lin Y-C, et al: Immunoglobulin heavy-chain switching may be directed by prior induction to transcripts from constant-region genes. *Proc Natl Acad Sci USA* 85:7704–7708, 1988.

83. Rothman P, Lutzker S, Cook W, et al: Mitogen plus interleukin 4 induction of Cε transcripts in B lymphoid cells. *J Exp Med* 168:2385–2389, 1988.

84. Lutzker S, Rothman P, Pollock R, et al: Mitogen- and IL-4-regulated expression of germ-line Ig γ2b transcripts: evidence for directed heavy chain class switching. *Cell* 53:177–184, 1988.

85. Ishizaka K: Regulation of IgE synthesis. *Annu Rev Immunol* 2:159–182, 1984.

86. Huff TF: IgE-binding factors and the regulation of the IgE response. In Strober W, Lamm ME, McGhee JR, James SP: *Mucosal Immunity and Infections at Mucosal Surfaces.* New York, Oxford University Press, 1988, pp 46–55.

87. Strober W, Hague NE, Lum LG, et al: IgA-Gc receptors on mouse lymphoid cells. *J Immunol* 121:2440–2445, 1978.

88. Lum LG, Muchmore AV, Keren D, et al: A receptor for IgA on human T lymphocytes. *J Immunol* 122:59–65, 1979.

89. Kiyono H, McGhee JR, Mosteller LM, et al: Murine Peyer's patch T cell clones characterization of antigen-specific helper T cells for immunoglobulin A responses. *J Exp Med* 156:1115–1130, 1982.

90. Kiyono H, Cooper MD, Kearney JF, et al: Isotype specificity of helper T cell clones. Peyer's patch Th cells preferentially collaborate with mature IgA B cells for IgA responses. *J Exp Med* 159:798–811, 1984.

91. Kiyono H, Mosteller-Barnum LM, Pitts AM, et al: Isotype-specific immunoregulation IgA-binding factors produced by Fcα receptor-positive T cell hybridomas regulate IgA responses. *J Exp Med* 161:731–747, 1985.

92. Williams KR, Lynch RG: Tumor models of isotype-specific regulation. In Strober W, Lamm ME, McGhee JR, James SP: *Mucosal Immunity and Infections at Mucosal Surfaces.* New York, Oxford University Press, 1988 pp 74–79.

93. Hoover RG, Lynch RG: Isotype-specific suppression of IgA: suppression of IgA responses in Balb/c mice by Tα cells. *J Immunol* 130:521–523, 1983.

94. Müller S, Hoover RG: T cells with Fc receptors in myeloma; suppression of growth and secretion of MOPC-315 by Tα cells. *J Immunol* 134:644–647, 1985.

95. Adachi M, Yodoi J, Noro N, et al: Murine IgA binding factors produced by FcαR(+) T cells: role of FcγR(+) cells for the induction of FcαR and formation of IgA-binding factor in Con A-activated cells. *J Immunol* 133:65–71, 1984.

96. Noro N, Adachi M, Yasuda K, et al: Murine IgA binding factors (IgA-BF) suppressing IgA production: chracterization and target specificity of IgA-BF. *J Immunol* 136:2910–2916, 1986.

97. Sarfati M, Rubio-Trujillo M, Wong K, et al: Induction of IgA-specific suppressor activity in human T-lymphocyte cultures. *Cell Immunol* 90:85–91, 1985.

98. Williams KR, Lynch RG: A clonal model for T lymphocytes bearing Fc receptors for IgA. *J Cell Biochem* (suppl) 8A:265, 1985.

99. Roman S, Moore JS, Darby C, et al: Modulation of Ig gene expression by Ig binding factors. Suppression of α-H chain and λ-2-L chain mRNA accumulation of MOPC-315 by IgA-binding factor. *J Immunol* 140:3622–3630, 1986.

100. Strober W, James SP: The interleukins. *Pediatr Res* 24:549–557, 1988.

101. Harriman GR, Strober W: The immunobiology of IL-5. *The Year in Immunol* 5:160–177, 1988.

102. Campbell HD, Tucker WQJ, Hort Y, et al: Molecular cloning, nucleotide sequence and expression of the gene encoding human eosinophil differentiation factor (interleukin 5). *Proc Natl Acad Sci USA* 84:6629–6633, 1987.

103. Harada N, Kikuchi Y, Tominaga A, et al: BCGFII activity on activated B cells on a purified murine T cell replacing factor (TRF) from a T cell hybridoma (B151K12). *J Immunol* 134:3944–3951, 1985.

104. Kagnoff MF, Arner LS, Swain SL: Lymphokine-mediated activation of a T cell-dependent IgA anti-polysacchardie response. *J Immunol* 131:2210–2214, 1983.

105. Coffman RL, Shrader B, Carty K, et al: A mouse T cell production that preferentially enhances IgA production. I. Biologic characterization. *J Immunol* 139:3685–3690, 1987.

106. Harriman GR, Kunimoto DY, Elliott JF, et al: The role of IL-5 in IgA B cell differentiation. *J Immunol* 140:3033–3039, 1988.

107. Beagley KW, Eldridge JH, Kiyono H, et al: Recombinant murine IL-5 induces high rate IgA synthesis in cycling IgA-positive Peyer's patch B cells. *J Immunol* 141:2035–2042, 1988.

108. Matsumoto M, Tominaga A, Harada N, et al: Role of T cell-replacing fact (TRF) in the murine B cell differentiation. Induction of increased levels of expression of secreted type IgM mRNA. *J Immunol* 138:1836–1833, 1987.

109. Murray PD, Swain SL, Kagnoff MP: Regulation of the IgM and IgA anti-dextran B1355S response: synergy between IFN-γ, BCGF II and IL-2. *J Immunol* 135:4015–4020, 1985.

110. Swain SL: Role of BCGF II in the differentiation to antibody secretion of normal and tumor B cells. *J Immunol* 134:3934–3943, 1985.

111. Kunimoto RY, Nordan RP, Strober W: IL-6 is a potent co-factor of IL-1 in IgM synthesis and of IL-5 in IgA synthesis. *FASEB J* 3:A1367, 1988.

112. Cherwinski HM, Schumacher JH, Brown KD, et al: Two types of mouse helper T cell clones. III. Further differences in lymphokine synthesis between Th1 and Th2 clones revealed by RNA hybridization, functionally monospecific biosassays, and monoclonal antibodies. *J Exp Med* 166:1229–1244, 1987.

113. Strober W, Richman LK, Elson CO: The regulation of gastrointestinal immune responses. *Immunol Today* 2:156–161, 1981.

114. Mowat AM: The regulation of immune responses to dietary protein antigens. *Immunol Today* 8:93–98, 1987.

115. Richman LK, Cheller JM, Brown WR: Enterically induced immunologic tolerance. I. Induction of suppressor T lymphocytes by intragastric administration of soluble proteins. *J Immunol* 121:2429–2434, 1978.

116. Bruce MG, Ferguson A: Oral tolerance to ovalbumin in mice: studies of chemically modified and "biologically filtered" antigen. *Immunology* 57:627–630, 1986.

117. Kuchroo VK, Minami M, Diamond B, Dorf ME: Functional analysis of cloned macrophage hybridomas. VI. Differential ability to induce immunity or suppression. *J Immunol* 141:10–16, 1988.

118. Kiyono H, Balb JL, Michalek SM, et al: Cellular basis for elevated IgA responses in C3H/HeJ mice. *J Immunol* 125:732–737, 1980.

119. Michalek SM, Kiyono H, Wannemuehler NJ, et al: Lipopolysaccharide (LPS) regulation of the immune response: LPS influence on oral tolerance induction. *J Immunol* 128:1992–1998, 1982.

120. Reynolds JD: Evidence of extensive lymphocyte death in sheep Peyer's patches. I. A comparison of lymphocyte production and export. *J Immunol* 136:2005–2010, 1986.

121. Richman LK, Graeff AS, Yarchoan R, et al: Simultaneous induction of antigen-specific IgA helper T cells to IgG suppressor T cells in the murine Peyer's patches after protein feeding. *J Immunol* 126:2079–2083, 1981.

122. Gershon RK, Eardley DD, Durum S, et al: Contrasuppression: a novel immunoregulatory activity. *J Exp Med* 153:1533–1546, 1981.

123. Green DR, St Martin S: Suppression and contrasuppression in the regulation of gut-associated immune responses. *Ann NY Acad Sci* 409:284–291, 1983.

124. Kitamura K, Kiyono H, Fujihashi K, et al: Contrasuppression cells that break oral tolerance are antigen-specific T cells distinct from T helper (L3T4+), T suppressor (Lyt-2+), and B cells. *J Immunol* 139:3251–3259, 1987.

125. Kitamura K, Kiyono H, Fujihashi K, et al: Isotype-specific immunoregulation, systemic antigen induces splenic T contrasuppressor cell which support IgM and IgG subclass but not IgA responses. *J Immunol* 140:1385–1392, 1988.

CHAPTER 9

Oral Immunization and Oral Tolerance

MAUREEN G. BRUCE

CHARLES O. ELSON

INTRODUCTION

The intestine is a rich source of lymphoid cells, which are in close contact with the many antigens constantly entering and, in the case of bacteria, colonizing the gastrointestinal tract. This ubiquitous presence of antigen leads to the induction of a variety of local and systemic immune responses, which can be broadly classified as either oral immunization or oral tolerance. In the intestine, immune responses are induced and regulated in specialized areas of tissue known as gut-associated lymphoid tissue, or GALT. This is comprised of lymphoid follicles or Peyer's patches, lymphocytes in the lamina propria, and lymphocytes within the epithelium of the intestinal mucosa (Fig. 9–1).

ORAL IMMUNIZATION

When antigen feeding induces a state of oral immunization, IgA is secreted at mucosal surfaces.[1] Experiments in rodents have shown that following oral immunization with bacterial or viral antigens, an IgA antibody response can be induced in saliva, colostrum, milk, and tears and in the secretions of the lower respiratory tract and genital tract. The secretory IgA (SIgA) response can occur in the absence of serum antibody. In some oral immunization regimes in which IgG antibodies were found in secretions following oral immunization, serum IgG antibodies were also observed. It is not known whether the IgG in secretions was produced locally or diffused into the mucosal site from blood. Bacterial antigens that have been fed to animals include *Escherichia coli* and *Streptococcus mutans*. Oral immunization with *S. mutans* or glycosyltransferase of *S. mutans* affords protection from dental

171

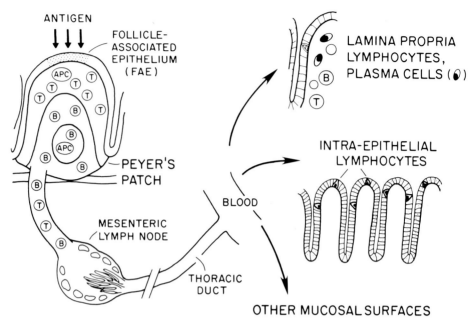

Figure 9 – 1 The intestinal immune system: The organization of gut-associated lymphoid tissue into three major compartments; Peyer's patches, intraepithelial lymphocytes, and lamina propria lymphocytes. (From Elson CO: The immunology of inflammatory bowel disease. In Kirsner JB, Shorter RG: *Inflammatory Bowel Disease,* ed 3. Philadelphia, Lea & Febiger, 1988, p. 97, with permission.)

caries.[2,3] Viral vaccines that have been orally administered to animals include live respiratory syncytial virus and live influenza virus. The latter was found to protect mice against challenge with virulent virus.

In humans, oral immunization is difficult to achieve with many antigens and in particular with nonviable vaccines. However, results from a number of clinical trials indicate that oral immunization with certain antigens is also effective in humans and may be administered to people of all ages with little risk of adverse side effects. Oral immunization trials have been conducted using bacterial antigens, including *E. coli, S. mutans, Hemophilus influenzae,* and cholera.[4] Viral vaccines that have been tested include poliovirus, adenovirus, and influenza. Live vaccines induce IgA in secretions and in serum whereas oral immunization with killed vaccines leads to IgA in secretions only. Multiple doses of oral vaccine seem to be more efficient in inducing a mucosal response, and orally induced antibody reaches peak titer more slowly than parenterally induced serum antibody. This may be influenced by the length of time when antigen is present in the intestine; animal experiments indicate that longer exposure to antigen at the intestinal mucosa may result in a quicker response. Information is lacking regarding the duration of the human secretory antibody response following oral immunization. In one study, salivary IgA to *S. mutans* was short-lived, while a trial in children showed that anti-influenza IgA induced by killed vaccine remained elevated for 6 months.

Priming of the Mucosal IgA Response

Antigen entering Peyer's patches initiates the induction of a local secretory antibody response by plasma cells in the lamina propria, which is predominantly of the IgA isotype. IgA synthesized by plasma cells binds to epithelial cells by means of a specialized molecule known as secretory component and is transported across the intestinal epithelium into the lumen with secretory component still attached. This secreted form of the antibody is thus described as secretory IgA,[5] and this response is T cell-dependent. The differentiation of B cells into IgA-secreting plasma cells requires changes in immunoglobulin gene expression known as isotype switching. This may depend on the action of a specialized T cell known as a switch T cell, or may be effected via the soluble products of T cells known as lymphokines. This is an active area of research at present and, while as yet an IgA switch T cell has not been fully characterized, it is clear that T cells isolated from Peyer's patches promote IgA responses of a high magnitude in vitro.[6]

ORAL TOLERANCE

Oral tolerance describes the state of antigen-specific hyporesponsiveness of humoral or cellular immunity induced by antigen feeding prior to systemic immunization. This is a long-recognized phenomenon said to have been utilized by American Indians, who are thought to have fed their young *Rhus* leaves to prevent them from getting contact sensitivity from "poison ivy".[7] The first reports of the induction of oral tolerance under laboratory conditions were published in 1911[8,9] and described the prevention of systemic anaphylaxis in guinea pigs by previous antigen feeding. Later experiments on the induction of tolerance by feeding contact-sensitizing agents led to the description of orally induced hyporesponsiveness as the Sulzberger-Chase phenomenon.[10] Since these early observations, oral tolerance has been demonstrated in various species of experimental animals including mice (Fig. 9–2), rats, rabbits, and guinea pigs after the feeding of many different antigens such as heterologous erythrocytes, inactivated bacteria or viruses, and soluble protein antigens.[11] Oral tolerance may be induced in the host directly or, in the case of young animals, may be transferred from a tolerized mother to her young by suckling.[12,13] Certain effector limbs of immunity such as delayed-type hypersensitivity (DTH) and immediate hypersensitivity (IgE responses) are more readily subject to profound and long-lasting suppression following even a single oral exposure to antigen.[11]

In spite of the existence of a large literature describing oral tolerance in animals, its occurrence in humans is largely unproven, due mainly to difficulties in designing ethical and well-controlled experiments on human subjects who have already been exposed to many antigens via the gastrointestinal tract. However, there is some evidence to suggest that oral tolerance does occur in man: in one study, exposure to a contact-sensitizing agent via the buccal mucosa prior to subsequent skin challenge led to unresponsiveness in more than one-half of the group under study.[14] In another series of experiments on human volunteers, serum antibodies to bovine serum albumin (BSA) were measured before and after test feeding of large amounts of this antigen. Those subjects who had anti-BSA antibodies before eating BSA

A.

Feed antigen

Later: immunize with
antigen and
measure response

B.

Feed antigen

Transfer cells

Immunize with
antigen

Measure response

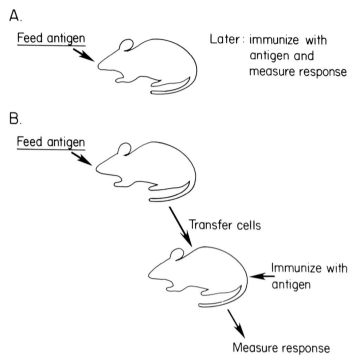

Figure 9-2 Experimental protocols used for the demonstration of oral tolerance: **A:** Mice are fed antigen and then immunized systemically, and the response is measured. **B:** Mice are fed antigen and then cells (or serum) are transferred to syngeneic recipients, which are immunized, and the response is measured (From Elson CO: Induction and control of the gastrointestinal immune response. *Scand J. Gastroenterol* 20:1–15, 1985. With permission.)

showed a rise in their serum anti-BSA titers. A similar response pattern was observed when some subjects were given an additional parenteral injection of BSA; again only those who had previously demonstrated serum antibodies to BSA responded to the immunization. The subjects who did not have anti-BSA antibodies before or after the test feed did not respond to subsequent intradermal immunization; they were tolerant.[15] Hopefully, the elucidation of oral tolerance mechanisms in animals will allow testing for the presence of similar immune effector mechanisms in humans.

Mucosal Priming With Systemic Suppression

In several series of experiments using both soluble and particulate antigens, it has been reported that antigen feeding can induce oral tolerance with concomitant priming of the mucosal IgA response. One report demonstrated the presence of antigen-specific helper T cells for IgA together with antigen-specific suppressor cells for IgA in the Peyer's patches of mice given a single oral dose of ovalbumin 8 days previously.[16] This may be one of the immune mechanisms by which antigen feeding elicits mucosal IgA and systemic suppression. However, in experiments in which secretory IgA was measured directly in intestinal washings of antigen-fed mice, evidence has been obtained indicating that the mucosal IgA response may also be subject to suppression following antigen feeding: Oral administration of proteins to mice (which induced systemic tolerance) did not elicit secretory IgA in intestinal washings. It was further observed that, in contrast to most proteins, cholera toxin (CT) feeding did not induce oral tolerance but instead stimulated a strong intestinal IgA response and a serum IgG response. From these results it was hypothesized that CT feeding leads to the induction of a different regulatory pathway in GALT than that induced by other ingested proteins. In order to test this hypothesis, mice were fed either keyhole limpet hemocyanin (KLH) alone or KLH and CT together and were subsequently immunized parenterally with KLH. The mice fed KLH alone developed oral tolerance, while those fed KLH plus CT were not tolerized but rather made serum and secretory antibody responses to KLH.[17,18] Thus CT is able to alter the normal regulatory environment of the intestine.[6] It would therefore seem that the suppression induced by feeding protein antigens affects not only systemic immunity but extends also to the local intestinal antibody response.

MECHANISMS OF ORAL TOLERANCE

Various effector mechanisms have been described in orally tolerized animals. The induction of a particular immunosuppressive mechanism depends on such parameters as the nature of the orally administered antigen, the immune status of the host, and the age at which antigen is first ingested. Some of the more well-defined effector mechanisms will be described in this section.

Suppressor Cells

The activation of suppressor cells by feeding antigens has been well documented in several series of in vivo and in vitro experiments. For example, feeding sheep erythrocytes induces T cell-mediated feedback suppression of systemic humoral immunity, and this active suppression may be accompanied by additional suppressive mechanisms such as serum antibody or immune complexes.[6]

In experiments on oral tolerance to contact sensitizing agents, multiple suppressor mechanisms may be induced. For example, a large oral dose of contact sensitizing agent administered to mice prior to skin sensitization suppresses contact sensitivity; suppressor B cells have been demonstrated in these mice by means of cell transfer experiments. However, these cells may not be actively mediating the immune suppression, since they have been detected in sensitized mice as well and because the induction of oral tolerance in these animals is prevented by adult thymectomy. When oral tolerance is induced by feeding low doses of sensitizing agent, suppression may be prevented by injection with cyclophosphamide 2 days prior to feeding at doses that have been shown to abrogate suppressor cell activity. This implies that a suppressor cell is induced by feeding low doses of contact sensitizing agent.[6] Further work in this area has shown that following the ingestion of a contact sensitizing agent, specific suppressor T cells signal a second population of T cells via a soluble factor and cause these cells to release a nonspecific suppressor factor that acts on effector cells responsible for contact sensitivity expression.[19]

Suppressor T cells (Ts) have also been demonstrated in oral tolerance to protein antigens,[11] although the cellular interaction pathways involved are not as well described as those occurring in response to feeding with sheep erythrocytes. Oral tolerance to the soluble protein ovalbumin (OVA) is readily induced by feeding a single large dose of this antigen prior to systemic immunization and both humoral (serum antibody) and cell-mediated immunity (DTH), are suppressed. Treatment of mice with cyclophosphamide (CY) or 2'-deoxyguanosine before OVA feeding depletes suppressor cells and abrogates oral tolerance to OVA. Suppression of CMI is more readily prevented by CY pretreatment, and, similarly, adoptive transfer of spleen cells from OVA-fed mice consistently leads to suppression of CMI in recipients.[11] These observations have led to the hypothesis that Ts cells are active in suppression of DTH by OVA feeding, while antibody responses are suppressed by some additional mechanisms. It is thus important to distinguish between orally induced suppression of humoral as compared with cellular responses because the governing regulatory mechanisms are probably distinct and independent of each other. The site of activation of Ts cells following antigen feeding has not yet been clearly defined. Although there is some evidence to suggest that Ts cells for humoral responses are activated in Peyer's patches and then migrate to the mesenteric lymph node and spleen, intestinally processed antigen (see below) can cause activation of Ts cells that suppress DTH following parenteral injection, indicating that Ts cells can be activated at sites distant from the intestine. As described in other models of systemic tolerance, I-J[+] cells[20] may be important, since treatment of mice with anti-I-J antiserum prevents the induction of oral tolerance. However it is not known at present whether I-J is expressed on a Ts cell or on an antigen-presenting cell involved in immune suppression.[21]

Antigen Processing by the Intestine

The physiologic handling of proteins in the intestine has been found to be important in the suppression of DTH by antigen feeding. This has been studied in mice by means of serum transfer experiments: serum is collected from mice 1 hour after feeding a single tolerizing dose of OVA. One hour was chosen as the time required for gastric emptying and absorption of the ingested protein into the systemic circulation. The serum is transferred via i.p. injection to recipient mice, which are subsequently immunized with OVA. These recipients have suppressed DTH upon subsequent parenteral immunization with OVA but mount a normal serum antibody response to this antigen.[22] This again illustrates differences in regulatory mechanisms governing the suppression of different limbs of immunity. The active species in tolerogenic serum was OVA, which was detectable by enzyme-linked immunosorbent assay (ELISA) and which had a molecular weight approximately equal to native OVA. Removal of OVA from the serum by absorption with anti-OVA antibody bound to Sephadex removed the suppressive activity of the serum. The suppression induced by serum transfer was dependent on prior feeding of the antigen, since serum obtained from mice at 1 hour following either i.p. or i.v. injection of OVA was not suppressive. In addition, tolerance induced by serum transfer was not dependent merely on the dose of antigen transferred, because systemic injections of antigen in amounts similar to those previously measured in tolerogenic serum did not induce suppression. Furthermore, the tolerogenic effect of serum OVA could not be reproduced by injection of either denatured or deaggregated forms of the antigen: denatured OVA was not tolerogenic; deaggregated OVA induced profound suppression of both DTH and antibody responses.[23,24] From these results, therefore, it was proposed that, following antigen ingestion and its subsequent digestion and absorption, antigen is present in tolerogenic form in the circulation. The sequence of events leading to the appearance of the tolerogenic form of OVA in serum has been termed intestinal antigen processing.

Antibody and Immune Complexes

Specific humoral antibody and IgA-antigen immune complexes have been implicated in orally induced suppression of anti-sheep erythrocyte plaque-forming cell (PFC) responses. Oral tolerance induced in mice by repeated feeding with sheep erythrocytes could be transferred to unfed mice by serum collected some days after antigen feeding. Although immune complexes of IgA and sheep erythrocytes were at first believed to be responsible, the results of further experiments indicated that the suppression was associated with the presence of IgG anti-sheep erythrocyte antibody. There was also some evidence of an anti-idiotypic antibody circulating in the serum of sheep erythrocyte-fed mice.[25,26]

Clonal Inactivation/Deletion

Experiments on oral tolerance to OVA have shown that the humoral response can be restored by stimulating antigen-specific B cells with antigen plus either lipopolysaccharide (LPS) or an alternative carrier molecule. This demonstrates that B cells are able to respond and that the tolerance is due to a state of T-cell unresponsiveness in these animals. Functional T-cell anergy may be the result either of deletion of antigen-specific T-cell clones or of specific clonal inactivation. Since in some experiments T-cell unresponsiveness was shown to return eventually in antigen-fed mice, it seems unlikely that clonal deletion is involved. Mechanisms of clonal anergy are not as yet well understood. Two current hypotheses are that either unresponsiveness is induced via the direct interaction of T-helper cells with antigen or that the effect is mediated by the action of suppressor cells.[11]

Intestinal Flora

Being able to mount a response to bacterial antigens in the intestine may be important in suppressing immunity to subsequently ingested antigens, since rats and mice are known to possess nonspecific suppressor cells that have been induced in response to their intestinal bacterial flora: germ-free animals are lacking in these cells unless they are colonized with a normal flora.[27-29] The nonspecific suppressor cell observed in rats is a macrophage-like cell that is adherent and phagocytic. In the mouse the suppressor is a T cell that can suppress the mitogenic response to bacterial LPS. Mice that are genetically determined nonresponders to LPS and are lacking in this suppressor T-cell activity also exhibit a defect in oral tolerance to sheep erythrocytes when fed with this antigen; instead of developing specific T-suppressor cells, these mice are primed for both cellular and humoral responses to this antigen. This mechanism does not seem to operate in the response to soluble proteins, however, because LPS-unresponsive mice are tolerized by OVA feeding.[12] This emphasizes an important feature of orally induced immune regulation — different regulatory mechanisms may be induced in response to different types of fed antigen. This in turn may have implications for the role of antigen handling in the intestine in determining the immunologic outcome of antigen feeding.

Specialized Antigen-Presenting Cells

While strictly speaking antigen-presenting cells have not been described as playing a direct role in mechanisms of oral tolerance, research on systemic immune responses has emphasized the importance of antigen-presenting cells in immune regulation. Likewise, in oral tolerance, the role of cells of the reticuloendothelial system (RES) has been observed in mice treated with a variety of agents known to cause activation of the RES. These include injection of estrogen, muramyl dipeptide adjuvant, and allogeneic lymphocytes (to induce graft-versus-host reaction). Each one of these treatments enhanced the activity of antigen-presenting cells and prevented the induction of DTH oral tolerance to OVA.[11] Thus oral immunization is favored when antigen-presenting cells become activated.

GENETIC CONTROL OF ORAL TOLERANCE

Elucidation of the genetic basis of oral tolerance in animals is of potential importance in understanding the immunopathogenesis of certain gastrointestinal diseases such as celiac disease, which reflects intestinal hypersensitivity to gliadin and shows strong association with certain major histocompatibility complex (MHC) class II gene loci. It has been reported that the induction of oral tolerance may be subject to control by genes of the murine MHC (H-2) gene locus.[11,30] One study carried out in two MHC congenic inbred strains of mice that differ markedly in their susceptibility to oral tolerance induction explored whether this difference was due to differences in the intestinal processing of OVA or was related to differences in systemic immune responsiveness: BALB/c mice fed with OVA develop profound suppression of the systemic DTH response and marked suppression of specific serum IgG. In contrast, OVA-fed BALB/B mice have normal DTH and serum IgG levels following immunization. Furthermore, serum from OVA-fed BALB/c mice suppresses DTH when transferred to syngeneic recipients but is not tolerogenic in BALB/B recipients that have normal DTH and enhanced serum antibody responses. In the converse experiment, serum transferred from OVA-fed BALB/B donors to BALB/B recipients is not suppressive but rather enhances DTH, whereas BALB/c recipients of the same serum show suppression of DTH. Therefore the defect in oral tolerance induction in BALB/B mice is not due to inappropriate antigen processing in the intestine but rather seems the result of some defect in the immune recognition of tolerogenic OVA in BALB/B strain mice.[31]

POSSIBLE CLINICAL RELEVANCE

Mucosal Delayed-Type Hypersensitivity

Delayed-type hypersensitivity in the intestinal mucosa is characterized by a typical enteropathy, which includes increases in numbers of intraepithelial lymphocytes, and by crypt cell proliferation; in some cases it can be accompanied by varying degrees of villous atrophy. These typical features are characteristic of the intestinal damage seen in certain clinical disorders such as celiac disease and cow's milk protein intolerance, which arise as a result of sensitivity to food antigens.[32-34] Similar enteropathic changes in the intestinal mucosa can be induced in mice under conditions in which cell-mediated immunity is activated, such as during allograft rejection[35] or during a mild graft-versus-host reaction.[36] In both of these examples, concomitant antigen feeding according to a tolerizing regimen does not induce oral tolerance.

The relevance of oral tolerance as a homeostatic mechanism preventing the induction of tissue-damaging intestinal hypersensitivity has become apparent from experiments examining effects on the intestine when oral tolerance is abrogated. For example, treatment of mice with cyclophosphamide or 2'-deoxyguanosine prior to oral challenge with antigen is known to prevent the induction of oral tolerance. Mice given this treatment also develop delayed-type hypersensitivity in the intestinal mucosa.[37,38] Similarly, and perhaps of more clinical relevance, neonatal mice fed a large dose of OVA on the first day of life do not become tolerant to this antigen. Furthermore, if mice are fed OVA when they are 1 day old and are then challenged with this antigen in adult life, changes occur in the gut that are consistent with the induction of a local CMI reaction in the intestinal mucosa.[39] These results illustrate the possible damaging immunologic consequences of introducing large amounts of foreign protein into the intestine at a time when the normal immunoregulatory mechanisms are not yet fully developed.

Oral Desensitization

Since failure of oral tolerance mechanisms may lead to the induction of hypersensitivity reactions to food antigens, the re-establishment of tolerance in sensitized individuals would obviously be of benefit. To date there has been little research in this important area, and this has been confined mainly to studies on humoral immunity. In early reports, the systemic antibody responses of immunized animals were found to be enhanced by antigen feeding[40,41]; however, subsequent work by others has demonstrated that antibody responses in immunized hosts can be suppressed by multiple oral administrations of antigen.[42-44] More recently, it has been reported that suppression of DTH to OVA in animals already expressing this response may be achieved by feeding a single tolerizing dose (25 mg) of this antigen.[45] In this study, orally induced suppression of DTH occurred irrespective of whether OVA was fed 7 days before, at the same time as, or up to 14 days after immunization. It will be of interest to determine the length of time following immunization at which antigen feeding will cause suppression of DTH. This initial study indicates that suppression is most profound when antigen is fed close to the time of primary immunization.

The mechanism of oral desensitization is not yet fully characterized; however, further experiments have shown that, in contrast to classical oral tolerance, suppression of DTH induced in immunized animals by antigen feeding is not sensitive to the action of 2'-deoxyguanosine. In addition, orally induced tolerance in immunized mice is not transferred to immunized recipients with spleen cells collected after antigen feeding. Thus the mechanism of post immunization suppression by antigen feeding does not operate solely via the OVA-specific suppressor cells that mediate classical oral tolerance to this antigen. Instead, it has been proposed that oral administration of antigen to immune mice may lead to a state of functional anergy in the T cells responsible for DTH or, alternatively, that phenotypic anergy is observed as a result of effector cells being unable to migrate to the site of antigen challenge. An interesting feature of this experimental system is that spleen cells from preimmunized, antigen-fed mice contain a population of cells that induce antigen-specific suppression when transferred into immunologically naive animals. It is tempting to speculate that every oral encounter with antigen causes activation of such suppressor-inducer cells but that an appropriate immunoregulatory mechanism is induced in the host under the influence of additional factors such as the host immune status at the time of feeding.

REFERENCES

1. Bergmann KC, Waldman RH. Stimulation of secretory antibody following oral administration of antigen. *Rev Infect Dis* 10:939–950, 1988.
2. Michalek SM, McGhee JR, Mestecky J, et al. Ingestion of *Streptococcus mutans* induces secretory immunoglobulin A and caries immunity. *Science* 192:1238–1240, 1976.
3. Smith DJ, Taubman MA, Ebersole JL. Effect of oral administration of glucosyltransferase antigens on experimental dental caries. *Infect Immun* 26:82–89, 1979.
4. Clemens JD, Sack DA, Harris JR, et al. Field trial of oral cholera vaccines in Bangladesh. *Lancet* ii:124–127, 1986.
5. Brandtzaeg P, Valnes K, Scott H, et al. The human gastrointestinal secretory immune system in health and disease. *Scand J Gastroenterol* 20:17–38, 1985.
6. Elson CO. Induction and control of the gastrointestinal immune response. *Scand J Gastroenterol* 20:1–15, 1985.
7. Dakin R. Remarks on a cutaneous affection produced by certain poisonous vegetables. *Am J Med Sci* 4:98–100, 1829.
8. Wells HG. Studies on the chemistry of anaphylaxis. III. Experiments with isolated proteins, especially those of the hen's egg *J Infect Dis* 9:147–171, 1911.
9. Wells HG, Osborne TB. The biological reactions to vegetable proteins. I. Anaphylaxis. *J Infect Dis* 8:66–124, 1911.
10. Chase MW. Inhibition of experimental drug allergy by prior feeding of the sensitizing agent. *Proc Soc Exp Biol Med* 61:257–259, 1946.
11. Mowat A McI. Regulation of immune responses to dietary protein antigens. *Immunology Today* 8:93–98, 1987.
12. Jarrett EEE, Hall E. Selective suppression of IgE responses by maternal influence. *Nature* 280:145–147, 1979.
13. Peri BA, Rothberg RM. Specific suppression of antibody production in young rabbit kits after maternal ingestion of bovine serum albumin. *J Immunol* 127:2520–2525, 1981.
14. Lowney ED. Immunologic unresponsiveness to a contact sensitizer in man. *J Invest Dermatol* 51:411–417, 1968.
15. Korenblat PE, Rothberg RM, Minden P, et al. Immune responses of human adults after oral parenteral exposure to bovine serum albumin. *J Allergy* 41:226–235, 1968.
16. Richman LK, Graeff AS, Yarchoan R, et al. Simultaneous induction of antigen specific IgA helper T cells and IgG suppressor cells in the murine Peyer's patch after protein feeding. *J Immunol* 126:2079–2083, 1981.
17. Elson CO, Ealding W. Cholera toxin feeding did not induce oral tolerance in mice and abrogated oral tolerance to an unrelated protein antigen. *J Immunol* 133:2892–2897, 1984.

18. Elson CO, Ealding W. Generalized systemic and mucosal immunity in mice after mucosal stimulation with cholera toxin. *J Immunol* 132:2736–2742, 1984.

19. Gautam SC, Battisto JR. Orally induced tolerance generates an efferently acting suppressor T cell and an acceptor T cell that together down regulate contact sensitivity. *J Immunol* 135:2975–2983, 1985.

20. Murphy DB. The I-J puzzle. *Annu Rev Immunol* 5:405–427, 1987.

21. Dorf ME, Benacerraf B. Suppressor cells and immunoregulation. *Annu Rev Immunol* 2:127–158, 1984.

22. Strobel S, Mowat A McI, Drummond HE, et al. Immunological responses to fed protein antigens in mice. II. Oral tolerance for CMI is due to activation of cyclophosphamide-sensitive cells by gut processed antigen. *Immunology* 49:451–455, 1983.

23. Bruce MG, Ferguson A. Oral tolerance to ovalbumin in mice: studies of chemically modified and of "biologically filtered" antigen. *Immunology* 57:627–630, 1986.

24. Bruce MG, Ferguson A. The influence of intestinal processing on the immunogenicity and molecular size of absorbed, circulating ovalbumin in mice. *Immunology* 59:295–300, 1986.

25. Kagnoff MF. Effects of antigen feeding on intestinal and systemic immune responses. III. Antigen-specific serum-mediated suppression of humoral antibody responses after antigen feeding. *Cell Immunol* 40:186–203, 1978.

26. Chalon MP, Mine RW, Vaerman JP. *In vitro* immunosuppressive effect of serum from orally immunized mice. *Eur J Immunol* 9:747–751, 1979.

27. Mattingly JA, Eardley DD, Kemp JD, et al. Induction of suppressor cells in rat spleen: influence of microbial stimulation. *J Immunol* 122:787–790, 1980.

28. McGhee JR, Kiyono H, Michalek SM, et al. Lipopolysaccharide (LPS) regulation of the immune response: T lymphocytes from normal mice suppress mitogenic and immunogenic responses to LPS. *J Immunol* 124:1603–1611, 1980.

29. Kiyono H, Babb JL, Michalek SM, et al. Cellular basis for elevated IgA responses in C3H/HeJ mice. *J Immunol* 125:732–737, 1980.

30. Stokes CR, Swarbrick ET, Soothill JF. Genetic differences in immune exclusion and partial oral tolerance to ingested antigens. *Clin Exp Immunol* 52:678–684, 1984.

31. Mowat A McI, Lamont AG, Bruce MG. A genetically determined lack of oral tolerance to ovalbumin is due to failure of the immune system to respond to intestinally derived tolerogen. *Eur J Immunol* 17:1673–1676, 1987.

32. Ferguson A, Murray D. Quantitation of intraepithelial lymphocytes in human jejunum. *Gut* 12:988–994, 1971.

33. Ferguson A, McLure JP, Townley RR. Intraepithelial lymphocyte counts in small intestinal biopsies from children with diarrhoea. *Acta Pediatr Scand* 65:541–546, 1976.

34. Phillips AD, Rice SJ, France NE, et al. Small intestinal intraepithelial lymphocyte levels in cow's milk protein intolerance. *Gut* 20:509–512, 1979.

35. McDonald TT, Ferguson A. Hypersensitivity reactions in the small intestine. II. Effects of allograft rejection on mucosal architecture and lymphoid cell infiltrate. *Gut* 17:81–91, 1976.

36. Mowat A McI, Ferguson A. Intraepithelial lymphocyte count and crypt cell hyperplasia measure the mucosal component of the graft-versus-host reaction in mouse small intestine. *Gastroenterology* 83:417–423, 1982.

37. Mowat A McI, Strobel S, Drummond HE, et al. Immunological responses to fed protein antigens in mice. I. Reversal of oral tolerance to ovalbumin by cyclophosphamide. *Immunology* 45:105–113, 1982.

38. Mowat AMcI. Depletion of suppressor T cells by 2'-deoxyguanosine abrogates tolerance

in mice fed ovalbumin and permits the induction of intestinal delayed-type hypersensitivity. *Immunology* 58:179–184, 1986.

39. Strobel S, Ferguson A. Immune responses to fed protein antigens in mice. Systemic tolerance or priming is related to age at which antigen is first encountered. *Pediatr Res* 18:588–594, 1984.

40. Hanson DG, Vaz NM, Rawlings LA, et al. Inhibition of specific immune responses by feeding protein antigens. II. Effects of prior passive and active immunization. *J Immunol* 122:2261–2266, 1977.

41. Titus RG, Chiller JM. Orally induced tolerance. Definition at the cellular level. *Int Arch Allergy Appl Immunol* 65:323–338, 1981.

42. Lafont S, Andre C, Andre F, et al. Abrogation by subsequent feeding of antibody responses, including IgE, in parenterally immunized mice. *J Exp Med* 155:1573–1578, 1982.

43. Bloch KJ, Perry R, Bloch M, et al. Induction of (partial) systemic tolerance in primed rats subjected to prolonged oral administration of antigen. *Ann NY Acad Sci* 409:787–788, 1983.

44. Saklayan M, Pesce AJ, Pollack V, et al. Ileum is the effector site for induction of oral tolerance. *Fed Proc* 45:944A, 1984.

45. Lamont AG, Bruce MG, Watret K, et al. Suppression of an established DTH response to ovalbumin in mice by feeding antigen after immunization. *Immunology* 64:135–139, 1988.

46. Elson CO. The immunology of inflammatory bowel disease. In Kirsner JB, Shorter RG: *Inflammatory Bowel Disease.* ed 3. Philadelphia, Lea & Febiger, 1988, p 97.

CHAPTER 10

Neuroendocrine Regulation of the Mucosal Immune System

KENNETH CROITORU
PETER B. ERNST
ANDRZEJ M. STANISZ
RON H. STEAD
JOHN BIENENSTOCK

INTRODUCTION

Clinicians and gastroenterologists, who treat intestinal disease, are often faced with patients who have subjective discomforts and intestinal disease that are influenced by stress. These observations have led to the concept of a brain-gut axis in which the nervous system can also influence gastrointestinal physiology, i.e., absorption, secretion, and motility.[1] Since psychological stress can also influence the symptoms of inflammation in such diseases as inflammatory bowel disease (IBD) and asthma, the concept of neural influences on intestinal function has now been extended to include the regulation of the immune response of the gut. The study of the morphologic, physiological, and molecular basis of this interaction has become the subject of intensive research.

The interaction between the diffuse neuroendocrine system and the nervous system with the immune system is not a novel idea. There is a great deal of evidence for the hormonal influence on various aspects of the immune response.[2-6] Corticosteroids, which have been shown to have a generally depressive effect on the immune response, have proved highly useful therapeutically.[7] Other examples that are perhaps more pertinent to the mucosal immune response include testosterone, which has an influence on the synthesis and secretion of IgA in the eye,[8] and other sex hormones such as estradiol, which can modulate IgA secretion, IgA lymphoblast migration, and epithelial cell expression of secretory component.[9-11] These latter effects have been seen in mucosal tissues, the main site of IgA production and secretion.[12,13]

This work was supported by the Canadian Foundation for Ileitis and Colitis, the Medical Research Council of Canada, and the Canadian Arthritis and Rheumatism Society.

The notion that the nervous system may contribute to the pathophysiology of inflammation[14] and therefore to the pathogenesis of inflammatory diseases is illustrated by conditioning experiments, in which, for example, the immunosuppressive effects of cyclophosphamide, combined with an inert substance such as saccharin, can be conditioned such that the immunologic events can be reproduced with the conditioned stimulus alone.[15,16] The relationship between the nervous system and the immune response is further illustrated by the phenomenon of neurogenic inflammation, involving the axon reflex, represented by nerve, mast cell, and capillary interaction.[17,18] Such studies suggest the existence of important communication between these seemingly unrelated organ systems.

The bidirectional communication between the immune and nervous system is also illustrated by the finding that antigenic stimulation can increase the firing rate of neurons in the hypothalamus.[19] Blalock has suggested that the immune system can act as a sensory afferent organ for the central nervous system (CNS), surveying and discriminating the constant onslaught of new molecules with which the body is faced.[20-22]

The various mechanisms involved in the regulation of both the local humoral and cellular immune responses have been well reviewed.[23,24] Such a regulatory control of the local immune response is necessary, if one considers the onslaught of foreign antigens and organisms to which the mucosa is exposed. As the interest in the interaction between the neuroendocrine system and the systemic immune system has grown, it has also become apparent that such interactions play important regulatory roles in the intestinal mucosa.

Mucosal surfaces are especially well designed to allow for interactions to occur between nerves and the cells of the immune system. The intestine contains $10^7 - 10^8$ nerve cell bodies, a number comparable to that found in the spinal cord.[25] In addition to being highly innervated, the intestinal mucosa contains significant amounts of the neuropeptide neurotransmitters.[26,27] This would allow the neuroendocrine system, through the local release of these chemical messengers, to affect rapidly a population of lymphocytes and immune effector cells, which are widely dispersed over a large surface area.

Abnormalities in the nerve-immune interactions may also be important in disease pathogenesis. Altered levels of neuropeptides have been described in inflammatory diseases involving mucosal surfaces, including inflammatory bowel disease[28-30] and asthma.[5] Vasoactive intestinal peptide (VIP), for example, has been shown to be increased in intestinal tissues adjacent to or directly involved by Crohn's disease.[31] There is also an apparent hyperplasia of VIP-containing nerves in these tissues,[31,32] although conflicting reports exist.[33,34] Tissues from patients with ulcerative colitis, on the other hand, contain normal or lower levels of VIP.[32] Substance P (SP) has not been consistently shown to be altered in IBD,[33] although recent studies have demonstrated elevated levels in tissue from left-sided ulcerative colitis,[34] and an increase in the expression of substance P receptors on small vessels in the intestine of patients with both ulcerative colitis and Crohn's disease.[35]

Our own interest in the mucosal immune system has led us to examine the relation between nerves, neurotransmitters, and the local intestinal immune response. In this chapter, we review the anatomic basis for nerve-immune interactions and describe some of the work elucidating the molecular mechanisms involved. For extensive reviews on the interactions between the nervous system and the systemic immune response, we refer the reader to other recent publications.[5,36] We concentrate more on the functional interactions that have been described in the intestine.

THE NEUROENDOCRINE SYSTEM

The neuroendocrine system in the gastrointestinal tract includes specialized epithelial cells and the intrinsic and extrinsic nervous system, which produce and secrete neurotransmitter regulatory peptides.[37] These cells make up part of the "diffuse neuroendocrine system," which can also be found in the respiratory tract and many peripheral lymphoid tissues.[38]

Regulatory peptides or neuropeptides are produced by autonomic nerves, sensory nerves, and cells belonging to the amine precursor uptake and decarboxylation (APUD) system.[39,40] The characteristic intracytoplasmic dense core granules allow for their classification. In addition, some of these cells have cytoplasmic extensions that extend toward the basement membrane, suggesting a paracrine function.[38] Other possible sources of neuropeptides in the gut include cells not normally considered part of the nervous or APUD systems, such as mast cells, macrophages, basophils, leukocytes,[41] and eosinophils.[42] Clearly the mucosal localization of these neuropeptides suggests that their release locally could directly affect both epithelial cell and lymphocyte function.

Innervation of Lymphoid Tissues

To allow for interactions between the nervous system and the immune system, one must consider the anatomic relations between nerves and the lymphoid compartments. Such a relationship is necessary for the local delivery of chemical messengers to lymphoid cells, under the control of higher neural influences.

Nerves have clearly been demonstrated within primary and secondary lymphoid organs, including the bone marrow, thymus, tonsils, spleen, and lymph nodes.[43,44] These nerves seem to predominate in T-cell zones of lymphoid aggregates and contain the neurotransmitters noradrenaline and acetylcholine, and various neuropeptides.[45] Felten et al. have demonstrated intimate adrenergic nerve membrane-lymphocyte membranes association,[46] while others have shown the thymus to contain both sympathetic and parasympathetic innervation.[47] In addition, VIP-containing nerves form a finely branched network within the thymic cortex, a region involved in T-cell development.[48]

Innervation of Gut-Associated Lymphoid Tissues (GALT)

The extensive network of the enteric nervous system is integrated with the sympathetic and parasympathetic nervous systems and sensory afferent nerves. The enteric nerve cell bodies lie within the myenteric and submucosal plexi; their processes ramify throughout the intestinal wall[27,49,50] and extend to, contact or lie subadjacent to the epithelial endocrine and nonendocrine cells.[38] In rat respiratory mucosa, nerves have been identified within the epithelium.[51] Free axons have also been demonstrated within Peyer's patches.[52] Within the lamina propria, many nerves contain the neuropeptides, substance P, VIP, cholecystokinin, and somato-statin.[53,54] The majority of these nerves were intrinsic in origin.

VIP-containing nerves are abundant in areas surrounding blood vessels adjacent to the postcapillary venules, the site of lymphocyte traffic out of the systemic circulation into the mucosa.[55] The abundance of VIP-containing nerves in the colonic mucosa has led to the postulation that these nerves serve a sensory role.[56-58] The cell bodies for substance P-containing nerves are found in the myenteric plexus[59,60] and are less dense in submucosal plexus.[61-63] It is also clear that there is considerable species variation in the distribution of the neuropeptide-containing nerves in the gut.[27]

This anatomic organization of nerves and neuroendocrine cells within intestinal lymphoid tissue, as in peripheral lymphoid tissues, can allow for the modulation of inflammatory events by the chemical mediators released. These effects could result from direct interaction with target cells locally. Alternatively, neuropeptides may have indirect effects, for example, by influencing capillary permeability and endothelial cell receptor expression. This could influence the binding of lymphocytes to vessel walls and effect their subsequent emigration into mucosal tissues.

NEUROPEPTIDE RECEPTORS ON LYMPHOCYTES

The demonstration of neuropeptide receptors on lymphocytes has added credence to the notion that functional interactions between immune effector cells and nerves can exist. There are numerous studies describing such receptors specific for the different neuropeptides on lymphocytes (Table 10–1).

Specific cell surface receptors for substance P have been described on human lymphocytes, predominately T-helper cells;[63,64] recently a monoclonal antibody to this receptor has been described.[65] Murine lymphocytes of both B and T phenotypes bear substance-P receptors, although cells isolated from Peyer's patches have significantly greater numbers than those isolated from spleen.[66]

Receptors for somatostatin on both murine T and B cells have also recently been described.[67] Again there is an organ-related difference in that a greater percentage of cells from the Peyer's patch bind somatostatin, compared with spleen. In addition, a greater number of the Lyt2+ (CD8) cells bind somatostatin, as opposed to the L3T4 (CD4) cells. The predominance of somatostatin receptors on cells with the T-suppressor/cytotoxic phenotype suggests a possible mechanism for the depressive effect of somatostatin on lymphocyte function.

VIP receptors have been described on human,[68,69] murine,[70,71] and rat lymphocytes.[72] Such studies examining the distribution and characteristics of the specific neuropeptide receptors on lymphocytes can help us to understand the differential effects on the immune response. Site and organ-specific differences may also allow us to explain the specific effects seen in the intestinal immune response.

NEUROPEPTIDE EFFECTS ON LYMPHOCYTES

Important differences may depend on dose, time of exposure, culture condition, organ, and species.[73,74] In addition, there may be cell cycle-dependent influences.[75] This may account for discrepancies seen in different in vitro studies.[76,77] When

Table 10–1 NEUROPEPTIDE RECEPTORS DESCRIBED ON IMMUNE EFFECTOR CELLS[a]

Neuropeptide	Cell/source	Receptor	K_D	Receptor no.	Reference
VIP	Human PBMNC	+	>25		68
		+	<0.25		69
	Murine				
	T Lymphocytes	+	5		71
	Spleen	+			
	MLN	+			
	PP	+			
	Thymus	−			
	Rat				72
	Lymphocyte	+			
	Human				
	MOLT-4	+	7.3	15,000	70
	T lymphocytes	+	0.47	1,700	127
SP	Human				
	PBMNC	+	185	7,035	63
	CD4+	+(18)			
	CD8+	+(10)			
	IM-9	+	0.65	22,000	64, 128
	Murine				
	Spleen	+(68)	0.68	190	66
	PP	+(40)		647–1,000	
	CD4+	+			
	CD8+	+			
	B cells	+			
	IgG/M/A				
SOM	Human PBMNC	+	1.4	500	129
	Murine				
	MOPC 315	+(68)	1.6	40,733	130
	PP	+(47)			67
	T cells	+(80–90)			
	B cells	+(80)			
	Spleen				
	T cells	+(30–50)			
	B cells	+(30)			

[a] +, present; −, absent (% positive); K_D, dissociation constant 10^{-9} M; PBMNC, peripheral blood mononuclear cells; MLN, mesenteric lymph node; PP, Peyer's patch.

examining the in vivo effects of neuropeptides, on the other hand, one must further consider a multiplicity of cell interactions in addition to the direct effects on the cell whose function is being examined. With this in mind, some of these functional effects are examined.

Various neuropeptides have been shown to influence a host of immune reactions, including B-lymphocyte proliferation and antibody synthesis,[78,79] T-lymphocyte proliferation,[74,77,80] natural killer cell function,[81,82] and macrophage activity.[83] The microanatomic relationship between intestinal mucosal mast cells and enteric nerves[84] has been studied. Sixty-seven percent of rat mucosal mast cells were associated with subepithelial nerves identified by staining with antibody specific for neuron-specific enolase. We also showed that 61% of the mucosal mast cell population were associated with substance P-containing nerves, and that calcitonin gene-related peptide (CGRP) was present also in axons adjacent to these cells. Electron microscopy confirmed this relationship in random villus sections, revealing that 31% of the mucosal mast cells were within 250 nm of axon profiles.

Proliferation

Lymphocyte proliferation is an indirect measure of antigen responsiveness, since many nonantigen-specific stimuli can alter this response. Nonetheless, proliferation does allow us to assess differences in polyclonal responses that can be influenced by neuropeptides (Table 10–2). This might occur through changes in cell cycling, resulting in altered sensitivity to the various mitogens. How these proliferative responses reflect physiologic efffects of the neuropeptides remains speculative.

Substance P enhanced human T-cell response to phytohemagglutinin (PHA) or concanavalin A (con A) by 40–60%.[80] In mice, substance P was shown to increase lymphocyte proliferation, as measured by [^{3}H]thymidine uptake in a mitogen (con A)-stimulated culture. This was true for both spleen and Peyer's patch lymphocytes.[85] Somatostatin inhibited PHA-induced proliferation of human peripheral blood mononuclear cells.[86] On murine lymphocytes derived from Peyer's patches, somatostatin had a similar inhibitory influence of up to 50%.[85] Inhibition of proliferation was also seen with VIP on T cells from mesenteric lymph nodes and spleen;[71] this process occurred via activation of cAMP.

Table 10–2   NEUROPEPTIDE EFFECTS ON LYMPHOCYTE PROLIFERATION[a]

Neuropeptide	Source	Mitogen	Effect	Reference
VIP	Murine			71
	MLN	Con A	−	
		PHA	−	
	Spleen	Con A	−	
		PHA	−	
	B cell	LPS	ø	
SOM	Human			
	PBMNC	PHA	−	86
	Murine			
	Spleen	Con A	−	85
	PP	Con A	−	
SP	Human			
	T cells	PHA	+	63
		Con A	+	
	Murine			
	Spleen	Con A	+	85
	MLN	Con A	+	
	PP	Con A	+	

[a] +, increase; −, decrease; ø, no change in mitogen-induced proliferation; VIP, vasoactive intestinal polypeptide; MLN, mesenteric lymph node; Con A, concanavalin A; PHA, phytohemagglutinin; LPS, lipopolysaccharide; SOM, somatostatin; PBMNC, peripheral blood mononuclear cells; PP, Peyer's patch; SP, substance P.

Mucosal Lymphocyte Traffic

As discussed in Chapter 5, VIP can influence the trafficking ability of lymphocytes destined for mucosal sites. Mesenteric lymph node cells preincubated with VIP alter the number of VIP receptors expressed. This treatment also produces an alteration in the binding of such cells to high endothelial venules, resulting in a decrease in the specific ability of these cells to localize to mucosal tissues.[87]

Similar effects on traffic were obtained in a sheep lymphocyte traffic model. The acute infusion of VIP into cannulated afferent lymphatics produced a decrease in the lymphocyte output into the efferent lymph.[88] Thus VIP seems to have an important regulatory effect on the traffic of lymphocytes into tissues. The effects of other neuropeptides on lymphocyte traffic have been less well studied.

Effect on Antibody Production

The effect of neuropeptides on intestinal antibody (Ab) secretion has also been examined (Table 10–3). Cholecystokinin (CCK), given to human volunteers, increases intestinal antibodies of the IgA, M, E, and D classes.[89,90] In an isolated loop of a rat intestine model, this group also showed that intravenous CCK resulted in a rise of intestinal lumenal IgA and IgG antibodies which, was blocked by the CCK antagonist proglumide. Furthermore, intragastric instillation of food produced a similar increase in intestinal antibody levels.[91] The mechanism of this increase in antibody levels is not clear. The response was extremely rapid, suggesting that de novo antibody synthesis and transport was not responsible. It seems likely to us that the process involves increased release, transport, or secretion of preformed antibody across the epithelium. Although these studies demonstrate changes in local Ab levels with CCK, they do not address the issue of a possible direct effect of neuropeptide on the Ab-producing cells.

Other studies have examined the ability of neuropeptides to affect antibody production more directly. Antibody synthesis by murine lymphocytes in a con A-stimulated culture system is stimulated by substance P and inhibited by somatostatin. Interestingly, in this study, the effect of substance P was more marked (three- to fourfold) on the cells derived from Peyer's patches, compared with splenocytes, suggesting an organ-specific effect. In addition, there was also a difference in the isotype affected, in that IgA was increased more than IgM, while there was little effect on IgG synthesis.[85] The VIP effect on immunoglobulin synthesis was also specific in an isotype- and organ-related manner. IgA was affected more than IgM or IgG, and the effect on Peyer's patch cells was inhibitory, while in spleen, it was stimulatory.[85] These studies demonstrate that Ab responses to neuropeptide, in a non-Ag-specific manner, may differ in different tissues.

Ag-specific antibody response to sheep red blood cells (SRBC) has been examined. In capsaicin-treated rats, lymph node anti-SRBC Ab was decreased by more than 80%. Capsaicin treatment depletes sensory peripheral nerves of substance P. The resulting decrease in Ab to SRBC could be restored if the antigen was given with substance P. This study supports a regulatory effect of this neuropeptide on an antigen-specific antibody response.[92]

To assess the response to neuropeptides in vivo, a series of experiments were carried out in which substance P was administered continuously for 7 days by subcutaneously implanted mini-osmotic pumps.[93] The pumps allowed the serum levels of substance P to be chronically maintained at a level two- to threefold higher

Table 10–3 EFFECT OF NEUROPEPTIDES ON ANTIBODY PRODUCTION[a]

Neuropeptide	Tissue	Effect	Reference
CCK	Human		
	intestinal secretion		89
	IgA, M, E, D	+	
	Rat		
	intestinal secretion		
	IgA, G	+	90
SP	Murine		
	in vitro[b]		
	Spleen		
	IgA	+	85
	IgM	−	
	PP		
	IgA	+++	
	IgM	+	
	in vivo[b]		
	Spleen & PP		
	IgA	+	93
	IgM	+	
SOM	Murine		
	in vitro[b]		
	Spleen & PP		
	IgA	−	85
	IgM	−	
	in vivo[b]		
	Spleen & PP		
	IgA	+	94
VIP	Murine		
	in vitro[b]		
	Spleen		
	IgA	+	85
	PP		
	IgA	−	
	IgM	+	

[a] +, increase; −, decrease in antibody production; CCK, cholecystokinin; SP, substance P; PP, Peyer's patch; SOM, somatostatin; VIP, vasoactive intestinal polypeptide.

[b] Con A-stimulated cultures (1 μm/ml).

than normal. Peyer's patch and spleen lymphocytes of animals treated with these pumps showed an increase in both proliferative ability and antibody-producing capacity, again predominately for IgA. Thus the in vivo experiments reflected accurately the observations previously noted in vitro with substance P. Somatostatin, on the other hand, administered in vivo, caused an increase in proliferation and antibody production.[94]

Recent work has demonstrated a "dual" or bidirectional response to somatostatin in vitro, with both stimulatory effects and inhibitory effects, depending on the specific experimental conditions, such as dose and time of exposure.[76] Such "dual" effects have also been seen with other neuropeptides.[73,77] This finding suggests that some of the influences of neuropeptides on immune function may involve complex pathways and multiple intermediate signals. Somatostatin in vivo, for example, may be acting on lymphocytes indirectly via its effect on other hormones or neuropeptides. The mechanism of the isotype-specific response is unexplained. It may simply reflect the fact that there are more IgA-committed B and T cells in Peyer's patches, as opposed to other isotypes. It remains to be shown where in the regulatory network the neuropeptides are having their effects. With the evidence for high-affinity receptors on B and T cells, substance P could be affecting B cells directly or indirectly through T-cell cytokine production, such as IL4, IL5, or IL6, or via T-suppressor or -contrasuppressor cell activation.

These experiments not only serve to highlight differences between the neuropeptides, but also illustrate differences related to the tissue of origin of the responding lymphocyte. Since neuropeptides are prevalent in intestinal tissues, it would seem that gut-specific effects may be the more significant interaction. This points to the importance of examining directly those lymphocytes of the intestinal immune system. In addition, these studies suggest that the effect of neuropeptides on the mucosal immune system may also occur through effects on other nonimmune cells such as epithelium or vascular endothelium, in addition to direct effects on lymphocytes or Ag-presenting or -processing cells. Changes in epithelial or vascular permeability can, for example, effect the access of Ag to the immune effector cells.

Cytotoxicity

The effect of neuropeptides on cells with cytotoxic activity has been addressed in only a few studies (Table 10–4). Mathews et al.[81] demonstrated that β-endorphin and methionine-enkephalin can increase human peripheral blood natural killer (NK) activity. More recently, NK activity of human peripheral blood lymphocytes was shown to be modulated in vitro by VIP. The effect was dependent on whether the cells were preincubated with VIP, in which case a stimulatory effect was seen, or coincubated for the duration of the cytotoxic assay, in which case an inhibitory effect was seen. The inhibitory effect of VIP was not related to its ability to activate the adenylate cyclase system.[82]

Table 10–4 NEUROPEPTIDE EFFECT ON CYTOTOXICITY (NK)[a]

Neuropeptide	Cell/source	Effect	Reference
VIP	Human PBMNC		82
	Coincubation	−	
	Preincubation	+	
SP	Murine		96
In vitro	Spleen	ø	
	IEL	+	
In vivo	Spleen	ø	
	IEL	++	

[a] +, increase; −, decrease; ø, no change in natural killer (NK) activity; VIP vasoactive intestinal polypeptide; SP, substance P; PBMNC, peripheral blood mononuclear cells; IEL, intraepithelial leukocytes.

In order to address the question of whether neuropeptides can exert an effect on the cytotoxic activity of intestinal lymphocytes, we examined the changes in NK activity of intraepithelial leukocytes (IEL). Our preliminary results suggest that substance P stimulated the NK activity of IEL, a population with diverse cytotoxic ability.[95] This effect was specific for the intestine, since there was only a minimal effect on the NK activity of spleen. Interestingly, substance P given by osmotic pump in vivo for 7 days also increased NK activity of IEL without affecting splenic NK activity.[96]

The organ specificity of this regulatory action of substance P, in vivo and in vitro, again illustrates the potential importance of these neuropeptides in regulating intestinal lymphocytes.

MAST CELLS

Mast cells in different sites are heterogeneous with respect to histochemical, biochemical, pharmacologic, and functional characteristics.[97,98] Major differences are exhibited between mast cells isolated from the peritoneal cavity and those found in the intestinal and respiratory mucosae in the rat.[99,100,101] Enerback[102] showed that mucosal mast cells could not be demonstrated following routine formalin fixation. Similar histochemical heterogeneity has been described in primates and most recently in humans.[103-105]

In rats, mucosal mast cells contain a unique rat mast cell protease II (RMCP II), as opposed to the serosal mast cell, which contains RMCP I.[97] These proteases are preformed and released upon degranulation and secretion. Antigen stimulation of mast cells causes the release of other potent mediators such as serotonin (5-HT), histamine, and products of arachidonic acid, either preformed and stored within the granules or newly formed following stimulation. The basis of histochemical heterogeneity appears to be the presence of heparin in the connective tissue mast cell and its absence in the mucosal mast cell, which instead contains and synthesizes chondroitin sulphate di-B.[99] A similar heterogeneity in terms of enzyme content has been shown for intestinal mucosal mast cells and other mast cells in the human.[105] In addition, the responsiveness to secretagogues, compound 48/80, bee venom peptide 401, neuropeptides, and endorphins differs in the two mast cell populations.[106] Of particular importance is the lack of effect of the antiallergic compounds sodium cromoglycate and theophylline on rat mucosal mast cells.[101] Doxantrazole, quercetin, and related flavonoids, on the other hand, are effective in inhibiting histamine release from both connective tissue as well as mucosal mast cells.

The presence of mast cells in peripheral nerves and associated with nerve regeneration has been known for many years and is reviewed extensively by Olsson.[107] It is also well established that mast cells are present in benign nerve sheath tumors including neurofibromata and in amputation neuromas in rodents and humans. Mast cells are found in glomus tumors, where they have been observed closely apposed to unmyelinated nerve fibers and sometimes exhibit various stages of degranulation. Scattered, mostly anecdotal references, also describe occasional mast cell/nerve relationships in the diaphragm, mesentery, normal skin, and myocardium; in the first two of these sites, substance P-containing nerves were observed close to mast cells.[108-111] Recently we have shown an extensive and intimate association of intestinal mucosal mast cells with subepithelial nerves in a careful morphometric study of both normal and inflamed rat intestine after nematode infection with *Nippostrongylus brasiliensis*.[84]

Kiernan[17] and Lembeck and Holzer[112] have suggested that mast cells and substance P-containing nerves may be involved in the axon reflex responsible for the flare reaction to noxious stimuli in the skin. Injection of substance P into skin mimics the response of local injection of histamine or the mast cell degranulation agent compound 48/80, and is inhibited by antihistamines.[113-115] Somatostatin was added to the list of neuropeptides capable of affecting histamine release from skin mast cells in situ.[116] Other in vivo experiments have shown that antidromic nerve stimulation can cause mast cell degranulation, neurogenic edema, and histamine-mediated modulation of neurotransmitter release. Many neuropeptides and endorphins effect histamine release from connective tissue mast cells, but only substance P, of all the neuropeptides tested, caused release from intestinal mucosal mast cells.[106]

Direct stimulation of the vidian nerve in patients caused morphologic mast cell changes and a significant decrease in tissue-based histamine.[117] Leff et al. showed that vagal stimulation caused an enhancement of secretion of histamine in the lung after challenge with ascaris antigen in natively allergic dogs.[118] One report showed a decrease in mast cell granularity in rat ileum following electric field stimulation.[119] These studies demonstrate that neural activity can cause mast cell stimulation. Other studies have provided evidence that the effects of mucosal mast cell mediators in ion transport may act in part through enteric nerves.[120,121] Weinreich has recently shown that antigen produces compound action potentials when placed in contact with the superior cervical ganglion removed from sensitized rats.[122]

Finally, in a classical conditioning paradigm, guinea pigs have shown an increased plasma histamine in response to the conditioning stimulus alone.[123] In another conditioning model, we have shown that an audiovisual stimulus coupled with antigen can condition on exposure to the stimulus without antigen for RMCP II elevations.[124] These data again strongly suggest that mucosal mast cells and nerves have a significant and purposeful interaction.

In coculture experiments using murine superior cervical ganglions (SCG) from newborn mice (1–2 days) and rat basophil leukemia (RBL-2H3) cells, it was apparent that neurite extensions appeared to be directed toward RBL cells and that these cells displayed a neurotropic influence. When neurite contacts with RBL were quantitated in culture, they increased with time to between 80 and 100%. We observed that when contacts were formed, they were maintained over periods of up to 100 hours' observation. Furthermore, the RBL cells displayed similar properties in this respect to freshly isolated peritoneal mast cells representative of connective tissue mast cells. RBL ceased to divide on contact and became highly granular, suggesting that the nerve contact had a differentiative effect on these mast cells.[125]

Electrophysiologic experiments involving microprobing of mast cells in contact with nerves and those in the same culture dishes not in contact showed that while the membrane potentials of RBL in all groups was the same, the input resistance (conductance) was significantly reduced by approximately 50% in those RBL that were "innervated".[125]

We believe from the evidence reviewed above that mast cells and local enteric nerves may form a purposeful interaction within the intestinal mucosa to form a homeostatic regulatory unit. Growth, chemotaxis, maturation, and differentiation

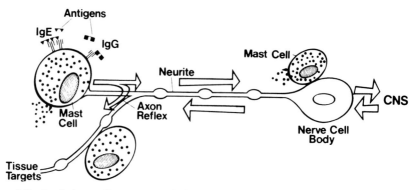

Figure 10–1 Schematic representation of the bidirectional interaction between mast cells and nerves.

of mast cells may be under local environmental regulation. Inflammation may alter such regulation, and the resulting mast cell hyperplasia commonly found associated with inflammation and repair could reflect in part an interaction between mast cells and nerves. While true axon reflexes have not been described in the intestine, we believe that they occur. Burnstock[126] talks about these as "sensorimotor" events, believing that the concept of axon reflexes may not be entirely valid and that purposeful passage of impulses generated at one site may be transmitted to another site through a motor afferent effector arm. Mast cells sensitized by IgE and in contact with nerves could act as a transducer of environmental signals for the central nervous system. This is diagrammatically shown in Figure 10–1.

CONCLUSIONS

It is clear that the neuropeptides, substance P, somatostatin, and VIP have profound effects on lymphocytes and their function. The description of the structural and molecular basis that allows this interaction to occur supports the concept that the nervous system (via neuropeptide neurotransmitters) can influence the local

Table 10–5 EFFECTS OF SUBSTANCE P

Immune
  Increased phagocytosis
  Macrophage activation
  Monocyte chemotaxis
  Increased lymphocyte proliferation
  Increased immunoglobulin production — IgA
  Increased intestinal NK activity
Nonimmune
  Smooth muscle contraction
  Vasodilatation
  Increased vascular permeability (skin)
  Increased secretion (respiratory/nasal mucosa)

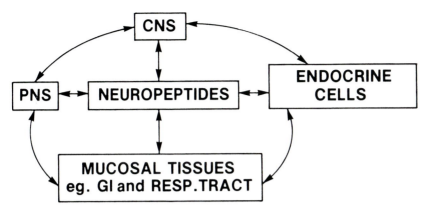

Figure 10−2 Interaction between the neuroendocrine system and the mucosal tissues, including the intestinal immune system, relies on neuropeptides as one of the important chemical messengers.

immune response in the intestinal mucosa. Taking substance P as an example, we have reviewed several of these effects. In addition to the effects of substance P on B, T, NK, and mast cells, we must also not lose sight of the fact that substance P can influence nonimmune cell functions of the intestine (Table 10−5). These nonimmune effects may be equally important in influencing the immune response that occurs in vivo when a food allergen or pathogenic organism is presented to the intestinal mucosa. The complexity of these interactions is only beginning to be dissected in an effort to build a unifying concept of the regulatory events that control the intestinal immune response.

Such studies may be especially relevant to gastrointestinal diseases characterized by chronic inflammation. It will now become important to identify how the interactions between the neuropeptides and the immune system and nonimmune elements of the intestine (Fig. 10−2) are related to the alterations in the immune response described in patients with inflammatory bowel disease. It is hoped that these endeavors will allow the development of new modalities of therapy directed at these regulatory molecules.

REFERENCES

1. Lundgren O: Nervous control of intestinal transport. *Baillieres Clin Gastroenterol* 2:85−106, 1988.
2. Ader R: *Psychoneuroimmunology.* New York, Academic Press, 1981.
3. Cosma J, Leonhardt H, Wekerk H: Hormonal coordination of the immune response. *Rev Physiol Biochem Pharmacol* 92:116, 1982.
4. Wybran J: Enkephalins and endorphins as modifiers of the immune system: present and future. *Fed Proc* 44:92−94, 1985.
5. Payan DG, McGillis JP, Goetzl EJ: Neuro-immunology. *Adv Immunol* 39:299−323, 1986.
6. Berczi I, Nagy E. The effect of prolactin and growth hormone on hemolymphonpoietic tissue and immune function. In Berczi I: *Hormone and Immunity.* Norwell, MTP Press Limited, 1987, p 145.

7. Claman HN: Corticosteroids, immunologic and anti-inflammatory effects. In Berczi I: *Hormone and Immunity.* Norwell, MTP Press Limited, 1987, p 38.

8. Sullivan DA: Endocrine control of the ocular secretory immune system. In Berczi I: *Hormone and Immunity.* Norwell, MTP Press Limited, 1987, p 54.

9. Wira CR, Colby EM: Regulation of secretory component by glucocorticoids in primary cultures of rat hepatocytes. *J Immunol* 134:1744–1748, 1985.

10. Kelly JK, Fox H: The local immunological defence system of the human endometrium. *J Reprod Immunol* 1:39–45, 1979.

11. Cox J, Ford WL: Lymphocyte traffic in pregnant or estrogen stimulated rats. *J Reprod Immunol* 6:167–176, 1984.

12. Weisz-Carrington P, Roux ME, McWilliams M, et al: Hormonal induction of the secretory immune system in the mammary gland. *Proc Natl Acad Sci USA* 75:2928–2932, 1978.

13. Murdoch AJM, Buckley CH, Fox H: Hormonal control of the secretory immune system of the human uterine cervix. *J Reprod Biol* 4:23–30, 1982.

14. Fearn HJ, Karady S, West GB: The role of the nervous system in local inflammatory responses. *J Pharm Pharmacol* 17:761–765, 1965.

15. Ader R, Cohen N: Behaviorally conditioned immunosuppression. *Psychosom Med* 37:333–340, 1975.

16. Ghanta VK, Hiramoto RN, Solvason HB, et al: Neural and environmental influences on neoplasia and conditioning of NK activity. *J Immunol* 135:848s–852s, 1985.

17. Kiernan JA: A pharmacological and histological investigation of the involvement of mast cells in cutaneous axon reflex vasodilatation. *Q J Exp Physiol* 60:123–136, 1975.

18. Foreman JC: Peptides and neurogenic inflammation. *Br Med Bull* 43:386–400, 1987.

19. Besedovsky HO, Felix D, Haas H: Hypothalamic changes during the immune response. *Eur J Immunol* 7:323–325, 1977.

20. Blalock JE: The immune system as a sensory organ. *J Immunol* 132:1067–1070, 1984.

21. Blalock JE, Smith EM: A complete regulatory loop between the immune and neuroendocrine systems. *Fed Proc* 44:108–111, 1985.

22. Carr DJJ, Blalock JE: A molecular basis for bi-directional communication between the immune and neuroendocrine system. In Cinader B and Miller RG: *Progress in Immunology* VI. Orlando, Academic Press, 1986, p 619.

23. Bienenstock J, Befus AD: The gastrointestinal tract as an immune organ. In Shorter R: *Gastrointestinal Immunity for the Clinician.* New York, Raven Press, 1985, p 1.

24. Elson CO, Kagnoff MF, Fiocchi C, et al: Intestinal immunity and inflammation: recent progress. *Gastroenterology* 91:746–768, 1968.

25. Furness JB, Costa M: Commentary: types of nerves in the enteric nervous system. *Neurosciences* 5:1–20, 1980.

26. Pernow B: Substance P. *Pharmacol Rev* 35:84–151, 1983.

27. Cooke HJ: Neurobiology of the intestinal mucosa. *Gastroenterology* 90:1057–1081, 1986.

28. Johnson AR, Erdos EG: Release of histamine from mast cells by vasoactive peptides. *Proc Soc Exp Biol Med* 142:1252–1256, 1973.

29. Lembeck F, Donnerer J, Colpaert FC: Increase of substance P in primary afferent nerves during chronic pain. *Neuropeptides* 1:175, 1981.

30. Besterman HS, Mallinson CN, Modigliani R, et al: Gut hormones in inflammatory bowel disease. *Scand J Gastroenterol* 18:845–852, 1983.

31. Bishop AE, Polak JM, Bryant MG, et al: Abnormalities of vasoactive intestinal polypeptide-containing nerves in Crohn's disease. *Gastroenterology* 79:853–860, 1980.

32. O'Morain C, Bishop AE, McGregor GP, et al: Vasoactive intestinal peptide concentrations and immunocytochemical studies in rectal biopsies from patients with IBD. *Gut* 25:57–61, 1984.

33. Sjolund K, Schaffalitzky de Muckadeli OB, Fahrekrug J, et al: Peptide-containing nerve fibres in the gut wall in Crohn's disease. *Gut* 24:724–733, 1983.

34. Koch TR, Carney JA, Go VLW: Distribution and quantitation of gut neuropeptides in normal intestine and inflammatory bowel diseases. *Dig Dis Sci* 32:369–376, 1987.

35. Mantyh CR, Gates TS, Zimmerman RP, et al: Receptor binding sites for substance P, but not substance K or neuromedin K, are expressed in high concentrations by arterioles, venules, and lymph nodules in surgical specimens obtained from patients with ulcerative colitis and Crohn disease. *Proc Natl Acad Sci USA* 85:3235–3239, 1988.

36. Besedovsky HO, Del Rey AE, Sorkin E: What do the immune system and the brain know about each other? *Immunol Today* 4:342–346, 1983.

37. Polak JM, Bloom SR: Regulatory peptides: key factors in the control of bodily functions. *Br Med J* 286:1461–1466, 1983.

38. Polak JM, Bloom SR: Regulatory peptides of the gastrointestinal and respiratory tracts. *Arch Int Pharmacodyn* 280 (Suppl):16–49, 1986.

39. Pearse AGE, Polak JM: Neural crest origin of the endocrine polypeptide (APUD) cells of the gastrointestinal tract and pancreas. *Gut* 12:783–788, 1971.

40. Papadaki L, Rode J, Dhillon AP, et al: Fine structure of a neuroendocrine complex in the mucosa of the appendix. *Gastroenterology* 84:490–497, 1983.

41. O'Dorisio MS: Neuropeptides and gastrointestinal immunity. *Am J Med* 81 (Suppl 6B):74–82, 1986.

42. Weinstock JV, Blum AJ, Fry G: Tachykinin production by granuloma eosinophils in murine schistosomiasis mansoni. *FASEB J* 2:A882, 1988.

43. Bulloch K: Nueroanatomy of lymphoid tissue: a review. In Guillemin R: *Neural Modulation of Immunity.* New York, Raven Press, 1985, p 111.

44. Felten DL, Felten SY, Carlson SL, et al: Noradrenergic and peptidergic innervation of lymphoid tissue. *J Immunol* 135:755s–765s, 1985.

45. Ackerman KD, Felten SY, Bellinger DL, et al: Noradrenergic sympathetic innervation of spleen and lymph nodes in relation to specific cellular components. In Cinader M, Miller RG: *Progress in Immunology* VI. Orlando, Academic Press, 1986, p 588.

46. Felten DL, Ackerman KD, Wiegard SJ, et al: Noradrenergic sympathetic innervation of the spleen. I. Nerve fibres associate with lymphocytes and macrophages in specific compartments of the splenic white pulp. *J Neurosci Res* 18:28–36, 1987.

47. Hammer JA: Innervations-verhaltnisse der krelorgane der Thymus bis in den 4 Tetalmonat. *Z Mikrosk Anat Forsch* 8:253, 1935.

48. Bulloch K, Pomerantz W: Autonomic nervous system innervation of thymic-related lymphoid tissue in wild-type and nude mice. *J Comp Neurol* 228:57–68, 1984.

49. Davison JS: Innervation of the gastrointestinal tract. In Christensen J, Wingate D: *A Guide to Gastrointestinal Motility.* Bristol, Wright, 1983, p 1.

50. Gabella G: Innervation of the gastrointestinal tract. *Int Rev Cytol* 59:129–1193, 1979.

51. Jeffrey P, Reid L: Intra-epithelial nerves in normal rat airways: a quantitative electron microscopic study. *J Anat* 114:35–45, 1973.

52. Pfoch M, Unsicker K: Electron microscopic study on the innervation of Peyer's patches of the Syrian hamster. *Z Zellforsch* 123:425–429, 1972.

53. Ekblad E, Winther C, Ekman R, et al: Projections of peptide-containing neurons in rat small intestine. *Neuroscience* 20:169–188, 1987.

54. Probert L, DeMey J, Polak JM: Distinct subpopulations of enteric p-type neurons contain substance P and vasoactive intestinal polypeptide. *Nature* 293:470–471, 1981.

55. Ottaway CA, Lewis DL, Asa SL: Vasoactive intestinal peptide-containing nerves in Peyer's patches. *Brain Behav Immun* 1:148–158, 1987.

56. Schultzberg M, Hokfelt T, Nilsson G, et al: Distribution of peptide- and catecholamine-containing neurons in the gastrointestinal tract of rat and guinea-pig: immunohistochemical studies with antisera to substance P, vasoactive intestinal polypeptide, enkephalins, somatostatin, gastrin/cholecystokinin, neurotensin and dopamine β-hydroxylase. *Neuroscience* 5:689–744, 1980.

57. Reinecke M, Schulter P, Yanaihara N, et al: VIP immunoreactivity in enteric nerves and endocrine cells of the vertebrate gut. *Peptides* 2:149–156, 1981.

58. Jessen DR, Polak JM, Van Noorden S, et al: Peptide-containing neurones connect the two ganglionated plexuses of the enteric nervous system. *Nature* 283:391–393, 1980.

59. Bishop AE, Polak JM, Lake BD, et al: Abnormalities of the colonic regulatory peptides in Hirschsprung's disease. *Histopathology* 5:679–688, 1981.

60. Pearse AGE, Polak JM: Immunocytochemical localization of substance P in mammalian intestine. *Histochemistry* 41:373–375, 1975.

61. Furness JB, Costa M, Keast JR: Choline acetyltransferase- and peptide-immunoreactivity of submucous neurons in the small intestine of the guinea-pig. *Cell Tissue Res* 237:329–333, 1984.

62. Nilsson G, Brodin E: Tissue distribution of substance P-like immunoreactivity in dog, rat and mouse. In von Evler US, Pernow B: *Substance P.* New York, Raven Press, 1977, p 49.

63. Payan DG, Brewster DR, Missirian-Bastian A, et al: Substance P recognition by subset of human T lymphocytes. *J Clin Invest* 74:1532–1539, 1984.

64. Payan DG, Brewster DR, Goetzl EJ: Stereospecific receptors for substance P on cultured human IM-9 lymphoblasts. *J Immunol* 133:3260–3265, 1984.

65. Organist ML, Harvey J, McGillis JP, et al: Characterization of a monoclonal antibody against the lymphoblast substance P receptor. *J Immunol* 139:3050–3054, 1987.

66. Stanisz AM, Scicchitano R, Dazin P, et al: Distribution of substance P receptors on murine spleen and Peyer's patch T and B cells. *J Immunol* 139:749–754, 1987.

67. Scicchitano R, Dazin P, Bienenstock J, et al: Distribution of somatostatin receptors on murine spleen and Peyer's patch T and B lymphocytes. *Brain Behav Immun* 1:173–184, 1987.

68. Wiik P, Opstad PK, Boyum A: Binding of vasoactive intestinal polypeptide (VIP) by human blood monocytes: demonstration of specific binding sites. *Reg Peptides* 12:145–153, 1985.

69. Ottaway CA, Bernaerts C, Chan B, et al: Specific binding of vasoactive intestinal peptide to human circulation mononuclear cells. *Can J Physiol Pharmacol* 61:664–671, 1983.

70. Beed EA, O'Dorisio MA, O'Dorisio TM et al: Demonstration of a functional receptor for vasoactive intestinal polypeptide on MOLT 4b T lymphoblasts. *Regul Pept* 6:1–12, 1983.

71. Ottaway CA, Greenberg G.R: Interaction of vasoactive intestinal peptide with mouse lymphocytes: specific binding and the modulation of mitogen responses. *J Immunol* 132:417–423, 1984.

72. Calvo JR, Mlinero P, Jimenez J, et al: Interaction of vasoactive intestinal peptide (VIP) with rat lymphoid cells. *Peptides* 7:177–181, 1986.

73. Scicchitano R, Bienenstock J, Stanisz AM: The differential effect with time of neuropeptides on the proliferative responses of murine Peyer's patch and splenic lymphocytes. *Brain Behav Immun* 1:231–237, 1987.

74. Soder O, Hellstrom PM: Neuropeptide regulation of human thymocyte, guinea pig T

lymphocyte and rat B lymphocyte mitogenesis. *Int Arch Allergy Appl Immunol* 84:205–211, 1987.

75. Scicchitano R, Stanisz AM, Payan DG, et al. Expression of substance P and somatostatin receptors on a T helper cell line. In Mestecky J, McGhee J, Bienenstock J, et al: *Recent Advances in Mucosal Immunology.* New York, Plenum Press, 1987, p 185.

76. Pawlikowski M, Stepien H, Kunert-Radek J, et al: Effect of somatostatin on the proliferation of mouse spleen lymphocytes *in vitro. Biochem Biophys Res Commun* 129:52–55, 1985.

77. Nordlind C, Mutt V: Influence of beta-endorphin, somatostatin, substance P and vasoactive intestinal peptide on the proliferative response of human peripheral blood T lymphocytes to mercuric chloride. *Int Arch Allergy Appl Immunol* 80:326–328, 1986.

78. Johnson HM, Smith EM, Torres BA, et al: Regulation of the in vitro antibody response by neuroendocrine hormones. *Proc Natl Acad Sci USA* 79:4171–4174, 1982.

79. Sandberg G, Ljungdahl A: Mitogenic responses of splenic B and T lymphocytes in neonatally capsaicin-treated mice. *Int Arch Allergy Appl Immunol* 81:343–347, 1986.

80. Pyan DG, Brewster DR, Goetzl EJ: Specific stimulation of human T lymphocytes by substance P. *J Immunol* 131:1613–1615, 1983.

81. Mathews PM, Froehlich CJ, Sibbitt WL, et al: Enhancement of natural cytotoxicity by beta-endorphin. *J Immunol* 130:1658–1662, 1983.

82. Rola-Pleszczynski M, Bolduc D, St Pierre S: The effects of vasoactive intestinal peptide on human natural killer cell function. *J Immunol* 135:2569–2573, 1985.

83. Bar-Shavit Z, Terry S, Blumerg S, et al: Neurotensin-macrophage interactions: specific binding and augmentation of phagocytosis. *Neuropeptides* 2:325–335, 1982.

84. Stead RH, Tomioka M, Quinonez G, et al: Intestinal mucosal mast cells in normal and nematode-infected rat intestines are in intimate contact with peptidergic nerves. *Proc Natl Acad Sci USA* 84:2975–2979, 1987.

85. Stanisz AM, Befus D, Bienenstock J: Differential effects of vasoactive intestinal peptide, substance P, and somatostatin on immunoglobulin synthesis and proliferation by lymphocytes from Peyer's patch, mesenteric lymph node and spleen. *J Immunol* 136:152–156, 1986.

86. Payan DG, Hess CA, Goetzl EJ: Inhibition by somatostatin of the proliferation of T lymphocytes and Molt-4 lymphoblasts. *Cell Immunol* 84:433–438, 1984.

87. Ottaway CA: In vitro alteration of receptors for vasoactive intestinal peptide changes the in vivo localization of mouse T cells. *J Exp Med* 160:1054–1069, 1984.

88. Moore TC, Spruck CH, Said SI: Depression of lymphocyte traffic in sheep by vasoactive intestinal peptide (VIP). *Immunology* 64:475–478, 1988.

89. Shah PC, Freier S, Park BH, et al: Pancreozymin and secetin enhance duodenal fluid antibody levels to cow's milk proteins. *Gastroenterology* 83:916–921, 1982.

90. Frier S, Lebenthal E, Frier M, et al: IgE and IgD antibodies to cow milk and soy protein in duodenal fluid: effects of pancreozymin and secretin. *Immunology* 49:69–75, 1983.

91. Frier S, Eran M, Faber J: Effect of cholecystokinin and of its antagonist, of atropine, and of food on the release of immunoglobulin A and immunoglobulin G specific antibodies in the rat intestine. *Gastroenterology* 93:1242–1246, 1987.

92. Helme RD, Eglezos A, Dandie GW, et al: The effect of substance P on the regional lymph node antibody response to antigenic stimulation in capsaicin-pretreated rats. *J Immunol* 139:3470–3474, 1987.

93. Scicchitano R, Bienenstock J, Stanisz AM: In vivo immunomodulation by the neuropeptide substance P. *Immunology* 63:733–735, 1988.

94. Stanisz AM, Scicchitano R, Bienenstock J: The regulation of the role of vasoactive peptide and other neuropeptides in immune response in vitro and in vivo. In Said S,

Mott V: *Vasoactive Intestinal Peptide and Related Peptides. Ann NY Acad Sci* 1988, 527:478–485.

95. Ernst PB, Befus AD, Bienenstock J: Leucocytes in the intestinal epithelium. An unusual immunological compartment. *Immunol Today* 6:50–55, 1985.

96. Croitoru K, Ernst PB, Bienenstock J: The effect of substance P (SP) and vasoactive intestinal polypeptide (VIP) on murine intestinal natural killer activity. *Gastroenterology* 94:A80, 1988.

97. Befus AD, Bienenstock J, Denburg JA: Mast Cell Heterogeneity. New York, Raven Press, 1986.

98. Bienenstock, J: Comparative aspects of mast cell heterogeneity in different species and sites. *Int Arch Allergy Appl Immunol* 77:126–129, 1985.

99. Stevens RL, Lee TDG, Seldin DC, et al: Intestinal mucosal mast cells from rats infected with *Nippostrongylus brasiliensis* contain protease-resistant chondroitin sulphate di-B proteoglycans. *J Immunol* 137:291–295, 1986.

100. Bienenstock J, Befus AD, Pearce F, et al: Mast cell heterogeneity: derivaton and function with emphasis on the intestine. *J Allergy Clin Immunol* 70:407–412, 1982.

101. Lee TDG, Shanahan F, Miller HRP, et al: Intestinal mucosal mast cells: isolation from rat lamina propria and purificaton using unit gravity velocity sedimentation. *Immunology* 55:721–728, 1985.

102. Enerback L: Mast cells in rat gastrointestinal mucosa. *Acta Pathol Microbiol Scand* 66:289–302, 1966.

103. Barrett KE, Szucs EF, Metcalfe DD: Mast cell heterogeneity in higher animals: A comparison of the properties of autologous lung and intestinal mast cells from nonhuman primates. *J Immunol* 137:2001–2008, 1986.

104. Befus AD, Goodacre R, Dyck N, et al: Mast cell heterogeneity in man. I. Histologic studies of the intestine. *Int Arch Allergy Appl Immunol* 76:232–236, 1985.

105. Schwartz LB, Bradford RR, Irani A-MA, et al: The major enzymes of human mast cell secretory granules. *Am Rev Respir Dis* 135:1186–1189, 1987.

106. Shanahan F, Denburg JA, Fox J, et al: Mast cell heterogeneity. Effects of neuroenteric peptides on histamine release. *J Immunol* 135:1331–1337, 1985.

107. Olsson Y: Mast cells in human peripheral nerves. *Acta Neurol scand* 47:357–359, 1971.

108. Weisner-Menzel L, Schulz B, Vakilzadeh F, et al: Electron microscopical evidence for a direct contact between nerve fibres and mast cells. *Acta Derm Venereol (Stockh)* 61:465–469, 1981.

109. Skofitsch G, Savitt JM, Jacovowitz DM: Suggestive evidence for functional unit between mast cells and substance P fibres in the rat diaphragm and mesentery. *Histochemistry* 82:5–8, 1985.

110. Newson B, Dahlstrom A, Enerback L, et al: Suggestive evidence for a direct innervation of mucosal mast cells. An electron microscopy study. *Neuroscience* 10:565–570, 1983.

111. Bienenstock J, Tomioka M, Matsuda H, et al: The role of mast cells in inflammatory processes: evidence for nerve/mast cell interactions. *Int Arch Allergy Appl Immunol* 82:238–243, 1987.

112. Lembeck F, Holzer P: Substance P as neurogenic mediator of antidromic vasodilation and neurogenic plasma extravasation. *Arch Pharmacl* 310:175, 1979.

113. Erjavec F, Lembeck F, Florjane-Irman T, et al: Release of histamine by substance P. *Naunyn-Schmiedebergs Arch Pharmacol* 317:67–70, 1981.

114. Hagermark O, Hokfelt T, Pernow B: Flare and itch induced by substance P in human skin. *J Invest Dermatol* 71:233–235, 1978.

115. Foreman JC, Jordan CC: Antagonism by neurotensin for the substance P-induced flare in human skin and its relationship to histamine release. *J Physiol* 328:58P–59P, 1982.

116. Piotrowski W, Foreman JC: Actions of substance P, somatostatin, and vasoactive intestinal polypeptide on rat peritoneal mast cells and in human skin. *Arch Pharmacol* 331:364, 1985.

117. Masini E, Rucci L, Cirri-Borghi MB, et al: Stimulation or resection of vidian nerve in patients with chronic hypertrophic non-allergic rhinitis. *Agents actions* 18:251–253, 1986.

118. Leff AR, Stimler NP, Munoz NM, et al: Augmentation of respiratory mast cell secretion of histamine caused by vagus nerve stimulation during antigen challenge. *J Immunol* 136:1066–1073, 1986.

119. Bani-Sacchi T, Barattini M, Bianchi S, et al: The release of histamine by parasympathetic stimulation in guinea-pig auricle and rat ileum. *J Physiol* 371:29–43, 1986.

120. Harari Y, Russell DA, Castro GA: Anaphylaxis-mediated Cl-secretion and parasite rejection in rat intestine. *J Immunol* 138:1250–1255, 1987.

121. Perdue MH, Chung M, Gall DG: The effect of intestinal anaphylaxis on gut function in the rat. *Gastroenterology* 86:391–397, 1984.

122. Weinreich D, Undem BJ: Immunological regulation of synaptic transmission in isolated guinea pig autonomous ganglia. *J Clin Invest* 79:1529–1532, 1987.

123. Russell M, Dark KA, Cummins RW, et al: Learned histamine release. *Science* 225:733, 1984.

124. MacQueen G, Marshall J, Perdue M, et al: Conditional secretion of rat mast cell protease II by mucosal mast cells. *Science* 243:83, 1989.

125. Blennerhassett MG, Bienenstock J: The innervation of mast cells *in vitro*. (submitted), 1988.

126. Burnstock G: The Airways. Neural Control in Health and Disease. Basel, Marcel Dekker, Inc., 1988, p 1.

127. Danek A, O'Dorisio MS, O'Dorisio TM, et al: Specific binding sites for vasoactive intestinal polypeptides on nonadherent peripheral blood lymphocytes. *J Immunol* 131:1173–1177, 1983.

128. Payan DG, McGillis JP, Organist ML: Characterization of the lymphocyte substance P receptor. *J Biol Chem* 261:14321–14329, 1986.

129. Bhathena SJ, Louie J, Schecter GP, et al: Identification of human mononuclear leukocytes bearing receptors for somatostatin and glucagon. *Diabetes* 30:127–131, 1981.

130. Scicchitano R, Dazin P, Bienenstock J, et al: The murine IgA-secreting plasmacytoma MOPC-315 expresses somatostatin receptors. *J Immunol* 141:937–941, 1988.

PART FOUR

IMMUNOPHYSIOLOGY

CHAPTER 11

Immunophysiology: Influence of the Mucosal Immune System on Intestinal Function

A. DEAN BEFUS

INTRODUCTION

Some of the fundamental physiologic principles underlying intestinal function have been elucidated through investigations of pathologic and/or adaptive changes that occur during infection or other disease processes. Tissue damage or adaptative changes may be initiated in numerous ways as a result of infection or because of some nutritional or other environmental stimulus. In this chapter, as the title implies, the major focus will be on stimuli originating from immune and inflammatory responses.

Local immune and inflammatory responses in the gastrointestinal tract recruit and/or activate a spectrum of cell types, each with a multiplicity of mediators. Among the actions of these mediators is the capacity to alter the ontogenic potential or physiologic responsiveness of intestinal cell populations. This field of *immunophysiology* has begun to emerge only recently, as some researchers have boldly moved to bridge the two disciplines of intestinal physiology and immunology. Unfortunately, these disciplines have largely evolved independently, and few workers have been conversant in both areas. Moreover, few research groups have been assembled with a view to integrating these disciplines, although this myopic state is starting to change, and it is easy to predict that the snowball effect is not too far in the future. The highly heterogeneous nature of the intestinal microenvironment in time and space, together with the array of cell types and mediators in the mucosal immune system, makes the study of the networks and cascades of intestinal immunophysiology particularly challenging. However, the diagnostic, prognostic, therapeutic, and intellectual rewards that will arise from these studies cannot be underestimated, and their application will not be restricted to the gastrointestinal tract.

It is my objective to provide an overview of immunophysiology as it relates to the gastrointestinal tract, particularly the small intestine. Because of the heterogeneity and complexity of potential interactions, I will initially provide a brief outline of the players in the mucosal immune system covered extensively elsewhere in this book. Thereafter, some of the major physiologic targets will be identified. I will present a generalized model of immunophysiologic cell interactions in intestinal function, based upon a recent review of analogous cell-cell interactions in hemopoiesis in the bone marrow microenvironment.[1] This model is highly simplified, for the purposes of conceptual development, and the in vivo complexity is far greater, with multiple reciprocities of mediators and cell responses. With this paradigm, examples of cells and mediators from the immune system interacting with intestinal targets such as the epithelium, smooth muscle, stroma, enteric nervous system, and vasculature will be discussed. Because of space limitations, it will not be possible to touch upon all of the exciting investigations that have recently appeared in the literature, and I apologize for the omissions. However, from the bases provided, it will be possible to identify where significant gaps exist in our knowledge and where new tools must be generated to facilitate research activities necessary to remove critical deficiencies.

Castro, Gall, Perdue, Collins, Baird, and their colleagues have been important players in the evolution of these types of study of intestinal function; to help orient the reader, reviews by Walker,[2] Gall and Perdue,[3] and Russell and Castro[4] are highly recommended. In addition, it is important to recognize that in investigations of respiratory physiology and pathophysiology, the role of immune and inflammatory mediators from multiple sources has been widely studied.[5-7]

MUCOSAL IMMUNE SYSTEM AND LOCAL PHYSIOLOGIC TARGETS

This book contains chapters prepared by the experts most knowledgeable on the plethora of cell types involved in mucosal immune and inflammatory responses. Accordingly, it is only necessary to provide a short list of the cells involved and refer briefly to those that have received most study. Specific examples of immunophysiologic interactions between the immune system and intestinal target cells will be outlined in more detail below.

Within the mucosal immune system there are distinct anatomic compartments including the lymphoid aggregates such as the Peyer's patches, appendix, and solitary nodules; the lamina propria; and the intraepithelial site that contains a large and diverse leukocyte population.[8-10]. The cell populations in each of these compartments are highly heterogeneous and collectively function differently from those in other compartments. Moreover, given the pleomorphic nature of the gastrointestinal tract and its immunologic and physiologic compartmentalization, it is paramount to conceptualize microenvironments, each with a local community of cell types that may be continually evolving in response to endogenous stimuli or foreign invaders. New cells may be attracted into the microenvironment and in turn generate mediators or signals through direct cell contact that induce new adaptations to maintain physiologic activity and functional harmony, despite adversity.

Of the spectrum of cell types in immune and inflammatory responses that may be critical in immunophysiologic adaptations to stimuli, T and B lymphocytes,

Table 11 – 1   IMMUNE AND INFLAMMATORY CELLS AND SOME OF THEIR MEDIATORS IN INTESTINAL IMMUNOPHYSIOLOGIC INTERACTIONS

Cell Types	Mediators
Lymphocytes	
T cells	Interleukins 2, 3, 4, 5, 6; granulocyte/macrophage-colony stimulating factor, interferons, lymphotoxin, neuropeptides
B cells	Immunoglobulins, antibodies
Mast cells	Histamine, 5-HT (in some species), proteases, proteoglycans, chemotactic factors, neuropeptides, tumor necrosis-like factor, lysosomal enzymes, adenosine, arachidonic acid metabolites, platelet-activating factor, oxygen radicals
Eosinophils	Major basic protein, eosinophil cationic protein, eosinophil-derived neurotoxin, neuropeptides, histaminase, peroxidase, lysosomal enzymes, arachidonic acid metabolites, platelet-activating factor, oxygen radicals
Macrophages	Interleukins 1, 6, tumor necrosis factor/cachectin, fibroblast activating factor, clotting factors, proteases, interferons, complement components, colony stimulating factors, arachidonic acid metabolites, platelet-activating factor, oxygen radicals
Neutrophils	Proteases, lactoferrin, lyosomal enzymes, oxygen radicals
Platelets	Platelet-derived growth (PGDF) factor, transforming growth factor-beta (TGF-β), epidermal growth factor (EGF), histamine, 5-HT (in some species), proteoglycans, proteases, oxygen radicals

mast cells, eosinophils, macrophages, neutrophils, and platelets must be considered major contributors (Table 11 – 1). These cells produce a multiplicity of mediators, including immunoglobulins, interleukins (IL) 1 to 6, interferons, and other cytokines such as tumor necrosis factor (TNF), lymphotoxin, clotting factors, colony stimulating factors, fibroblast activating factors, and platelet-derived growth factor. Lysosomal enzymes, additional proteases, vasoactive amines (histamine and 5-hydroxytryptamine; 5-HT), arachidonic acid metabolites, platelet activating factor (PAF), oxygen radicals, and even neuropeptides and hormones are also within the chemical repertoire of these cells (Table 11 – 1). Although many of these mediators are well known for their actions in host defence and tissue damage, few have been considered in the context of their actions on the physiology of intestinal targets such as the epithelium, with its wealth of cell types: smooth muscle, enteric nervous system, stromal elements, and the vasculature (Table 11 – 2).

SIMPLIFIED MODEL OF IMMUNOPHYSIOLOGY

Before reviewing many of the exciting examples of intestinal immunophysiologic interactions that have been uncovered recently, it is important to develop a simplified model of such interactions so that generalizations can be more easily seen, and

Table 11 – 2   PHYSIOLOGIC TARGETS IN INTESTINAL IMMUNOPHYSIOLOGY

Compartment	Cell Types
Epithelium	Intraepithelial leukocytes, digestive/absorptive enterocytes, goblet cells, Paneth's cells, neuroendocrine cells, nerve endings
Lamina propria	Mucosal immune system, vasculature, enteric nervous system, stromal/mesenchymal elements
Mucosal layers	Smooth muscle, vasculature, enteric nervous system, stromal/mesenchymal elements

future directions more clearly targeted. The model is not original but is derived from one presented by Torok-Storb in the context of the cellular interactions in hemopoiesis.[1] Some of the concepts championed by Stiles[11] on factors determining cellular responsiveness to stimuli, and the regulation of gene expression, are incorporated to aid in visualizing some of the underlying molecular determinants.

In embryogenesis and developmental biology, it is well recognized that precisely timed and orchestrated cellular interactions are key determinants in organogenesis and in the proliferation and differentiation of selected cell types. Unfortunately, in the gastrointestinal tract the complex cellular and molecular determinants of organ development and continued maintenance are poorly known (Fig. 11 – 1). Clearly, both positive and negative regulatory elements must be involved, and given the pleomorphic nature of the intestinal microenvironment, it is likely that gradients of inductive or inhibitory signals exist, for example in a crypt or villus as epithelial cells move towards the tip. Within this microenvironment there must be a wealth of continuously evolving growth and differentiation factors with the potential to alter responsiveness and gene expression in stem cells, progenitor cells, and more mature cells of various lineages. Some of these factors are derived from the mucosal immune system and its component immune and inflammatory reactions. Equally, these immune and inflammatory responses must be modulated by factors derived from, and cell contacts with, numerous other local cell types.

Figure 11 – 1 diagrams some of the potential interactions involved in the proliferation and differentiation of cells within the intestinal epithelium. Stem cells in the crypts are capable of self-renewal and can produce progeny with the potential to differentiate into all the separate intestinal epithelial cell lineages, with the exceptions of intraepithelial leucocytes (IEL). Neuroendocrine cells in the epithelium were thought to be primarily of neural crest origin, but presently an endodermal origin is more widely supported.[12] Their relationship to crypt stem cells is unclear, whereas IEL are of bone marrow origin[8] like other leukocytes and appear to move in the epithelium independently of the upward migration of the enterocytes.[13] Lineage commitment produces progenitor cells that are restricted in their potential to the expression of selected portions of their genome. Progenitors can express a spectrum of developmental or maturational states and thus exhibit both a heterogeneity in phenotypes relating to surface and intracellular properties and a responsiveness to proliferative and differentiation signals. Maturation of these progenitors further restricts gene expression and functional properties to end-stage phenotypes.

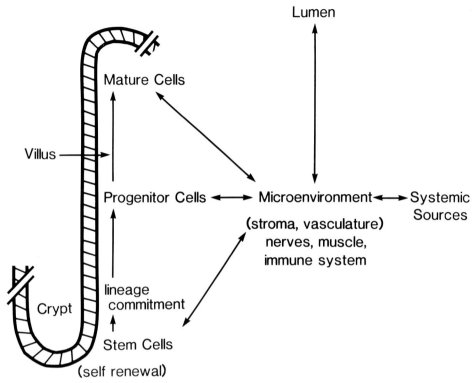

Figure 11–1 Model of immunophysiologic interactions in the proliferation and differentiation of intestinal epithelial cells.

The microenvironment imposes constant controls upon these stages in cell ontogeny and itself is in constant flux as local, lumenal, and systemic influences exert their effects on the network. In the unfolding of this model for the task at hand, emphasis will be placed upon the immune and inflammatory influences. Immune and inflammatory cells can be stimulated to infiltrate the local microenvironment and induce the production of, or produce by themselves, localized concentrations of cytokines sufficient to influence target cell responsiveness, proliferation, or differentiation. Unraveling these types of cellular interactions is most challenging because of the overall complexity and sampling problems presented by the microheterogeneity of the gastrointestinal tract. To some extent the developmental processes must be controlled by the random nature of the events. However, the complexity of the environment also suggests that there must be some preprogramming of selected responses and regulatory mechanisms.

In the lamina propria and muscle layers (Table 11–2), the physiologic targets are not directly analogous to the epithelium, because of the apparent lack of such ordered and predictable differentiation events as in the epithelium. With the exception of the leukocytes, there appear to be few stem cells in the lamina propria or muscle layers; the majority of the cells must be categorized as progenitors or mature cells. Thus lineage commitment decisions must presently be considered to be unusual in the lamina propria and muscle layers, and the important regulatory events must involve effects on responsiveness and gene expression in progenitor and mature cell types.

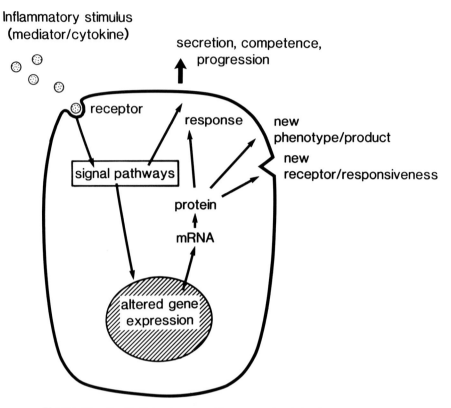

Figure 11–2   Cellular bases of immunophysiologic responses.

At the level of an individual cell the immune or inflammatory stimulus may act by initiating one or more of many pathways (Fig. 11–2). The signal must be received by a surface receptor or in some other way. This in turn activates messenger pathways that may directly generate some response such as secretion, contraction, etc., or may induce the expression of a new set of genes crucial to an adaptive response to the initial stimulus. The altered gene expression may induce new surface receptors or other functional proteins, or may generate a specific response to ongoing environmental stimuli. Stem cells may be driven to lineage commitment by such changes in gene expression, whereas progenitors may alter their proliferative rates or functional repertoire. Stiles[11] used the term *competence* to describe the state in which some stimulus renders the cell responsive to some other stimulus. *Progression* refers to movement through the cell cycle as a result of the stimulus, or to movement through the lineage pathway once activated (Fig. 11–2).

IMMUNOPHYSIOLOGIC INTERACTIONS

Epithelium

Stem Cells
Epithelial stem cells near the base of the crypts may be influenced by immune and inflammatory reactions in two major ways other than direct cytotoxicity. First,

stem cell proliferation may be regulated, and second, lineage commitments may be influenced. In a number of immune and inflammatory reactions to infectious agents there is evidence for enhanced cell proliferation in the crypts, which presumably includes stem cells.[14] The thymus dependency of partial villus atrophy in some intestinal infections could be explained by some inhibitory action of T lymphocytes on stem cell proliferation. However, other explanations such as increased loss from the villus tip mediated by T cells, are also possible. In addition, MacDonald and Spencer[15] recently established that the treatment of explants of human fetal intestine with pokeweed mitogen produced a striking crypt cell hyperplasia together with villus atrophy. T-cell activation in the lamina propria of the explants, as evidenced by IL-2 production and CD25 (IL-2 receptor) expression, correlated with these events. The mechanisms underlying increased mitotic rates in crypts are unknown, but it may be that cytokines released from T lymphocytes or macrophages have a direct effect on stem cell or early progenitor cell proliferation. Unfortunately, recombinant IL-2 and gamma-interferon had little effect on mucosal morphology in the intestinal explants.[15] Granulocyte/macrophage colony-stimulating factor (GM-CSF) thought to be produced by IEL T cells[16] should be tested for such activity.

Goblet cell hyperplasia is also a feature of some parasitic infections. With *Nippostrongylus brasiliensis* infection, Miller and colleagues established that T cells from the thoracic duct of sensitized rats could transfer the ability to generate goblet cell hyperplasia in newly infected rats.[17] The selective increase in one epithelial cell lineage could have many explanations; one attractive hypothesis is that activated T cells from the intestinal mucosa produce a factor(s) that enhances stem cell commitment to the goblet cell lineage. Whether this factor(s) or other factors are capable of modulating the relative frequency of lineage commitments for Paneth's, enteroendocrine, or columnar epithelial cells in the villus, or microfold (membrane) M cells in the lymphoepithelium overlying the mucosal lymphoid aggregates, remains to be determined.

Progenitor Cells and Their Maturation

Columnar Enterocytes

Some inflammatory mediators produce a rapid response in columnar epithelial cells. Perdue et al.[18] established that intraluminal antigen challenge in sensitized rats caused a rapid and marked reduction in water, Na^+, K^+, and Cl^- absorption from the jejunum. This response was antigen-specific and dependent upon previous sensitization. The malabsorption correlated with a reduction in mucosal histamine and local mucosal mast cells. Although epithelial damage was prominent, enhanced mucus release from goblet cells did not occur.[19] The authors postulated that IgE-mediated mast cell degranulation released histamine and other mediators that induced abnormalities in absorptive function.

Baird et al.[20] studied the responses to antigen challenge in the colon and ileum of guinea pigs sensitized to cow's milk. Interestingly, the responses in these two portions of the intestine differed. Challenge of both tissues with antigen caused an inwardly directed, transient short circuit current (SCC). The mediators involved in the colon were arachidonic acid metabolites and histamine (H1 receptor-mediated), and Cl^- ions were the major carriers of the current. By contrast, in the ileum 5-HT was the major relevant mediator. The authors were unable to identify the nature of the ions involved in the current developed. There was an overall secretion of fluid into the ileal lumen. Unlike the studies in rats, IgG and not IgE containing fractions of immune serum transferred the response to naive guinea pigs.[21] Selected 5-HT receptor antagonists were employed to establish that type 3 (neuronal) receptors were critical in the response.[22] Moreover, the neurotoxin tetrodotoxin blocked the response to exogenous 5-HT and to antigen challenge.

In contrast to the work of Baird and colleagues, Cooke et al.[23] showed that exogenous histamine increases SCC in the guinea pig ileum and stimulates Cl^- secretion. The action of histamine was mediated in part by H1 receptors on enterocytes, but also by H1 receptors on the enteric nervous system. Thus the same response in the epithelium may be generated by different mediators in different experimental systems.

Russell[24] studied the jejunal SCC response to antigen challenge in guinea pigs sensitized by infection with the nematode *Trichinella spiralis*. It was concluded that antigen stimulated Cl^- secretion and that there was a biphasic time course in the changes in SCC. The initial phase was inhibited by the H1 antagonist diphenhydramine, whereas the second phase was inhibited by indomethacin, the cyclooxygenase/prostaglandin synthetase inhibitor. Castro and coworkers[25] extended these observations to the rat and found that phase I of the biphasic change in SCC was mimicked by exogenous histamine or 5-HT and blocked by their antagonists. Phase II was mimicked by exogenous prostaglandin E_2 (PGE_2) and blocked by an inhibitor of prostaglandin synthesis.

Moreover, the neurotoxin tetrodotoxin had a marked inhibitory effect on the phase I response, but had little effect on the phase II response. The response was tranferred by immune serum with a high titer of late-acting (48 hour) passive cutaneous anaphylaxis antibody that was heat-sensitive and thus probably IgE.[26] In summary, in the parasitized rat jejunum, 5-HT, histamine and PGE_2 act together in antigen-induced alterations in SCC in the epithelium; part of this action is neurally mediated.

In rats sensitized with egg albumin, Perdue and Gall[27] showed a biphasic SCC response to antigen challenge. Interestingly, in contrast to the results of Castro and coworkers with parasitized rats, in this antigen-sensitized model the neurotoxin tetrodotoxin depressed the second phase but had little effect on the first phase. This suggests that in different experimental models the magnitude and time course of neurogenic control of immunophysiologic responses is variable.

The mast cell-stabilizing drug doxantrazole, which inhibits both mucosal mast cells and mast cells elsewhere, such as in the peritoneal cavity,[28] inhibited Cl^- secretion in both the rat jejunum[29] and colon.[30] Thus it appears that in intestinal anaphylaxis, mast cell secretion of mediators such as histamine and 5-HT can have marked and rapid effects on the physiologic activity of columnar epithelial cells. However, given the spectrum of mediators produced by mast cells (Table 11–1) and their ability to recruit and activate other cell types containing other potent mediators, it seems that many other mediators may alter epithelial physiology. Moreover, it is possible that epithelial cells themselves can be induced to produce important mediators that alter their physiology. For example, it is well recognized that respiratory epithelial cells produce a spectrum of arachidonic metabolites that varies from one species to another.[31] These mediators can influence ion movements in the respiratory epithelium. It is likely that similar events occur in the intestine and can be modified by immune and inflammatory responses.

The approach employed by Wasserman and colleagues, in which the cultured epithelial cell line T_{84} was systematically tested in vitro with histamine and various pharmacologic agents, is most promising to facilitate detailed analysis of the effects of various inflammatory mediators and cytokines on epithelial physiology.[32] This cell line was also employed by Nash and colleagues[33] to assess the effects of granulocytes on barrier function in an epithelium. Barrier function was impaired and focal injury was evident when granulocytes were incubated with an epithelial monolayer in the presence of a chemotactic gradient. Kohan and Schreiner[34] recently established that IL-1 increases the uptake of sodium and sodium-linked methylglucoside and aspartate uptake, but not leucine or arginine uptake by primary cultures of murine renal proximal tubule epithelium. It is intriguing to speculate that analogous effects occur with intestinal epithelium. Although such approaches will be highly productive, it is critical that observations with cultured cell lines be confirmed using in vivo-derived cells and tissues derived from a number of experimental models.

In addition to the immediate responses induced by immune and inflammatory mediators interacting with columnar enterocytes (see Fig. 11–2), there are those responses that probably involve the transcription and translation of new genes following stimulation with mediator(s). Such speculation is well founded because there is evidence that IEL produce an interferon-like factor that induces the expression of class II major histocompatibility complex molecules on epithelial cells[35] (Table 11–3). What role these molecules play on epithelial cells is not fully clear, although it is evident that they are important in antigen presentation to the immune system.[36] Perhaps their expression allows for other forms of cell-to-cell communication in the epithelium, as in the immune system.

More recently Brandtzaeg and coworkers have established that both interferon gamma[37] and TNF[38] induce the expression of secretory component in epithelial cells (Table 11–3). Secretory component is a quintessential factor in the transport of secretory IgA into the intestinal lumen, and epithelial cells in the crypt are the major intraintestinal source of this factor. These observations suggest that immune and inflammatory responses generate mediators that up-regulate the expression of this epithelial component critical to the most effective functioning of the mucosal immune system. It seems probable that other mediators and cytokines influence enterocyte responses and gene expression important in adaptive responses to infectious agents or other antigenic challenges. Furthermore, it is particularly intriguing that a number of human epithelial tumor cells have recently been shown to synthesize TNF themselves.[39] If intestinal epithelial cells can be induced to express TNF by inflammatory or other stimuli, the impact of this mediator in the microenvironment could be crucial in local physiologic activities and host defences.

Table 11–3 IMMUNE AND INFLAMMATORY MEDIATORS ALTER GENE EXPRESSION IN INTESTINAL EPITHELIAL CELLS

Mediator	Expression
Interferon gamma	Class II molecules, secretory component
Tumor necrosis factor	Secretory component
?	Wheat germ agglutinin binding depressed

In parasitized rats, Castro and Harari[40] demonstrated that infection induced a long-lived alteration in the wheat germ agglutinin binding capacity of the intestinal brush border. The basis of this alteration in lectin binding was not established, but the observation suggests that an alteration was induced in columnar enterocyte development that persisted long after the parasite had left the intestine and the epithelium had been renewed many times. This "memory" cannot be easily explained at present, but it is interesting to speculate that the memory inherent in the immune system influenced the continuing process of epithelial renewal (Table 11–3).

Goblet Cells
The immunophysiologic investigations of goblet cells have largely been restricted to the actions of inflammatory mediators as mucus secretagogues (Table 11–4). Moreover, mucus secretion from the respiratory tract has been more extensively investigated than that from the gastrointestinal tract, in large part because of the ability to employ short-term cultures of human and dog tracheal epithelium.[41] Studies of intestinal goblet cells have employed in vivo systems, in vitro organ cultures, and also isolated epithelial sheets,[42] but there are few reports of the effects of specific inflammatory mediators.

It has been known for more than two decades that some intestinal infections stimulate goblet cell hyperplasia.[43] More recently, evidence has accumulated that sensitized T lymphocytes are involved in this hyperplasia,[17,44] and that mucus secretion entraps the parasites and is strongly associated with a phenomenon called immune exclusion and/or rapid expulsion.[44,45] The precise mediators involved in the mucus secretion in these rat experimental models are unknown, although Miller[46] nicely reviewed some of the potential secretagogues.

Immune and inflammatory responses have also been associated with intestinal mucus secretion in models not employing infectious agents. Walker et al.[47] established that the injection of preformed immune complexes into the duodenum of rats induced goblet cell disruption and the release of radiolabeled mucus products into the lumen. Subsequently, this same team of researchers demonstrated that infusion of antigen into the intestine of orally immunized rats induced mucus discharge, but that rats immunized systemically in a manner designed to produce a strong IgG response did not release increased amounts of mucus upon local antigen challenge.[48] However, when the rats were immunized in a manner designed to

Table 11–4 MUCUS SECRETAGOGUES OF IMMUNE AND INFLAMMATORY ORIGIN

Histamine
5-HT
prostaglandins E_1, F_2 alpha, D_2, I_2, A_2
5-, 8-, 9-, 11-, or 15- Hydroxyeicosatetraenoic acid
5- and 9- Hydroperoxyeicosatetraenoic acid
Leukotriene C_4, D_4
Macrophage or monocyte mucus secretagogue
Lymphoblastoid cell mucus secretagogue
C_3a, C_5a

induce IgE responses and intestinal anaphylaxis upon local antigen challenge, significant mucus secretion occurred.[49] Unfortunately, there is little direct information about the mediators involved in any of these goblet cell responses to antigen challenge in the intestine.

However, from other studies in the intestine[50] and from those in the respiratory tract, one can speculate about some of the underlying mechanisms. Histamine can induce mucus secretion in the dog stomach[51] and in the respiratory tract of a number of species.[41] Moreover, 5-HT[50]; prostaglandins E_1, F_2 alpha, D_2, I_2, and A_2, but not E_2; mono-hydroxy- and hydroperoxy-eicosatetraenoic acids; leukotriene C_4 and D_4[41]; a macrophage and monocyte mucus secretagogue[52]; C3a and C5a fragments of the complement cascade[53]; and a factor(s) from human lymphoblastoid cells[54] stimulate mucus release (Table 11–4). Indeed, it appears that some of these factors are interactive in their effects on mucus release; e.g., histamine and leukotriene C_4.[55]

It is well known that cholinergic and alpha-adrenergic innervation regulate mucus secretion in the airways and that substance P and vasoactive intestinal peptide (VIP) may also be involved.[41] The effects on mucus secretion of cholinergic innervation in the intestine have been well studied by Neutra and coworkers.[42,56–58] Both cholinergic and noncholinergic elements of the enteric nervous system regulate goblet cell secretion within the crypts of the ileum and colon. However, goblet cells higher up the villi, rather than in the crypts, are unresponsive to these stimuli induced by electric field stimulation. [58]

In a manner analogous to the nerve-immune/inflammatory interactions in the immunophysiology of the columnar enterocytes, it is likely that in the stimulation of goblet cell secretion such interactions occur. These may include the reciprocal interactions between the nervous and immune systems,[59–63] the production of neurotransmitters by the immune system,[59,64] or direct interactions at the level of the goblet cell. These various possibilities must be explored.

As indicated above, there is little information on the immunophysiology of commitment to the goblet cell lineage from the stem cell in the crypt, although Miller and Nawa[17] established that sensitized T lymphocytes can stimulate goblet cell hyperplasia in some unknown manner. There is an equal dearth of information about the regulation of gene expression in goblet cell progenitors. It is likely that a spectrum of inflammatory mediators, neurotransmitters, hormones, or cytokines influence gene expression, but this remains to be tested. The observations that there is marked heterogeneity in goblet cell phenotype[65] and that infection can alter the properties of mucus[44] suggest that this will be a highly productive field for investigation. The availability of monoclonal antibodies to distinguish different goblet cell phenotypes[65] is an important step toward the experimental systems necessary for these investigations.

Other Cells; Neuroendocrine and Paneth's
Knowledge of factors controlling the lineage commitment, differentiation, maturation, and function of neuroendocrine and Paneth's cells in the intestinal epithelium is limited. Nevertheless, the hypothesis that immune and inflammatory responses generate messages that modulate the development and functions of these cells is attractive. Given restrictions in space, the approaches necessary to probe this hypothesis will not be discussed here. In vivo and in vitro systems similar to those used for other epithelial cells would provide powerful starting points.

Smooth Muscle

It is well recognized that some inflammatory mediators such as histamine,[66] 5-HT,[67] leukotrienes,[68] and prostaglandins[69] effect intestinal smooth muscle and overall motility, but there has not been a systematic attempt to evaluate the effects of many other mediators or cytokines. Recently, some research workers have begun to describe alterations in smooth muscle activity associated with immune and inflammatory events in the intestinal tract using parasitic infections, a model of intestinal anaphylaxis, or toxic colitis. The observed abnormalities are interesting, and the models provide important tools to investigate the role of inflammatory mediators and cytokines in the evolution of these pathologic changes. Presumably the changes reflect both immediate responses to stimuli in the smooth muscle, as well as more long-term changes in gene expression (Fig. 11–2). However, confirmation of this hypothesis must await further experimentation.

Using rats previously infected with the nematode *T. spiralis,* Palmer and Castro[70] identified reduction in the frequency of slow waves, spike potentials, and migrating myoelectric complexes shortly after reinoculation of worms. Using an intestinal anaphylaxis model, Scott and coworkers[71] established that antigen-challenged, sensitized rats developed diarrhea, exhibited alterations in the intestinal motility pattern, lost migrating myoelectric complexes, and experienced an increased frequency of clustered contractions proceeding in an aboral direction. The mediators responsible for these changes were not identified, although the authors suggested that mediators produced by mast cells as a result of antigen-IgE interactions would be probable candidates.

Changes in muscle characteristics in inflamed states have also been investigated in vitro.[72-77] Parasitic infection induces a state of hyperresponsiveness to cholinergic stimuli and to 5-HT,[72-74] expressed as an increase in the maximum tension generated by jejunal longitudinal muscle when stimulated with the appropriate agonist. With *T. spiralis* infection, there was also a left shift in the dose-response curve to 5-HT.[74] These changes were reversible and returned to normal responsiveness after the infections were cleared.[74] However, the smooth muscle remains sensitive to antigen-induced contractions for at least 3 months, and 5-HT appears to be the primary mediator of contraction.[75] On the bases of inhibition of the response to antigen with the mast cell-stabilizing drug doxantrazole and mast cell hyperplasia in the smooth muscle, the authors proposed that mast cell degranulation is the underlying mechanism of the antigen-induced muscle contraction; they were unable to identify a neurogenic component.

Muller and colleagues[76] explored the pharmacologic bases of the hyperresponsiveness to cholinergic stimulation and established that in *T. spiralis*-infected rats there was a reduction in the number of muscarinic receptor sites in jejunal longitudinal muscle. The affinity of the remaining sites was normal. Most interestingly, there was a 90% reduction in an enzyme marker of the Na^+-K^+ pump (K^+-stimulated, ouabain-sensitive, p-nitrophenylphosphatase) in the plasma membranes of muscle from infected rats compared with uninfected animals.[76] The authors proposed that suppression of the electrogenic Na pump is an important factor in the hyperresponsiveness of jejunal muscle in parasitized rats.

In rabbits with toxic colitis, colonic muscle generates weakened tensions, lowered electrochemical potential, and decreased membrane resistance.[77] This is clearly a different type of response in an intestinal inflammatory condition than in the rat models outlined above and requires further investigation.

How inflammatory responses induce states of hyperresponsiveness in intestinal smooth muscle such as described above, or in bronchial smooth muscle in asthma[78] remains to be elucidated. Exogenous prostaglandin F_2 alpha, leukotriene B_4, and PAF can all induce bronchial hyperresponsiveness. The neutrophil appears to be closely involved, because experiments designed to deplete neutrophils exhibited no hyperreactivity.[79] The results of experiments designed to investigate the mechanisms of intestinal smooth muscle hyperreactivity should prove to be enlightening and to help identify new therapeutic approaches to intestinal diseases.

Enteric Nervous System

The enteric nervous system is a major division of the autonomic system that also includes the parasympathetic and sympathetic components. The enteric division is "an independent integrative nervous system that consists of two ganglionated plexuses, the myenteric and submucosal plexuses, that function to coordinate the activity of the gastrointestinal musculature, vasculature, transporting epithelium, enteroendocrine cells, and immune elements." [80] Unfortunately, at present there is little direct information pertaining to the influences of local mucosal immune and inflammatory responses on the responsiveness, or development and maintenance, of the enteric nervous system. However, I would like to provide a general overview of the arena and outline some of the research directions likely to be fruitful.

The exciting field of neuroimmunology has had a recent rejuvenation as it has moved into more cellular and molecular approaches employing the most up-to-date methods in immunology and cell biology. This has been more extensively reviewed in Chapter 10 and will not be elaborated further. It is well recognized that immune responses are markedly influenced by neuropeptides[61] and that lymphoid tissues in mucosae and elsewhere have a comprehensive innervation.[62]

Products of immune and inflammatory responses such as histamine and 5-HT can act as neurotransmitters.[81] Moreover, it is now widely recognized that many cells in the immune system make neuropeptides such as opioids, substance P, VIP, and somatostatin,[59,61,64,82] which modulate nervous function and act on many other cells expressing the appropriate receptors.[83] It has also become clear that IL-1 and -3 can be produced by cells of the nervous system and that specific receptors for these cytokines exist in selected portions of the nervous system.[84-86] For example, Breder et al.[84] demonstrated that nerve fibers containing IL-1 beta were present as a network throughout the human hypothalamus, but no cell bodies positive for IL-1 beta were found in the hypothalamus or elsewhere in the brain. They postulated that circulating IL-1 may stimulate IL-1-bearing neurons in the hypothalamus, which in turn employ IL-1 and other neurotransmitters to modify central and peripheral responses. It is tempting to generalize that this type of immune/nervous integration is of fundamental significance in normal physiologic homeostasis throughout the body.[59] It has been recently postulated that a disturbance in the hypothalamo-hypophyseal axis of immunoendocrine pathways is the underlying mechanism in spontaneous autoimmune thyroiditis in Obese chickens and that this defect is associated with an endogenous virus in these birds.[87] Is it possible that some intestinal diseases are associated with alterations in the local immunophysiologic communications networks?

Abnormalities in the distribution of neuropeptides and their receptors have been identified in intestinal tissues in inflammatory bowel disease,[88,89] but whether these changes are of etiologic significance in the disease or secondary to the local pathologic reactions is unknown. Interestingly, infection with the nematode *T. spiralis* results in an impairment in acetylcholine release from the myenteric plexus in rats.[90] Worm antigen did not alter acetylcholine release from sensitized rats, so the mechanisms underlying this defect in infected rats are unclear. The possibility that immune and inflammatory responses are responsible is intriguing.

Perhaps the best example of how immune and inflammatory responses can alter a neurogenic response is the recent description of how, through the action of mast cells, substance P modulates the cutaneous vasodilation induced by calcitonin gene-related peptide (CGRP).[91] CGRP alone induces a prolonged vasodilation, but when administered with substance P, the response is attenuated. The authors provided evidence that substance P induces mast cell degranulation in the local microenvironment, and mast cell proteases break down CGRP, thereby shortening its duration of action. This is an interesting example of how coexisting neuropeptides[92] may interact through a cell of the immune system. Caughey et al.[93] also recently established that mast cell-derived tryptase and chymase can degrade neuropeptides. Tryptase cleaved VIP but had no effect on substance P, whereas chymase cleaved both neuropeptides. Given that in humans tryptase is found selectively in a mast cell population largely restricted to mucosal surfaces, whereas chymase is present in mast cells in all tissues,[94] the degradation of substance P by mast cells may be highly dependent upon the phenotype of the mast cell population in the local microenvironment.

It is clear that investigations of the actions of immune and inflammatory mediators on the enteric nervous system are likely to uncover a wealth of cellular and molecular pathways of great significance in the maintenance of intestinal homeostasis and the adaptations necessary under adverse conditions. Few mediators have been explored to date, and some of the lipid ones may be particularly important.[63] It will be challenging to develop experimental models to stimulate the intestinal environment for these types of investigations, and recent successful attempts to culture portions of the enteric nervous system hold much promise for such studies of cellular and molecular interactions.[95]

Vasculature

The vasculature of the gastrointestinal tract is morphologically complex, and its physiology is elaborately controlled by a variety of neurogenic and other mediators.[96-98] Some of the principal cell types in the vasculature include pericytes, smooth muscle, and endothelial cells. For the purposes of this overview, I will not attempt to discuss all the vascular control mechanisms, but instead will focus on the endothelium and some more recent examples of alterations in intestinal blood flow induced by inflammatory mediators.

The vascular endothelium has a variety of functions central to the regulation of blood flow, permeability, coagulation, and the adherence, activation, and function of leukocytes and platelets. The endothelium releases two important vasodilators, prostacyclin and endothelium-derived relaxing factor (EDRF), and catabolizes a number of vasoactive moities including catecholamines, angiotensin, bradykinin, and prostaglandins.[99] EDRF is produced largely by arterial endothelial cells and appears to act over short distances on local smooth muscle cells or pericytes. It relaxes vascular smooth muscle, inhibits platelet aggregation and adhesion, and stimulates platelets to disaggregate. There is strong evidence that EDRF is nitrous oxide.[99]

The role that immune and inflammatory mediators might play in the production or action of EDRF remains to be investigated, but it is attractive to speculate that certain mediators possess powerful influences. Recently Kaiser et al.[100] established that infection with the canine heartworm *Dirofilaria immitis* induced alterations in endothelial cell-mediated arterial dilatation in dogs. Infected dogs exhibited a depressed dilatation response to increased flow that correlated with the number of female worms. Moreover, infected dogs were hyporesponsive to the vasodilatory stimulus acetylcholine, and, unlike in uninfected dogs, indomethacin depressed the response to acetylcholine in infected dogs. Thus infection, and perhaps the associated immune and inflammatory responses, alter the regulation of vascular tone and the impact of arachidonic acid metabolites on this adaptive response. What mediators are involved in these alterations remains to be investigated, as does the extent to which this effect may be seen in other infections and in selected target organs. Perhaps it is but one example of the immunophysiology of the adaptive abilities of the vasculature.

It must also be recognized the endothelium is not a homogenous layer throughout the vasculature, but that there are microenvironmental specializations such as the high endothelium of postcapillary venules.[98] These high endothelial venules (HEV) are found in lymph nodes, Peyer's patches, bronchus-associated lymphoid tissue and granuloma and other inflammatory sites, but not in the spleen or lamina propria of the intestine. They are specialized sites for the emigration of lymphocytes from the blood into the tissues, and the nature of the surface receptors involved has been subject to much study.[101] Why inflammation stimulates the formation of HEV is not entirely clear, although IL-2 and gamma-interferon may be involved.[102]

The absence of HEV in the lamina propria of the intestine is puzzling, because it is well recognized that lymphocytes enter the intestinal wall from the circulation in sites other than the postcapillary venules of the Peyer's patches. Jeurissen et al.[103] shed light on this puzzle when they demonstrated that, although HEV could not be identified in the intestinal lamina propria on morphologic grounds, using a monoclonal antibody, MECA-325, which recognizes HEV in lymph nodes but not the critical homing receptor, they identified MECA-325+ venules between the crypts. These MECA-325+ venules had a low profile endothelium, but were shown to be sites of lymphocyte migration. Clearly these specialized venules in the intercryptal regions of the lamina propria bear some of the properties of HEV without sharing their morphologic character. How these venules might be selectively influenced by immune and inflammatory mediators must be evaluated; clearly they appear to be selected as targets for inflammatory mediators in vascular permeability also.[104]

It is interesting to note that injection of recombinant human TNF into rats induces ischemic bowel necrosis (Fig. 11–3) and is associated with increased height of the endothelium of small vessels near the crypts and increased adherence of mononuclear and neutrophilic cells to the endothelial surface.[105] It appears that the bowel necrosis induced by TNF is mediated by the subsequent release of PAF,[106] which in turn stimulates release of the vasoconstrictor leukotriene C_4. Leukotriene C_4 is a short-acting vasoconstrictor, but the long-acting vasoconstrictor norepinephrine is also released,[107] which maintains a prolonged ischemia and induces the bowel necrosis. Why this initial injection of TNF or PAF does not yield a compensatory vasodilation induced by mediators such as prostaglandin E_2, histamine, EDRF, acetylcholine, or opiates remains a mystery.

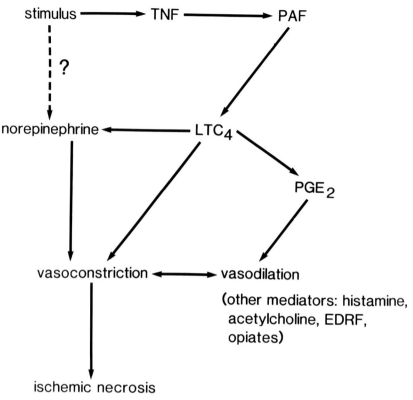

Figure 11–3 Cascade of factors in ischemic bowel necrosis.

Mesenchymal Elements

The mesenchymal elements in the gastrointestinal tract include a number of cell types that make up the stromal or connective tissue elements such as fibroblasts, smooth muscle cells, and myofibroblasts. These cells form a supporting framework of the organ, and other cell types are distributed throughout its spaces, e.g., immune elements, enteric nervous system, and vasculature. Although it is not a field that has been widely explored, the reciprocal interactions between the mesenchymal elements and these other cell systems are of fundamental importance in the development and maintenance of the integrity of the gastrointestinal tract. In chronic inflammatory diseases such as Crohn's disease, this framework can be seriously disrupted, in a manner analogous to fibrotic lung diseases.[108] In an understanding of the cellular and molecular components of these changes lie innovative therapeutic approaches to some of these inflammatory changes.

Myofibroblasts form a subepithelial and pericryptal supporting network below the epithelial basal lamina of the small intestine and colon. In addition, there are stellate-shaped cells in close contact with each other and with the extracellular matrix that form a three-dimensional network within the villar lamina propria. These myofibroblasts contain isotropomyosin, isomyosin, and actin, all cytoskeletal and contractile proteins.[109] These proteins are present in these cells in quantities greater than in fibroblasts, but less than that in smooth muscle cells. Joyce et al.[109] concluded that these observations suggest a "smooth muscle-like, contractile function for these cells and indicate that this cellular network may provide a supportive tonus for the epithelium, as well as provide the force needed for active movement of the villus, expulsion of crypt secretion products, and propulsion of absorption products in the lamina propria, the microvasculature, and lacteals of the intestinal villus."

In chronic inflammatory and scarring diseases, the mechanisms that modulate the stromal elements, particularly the fibroblasts, are beginning to be identified.[110-113] Given the increasingly recognized phenotypic overlap among stromal cell types,[109] it may be that the categories employed to distinguish cell types are highly artificial and that the complex pathways of cellular interactions do not clearly distinguish among the stromal smooth muscle, fibroblasts, and myofibroblasts. For example, in addition to the sharing of contractile elements, it appears that human intestinal smooth muscle, like fibroblasts, is an important source of collagen synthesis relevant to intestinal strictures.[114]

One of the tripartite divisions of cellular and molecular interactions that has been investigated in fibrotic responses is the relationship among fibroblasts, mast cells, and macrophages.[110,112,115-117] Histologic studies established that changes occur in the distribution and abundance of mast cells in the evolution of wound healing.[118] Recently, Kirkpatrick and Curry[119] investigated the ultrastructure of mast cell-perineural fibroblast interactions and reported on observations of potential vesicular exchange between the two cell types. Many other reports exist of such contact, exchange, and bidirectional interactions between mast cells and fibroblasts.[120,121] Fibrotic responses are regularly associated with hyperplasia of mast cells,[122] and numerous functional mast cell-fibroblast interactions have been identified. Histamine promotes fibroblast proliferation through H2 receptors and in a manner that is highly dependent upon the phase of the cell cycle of the targeted fibroblast.[123] Heparin down-regulates collagen and other protein synthesis in intestinal smooth muscle cells, and perhaps the same is true of fibroblasts.[124] Fibroblasts endocytose mast cell granules[121] and degrade their components.[117,121] In turn fibroblasts provide important, still unknown, messages that sustain mast cell growth and survival.[115]

Macrophages can modulate the function of fibroblasts and mast cells[110,112] and are influenced by products of these cells also. IL-1 and other macrophage products can stimulate mast cell secretion.[116,125] IL-1 and other fibroblast-activating factors derived from macrophages can modify fibroblast growth and expression of selected genes.[110-112] The type of reciprocal interactions outlined here are likely to be an ongoing part of normal physiologic events in the intestinal microenvironment. In disease states, the delicate balance that preserves normal integrity is disturbed. Because of the complexity of interactions, it will be most challenging to dissect the site of perturbation and intervene successfully.

REVOLUTIONARY EXPECTATIONS FOR IMMUNOPHYSIOLOGY?

It is critical in attempting to understand the complexity of organization of the gastrointestinal tract to start from the premise that immunologic responses are constantly ongoing, and not merely lying dormant until some serious infection or other challenge appears. The stimuli that are responsible for this activity are multiple, but the rapidly expanding information base in neuroimmunology suggests that neuropeptides and other neurotransmitters are major players. Various signals, not only direct antigenic stimulation, must activate the immunophysiologic pathways central to the continual adaptive state of integration of epithelial, smooth muscle, vascular, nervous, stromal, and immune functions. Pathways are bidirectional; physiologists must expand their exploration of the roles of factors generated by the immune system, as well as direct effects on immunologic pathways. Immunologists must explore multiple physiologic activation systems for immune and inflammatory responses, as well as diversify their concepts of target sites for immune responses. Interdisciplinary studies must be fostered and a new level of innovative research groups developed. Their mandate must be to break the long-standing barriers imposed by classical discipline boundaries and the existing research infrastructure.

The spectrum of cellular and molecular pathways involved in the complexity of interactions that have been outlined in the context of this review is frightening. Not only is the extent of research activity needed to approach this complexity using

INTESTINAL IMMUNOPHYSIOLOGY

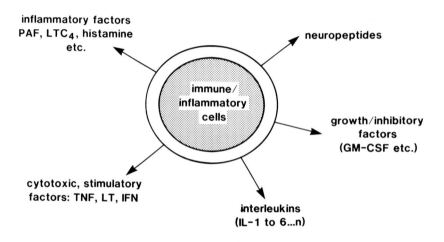

inflammatory factors
PAF, LTC$_4$, histamine
etc.

neuropeptides

immune/
inflammatory
cells

growth/inhibitory
factors
(GM–CSF etc.)

cytotoxic, stimulatory
factors: TNF, LT, IFN

interleukins
(IL–1 to 6...n)

TARGETS:

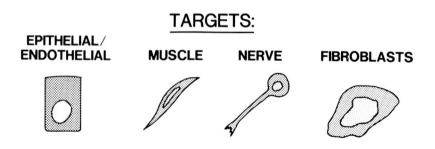

EPITHELIAL/
ENDOTHELIAL   MUSCLE   NERVE   FIBROBLASTS

RESPONSES: growth, differentiation, secretion, transmission,
factor production, responsiveness, contraction

Figure 11–4 Immune and inflammatory mediators and physiologic targets in the intestine.

a reductionist strategy almost infinite, but the challenge of developing more holistic approaches is at the present time almost unrealistic. Each of the mediators has multiple biologic activities. In this review my focus was on a restricted group of immune and inflammatory mediators and physiologic targets (Fig. 11–4), but when one considers other molecular messages such as platelet-derived growth factor[126] or epidermal growth factor, transforming growth factors, etc., and the cell sources and physiologic and pathophysiologic activities, the vision of the complexity begins to approach a state that more realistically approximates the in vivo situation. The immune system cannot be viewed in a manner devoid of other microenvironmental components.

Despite the serious concerns about the complexity of the intestinal environment and the difficulty in unraveling its mysteries, it is appropriate to be optimistic because of the evolution of a more holistic view of this environment and the development of new tools to explore the interface areas outlined above. The ongoing maturation of mucosal immunology and intestinal physiology continues to provide a new base of knowledge to define the potential mechanisms of interaction and identify new experimental systems to wed the hitherto largely separate disciplines. The availability of highly purified cell types, new cell culture systems[95] and purified or recombinant cytokines provides almost endless opportunities for reductionist-type experimentation to define possible in vivo interactions. Clearly, further improvements in these types of tools for in vitro experimentation are needed, such as monoclonal antibodies for specific markers on epithelial stem cells or on progenitor and mature cells of the spectrum of lineages present in the intestinal tract. Such markers and defined culture systems for the various lineages will facilitate studies on the signals that modulate competency, progression, and responsiveness (Fig. 11–2). In vivo studies of gene expression in the normal and inflamed gastrointestinal tract must be pursed vigorously in a number of experimental models and with human tissues. Gene probes must be used that include those to map the expression of the spectrum of immune and inflammatory mediators and cytokines, as well as those, still largely unavailable, that will define cell lineage commitments, and functional states. Within this type of exploration lies a wealth of knowledge that will spearhead the immunophysiologic revolution. It is an exciting time for students involved in the evolution of knowledge of gastrointestinal function.

REFERENCES

1. Torok-Storb B: Cellular interactions. *Blood* 72:373–385, 1988.
2. Walker WA: Immunoregulation of small intestinal function. *Gastroenterology* 86:577–579, 1984.
3. Gall DG, Perdue MH: Experimental models of intestinal allergy. *Front Gastrointest Res* 13:45–54, 1986.
4. Russell DA, Castro GA: Physiology of the gastrointestinal tract in the parasitized host. In Johnson LR: *Physiology of the Gastrointestinal Tract*, ed 2. New York, Raven Press, 1987, p 1749.
5. Holgate ST, Robinson C, Church MK, et al: The release of inflammatory mediators in asthma. *Clin Immunol Rev* 4:241–288, 1985.
6. McDonald DM: Neurogenic inflammation in the respiratory tract: actions of sensory nerve mediators on blood vessels and epithelium of the airway mucosa. *Am Rev Respir Dis* 136:S65–S72, 1987.

7. Leff AR: Endogenous regulation of bronchomotor tone. *Am Rev Respir Dis* 137:1198–1216, 1988.

8. Ernst P, Befus AD, Bienenstock J: Leukocytes in the intestinal epithelium: a unique and heterogeneous compartment. *Immunol Today* 6:50–55, 1985.

9. MacDonald TT, Dillon SB: Chemical mediators of cellular communication. In Heyworth MF, Jones AL: *Immunology of the Gastrointestinal Tract and Liver,* ed 1. New York, Raven Press, 1988, p 47.

10. Butzner JD, Befus D: Interactions among intraepithelial leucocytes and other epithelial cells in the intestinal development and function. In Lebenthal M: *Human Gastrointestinal Development* New York, Raven Press, 1989, in press.

11. Stiles CD: The biological role of oncogenes — insights from platelet-derived growth factor: Rhoads memorial award lecture. *Cancer Res* 45:5215–5218, 1985.

12. Solcia E, Capella C, Buffa R, et al: Endocrine cells of the digestive system. In Johnson LR: *Physiology of the Gastrointestinal Tract,* ed 2. New York, Raven Press, 1987, p. 111.

13. Darlington D, Rogers AW: Epithelial lymphocytes in the small intestine of the mouse. *J Anat* 100:813–830, 1966.

14. MacDonald TT, Ferguson A: Small intestinal epithelial cell kinetics and protozoal infection of mice. *Gastroenterology* 74:496–500, 1978.

15. MacDonald TT, Spencer J: Evidence that activated mucosal T cells play a role in the pathogenesis of enteropathy in human small intestine. *J Exp Med* 167:1341–1349, 1988.

16. Dillon SB, MacDonald TT: Functional characterization of Con A-responsive Lyt2-positive mouse small intestinal intraepithelial lymphocytes. *Immunology* 59:389–396, 1986.

17. Miller HRP, Nawa Y, Parish CR: Intestinal goblet cell differentiation in *Nippostrongylus*-infected rats after transfer of fractionated thoracic duct lymphocytes. *Int Arch Allergy Appl Immunol* 59:281–285, 1979.

18. Perdue MH, Chung M, Gall DG: Effect of intestinal anaphylaxis on gut function in the rat. *Gastroenterology* 86:391–397, 1984.

19. Perdue MH, Forstner JF, Roomi NW, et al: Epithelial response to intestinal anaphylaxis in rats: goblet cell secretion and enterocyte damage. *Am J Physiol* 247:G632–G637, 1984.

20. Baird AW, Coombs RRA, McLaughlan P, et al: Immediate hypersensitivity reactions to cow milk proteins in isolated epithelium from ileum of milk-drinking guinea-pigs: comparisons with colonic epithelia. *Int Arch Allergy Appl Immunol* 75:255–263, 1984.

21. Baird AW, Barclay WS, Blazer-Yost BL, et al: Affinity purified immunoglobulin G transfers immediate hypersensitivity to guinea pig colonic epithelium in vitro. *Gastroenterology* 92:635–642, 1987.

22. Baird AW, Cuthbert AW: Neuronal involvement in type 1 hypersensitivity reactions in gut epithelia. *Br J Pharmacol* 92:647–655, 1987.

23. Cooke HJ, Nemeth PR, Wood JD: Histamine action on guinea pig ileal mucosa. *Am J Physiol* 246:G372–G377, 1984.

24. Russell DA: Mast cells in the regulation of intestinal electrolyte transport. *Am J Physiol* 251:G253–G262, 1986.

25. Castro GA, Harari Y, Russell D: Mediators of anaphylaxis-induced ion transport changes in small intestine. *Am J Physiol* 253:G540–G548, 1987.

26. Harari Y, Russell DA, Castro GA: Anaphylaxis-mediated epithelial Cl⁻ secretion and parasite rejection in rat intestine. *J Immunol* 138:1250–1255, 1987.

27. Perdue MH, Gall DG: Rat jejunal mucosal response to histamine and anti-histamines in vitro. Comparison with antigen-induced changes during intestinal anaphylaxis. *Agents Actions* 19:5–9, 1986.

28. Pearce FL, Befus AD, Gauldie J, et al: Mucosal mast cells. II. Effects of anti-allergic compounds on histamine secretion by isolated intestinal mast cells. *J Immunol* 128:2481–2486, 1982.

29. Perdue MH, Gall DG: Intestinal anaphylaxis in the rat: jejunal response to in vitro antigen exposure. *Am J Physiol* 250:G427–G431, 1986.

30. Forbes D, Patrick M, Perdue M, et al: Intestinal anaphylaxis: in vivo and in vitro studies of the rat proximal colon. *Am J Physiol* 255:G201–G205, 1988.

31. Eling TE, Henke D, Danilowicz R: Arachidonic acid metabolism in respiratory epithelial cells. *Gen Pharmacol* 19:313–316, 1988.

32. Wasserman SI, Barrett KE, Huott PA, et al: Immune-related intestinal Cl⁻ secretion. I. Effect of histamine on the T_{84} cell line. *Am J Physiol* 254:G53–G62, 1988.

33. Nash S, Stafford J, Madara JL: Effects of polymorphonuclear leukocyte transmigration on the barrier function of cultured intestinal epithelial monolayers. *J Clin Invest* 80:1104–1113, 1987.

34. Kohan DE, Schreiner GF: Interleukin 1 modulation of renal epithelial glucose and amino acid transport. *Am J Physiol* 254:F879–F886, 1988.

35. Cerf-Bensussan N, Quaroni A, Kurnick JT, et al: Intraepithelial lymphocytes modulate Ia expression by intestinal epithelial cells. *J Immunol* 132:2244–2252, 1984.

36. Bland P: MHC class II expression by the gut epithelium. *Immunol Today* 9:174–178, 1988.

37. Soolid LM, Kvale D, Brandtzaeg P, et al: Interferon-gamma enhances expression of secretory component, the epithelial receptor for polymeric immunoglobulins. *J Immunol* 138:4303–4306, 1987.

38. Kvale D, Lovhaug D, Sollid LM, et al: Tumor necrosis factor-alpha up-regulates expression of secretory component, the epithelial receptor for polymeric Ig. *J Immunol* 140:3086–3089, 1988.

39. Spriggs DR, Imamura K, Rodriguez C, et al: Tumor necrosis factor expression in human epithelial tumor cell lines. *J Clin Invest* 81:455–460, 1988.

40. Castro GA, Harari Y: Intestinal epithelial membrane changes in rats immune to *Trichinella spiralis*. *Mol Biochem Parasitol* 6:191–204, 1982.

41. Kaliner M, Shelhamer JH, Borson B, et al: Human respiratory mucus. *Am Rev Respir Dis* 134:612–621, 1986.

42. Phillips TE, Phillips TH, Neutra MR: Regulation of intestinal goblet cell secretion. III. Isolated intestinal epithelium. *Am J Physiol* 247:G674–G681, 1984.

43. Wells PD: Mucin-secreting cells in rats infected with *Nippostrongylus brasiliensis*. *Exp Parasitol* 14:15–22, 1963.

44. Koninkx JFJG, Mirck MH, Hendriks HGCJM, et al: *Nippostrongylus brasiliensis:* histochemical changes in the composition of mucins in goblet cells during infection in rats. *Exp Parasitol* 65:84–90, 1988.

45. Miller HRP, Huntley JF, Wallace GR: Immune exclusion and mucus trapping during the rapid expulsion of *Nippostrongylus brasiliensis* from primed rats. *Immunology* 44:419–429, 1981.

46. Miller HRP: Gastrointestinal mucus, a medium for survival and for elimination of parasitic nematodes and protozoa. *Parasitology* 94:S77–S100, 1987

47. Walker WA, Wu M, Block KJ: Stimulation by immune complexes of mucus release from goblet cells of the rat small intestine. *Science* 197:370–372, 1977.

48. Lake AM, Bloch KJ, Neutra MR, et al: Intestinal goblet cell mucus release. II. In vivo stimulation by antigen in the immunized rat. *J Immunol* 122:834–837, 1979.

49. Lake AM, Bloch KJ, Sinclair KJ, et al: Anaphylactic release of intestinal goblet cell mucus. *Immunology* 39:173–178, 1980.

50. Forstner JF: Intestinal mucins in health and disease. *Digestion* 17:234–263, 1978.

51. Kowalewshi K, Pachkowski T, Secord DC: Mucinous secretion from canine Heidenhain pouch after stimulation with food, pentagastrin and histamine. *Eur Surg Res* 8:536–544, 1976.

52. Marom Z, Shelhamer JH, Kaliner M: Human monocyte-derived mucus secretagogue. *J Clin Invest* 75:191–198, 1985.

53. Marom Z, Shelhamer J, Berger M, et al: Anaphylatoxin C3a enhances mucous glycoprotein release from human airways in vitro. *J Exp Med* 161:657–668, 1985.

54. Kulemann-Kloene H, Krag SS, Bang FB: Mucus secretion-stimulating activity in human lymphoblastoid cells. *Science* 217:736–737, 1982.

55. Johnson HG, Chinn RA, Morton DR, et al: Diphenhydramine blocks the leukotriene-C_4 enhanced mucus secretion in canine trachea in vivo. *Agents Actions* 13:1–4, 1983.

56. Specian RD, Neutra MR: Regulation of intestinal goblet cell secretion. I. Role of parasympathetic stimulation. *Am J Physiol* 242:G370–G379, 1982.

57. Neutra MR, O'Malley LJ, Specian RD: Regulation of intestinal goblet cell secretion. II. A survey of potential secretagogues. *Am J Physiol* 242:G380–G387, 1982.

58. Phillips TE, Phillips TH, Neutra MR: Regulation of intestinal goblet cell secretion. IV. Electrical field stimulation in vitro. *Am J Physiol* 247:G682–G687, 1984.

59. Weigent DA, Blalock JE: Interactions between the neuroendocrine and immune systems: common hormones and receptors. *Immunol Rev* 100:79–108, 1987.

60. Besedovsky HO, del Rey A, Sorkin E, et al: Immunoregulatory feedback between interleukin-1 and glucocorticoid hormones. *Science* 233:652–654, 1986.

61. Stead RH, Bienenstock J, Stanisz AM: Neuropeptide regulation of mucosal immunity. *Immunol Rev* 100:333–359, 1987.

62. Felten DL, Felten SY, Bellinger DL, et al: Noradrenergic sympathetic neural interactions with the immune system: structure and function. *Immunol Rev* 100:225–260, 1987.

63. Greene R, Fowler J, MacGlashan D, Jr, et al: IgE-challenged human lung mast cells excite vagal sensory neurons in vitro. *J Appl Physiol* 64:2249–2253, 1988.

64. Weinstock JV, Blum A, Walder J, et al: Eosinophils from granulomas in murine schistosomiasis mansoni produce substance P. *J Immunol* 141:961–966, 1988.

65. Podolsky DK, Fournier DA, Lynch KE: Human colonic goblet cells: demonstration of distinct subpopulations defined by mucin-specific monoclonal antibodies. *J Clin Invest* 77:1263–1271, 1986.

66. Konturek SJ, Siebers R: Role of histamine H_1 and H_2 receptors in myoelectric activity of small bowel in the dog. *Am J Physiol* 238:G50–G56, 1980.

67. Ormsbee HS, Fondocaro JD: Action of serotonin on the gastrointestinal tract. *Proc Soc Exp Biol Med* 178:333–338, 1985.

68. Lewis RA, Austen KF: The biologically active leukotrienes: biosynthesis, metabolism, receptors, functions and pharmacology. *J Clin Invest* 73:889–897, 1984.

69. Koch KL, Dwyer A, Jeffries GH: Dose-response effects of indomethacin and PGE_2 on electromechanical activity of in vivo rabbit ileum. *Am J Physiol* 250:G135–G139, 1986.

70. Palmer JM, Castro GA: Anamnestic stimulus-specific myoelectric responses associated with intestinal immunity in the rat. *Am J Physiol* 250:G266–G273, 1986.

71. Scott RB, Diamant SC, Gall DG: Motility effects of intestinal anaphylaxis in the rat. *Am J Physiol* 255:G506–G511, 1988.

72. Farmer SG, Brown JM, Pollock D: Increased responsiveness of intestinal and vascular smooth muscle to agonists in rats infected with *Nippostrongylus brasiliensis*. *Arch Int Pharmacodyn Ther* 263:217–227, 1983.

73. Fox-Robichaud A, Collins SM: Altered calcium handling properties of jejunal smooth muscle from the nematode-infected rat. *Gastroenterology* 91:1462–1469, 1986.

74. Vermillion DL, Collins SM: Increased responsiveness of jejunal longitudinal muscle in *Trichinella*-infected rats. *Am J Physiol* 254:G124–G129, 1988.

75. Vermillion DL, Ernst PB, Scicchitano R, et al: Antigen-induced contraction of jejunal smooth muscle in the sensitized rat. *Am J Physiol* 255:G701–708, 1988.

76. Muller MJ, Huizinga JD, Collins SM: Altered smooth muscle contraction and sodium pump activity in the inflamed rat intestine. *Am J Physiol* in press.

77. Cohen JD, Kao HW, Tan ST, et al: Effect of acute experimental colitis on rabbit colonic smooth muscle. *Am J Physiol* 251:G538–G545, 1986.

78. Hargreave FE, Ryan G, Thomson NC, et al: Bronchial responsiveness to histamine and methacholine in asthma: measurement and clinical significance. *J Allergy Clin Immunol* 68:347–355, 1981.

79. Chung KF, Aizawa H. Leikauf GD, et al: Airway hyperresponsiveness induced by platelet-activating factor: role of thromboxane generation. *J Pharmacol Exp Ther* 236:580–584, 1986.

80. Cooke HJ: Complexities of nervous control of the intestinal epithelium. *Gastroenterology* 94:1087–1089, 1988.

81. Bloom FE: Neurotransmitters: past, present, and future directions. *FASEB J* 2:32–41, 1988.

82. O'Dorisio MS, Wood CL, O'Dorisio TM: Vasoactive intestinal peptide and neuropeptide modulation of the immune response. *J Immunol* 135:792s–796s, 1985.

83. O'Dorisio MS: Biochemical characteristics of receptors for vasoactive intestinal polypeptide in nervous, endocrine, and immune systems. *Fed Proc* 46:192–195, 1987.

84. Breder CD, Dinarello CA, Saper CB: Interleukin-1 immunoreactive innervation of the human hypothalamus. *Science* 240:321–324, 1988.

85. Frei K, Bodmer S, Schwerdel C, et al: Astrocytes of the brain synthesize interleukin 3-like factors. *J Immunol* 135:4044–4047, 1985.

86. Farrar WL, Hill JM, Harel-Bellan A, et al: The immune logical brain. *Immunol Rev* 100:361–378, 1987.

87. Kroemer G, Brezinschek H-P, Faessler R, et al: Physiology and pathology of an immunoendocrine feedback loop. *Immunol Today* 9:163–165, 1988.

88. Koch TR, Carney JA, Go VLW: Distribution and quantitation of gut neuropeptides in normal intestine and inflammatory bowel diseases. *Dig Dis Sci* 32:369–376, 1987.

89. Mantyh CR, Gates TS, Zimmerman RP, et al: Receptor binding sites for substance P, but not substance K or neuromedin K, are expressed in high concentrations by arterioles, venules, and lymph nodules in surgical specimens obtained from patients with ulcerative colitis and Crohn disease. *Proc Natl Acad Sci USA* 85:3235–3239, 1988.

90. Collins SM, Blennerhassett PA, Blennerhassett MG, et al: Impaired acetycholine release from the myenteric plexus of *Trichinella*-infected rats. Submitted.

91. Brain SD, Williams TJ: Substance P regulates the vasodilator activity of calcitonin gene-related peptide. *Nature* 335:73–75, 1988.

92. Hokfelt T, Millhorn D, Seroogy K, et al: Coexistence of peptides with classical neurotransmitters. *Experientia* 43:768–780, 1987.

93. Caughey GH, Leidig F, Viro NF, et al: Substance P and vasoactive intestinal peptide degradation by mast cell tryptase and chymase. *J Pharmacol Exp Ther* 244:133–137, 1988.

94. Irani AA, Schechter NM, Craig SS, et al: Two types of human mast cells have distinct neutral protease compositions. *Proc Natl Acad Sci USA* 83:4464–4468, 1986.

95. Korman LY, Nylen ES, Finan TM, et al: Primary culture of the enteric nervous system from neonatal hamster intestine. Selection of vasoactive intestinal polypeptide-containing neurons. *Gastroenterology* 95:1003–1010, 1988.

96. Granger DN, Richardson PDI, Kvietys PR, et al: Intestinal blood flow. *Gastroenterology* 78:837–863, 1980.

97. Bohlen HG: Regional vascular behavior in the gastrointestinal wall. *Fed Proc* 43:7–15, 1984.

98. Movat HZ: The Inflammatory Reaction, ed 1. Amsterdam, Elsevier, 1985, p 9.

99. Moncada S, Radomski MW, Palmer RMJ: Endothelium-derived relaxing factor: identification as nitric oxide and role in the control of vascular tone and platelet function. *Biochem Pharmacol* 37:2495–2501, 1988.

100. Kaiser L, Williams JF, Meade EA, et al: Altered endothelial cell-mediated arterial dilation in dogs with *D. immitis* infection. *Am J Physiol* 253:H1325–H1329, 1987.

101. Streeter PR, Berg EL, Rouse BTN, et al: A tissue-specific endothelial cell molecule involved in lymphocyte homing. *Nature* 331:41–46, 1988.

102. Duijvestijn A, Hamann A: Mechanisms and regulation of lymphocyte migration. *Immunol Today* 10:23–28, 1989.

103. Jeurissen SHM, Duijvestijn AM, Sontag Y, et al: Lymphocyte migration into the lamina propria of the gut is mediated by specialized HEV-like blood vessels. *Immunology* 62:273–277, 1987.

104. Grega GJ, Adamski SW: The role of venular endothelial cells in the regulation of macromolecular permeability. *Microcirc Endothelium Lymphatics* 4:143–167, 1988.

105. Patton JS, Peters PM, McCabe J, et al: Development of partial tolerance to the gastrointestinal effects of high doses of recombinant tumor necrosis factor-alpha in rodents. *J Clin Invest* 80:1587–1596, 1987.

106. Sun X-M, Hsueh W: Bowel necrosis induced by tumor necrosis factor in rats is mediated by platelet-activating factor. *J Clin Invest* 81:1328–1331, 1988.

107. Hsueh W, Gonzalez-Crussi F, Arroyave JL: Sequential release of leukotrienes and norepinephrine in rat bowel after platelet-activating factor: a mechanistic study of platelet-activating factor-induced bowel necrosis. *Gastroenterology* 94:1412–1418, 1988.

108. Goldstein RH, Fine A: Fibrotic reactions in the lung: the activation of the lung fibroblast. *Exp Lung Res* 11:245–261, 1986.

109. Joyce NC, Haire MF, Palade GE: Morphologic and biochemical evidence for a contractile cell network within the rat intestinal mucosa. *Gastroenterology* 92:68–81, 1987.

110. Claman HN: Mast cells, T cells and abnormal fibrosis. *Immunol Today* 6:192–195, 1985.

111. Turck CW, Dohlman JG, Goetzl EJ: Immunological mediators of wound healing and fibrosis *J Cell Physiol (Suppl)* 5:89–93, 1987.

112. Morhenn VB: Keratinocyte proliferation in wound healing and skin diseases. *Immunol Today* 9:104–107, 1988.

113. Thomas KA: Fibroblast growth factors. *FASEB J* 1:434–440, 1987.

114. Graham MF, Drucker DEM, Diegelmann RF, et al: Collagen synthesis by human intestinal smooth muscle cells in culture. *Gastroenterology* 92:400–405, 1987.

115. Ginsburg H, Ben-Shahar D, Ben-David E: Mast cell growth on fibroblast monolayers: two cell entities. *Immunology* 45:371–380, 1982.

116. Liu MC, Proud D, Lichtenstein LM, et al: Human lung macrophage-derived histamine-releasing activity is due to IgE-dependent factors. *J Immunol* 136:2588–2595, 1986.

117. Subba Rao PV, Friedman MM, Atkins FM, et al: Phagocytosis of mast cell granules by cultured fibroblasts. *J Immunol* 130:341–349, 1983.

118. Whitting HW: The tissue mast cell and wound healing. *Int Rev Gen Exp Zool* 4:131–168, 1969.

119. Kirkpatrick CJ, Curry A: Interaction between mast cells and perineurial fibroblasts in neurofibroma: new insights into mast cell function. *Pathol Res Pract* 183:453–458, 1988.

120. Greenberg G, Burnstock G: A novel cell-to-cell interaction between mast cells and other cell types. *Exp Cell Res* 147:1–13, 1983.

121. Atkins FM, Friedman MM, Subba Rao PV, et al: Interactions between mast cells, fibroblasts and connective tissue components. *Int Arch Allergy Appl Immunol* 77:96–102, 1985.

122. Goto T, Befus D, Low R, et al: Mast cell heterogeneity and hyperplasia in bleomycin-induced pulmonary fibrosis of rats. *Am Rev Respir Dis* 130:797–802, 1984.

123. Jordana M, Befus AD, Newhouse MT, et al: Effect of histamine on proliferation of normal human adult lung fibroblasts. *Thorax* 43:552–558, 1988.

124. Graham MF, Drucker DEM, Perr HA, et al: Heparin modulates human intestinal smooth muscle cell proliferation, protein synthesis, and lattice contraction. *Gastroenterology* 93:801–809, 1987.

125. Subramanian N, Bray MA: Interleukin 1 releases histamine from human basophils and mast cells in vitro. *J Immunol* 138:271–275, 1987.

126. Ross R, Raines EW, Bowen-Pope DF: The biology of platelet-derived growth factor. *Cell* 46:155–169, 1986.

SECTION B

IMMUNOPATHOLOGY OF THE LIVER AND GASTROINTESTINAL TRACT

PART **FIVE**

THE LIVER AND BILIARY TRACT

CHAPTER 12

Primary Biliary Cirrhosis and Sclerosing Cholangitis

STEPHEN P. JAMES

PRIMARY BILIARY CIRRHOSIS

Primary biliary cirrhosis (PBC) is a chronic disease of unknown etiology, which primarily affects middle-aged women and is characterized pathologically by inflammation and necrosis of intrahepatic bile ducts. The destruction of intrahepatic bile ducts causes chronic cholestasis, with its multiple clinical manifestations, and may progress to biliary cirrhosis and death.[1] The etiology of PBC is unknown. There is no evidence to implicate an infectious agent or an environmental factor such as a toxin. Syndromes resembling PBC may follow administration of drugs such as chlorpromazine, but no drug or drugs have been causally associated with PBC. Impaired activity of the hepatic sulfoxidation pathway has been suggested as a possible underlying metabolic defect, but this abnormality may be secondary.[2] Because of the histologic features of the disease, the occurrence of autoantibodies, and the frequent association with systemic autoimmune diseases, it is thought that immune mechanisms play a primary role in the pathogenesis of the disease, although this hypothesis remains to be proved.

Epidemiology and Genetics

The point prevalence of PBC has been estimated to be 2.3 to 14.4 per 100,000 in Great Britain.[3] The variation in prevalence may be due to the more frequent diagnosis of asymptomatic patients in urban areas. Although clustering of cases was reported in one report,[4] this was not confirmed by another study.[3] The distribution of the disease is worldwide and occurs in all races. The age at diagnosis is most commonly in the fifth and sixth decades, but the age at diagnosis varies widely from the early 20s to the 9th decade. Approximately 90% of patients are female.

Multiple familial occurrence of PBC is rare, having been reported in sisters,[5] in mothers and daughters,[6] once in brothers,[7] and once in twins.[8] There is no known significant HLA association with PBC.[9] Family members of patients with PBC have been reported to have an increased incidence of immunoglobulin abnormalities[10,11] and abnormalities of suppressor cell function,[12] suggesting the possibility that hereditary immunologic characteristics may predispose to the disease.

Clinical Features

The clinical features of PBC have been reviewed in detail[1,13,14] (Table 12–1). Typically, the disease symptoms have an insideous onset and commonly include pruritus, fatigue, increased skin pigmentation, arthralgias, dryness of the mouth and eyes, and Raynaud's phenomenon. Jaundice and GI bleeding are uncommon presentations. Common physical findings include hepatomegaly, splenomegaly, skin hyperpigmentation due to melanin deposition, excoriations, xanthomata, xanthelasma, and spider telangiectasia. Late in the course of the disease, deep jaundice, petechiae and purpura, and signs of hepatic encephalopathy occur due to advanced liver disease. Symptoms and signs of some of the associated syndromes (see below) may be the presenting manifestations. In asymptomatic patients it is not unusual for the physical examination to be entirely normal. Patients have been described with positive antimitochondrial antibody (AMA) and histologic features of PBC on liver biopsy, but without symptoms of liver disease or abnormalities of liver enzymes.[15] These patients appear to represent the very early spectrum of the disease, since some may eventually develop more significant manifestations of PBC.

Common laboratory abnormalities include elevation of the serum alkaline phosphatase and gamma-glutamyl transpeptidase. Total bilirubin is normal early in the disease, and progressively rises with advancing disease. Mild-to-moderate elevations of serum aminotransferases are found. Hypercholesterolemia and lipoprotein abnormalities are frequent. Urine copper and ceruloplasmin are elevated.

Table 12–1 TYPICAL FEATURES OF PRIMARY BILIARY CIRRHOSIS

Etiology	Unknown
Epidemiology	Predominantly middle-aged women
Genetics	No known HLA association; familial cases occur but rarely
Symptoms	Pruritis, fatigue, arthralgias, dry eyes, hyperpigmentation
Physical findings	Hepatomegaly, splenomegaly, hyperpigmentation, excoriations, xanthelasma
Laboratory	Increased alkaline phosphatase, bilirubin, cholesterol
	Antimitochondrial antibodies usually present in high titer
Liver biopsy	Early: nonsupportive destructive cholangitis; late: biliary cirrhosis
Cholangiography	Normal in early disease; nonspecific changes due to cirrhosis late in disease
Prognosis	Mean survival 11 years; asymptomatic patients may have normal survival
Treatment	Supportive: cholestyramine, fat-soluble vitamins
	Azathioprine or colchicine may be of benefit
	Liver transplantation for advanced disease

Abnormalities found with advanced liver disease, such as hypoalbuminemia and prolonged prothrombin time, occur with hepatocellular decompensation. Cholangiography shows normal biliary ducts, except when cirrhosis is present, which may cause nonspecific irregularity and tortuosity of small intrahepatic bile ducts. Serum total IgM is often elevated (see below). The AMA test (see below) is positive in more than 90% of patients and is the only relatively specific diagnostic test other than liver biopsy.

Associated Autoimmune Syndromes

PBC has been associated with a number of autoimmune syndromes (Table 12–2). Keratoconjunctivitis sicca is probably the most commonly associated syndrome, which is often asymptomatic or present in a very mild form.[16] Several forms of arthritis are frequently found. Most often patients have a seronegative nondestructive arthritis affecting small joints, and less often there is evidence of joint destruction.[17] True rheumatoid arthritis has been associated with PBC but may not be more common than the fortuitous association of two diseases. Scleroderma, either as the complete syndrome or as the CRST variant, is also associated with PBC.[18] It has been observed that this syndrome with PBC is often associated with keratoconjunctivitis sicca and anticentromere antibodies.[19] Evidence of hypothyroidism is common, and autoimmune thyroiditis may be the presenting manifestation of PBC.[20] Subclinical alveolitis, with increased CD4 T cells in bronchoalveolar lavage fluid, has been found in patients with PBC, suggesting that a pathologic process similar to sarcoidosis may occur in the lung in PBC.[21] Other associations have been reported uncommonly and may represent fortuitous associations. They include systemic lupus erythematosus, dermatomyositis, gluten-sensitive enteropathy, bullous phemphigoid, pyderma gangrenosum, lichen planus, cutaneous vas-

Table 12–2 SYNDROMES ASSOCIATED WITH PRIMARY BILIARY CIRRHOSIS

Common
    Keratoconjunctivitis sicca
    Seronegative, nondestructive arthritis
    Altered thyroid function
    Scleroderma (usually CREST variant)
    Raynaud's phenomenon

Uncommon
    Pulmonary fibrosis
    Glomerulonephritis
    Dermatomyositis
    Hemolytic anemia
    Pyoderma gangrenosum
    Polymyalgia rheumatica
    Bullous phemphigoid
    Myasthenia gravis
    Lichen planus
    Systemic lupus erythematosus
    Lichen planus

culitis with membranous glomerulonephritis, polymyalgia rheumatica, hemolytic anemia, interstitial lung disease, and myasthenia gravis.

Liver Pathology

The liver histopathologic abnormalities in PBC are relatively specific. The histologic features have been classified into four stages,[22] but these may overlap. The earliest and most specific lesions identified (stage I) show chronic inflammation and necrosis of intrahepatic bile ducts, which are infiltrated with lymphocytes and may be surrounded with granulomas. In stage II, bile ductules proliferate, mononuclear infiltration of portal areas is prominent, and some portal fibrosis may be evident. In stage III, there is a reduction in the portal inflammatory infiltrate, bile ducts are absent from portal triads, and there is an increase in portal fibrosis. Stage IV is characterized by biliary cirrhosis with a paucity of bile ducts and increased hepatic copper. thus the histopathologic features of PBC consist of a chronic inflammatory process associated with destruction and disappearance of intrahepatic bile ducts and progressive portal fibrosis, leading to biliary cirrhosis. Hepatocellular necrosis is not a prominent feature, although in occasional cases piecemeal necrosis surrounding portal tracts may resemble autoimmune chronic active hepatitis; in rare cases there is an associated clinical syndrome with features of both chronic active hepatitis and primary biliary cirrhosis.[23]

Immunofluorescence studies have shown that plasma cells in the portal infiltrates stain predominantly for IgM.[24] Deposition of IgM and complement has been observed in portal areas.[25] There is increased expression of HLA-DR antigens of bile duct epithelial cells, an abnormality that appears to be unusual in other liver diseases.[26] The portal infiltrates are composed primarily of T cells, which have a higher proportion of CD4-positive cells than in viral hepatitis, but CD8-positive T cells may be found in close proximity to some bile ducts.[27-30]

Immunologic Studies

Serum Immunoglobulins

Polyclonal elevation of serum immunoglobulins is found in most patients with PBC as the disease progresses,[1] although immunoglobulin levels may be normal early in the disease (Table 12–3). There is frequently a disproportionate elevation of IgM, a feature that distinguishes PBC from other chronic hepatic diseases. One explanation of the striking IgM elevation found in some patients is that low molecular weight (monomeric) is often found in PBC, which may falsely elevate IgM levels, as determined by radial immunodiffusion.[31] The presence of monomeric IgM is not, however, specific for PBC. Elevation of serum total and secretory IgA is also found in PBC,[32] but this finding is also common in other liver diseases such as alcoholic liver disease. A case has been reported with PBC and selective IgA deficiency indicating that IgA is not required as an immune effector mechanism for the pathogenesis of PBC.[33] The elevated immunoglobulin levels in PBC are usually due to polyclonal increases in immunoglobulins, but production of oligoclonal antibodies is occasionally found, and, in some cases, these monoclonal antibodies have been shown to have specificity for mitochondrial antigens.[34] Although patients with PBC have hypergammaglobulinemia, their antibody responses to immunization are diminished. Fox et al.,[35,36] using the antigen keyhole limpet hemocyanin

Table 12-3 IMMUNOLOGIC ABNORMALITIES IN PRIMARY BILIARY CIRRHOSIS

Humoral Immune Abnormalities
  Hypergammaglobulinemia, particularly IgM
  Autoantibodies
    Antimitochondrial antibodies (M2 nearly specific for PBC)
    Nonspecific: SMA, LMA, anti-LSP, ANA, rheumatoid factor, antithyroid antibodies,
      others
  Immune complex-like materials in serum
  Increased complement catabolism
  Decreased Kupffer cell-mediated clearance of C3b containing immune complexes

Cellular Immune Abnormalities
  Skin test anergy
  Diminished T-cell proliferative responses
  Diminished natural killer cell activity
  Abnormal function of immunoregulatory T cells
    Diminished autologous MLR
    Decreased suppressor T-cell function
  Morphologic: infiltration of liver with T4-positive cells, plasma cells, and T8-positive
    T cells in close proximity to damaged bile ducts

(KLH), found that on the average the primary antibody response was diminished in patients with PBC. Thomas et al.[37] found that while the primary antibody response to the antigen ϕX174 was normal in patients with PBC, the secondary antibody response was diminished; in addition, a greater proportion of the response was of the IgM class, compared with the IgG class, than the response in normal individuals. Similarly, patients with PBC have an accentuated secondary IgM response to tetanus toxoid immunization.[38] These observations suggest an abnormality in vivo of immunoglobulin class switching.

Mitochondrial Antibodies
The discovery of autoantibodies that react with mitochondria in the sera of patients with PBC, as detected by indirect immunofluorescence microscopy, was the first important laboratory evidence that PBC is an autoimmune disease.[39] The antigens recognized by mitochondrial antibodies are heterogeneous and are neither organ- nor species-specific. Nine separate groups of antigens, designated M1 to M9, have been described.[40] Varying patterns of reactivity by immunofluorescence have been associated with different diseases, including rheumatologic diseases, syphilis, myocarditis, and the pseudolupus syndrome. Reactivity with the inner mitochondrial M2 antigen is most specific for PBC. Antibodies to this antigen are present in most cases of PBC, and, conversely, antibodies to this antigen are found only occasionally in low titer in other diseases.[41] Reactivity to other mitochondrial antigens is found in PBC. Antibodies to M4 are found in patients with the PBC-chronic active hepatitis overlap syndrome, and antibody to M8 correlates with rapidly progressive disease. To date, extensive biochemical characterization has only been carried out with the M2 antigen. By Western blot, sera from most patients with PBC react with three major M2 peptides, of 70, 45, and 39 kD.

Gershwin et al. isolated and sequenced a rat liver cDNA encoding a fusion peptide that reacted with sera from PBC patients and absorbed reactivity to the 70-kD antigen.[42] In other recent studies it was shown that PBC sera react with the purified E2 subunit of pyruvate dehydrogenase, and the sequence of this peptide in *Escherichia coli* has sequence homology with the previously described fusion peptide.[43] Thus it appears likely that the major autoantigen of PBC has been identified as being a subunit of a critical enzyme pathway. Since this enzyme is present in all cells, the role that antibodies to the enzyme play in the disease is still uncertain. As suggested by Gershwin,[42] the availability of very specific molecular methods will now allow for further progress in determining whether there are cross-reactive antigens of biliary epithelia, whether there is T-cell reactivity to this antigen, and whether the autoantibodies arise as a cross-reaction to bacterial products. Interestingly, antibodies to the 70-kD fusion autoantigen are primarily IgG3 and IgM, which is of interest since antibodies of these classes typically arise as a result of viral infection.[44]

Other Autoantibodies
Many other autoantibodies have been described in PBC, but these are not specific for this disease. Smooth muscle antibodies are found in the serum of 20 to 50% of patients,[45] but titers are usually lower than in patients with diseases characterized by prominent hepatocellular necrosis, such as chronic active hepatitis. Antibodies to cytoskeleton components, which contain actin to which smooth muscle antibodies bind, are also found in PBC.[46] In one study, the majority of patients with PBC had antibodies in serum that reacted with bile ducts,[24] however, this reactivity is not specific for PBC and may be due to the presence of smooth muscle antibodies. MacSween et al.[47] found that 35% of patients with PBC have antibodies that react with rabbit liver bile canaliculi, as detected by indirect immunofluorescence; some, but not all of these sera also react with human bile canaliculi. Approximately two-thirds of sera containing bile canalicular antibodies in this study did not contain smooth muscle antibodies, suggesting that these antibodies are different. However, Kurki et al.[48] found that the reactivity of smooth muscle containing sera against bile canaliculi could be absorbed with purified actin, indicating that the antibile canalicular antibody was probably identical to smooth muscle antibody. Bile canalicular staining is also nonspecific for PBC.

Using a sensitive radioimmunoassay, it has been shown that about one-half of patients with PBC have antibodies reactive with an antigen prepared from human liver cell membranes [liver-specific protein (LSP)].[49] Although the specificity of the antigen preparation used in these studies has been questioned, it has been suggested that this antigen may be a target of immunologically mediated cellular injury in patients with chronic active hepatitis and PBC. Antibodies reactive with liver membrane antigens have also been detected by radioimmunoassay in about one-third of patients with PBC,[50] usually at a much lower titer than in chronic active hepatitis. In one study the presence of this antibody correlated with the presence of piecemeal necrosis of hepatocytes in PBC, suggesting that this antibody may play a role in hepatocyte damage in this disease. Antinuclear antibodies are found in about one-third to one-half of patients. The presence of the multiple nuclear dot pattern correlated with the presence of sicca syndrome,[51] and the presence of anticentromere antibodies correlated with the presence of sclerodactyly.[52] The pattern of autoantibody reactivity in PBC differs from that of primary

Sjögren's syndrome in that patients with the latter, but not the former, have reactivity to small ribonucleoproteins by radioimmune assay (RIA).[53] Other autoantibodies commonly found in PBC include rheumatoid factor (about two-thirds of patients),[54] antithyroid antibodies,[55] antinative DNA,[56] antiribosomal antibodies,[57] and antihistone antibodies.[58]

Whatever the significance of autoantibodies in PBC, it is unlikely that they all play a primary role in the pathogenesis of the bile duct lesions. First, the titer of autoantibodies does not correlate with activity of disease, and patients with otherwise typical PBC may not have detectable AMA. Second, none of the autoantibodies described to date is entirely disease-specific, each having been found in a variety of other hepatic and nonliver diseases. It is possible, nonetheless, that such antibodies may play a secondary role in tissue injury. The pathogenic mechanism by which autoantibodies are formed in PBC is no better understood in this disease than it is in other autoimmune states. It is possible that their occurrence relates to a fundamental abnormality in immune regulation, or that they arise due to cross-reactivity to some primary etiologic agent.

Immune Complexes

The discovery of the important role of circulating immune complexes in other human diseases lead to a search for them in liver diseases. Circulating immune complex-like materials have been reported to be present in PBC in several studies. Patients have serum substances reactive in the Raji cell radioimmunoassay for immune complexes:[59,60] a correlation was found between the presence of immune complex-like material and the severity of portal inflammation and the presence of autoimmune syndromes. In addition, materials reactive in the ^{125}I-C1q binding assay for immune complexes[61] have been found. Many patients with PBC have been shown to have cryoprecipitable material in serum, which, although not containing complement components, is able to activate complement, suggesting the presence of antigen-antibody complexes in the cryoprecipitates.[62] One unconfirmed report found evidence of antigens derived from bile in circulating immune complexes,[63] and another found evidence that they contained antimitochondrial antibodies.[64] Patients with PBC have been found to have a defect in Kupffer cell-mediated clearance of C3b-coated immune complexes[65] in the liver. Similarly, C3b receptor-mediated phagocytic function of neutrophils has been shown to be defective in patients with PBC.[66] The cause of this abnormality is unknown, but it might account for accumulation of immune complex-like materials in serum that are normally cleared by the liver. In contrast to these findings, in another carefully conducted study, using several well-defined methods, little evidence for circulating immune complexes was found in patients with PBC[67] when fresh serum specimens were used. Part of the difficulty in defining the presence of circulating immune complexes in PBC might be due to abnormal properties of IgM in PBC, which has been shown to have the capacity to fix complement in the apparent absence of antigen binding and to be more readily cryoprecipitable.[68] Other arguments against an immune complex-mediated pathogenesis of PBC are the absence of typical histopathologic features of immune complex deposition in the liver, and the low frequency of associated immune complex-mediated syndromes such as vasculitis and glomerulonephritis. Obviously the hypothesis that circulating immune complexes play a role in liver injury, or in extrahepatic manifestations of PBC awaits more definitive evidence of circulating antigen-antibody complexes in PBC.

Complement Abnormalities

Because antibody-mediated tissue injury may play a primary or secondary role in tissue injury in PBC, a number of studies have focused on the function of the complement system in this disease. The investigation of serum complement in liver disease is complicated by the fact that a number of complement components are synthesized in the liver, and therefore altered levels of complement components may be secondary to the liver disease itself. In studies of complement turnover using ^{125}I-labeled purified C3, it was found that patients with PBC have an increased fractional catabolic rate of C3, as well as evidence of an increased extravascular-to-intravascular pool.[69] Similarly, the fractional catabolic rate of C1q is increased in patients with PBC.[70] These findings are not simply due to the presence of liver disease, since patients with HBsAg-negative chronic active hepatitis do not have these abnormalities. Patient sera have been shown to contain elevated levels of C3, decreased levels of C4, and circulating conversion products of C3. More recently, activation of the classical complement pathway has been demonstrated by the finding of C1r, C1s, C1 inactivator complexes in serum of patients, but no evidence of activation of the alternative pathway was found.[17] The mechanisms by which the classical complement pathway is activated in PBC are unknown; these findings are compatible with the presence of antigen-antibody complexes that might be formed in the disease, but they might also be due to abnormal properties of serum proteins, such as that referred to above for serum IgM.

Lymphocyte Populations in Peripheral Blood

Patients with PBC often have a decrease in the absolute number of total circulating lymphocytes,[72] which is a nonspecific feature of liver disease. The proportion of CD3$^+$ T cells is either normal or decreased. The proportion of B cells is normal. The CD4 and CD8 subpopulations of T cells are highly variable. In some studies no differences were found compared with controls, while in others the proportion of CD4-positive cells was diminished.[73–75] In one study it was found that the proportion of CD4-positive cells was diminished in patients with less advanced disease, while the proportion of CD8-positive cells was diminished in patients with more advanced disease.[73] Since these monoclonal antibodies define heterogeneous populations of cells, it is not clear what implications these findings have for the pathogenesis of PBC; they may in part represent secondary changes due to liver disease. The proportion of null cells, as determined by an Fc binding assay, has been reported to be diminished in patients with PBC,[76] consistent with the presence of circulating immune complexes. In studies with monoclonal antibodies the proportions of anti-Leu7- and anti-CD16- [found on circulating natural killer (NK) cells] positive lymphocytes are normal in patients with PBC[77]; however, NK activity of peripheral blood lymphocytes was diminished, suggesting a functional impairment of NK cells in PBC. There is also evidence that B cells in peripheral blood of patients are more activated than normal, consistent with the observed hypergammaglobulinemia and presence of autoantibodies.[78]

Studies of Lymphocyte Function

More than one-half of patients with PBC have diminished or absent delayed-type skin test reactions to a variety of antigens, including PPD, KLH, and DNCB.[35,36,79] The mechanism of skin test anergy is unknown, but is probably a secondary effect of liver disease, since anergy correlates with stage of disease and is found in other liver diseases. Many patients have diminished in vitro lymphocyte proliferative responses to mitogens.[79] The diminished response may at least in part be due to serum inhibitory factors, in that extensively washed lymphocytes have normal responses, and patient sera inhibit the responses of normal lymphocytes. The nature of this inhibitory factor is presently unknown. It is of interest that inhibitory substances have been isolated from normal liver, and it is possible that inhibitory substances are released secondary to liver injury. The high concentrations of bile acids, cholesterol, and lipoproteins that are found in liver disease might also contribute to diminished lymphocyte responses.

Antigen-specific lymphocyte responses have also been examined. Lymphocytes from patients have been shown to produce migration inhibition factor in response to the liver membrane preparation liver-specific lipoprotein (LSP)[80] and in response to protein preparations from human bile.[81] These responses, however, are not specific for PBC. Again, this type of reactivity might represent secondary sensitization due to liver damage.

It is worthwhile to note that pathologic lesions closely resembling those of PBC are found in patients with chronic graft-versus-host-disease[82] and in chronic liver allograft rejection.[83] These findings suggest that immunologic mechanisms similar to those in graft rejection may play a role in PBC. Attempts have been made to determine whether patients have cell-mediated cytotoxicity against liver target cells. In a number of different experimental systems, patients have been found to have evidence of increased cytotoxicity against xenogeneic liver targets cells[84] but normal cytotoxicity against LSP-coated red cells[85] and against the PLC/PRF/5 hepatoma cell line.[86] Because of the design of these studies, it is likely that in each instance the cytotoxic reaction observed was not mediated by specific T-cell mechanisms, but by non-antigen-specific cytotoxic mechanisms. In studies of NK function, it has been found that patients have diminished NK cytotoxicity against typical NK target cells.[87] This decrease in function does not appear to be due to a decrease in the number of circulating cells having phenotypic markers of NK cells, but rather to a decrease in their functional activity.[77] Interestingly, in studies of antibody-dependent cell-mediated cytotoxicity, it has been found that patients have normal killing, indicating that this functional activity is not affected by the disease process. It is noteworthy that immunohistochemical studies of liver specimens have failed to show the presence of cells having a typical NK phenotype, but these results are not conclusive since the phenotypes of cytolytic cells might be different in tissue sites. In one study an attempt was made to determine whether patients circulating lymphocytes were capable of killing autologous liver target cells,[88] but the results were heterogeneous and did not indicate whether patients had increased or decreased killing in this assay system. As noted above, the increased proportion of CD8-positive T cells around injured bile ducts suggests the possibility that cytolytic T cells may play a specific role in tissue injury in this disease, but there are no clear-cut data to support this possibility as yet.

Because of the autoimmune associations of this disease, a number of studies have examined the question of whether immunoregulatory cell function is abnormal in PBC. Although the proportion of CD8-positive lymphocytes is usually normal, T cells from patients have a diminished ability to suppress pokeweed mitogen-stimulated immunoglobulin synthesis.[89] In addition, con A-activated lymphocytes from patients have a diminished capacity to mediate suppression of proliferative responses[90] or pokeweed mitogen-stimulated immunoglobulin synthesis. Interestingly, healthy relatives of patients with PBC have been shown to have a similar abnormality of suppressor cell function,[12] suggesting that this may be a genetic marker of disease predisposition. This abnormality, which has been identified in other diseases, has been suggested to play a role in hypergammaglobulinemia and the production of autoantibodies in PBC. It is possible that defective activation of suppressor cells might play a role in autoreactive T-cell-mediated cytotoxicity as well.

It has also been shown that patients with PBC have a diminished autologous mixed lymphocyte reaction,[91] which has also been found in a variety of other autoimmune diseases. It has been demonstrated that autoreactive cells have the ability not only to provide help for, but also suppress immunoglobulin synthesis *in vitro.* Thus autoreactive cells may play important immunoregulatory functions. Whether this defect is intrinsic, or secondary to liver disease has not yet been determined, but it may play a role in the altered immunoregulatory function mentioned above.

To summarize the immunologic abnormalities of PBC, the disease is characterized by the presence of non-organ-specific autoantibodies in serum, evidence of activation of the classical complement pathway, and alteration of the function of immunoregulatory T cells. As yet there is no definite evidence of primary immunologically mediated damage to the site of tissue injury, namely the intrahepatic bile ducts. It remains an important unanswered question as to whether the damage to bile ducts is a primary autoimmune event, or whether the inflammatory response is secondary to damage to bile ducts that occurs by some other mechanism. It is likely that there is an underlying genetic predisposition, as well as important hormonal effects, which interact with the immune system by mechanisms not yet understood.

Natural History and Response to Treatment

The prognosis for PBC is highly variable. Overall mean survival in a recent study was 11.9 years,[13] in contrast to earlier studies of primarily symptomatic patients in whom the average survival is only about 6 years; survival in patients who are asymptomatic at the time of diagnosis is very much better, not differing significantly from matched controls. The presence of granulomas, which are found in early disease and correlate inversely with fibrosis, is a good prognostic sign,[92] while increasing serum bilirubin and onset of symptoms and signs of portal hypertension are poor prognostic signs. The complications of PBC are many, including symptoms and signs associated with chronic cholestasis, such as pruritis, steatorrhea, hyperlipidemia, metabolic bone disease, and those complications related to cirrhosis and portal hypertension.[14]

No primary treatment of the underlying disease has proved to be uniformly successful in prolonging survival. At the moment, medical treatment is generally limited to supportive care, with cholestyramine and fat-soluble vitamins. Corticosteroid drugs have been shown to cause improvement in biochemical abnormalities in some patients, but these drugs are generally regarded as contraindicated for long-term treatment of PBC because they greatly exacerbate the metabolic bone disease to which these patients are prone. Although previous studies found no benefit of treatment with azathioprine, more recently treatment with this drug has been shown to prolong survival; however, this beneficial effect of the drug appears to be marginal.[93] D-penicillamine has been studied extensively, not only because it chelates copper and thus reverses the copper overload state associated with PBC, but also because of its anti-inflammatory properties. Despite initial favorable reports, experience with this drug after extended follow-up indicates that it causes no significant increase in survival and is associated with many potentially serious side effects.[94,95] A preliminary study of chlorambucil indicated that treatment with this drug is associated with decreased intrahepatic inflammation and improvement in some biochemical abnormalities, but its long-term usefulness is unknown.[96] Cyclosporin has been used in treatment of a small number of patients,[97] and its use is also associated with improvement in some clinical measurements of disease activity; however, significant renal toxicity developed in patients, possibly because the drug is metabolized in the liver, and its biological half-life may be significantly prolonged in liver disease. Levamisole was studied in a small preliminary trial, but it was without benefit.[98] Recent results of controlled trials suggest a beneficial effect on hepatic biochemistry and survival with colchicine treatment, but the drug did not appear to halt histologic progression of the disease.[99] One of the difficulties in developing improved treatments for the underlying inflammatory disease is that those patients who may be the best candidates for treatment are those with earlier, inflammatory stages of the disease, but these patients are often asymptomatic and may have an indolent, benign clinical course in the absence of any treatment. Advanced hepatic fibrosis and cirrhosis in PBC may not be amenable to treatment with anti-inflammatory drugs. For patients with advanced and deteriorating liver disease the best available treatment is hepatic transplantation.[100] Although recurrence of PBC in hepatic allografts has been reported, the features reported were probably due to chronic allograft rejection, which, interestingly, has features that closely resemble PBC.[101] More extensive follow-up of patients with hepatic transplantation for PBC has not revealed any evidence of recurrence of the disease in the allograft.[102] This observation is of great interest because it suggests either that the immunologic mechanisms contributing to the liver disease do not damage the allograft, or, more likely, that the immunosuppressive treatments used following transplantation effectively prevent emergence of the disease.

SCLEROSING CHOLANGITIS

Primary sclerosing cholangitis is a disease of unknown etiology characterized by inflammation and fibrosis of both intrahepatic and extrahepatic bile ducts[103,104] (Table 12–4). The disease occurs primarily in young men and is often found in association with inflammatory bowel disease (usually ulcerative colitis). The recognition of the disease has increased greatly since the advent of percutaneous and endoscopic cholangiography. This disease is frequently progressive and leads to biliary cirrhosis and death. There is a significant association with biliary cholangiocarcinoma,[105,106] and it has been suggested that sclerosing cholangitis may be regarded as a premalignant disease of the biliary system, just as ulcerative colitis may be associated with premalignant changes in the colon.

Clinical Features

The symptoms of sclerosing cholangitis are similar to other cholestatic liver diseases and include fatigue, pruritis, hyperpigmentation, xanthelasma, and jaundice.

Table 12-4 TYPICAL FEATURES OF IDIOPATHIC SCLEROSING CHOLANGITIS

Etiology	Unknown
Epidemiology	Predominantly young men; frequent association with inflammatory bowel disease
Genetics	HLA-B8; familial cases rare
Symptoms	Pruritis, fatigue
Physical findings	Often normal early; late: hepatomegaly, jaundice
Laboratory	High alkaline phosphatase, bilirubin; antimitochondrial antibodies absent
Histologic features	Liver: fibrous obliteration of intrahepatic and extrahepatic bile ducts
Cholangiography	Irregular, tortuous, beaded appearance of intrahepatic or extrahepatic bile ducts
Prognosis	Highly variable; may progress to biliary cirrhosis and death
Treatment	No medical treatment proved to arrest disease
	Supportive: cholystyramine; antibiotics for acute cholangitis
	Surgery for isolated high-grade obstruction
	Liver transplantation

Patients may also have symptoms of cholangitis with fever and abdominal pain. Symptoms of underlying inflammatory bowel disease may be prominent, but are often mild or absent. Unlike primary biliary cirrhosis, patients are usually young men, serum antimitochondrial antibody is nearly always absent, and extrahepatic syndromes such as keratoconjunctivitis sicca, arthritis, and thyroid disease are rare. The disease has been found in infants and young children with or without ulcerative colitis.[107]

Laboratory Abnormalities

The routine laboratory features of sclerosing cholangitis are similar to those of primary biliary cirrhosis,[108] described in detail above. Elevation of serum IgM is not as striking as in PBC, and serum antimitochondrial antibodies are nearly always absent. As in other cholestatic liver disease, copper accumulation may be striking in the liver, and laboratory tests of copper metabolism are abnormal. The most important laboratory test is cholangiography. Cholangiograms demonstrate variable degrees of narrowing of intrahepatic or extrahepatic bile ducts, with tortuosity and areas of dilatation, leading to a beaded appearance,[109] in contrast to primary biliary cirrhosis, in which the ducts appear normal until cirrhosis is prominent, in which case there may be narrowing and irregularity of intrahepatic bile ducts.

Pathology

The liver biopsy is usually abnormal; however, pathognomonic changes are not often seen. The portal tracts show expansion, with edema and fibrosis and relatively modest cellular infiltration. Later fibrous septa appear and finally biliary cirrhosis. The typical changes in the intrahepatic bile ducts are a fibrous-obliterative process in which segments of bile ducts are replaced by solid cords of connective tissue leading to an "onion skin" appearance. When the course is associated with bacterial cholangitis, numerous polymorphs may be present within and around bile ducts. When extrahepatic ducts are involved, the histologic appearance shows no unique pathognomonic features, revealing only fibrosis with a relatively modest inflammatory component. It has been suggested that the nonspecific hepatobiliary lesions identified in association with ulcerative colitis, previously alluded to as "pericholangitis," are in fact part of the spectrum of sclerosing cholangitis. The finding of portal inflammation and fibrosis in association with ulcerative colitis should indicate the need for careful examination of the biliary tree by cholangiography for evidence of sclerosing cholangitis.

Immunopathogenesis

The etiology of primary sclerosing cholangitis is unknown. Because of the association with inflammatory bowel disease, it has been suggested that absorption of bacteria or toxic materials from the intestine might be important in the etiology of the disease. However, sclerosing cholangitis appears to be a rare complication of ulcerative colitis, and there is no obvious correlation with the extent or severity of bowel disease. Sclerosing cholangitis may occur in patients with minimal ulcerative colitis. Furthermore, the course of the liver disease appears to be independent of the bowel disease. Patients who have undergone colectomy for ulcerative colitis may have relentless progression of the liver disease. Genetic factors have been suggested to be important, since the frequency of HLA-B8 is increased in this disease.[110] In addition, there have been rare reports of familial sclerosing cholangitis and ulcerative colitis.[111] Unlike PBC, sclerosing cholangitis is rarely associated with other autoimmune syndromes. The frequency of autoantibodies is much lower than in PBC. Cross-reactive antibodies reactive with colon and portal triads have been reported.[112] It has also been suggested that the disease may be related to an underlying disorder of fibrogenesis, since other unusual forms of fibrosis have been associated with the disease, including mediastinal fibrosis, Riedel's thyroiditis, orbital pseudotumor, and retroperitoneal fibrosis.[113-115] Because the disease is rare, relatively little is known concerning the immunology of the disease. Tests for circulating immune complexes have been reported to be positive in about 70% of patients, but the nature of these circulating immune complex-like materials is unknown, and their relationship to the pathogenesis of the disease is uncertain.[116] Peripheral blood lymphocytes show a higher than normal CD4/CD8 ratio in patients with sclerosing cholangitis. The autologous mixed lymphocyte reaction (MLR) is diminished in patients with sclerosing cholangitis, and there is an increased proportion of activated CD8 T cells following activation in the autologous MLR in vitro, suggesting the possibility of abnormal immunoregulatory mechanisms.[117] Phenotypes of T lymphocytes have been examined in hepatic tissues; while CD8-positive lymphocytes appear to infiltrate bile duct epithelium, CD4 lymphocytes tend to accumulate around other bile ducts.[118] Using a leukocyte migration inhibition test, it has been shown that some patients with sclerosing cholangitis may have leukocyte sensitivity to protein antigen preparations derived from human bile, suggesting that cellular reactivity to biliary epithelial cell-derived antigens might play a role in the disease.[81]

The occurrence of biliary cholangiocarcinoma in patients with sclerosing cholangitis suggests that the mechanisms that cause damage to bile ducts might also cause premalignant changes in the biliary epithelium, raising the possibility that the pathogenesis of sclerosing cholangitis may be related to ulcerative colitis, but with a different target epithelial cell, since ulcerative colitis is clearly associated with inflammation and dysplasia of colonic epithelial cells. Further progress in understanding the pathogenesis of ulcerative colitis might provide some future insights into the pathogenesis of sclerosing cholangitis.

Treatment

No form of medical treatment has been proved useful in retarding the progressive damage to bile ducts.[119] Medical management is currently limited to alleviation of complications of the disease, with such treatment as cholestyramine, fat-soluble vitamins, and antibiotics for episodes of acute cholangitis. Anti-inflammatory drugs have not been proved to have any predictable beneficial effect, and, as mentioned above, colectomy in patients with ulcerative colitis has not been predictably associated with a beneficial effect on the liver disease. For patients with localized areas of high-grade obstruction and symptomatic cholestasis or recurrent cholangitis, a variety of palliative surgical measures directed at the dominant area of obstruction may be useful.[120] Liver transplantation is the only effective treatment for patients with advanced hepatic decompensation.[100]

REFERENCES

1. Sherlock S, Scheuer PJ: The presentation and diagnosis of 100 patients with primary biliary cirrhosis. *N Engl J Med* 289:674–678, 1973.
2. Olomu AB, Vickers CR, Waring RH, Clements D, Babbs C, Warnes TW, Elias E: High incidence of poor sulfoxidation in patients with primary biliary cirrhosis. *N Engl J Med* 318:1089–1092, 1988.
3. Triger DR, Berg PA, Rodes J: Epidemiology of primary biliary cirrhosis. *Liver* 4:195–200, 1984.
4. Hamlyn AN, Macklon AF, James O: Primary biliary cirrhosis: geographical clustering and symptomatic onset seasonality. *Gut* 24:940–945, 1983.
5. Walker JG, Bates D, Doniach D, Ball PAJ, Sherlock S: Chronic liver disease and mitochondrial antibodies: a family study. *Br Med J* 1:146–148, 1972.
6. Fagan E, Williams R, Cox S: Primary biliary cirrhosis in mother and daughter. *Br Med J* 2:1195, 1977.
7. Brown R, Clark ML, Doniach D: Primary biliary cirrhosis in brothers. *Postgrad Med J* 51:110–115, 1975.
8. Chohan MR: Primary biliary cirrhosis in twin sisters. *Gut* 14:213–214, 1973.
9. Hamlyn AN, Adams D, Sherlock S: Primary or secondary sicca complex? Investigation in primary biliary cirrhosis by histocompatibility testing. *Br Med J* 281:425–426, 1980.
10. Galbraith RM, Smith M, Mackenzie RM, Tee De, Doniach D, Williams R: High prevalence of seroimmunologic abnormalities in relatives of patients with active chronic hepatitis or primary biliary cirrhosis. *N Engl J Med* 290:63–69, 1974.
11. Jaup BH, Zettergren LSW: Familial occurrence of primary biliary cirrhosis associated with hypergammaglobulinemia in descendents: a family study. *Gastroenterology* 78:549–555, 1980.
12. Miller KB, Sepersky RA, Brown KM, Goldberg MJ, Kaplan MM: Genetic abnormalities of immunoregulation in primary biliary cirrhosis. *Am J Med* 75:75–80, 1983.

13. Roll J, Boyer JL, Barry D, Klatskin G: The prognostic importance of clinical and histologic features in asymptomatic and symptomatic primary biliary cirrhosis. *N Engl J Med* 308:1–7, 1983.

14. Vierling JM: Primary biliary cirrhosis. In Zakim D, Boyer TD: *Hepatology*. Philadelphia, Saunders, 1982, pp 825–862.

15. James O, Macklon AF, Watson AJ: Primary biliary cirrhosis — a revised clinical spectrum. *Lancet* 1:1278–1281, 1981.

16. Culp KS, Fleming CR, Duffy J, Baldus WP, Dickson ER: Autoimmune associations in primary biliary cirrhosis. *Mayo Clin Proc* 57:365–370, 1982.

17. Lauritsen K, Diederichsen H: Arthritis in patients with antimitochondrial antibodies. *Scand J Rheumatol* 12:331–335, 1983.

18. Murray-Lyon IM, Thompson RPH, Ansell ID, Williams R: Scleroderma and primary biliary cirrhosis. *Br Med J* 1:258–259, 1970.

19. Powell FC, Schroeter AL, Dickson ER: Primary biliary cirrhosis and the CREST syndrome: a report of 22 cases. *Q J Med* 62:75–82, 1987.

20. Elta GH, Sepersky RA, Goldberg MJ, Connors CM, Miller KB, Kaplan MM: Increased incidence of hypothyroidism in primary biliary cirrhosis. *Dig Dis Sci* 28:961–965, 1983.

21. Wallaert B, Bonniere P, Prin L, Cortot A, Tonnel AB, Voisin C: Primary biliary cirrhosis. Subclinical inflammatory alveolitis in patients with normal chest roentgenograms. *Chest* 90:842–848, 1986.

22. Scheuer PJ: Liver Biopsy Interpretation, ed 3. London, Bailliere Tindall, 1980, pp 36–59.

23. Kenny RP, Czaja AJ, Ludwig J, Dickson ER: Chronic active hepatitis (CAH) with presence of antimitochondrial antibodies (AMA): a hybrid syndrome? *Gastroenterology* 84:1205, 1983 (abstr).

24. Paronetto F, Schaffner F, Popper H: Immunocytochemical and serologic observations in primary biliary cirrhosis. *N Engl J Med* 271:1123–1128, 1964.

25. Lindgren S, McKay J, Hansson I, Eriksson S: Evidence of increased intestinal synthesis and extracellular deposition of IgM in primary biliary cirrhosis. An immunofluorescence study of liver and small-intestinal biopsy specimens. *Scand J Gastroenterol* 19:97–104, 1984.

26. Ballardini G, Mirakian R, Bianchi FB, Pisi E, Doniach D, Bottazzo GF: Aberrant expression of HLA-DR antigens on bile duct epithelium in primary biliary cirrhosis: relevance to pathogenesis. *Lancet* 2:1009–1103, 1984.

27. Eggink HF, Houthoff HJ, Huitema S, Gips CH, Poppema S: Cellular and humoral immune reactions in chronic active liver disease. I. Lymphocyte subsets in liver biopsies of patients with untreated idiopathic autoimmune hepatitis, chronic active hepatitis B and primary biliary cirrhosis. *Clin Exp Immunol* 50:17–24, 1982.

28. Husby G, Blomhoff JP, Elgjo K, Williams RC Jr: Immunohistochemical characterization of hepatic tissue lymphocyte subpopulations in liver disease. *Scand J Gastroenterol* 17:855–860, 1982.

29. Pape GR, Rieber EP, Eisenburg J, Hoffmann R, Balch CM, Paumgartner G, Riethmüller G: Involvement of the cytotoxic/suppressor T-cell subset in liver tissue injury of patients with acute and chronic liver diseases. *Gastroenterology* 85:657–662, 1983.

30. Si L, Whiteside TL, Schade RR, Starzl TE, Van Thiel DH: T-lymphocyte subsets in liver tissues of patients with primary biliary cirrhosis (PBC), patients with primary sclerosing cholangitis (PSC) and normal controls. *J Clin Immunol* 4:262–272, 1984.

31. Fakunle YM, Aranguibel F, DeVilliers D, Thomas HC, Sherlock S: Monomeric IgM in chronic liver disease. *Clin Exp Immunol* 38:204–210, 1969.

32. Homburger HA, Casey M, Jacob GL, Klee GG: Measurement of secretory IgA in serum

by radioimmunoassay in patients with chronic nonalcoholic liver disease or carcinoma. *Am J Clin Pathol* 81:569–574, 1984.

33. James SP, Jones EA, Schafer DF, Hoofnagle JH, Varma RR, Strober W: Selective IgA deficiency associated with primary biliary cirrhosis in a family with liver disease. *Gastroenterology* 90:283–228, 1986.

34. Roux MEB, Florin-Christensen A, Arana RM, Doniach D: Paraproteins with antibody activity in acute viral hepatitis and chronic autoimmune liver diseases. *Gut* 15:396–400, 1974.

35. Fox RA, Dudley FJ, Sherlock S: The primary immune response to haemocyanin in patients with primary biliary cirrhosis. *Clin Exp Immunol* 14:473, 1973.

36. Fox RA, James DG, Scheuer PJ, Sharma O, Sherlock S: Impaired delayed hypersensitivity in primary biliary cirrhosis. *Lancet* 1:959–962, 1969.

37. Thomas HC, Holden R, Verrier Jones J, Peacock DB: Immune response to ƒX174 in man. 5. Primary and secondary antibody production in primary biliary cirrhosis. *Gut* 17:844, 1976.

38. Watmough D, French MA, Triger DR: Antibody responses to tetanus toxoid in patients with primary biliary cirrhosis. *J Clin Pathol* 70:683–686, 1987.

39. Walker JG, Doniach D, Roitt IM, Sherlock S: Serological tests in the diagnosis of primary biliary cirrhosis. *Lancet* 1:827–831, 1965.

40. Berg PA, Klein R: Immunology of primary biliary cirrhosis. *Baillieres Clin Gastroenterol* 1:675–706, 1987.

41. Mouritsen S, Demant E, Permin H, Wiik A: High prevalence of antimitochondrial antibodies among patients with some well-defined connective tissue diseases. *Clin Exp Immunol* 66:68–76, 1986.

42. Gershwin ME, Mackay IR, Sturgess A, Coppel RL: Identification and specificity of a cDNA encoding the 70 kd mitochondrial antigen recognized in primary biliary cirrhosis. *J Immunol* 138:3525–3531, 1987.

43. Yeaman SJ, Fussey SP, Danner DJ, James OF, Mutimer DJ, Bassendine MF: Primary biliary cirrhosis: identification of two major M2 mitochondrial autoantigens. *Lancet* 1:1067–1070, 1988.

44. Surh CD, Cooper AE, Coppel RL, Leung P, Ahmed A, Dickson R, Gershwin ME: The predominance of IgG3 and IgM isotype antimitochondrial autoantibodies against recombinant fused mitochondrial polypeptide in patients with primary biliary cirrhosis. *Hepatology* 8:290–295, 1988.

45. Wiedmann KH, Melms A, Berg PA: Anti-actin antibodies of IgM and IgG class in chronic liver diseases detected by fluorometric immunoassay. *Liver* 3:369–376, 1983.

46. Kurki P, Miettinin A, Salaspuro M, Virtanen I, Stenman S: Cytoskeleton antibodies in chronic active hepatitis, primary biliary cirrhosis, and alcoholic liver disease. *Hepatology* 3:297–302, 1983.

47. MacSween RNM, Armstrong EM, Gray KG, Mason M: Bile canalicular antibody in primary biliary cirrhosis and in other liver diseases. *Lancet* 1:1419, 1973.

48. Kurki P, Miettinin A, Linder E, Pikkarainen P, Yuoristo M, Salaspuro MP: Different types of smooth muscle antibody in chronic active hepatitis and primary biliary cirrhosis: their diagnostic and prognostic significance. *Gut* 21:878–884, 1980.

49. Tsantoulas D, Perperas A, Portman B, Eddleston ALWF, Williams R: Antibodies to a human liver membrane lipoprotein (LSP) in primary biliary cirrhosis. *Gut* 21:557–560, 1980.

50. Wiedmann KH, Bartholomew T, Brown D, Thomas HC: Liver membrane antibodies detected by immunoradiometric assay in acute and chronic virus-induced and autoimmune liver disease. *Hepatology* 4:199–204, 1984.

51. Kurki P, Gripenberg M, Teppo AM, Salaspuro M: Profiles of antinuclear antibodies in chronic active hepatitis, primary biliary cirrhosis and alcoholic liver disease. *Liver* 4:134–138, 1984.

52. Bernstein RM, Neuberger JM, Bunn CC, Callender ME, Hughes GR, Williams R: Diversity of autoantibodies in primary biliary cirrhosis and chronic active hepatitis. *Clin Exp Immunol* 55:553–560, 1984.

53. Whittingham S, Mackay IR, Tait BD: Autoantibodies to small nuclear ribonucleoproteins. A strong association between anti-SS-B (La), HLA-B8, and Sjögren's syndrome. *Aust NZ J Med* 13:565–570, 1983.

54. MacSween RNM, Berg PA: Autoimmune diseases of the liver. In Ferguson A, MacSween RNM: Imunological Aspects of the Liver and Gastrointestinal Tract. Baltimore, University Park Press, 1976, pp 345–386.

55. Schussler GC, Schaffner F: Increased serum thyroid hormone binding and decreased free hormone in chronic active liver disease. *N Engl J Med* 299:510–515, 1978.

56. Jain S, Markham R, Thomas HC, Sherlock S: Double-stranded DNA-binding capacity of serum in acute and chronic liver disease. *Clin Exp Immunol* 26:35–41, 1976.

57. Gerber MA, Shapiro JM, Smith H, Lebwohl O, Schaffner F: Antibodies to ribosomes in chronic active hepatitis. *Gastroenterology* 76:139–143, 1979.

58. Penner E, Muller S, Zimmermann D, Van Regenmortel MH: High prevalence of antibodies to histones among patients with primary biliary cirrhosis. *Clin Exp Immunol* 70:47–52, 1987.

59. Dienstag JL, Savarese AM, Cohen RB, Bhan AK: Circulating immune complexes in primary biliary cirrhosis: interactions with lymphoid cells. *Clin Exp Immunol* 50:7–16, 1982.

60. Gupta RC, Dickson ER, McDuffie FC, Bagenstoss AH: Immune complexes in primary biliary cirrhosis. Higher prevalence of circulating immune complexes in patients with associated autoimmune features. *Am J Med* 73:192–198, 1982.

61. Epstein O, DeVilliers D, Jain S, Potter BJ, Thomas HC, Sherlock S: Reduction of immune complexes and immunoglobulins induced by D-penicillamine in primary biliary cirrhosis. *N Engl J Med* 300:274–278, 1979.

62. Wands JR, Dienstag JL, Bhan AK, Feller ER, Isselbacher KS: Circulating immune complexes and complement activation in primary biliary cirrhosis. *N Engl J Med* 298:223–237, 1978.

63. Amoroso P, Vergani D, Wojcicka BM, McFarlane IG, Eddleston AL, Tee DE, Williams R: Identification of biliary antigens in circulating immune complexes in primary biliary cirrhosis. *Clin Exp Immunol* 42:95–98, 1980.

64. Penner EH, Goldenberg H, Albini B, Weiser MM, Milgram F: Immune complexes in primary biliary cirrhosis contain mitochondrial antigens. *Clin Immunol Immunopathol* 22:394–399, 1982.

65. Jaffe CJ, Vierling JM, Jones Ea, Lawley TJ, Frank MM: Receptor specific clearance by the reticuloendothelial system in chronic liver diseases: demonstration of defective C3b-specific clearance in primary biliary cirrhosis. *J Clin Invest* 62:1069–1077, 1978.

66. Lööf L, Hakansson L, Nyberg A, Venge P: Defective C3b receptor-mediate phagocytosis of neutrophils in patients with primary biliary cirrhosis. *Scand J Gastroenterol* 22:1169–1174, 1987.

67. Goldberg MJ, Kaplan MM, Mitamura T, Anderson CL, Matloff DS, Pinn VW, Agnello V: Evidence against an immune complex pathogenesis of primary biliary cirrhosis. *Gastroenterology* 83:677–683, 1982.

68. Lindgren S, Eriksson S: IgM in primary biliary cirrhosis. Physiochemical and complement activating properties. *J Lab Clin Med* 99:636–645, 1982.

69. Potter BJ, Elias E, Jones EA: Hypercatabolism of the third component of complement in patients with primary biliary cirrhosis. *J Lab Clin Med* 88:427--439, 1976.

70. Potter BJ, Elias E, Thomas HC, Sherlock S: Complement metabolism in chronic liver disease: catabolism of C1q in chronic active liver disease and primary biliary cirrhosis. *Gastroenterology* 78:1034–1040, 1980.

71. Lindgren S, Laurell AB, Eriksson S: Complement components and activation in primary biliary cirrhosis. *Hepatology* 4:9–14, 1984.

72. Thomas HC, Freni M, Sanchez-Tapias J, De Villiers D, Jain S, Sherlock S: Peripheral blood lymphocyte populations in chronic liver disease. *Clin Exp Immunol* 26:222–227, 1976.

73. Bhan AK, Dienstag JL, Wands JR, Schlossman SF, Reinherz EL: Alterations of T-cell subsets in primary biliary cirrhosis. *Clin Exp Immunol* 47:351–358, 1982.

74. Miller KB, Elta GH, Rudders RA, Kaplan MM: Lymphocyte subsets in primary biliary cirrhosis. *Ann Intern Med* 100:385–387, 1984.

75. Thomas HC, Brown D, Labrooy J, Epstein O: T cell subsets in autoimmune and HBV-induced chronic liver disease, HBs antigen carriers with normal histology and primary biliary cirrhosis: a review of the abnormalities and the effects of treatment. *J Clin Immunol* 2:57s–60s, 1982.

76. Sandilands GP, MacSween RNM, Gray KG, Holden RJ, Mills R, Reid FM, Thomas MA, Watkinson G: Reduction in peripheral blood K cells and activated T cells in primary biliary cirrhosis. *Gut* 18:1017–1020, 1977.

77. James SP, Jones EA: Abnormal natural killer cytotoxicity in primary biliary cirrhosis; evidence for a functional deficiency of cytolytic effector cells. *Gastroenterology* 89:165–171, 1985.

78. James SP, Jones EA, Hoofnagle JH, Strober W: Circulating activated B cells in primary biliary cirrhosis. *J Clin Immunol* 5:254–260, 1985.

79. Fox RA, Dudley FJ, Samuels M, Milligan J, Sherlock S: Lymphocyte transformation in response to phytohaemaglutinin in primary biliary cirrhosis: the search for a plasma inhibitory factor. *Gut* 14:89–93, 1973.

80. Miller J, Smith MGM, Mitchell CG, Reed WD, Eddleston ALWF, Williams R: Cell-mediated immunity to a human liver-specific antigen in patients with active chronic hepatitis and primary biliary cirrhosis. *Lancet* 2:296–297, 1972.

81. McFarlane IG, Wojcicka BM, Tsantoulas DC, Portmann BC, Eddleston ALWF, Williams R: Leukocyte migration inhibition in response to biliary antigens in primary biliary cirrhosis, sclerosing cholangitis, and other liver diseases. *Gastroenterology* 76:1333–1340, 1979.

82. Wick MR, Moore SB, Gastineau DA, Hoagland HC: Immunologic, clinical and pathologic aspects of human graft-versus-host disease. *Mayo Clin Proc* 48:603–612, 1983.

83. Vierling JM, Fennell RH. Histopathology of early and late human hepatic allograft rejection: evidence of progressive destruction of interlobular bile ducts. *Hepatology* 5:1076–1082, 1985.

84. Thompson AD, Cochrane AMG, McFarlane IG, Eddleston ALWF, Williams R: Lymphocyte cytotoxicity to isolated hepatocytes in chronic active hepatitis. *Nature* 252:721–722, 1974.

85. Votgen AJM, Hadzic N, Shorter RG, Summerskill WHJ, Taylor WF: Cell mediated cytotoxicity in chronic active liver disease: a new test system. *Gastroenterology* 74:883–889, 1978.

86. Dienstag JL, Bhan AK: Enhanced in vitro cell-mediated cytotoxicity in chronic hepatitis B virus infection: absence of specificity for virus-expressed antigen on target cell membranes. *J Immunol* 125:2269–2276, 1980.

87. Vierling JM, Nelson DL, Strober W, Bundy BM, Jones EA: In vitro cell-mediated cytotoxicity in primary biliary cirrhosis and chronic hepatitis: dysfunction of spontaneous cell-mediated cytotoxicity in primary biliary cirrhosis. *J Clin Invest* 60:1116–1128, 1977.

88. Geubel AP, Keller RH, Summerskill WHJ, Dickson ER, Tomasi TB, Shorter RG: Lymphocyte cytotoxicity and inhibition studied with autologous liver cells: observations in chronic active liver disease and the primary biliary cirrhosis syndrome. *Gastroenterology* 71:450–456, 1976.

89. James SP, Elson CO, Jones EA, Strober W: Abnormal regulation of immunoglobulin synthesis in vitro in primary biliary cirrhosis. *Gastroenterology* 79:242–254, 1980.

90. Alexander GJM, Nouri-Aria KT, Eddleston ALWF, Williams R: Contrasting relations between suppressor-cell function and suppressor-cell number in chronic liver disease. *Lancet* 1:1291–1293, 1983.

91. James SP, Elson CO, Waggoner JG, Jones EA, Strober W: Deficiency of the autologous mixed lymphocyte reaction in primary biliary cirrhosis. *J Clin Invest* 66:1305–1310, 1980.

92. Lee RG, Epstein O, Jauregui H, Sherlock S, Scheuer PJ: Granulomas in primary biliary cirrhosis: a prognostic factor. *Gastroenterology* 81:983–986, 1981.

93. Christensen E, Neuberger J, Crowe J, Altman DG, Popper H, Portmann B, Doniach D, Ranek L, Tygstrup N, Williams R: Beneficial effect of azathioprine and prediction of prognosis in primary biliary cirrhosis. *Gastroenterology* 89:1084–1091, 1985.

94. Dickson ER, Fleming TR, Wiesner RH, Baldus WP, Fleming CR, Ludwig J, McCall JT: Trial of D-penicillamine in advanced primary biliary cirrhosis. *N Engl J Med* 312:1011–1015, 1985.

95. Matloff DS, Alpert E, Resnick RH, Kaplan MM: A prospective trial of D-penicillamine in primary biliary cirrhosis. *N Engl J Med* 306:319–326, 1982.

96. Hoofnagle JH, Davis GL, Schafer DF, Peters MG, Avigan MI, Hanson RG, Pappas SC, Minuk GY, Dusheiko GM, Jones EA, MacSween RNM: Randomized trial of chlorambucil for primary biliary cirrhosis. *Hepatology* 4:1062, 1984 (abstr).

97. Routhier G, Epstein O, Janossy G, Thomas HC, Sherlock S, Kung PC, Goldstein G: Effects of cyclosporin A on suppressor and inducer T lymphocytes in primary biliary cirrhosis. *Lancet* 2:1223–1226, 1980.

98. Hishon S, Tobin G, Ciclitira PJ: A clinical trial of levamisole in primary biliary cirrhosis. *Postgrad Med J* 58:701–703, 1982.

99. Kaplan MM, Alling DW, Wolfe HJ, Zimmerman HJ, et al: A prospective trial of colchicine for primary biliary cirrhosis. *N Engl J Med* 315:1448–1454, 1986.

100. Maddrey WC, Van Thiel DH: Liver transplantation: an overview. *Hepatology* 8:948–959, 1988.

101. Neuberger J, Portmann B, Macdougall BRD, Calne RY, Williams R: Recurrence of primary biliary cirrhosis after liver transplantation. *N Engl J Med* 306:1–6, 1982.

102. Demetris AJ, Markus BH, Esquivel C, Van Thiel DH, Saidman S, Gordon R, Makowka L, Sysyn GD, Starzl TE: Pathologic study of liver transplantation for primary biliary cirrhosis. *Hepatology* 8:939–947, 1988.

103. Dickson ER, LaRusso NF, Wiesner RH: Primary sclerosing cholangitis. *Hepatology* 4:33s–35s, 1984.

104. LaRusso NF, Wiesner RH, Ludgwig J, MacCarty RL: Primary sclerosing cholangitis. *N Engl J Med* 310:899–903, 1984.

105. Akwari OE, Van Heerden JA, Adson MA, Foulk WT, Baggenstoss AH: Bile duct carcinoma associated with ulcerative colitis. *Rev Surg* 33:289–296, 1976.

106. Wee A, Ludwig J, Coffey RJ, LaRusso NF, Wiesner RH: Hepatobiliary carcinoma associated with primary sclerosing cholangitis and chronic ulcerative colitis. *Hum Pathol* 16:719–726, 1985.

107. Sisto A, Feldman P, Garel L, Seidman E, Brochu P, Morin CL, Weber AM, Roy CC: Primary sclerosing cholangitis in children: study of five cases and review of the literature. *Pediatrics* 80:918–923, 1987.

108. Wiesner RH, LaRusso NF, Ludwig J, Dickson ER: Comparison of the clinicopathologic features of primary sclerosing cholangitis and primary biliary cirrhosis. *Gastroenterology* 8:108–114, 1985.

109. Chapman RWG, Marburgh BA, Rhodes RM, Summerfield JA, Dick R, Scheuer PJ, Sherlock S: Primary sclerosing cholangitis: a review of its clinical features, cholangiography, and hepatic histology. *Gut* 21:870–877, 1980.

110. Chapman RW, Varghese Z, Gaul R, Patel G, Kokinon N, Sherlock S: Association of primary sclerosing cholangitis with HLA B8. *Gut* 24:38–41, 1983.

111. Quigley EMM, LaRusso NF, Ludwig J, RNM MacSween, Birnie GG, Watkiinson G: Familial occurrence of primary sclerosing cholangitis and ulcerative colitis. *Gastroenterology* 85:1160–1165, 1983.

112. Chapman RW, Cottone M, Selby WS, Shepherd HA, Sherlock S, Jewell DP: Serum autoantibodies, ulcerative colitis and primary sclerosing cholangitis. *Gut* 1:86–91, 1986.

113. Comings DE, Skub KB, Van Eyes J, Motulsky AG: Familial multifocal fibrosis, mediastinal fibrosis, sclerosing cholangitis, Riedel's thyroiditis, and pseudotumor of the orbit may be different manifestations of a single disease. *Ann Intern Med* 66:884–892, 1967.

114. Hellstrom HR, Perezstable EL: Retroperitoneal fibrosis with disseminated vasculitis and extrahepatic sclerosing cholangitis. *Am J Med* 40:184–187, 1966.

115. Wenger J, Gingrich GW, Mendeloff J: Sclerosing cholangitis — a manifestation of systemic disease. *Arch Intern Med* 116:590–514, 1965.

116. Bodenheimer HC, LaRusso NF, Thayer WR, Charland C, Staples P: Elevated circulating immune complexes in primary sclerosing cholangitis. *Hepatology* 3:150–154, 1981.

117. Lindor KD, Wiesner RH, LaRusso NF, Homburger HA: Enhanced autoreactivity of T-lymphocytes in primary sclerosing cholangitis. *Hepatology* 7:884–888, 1987.

118. Whiteside TL, Lasky S, Lusheng S, Van Thiel DH: Immunologic analysis of mononuclear cells in liver tissues and blood of patients with primary sclerosing cholangitis. *Hepatology* 5:468–474, 1985.

119. Lindor KD, Wiesner RH, LaRusso NF: Recent advances in the management of primary sclerosing cholangitis. *Semin Liver Dis* 7:322–327, 1987.

120. Lillemoe KD, Pitt HA, Cameron JL: Sclerosing cholangitis. *Adv Surg* 21:65–92, 1987.

CHAPTER **13**

Immunopathogenesis of Viral Hepatitis

VINCENT G. BAIN

GRAEME J. M. ALEXANDER

ADRIAN L. W. F. EDDLESTON

INTRODUCTION

Viral hepatitis is an important cause of acute morbidity and mortality as well as chronic illness, including cirrhosis, portal hypertension, and liver cancer. The term viral hepatitis encompasses liver infections caused by a number of different viruses; some (i.e., hepatitis A and B viruses) have been identified and characterized in detail, while others (the non-A, non-B viruses) have remained elusive.

Over the last two decades, scientists in many disciplines have intensively investigated viral hepatitis and the causative viruses. The virologist, immunologist, molecular biologist, pathologist, epidemiologist, and clinician have all played important roles. The study of non-A, non-B viral hepatitis, however, has been severely hampered by an inability to identify the virus or a specific antibody response; preliminary reports suggest that these initial obstacles may have been overcome.

This chapter reviews the progress made over the past two decades with emphasis on the commonest forms of viral hepatitis. The extensive coverage of hepatitis B virus reflects the particular interest of the scientific community in this widespread infection.

HEPATITIS A VIRUS

The clinical illness caused by hepatitis A virus (HAV) has long been known as short-incubation or infectious hepatitis, characterized by an incubation period of less than 40 days, transmission by the fecal-oral route, and failure to provide protective immunity against long-incubation hepatitis/serum hepatitis (HBV).[1] A

255

major breakthrough occurred in 1973 when Feinstone and coworkers detected HAV particles in human stool using electron microscopy.[2] As a result of their discovery, large quantities of stool-derived, purified HAV antigen became available, enabling the development of diagnostic tests for HAV antibody. Following frustrated attempts by many workers, Provost and Hilleman eventually established HAV in cell culture in 1979; since then HAV has been propagated in many different cell lines of human and monkey origin.[3]

In children, HAV causes an anicteric illness with diarrhea, nausea, and malaise as the predominant symptoms;[4] in adults, a more severe illness develops, with malaise, anorexia, jaundice, and, rarely, a fulminant course.[5] Chronic infection has not been well documented; if it exists, it must be rare.[6-8] Nevertheless, HAV is an important cause of morbidity particularly in developed countries, where progressively fewer adults have immunity due to declining childhood infection.[9]

Virology

HAV is a member of the picornavirus family and shares many features with the enteroviruses (Table 13-1). Its physical structure consists of a 27-nm, spherical, nonenveloped particle with icosahedral symmetry. Its genome, which was recently sequenced, consists of single-stranded RNA containing approximately 7,480 bases.[10,11] The genomic RNA has two purposes: it serves as a template for RNA replication, utilizing a viral RNA-dependent polymerase, and it encodes the various HAV proteins. In a strategy common to the picornavirus family, the RNA is translated into a large polypeptide subsequently cleaved into smaller functional peptides.

HAV replication remains incompletely understood but is believed to occur exclusively in the liver. After translation of viral proteins, viral particles are assembled in the hepatocyte cytoplasm, where they may be observed by electron microscopy within membrane-bound vesicles.[12] Following viral release by an unknown mechanism, residual membrane fragments are probably removed by the detergent action of bile acids in bile. Continued study of HAV-infected cell lines holds prom-

Table 13-1 CHARACTERISTICS OF HAV

Part	Characteristic
Virion	Spherical, nonenveloped
	27 nm
	Bouyant density, 1.34 gm/ml
Capsid	Cubic symmetry
	Four-capsid polypeptides (VP1-4)
Genome	Single-stranded RNA
	~7,480 bases
	(+) polarity
	3' polyadenylate tail
Viral proteins	VP1-4
	5' terminal protein (VPg)
	RNA-dependent polymerase
	Protease

ise for bettering our understanding of cellular uptake of virus, intracellular replication, and cellular release.

Following infection with HAV, an incubation period of 3–4 weeks precedes clinical illness, during which HAV is transported from the gastrointestinal tract to the liver by an as yet unknown mechanism. HAV replication in hepatocytes, followed by biliary excretion, leads to fecal shedding of infective virions for 1–2 weeks preceding the onset of jaundice (Fig. 13–1).

Approximately 4 weeks postinfection, serum transaminases peak, indicating hepatocellular necrosis, and a brief period of viremia occurs as the bilirubin begins to rise. By the time symptoms occur, specific IgM antibody is present in serum, providing a diagnostically useful indicator of acute HAV infection. Although the IgM levels peak and then fall off rapidly, sensitive antibody-capture assays continue to detect the antibody for 6 months.[13] High serum levels of total IgM are also seen in HAV infection; only a small fraction of the antibody, however, is virus-specific.[14,15] The IgG response immediately following the IgM response may last for many decades and is therefore useful in epidemiologic studies of prior HAV infection. As fecal viral shedding wanes, coproantibodies against HAV of the IgA class become detectable and persist for approximately 4 months;[16] presumably these function to shorten the duration of stool infectivity, and/or to provide local immunity against reinfection.

Immunopathology

The precise mechanism by which HAV induces hepatocellular necrosis is unknown. In general, a virus may damage the liver directly, inducing a cytopathic effect, or damage may be due to an immune-mediated attack against infected liver cells displaying viral antigens on the surface. Immune-mediated damage may occur by several mechanisms, including antibody-dependent cell-mediated cytotoxicity,

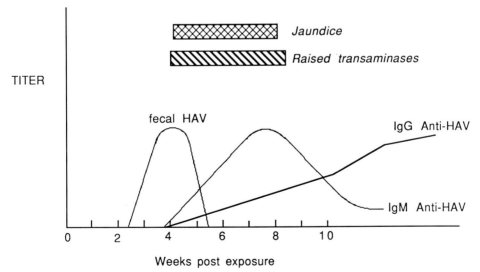

Figure 13–1 Typical clinical and serologic features of hepatitis A infection.

complement-dependent antibody-mediated lysis, and cytotoxicity secondary to natural killer (NK) cells or cytotoxic T lymphocytes.

Viruses with the capacity to interfere with vital cellular functions will produce a cytopathic effect usually defined by cellular changes observed in tissue culture; these include syncytium (giant cell) formation, abnormal cellular adhesion, inclusion body formation, or simply cell necrosis and lysis, the latter being most characteristic of enteroviruses. Indirect evidence that HAV exerts a cytopathic effect upon liver cells has been summarized by Friedman and Dienstag:[17]

1. HAV is classified among the enteroviruses, most of which have well-documented cytopathic effects.[18]

2. In some cell lines and animal models, HAV inoculation may be followed by evidence of liver cell injury within 1 week, a situation compatible with direct virally induced damage,[19,20] although this rapid effect was only observed with multiply passaged viral strains.

3. Lack of a healthy carrier state is consistent with a viral infection that has significant cytopathic potential.

Evidence has accumulated however, to suggest that HAV induces liver damage by mechanisms other than a direct cytopathic effect. The best evidence became available following the successful propagation of HAV in tissue culture in which HAV-infected cells from several lines failed to exhibit any cytopathic effects.[21-23] Unlike other picornaviruses, HAV does not significantly interfere with protein synthesis in the host cell; consequently the cells remain viable, and a persistent infection is established in tissue culture.[22,23] Other studies using human volunteers or primate models have established that fecal shedding of virus may precede the elevation of serum transaminases.[5] This finding suggests that HAV replication in hepatocytes, followed by virus release into biliary canaliculi, may occur in the absence of overt hepatic injury.

In the absence of a direct cytopathic effect by HAV, it is probable that the host immune response plays the pivotal role in the induction of hepatocellular necrosis. The humoral response produces antibodies with virus-neutralizing capability;[20,24-26] the effective use of immune serum globulin to prevent or blunt potential HAV infection further attests to this fact.[27] Temporally, biochemical and histologic evidence of hepatocellular damage follows the appearance of the anti-HAV response in serum.[5] These antibodies may recognize viral antigens on the hepatocyte membrane and participate in antibody-dependent cell-mediated cytotoxicity (ADCC) or complement-dependent cell lysis. The latter possibility was recently investigated using acute and convalescent anti-HAV sera and HAV-infected fibroblasts in an in vitro ^{51}Cr release cytotoxicity assay;[28] no complement-dependent antibody-mediated cytotoxicity against HAV-infected cells was found in this system.

The appearance of specific antibody may be unrelated to hepatocellular damage but may simply serve as a marker of a concurrent cellular immune response. This hypothesis is supported by a case report of HAV-induced hepatitis that preceded the anti-HAV response in a patient with drug-induced immunosuppression,[29] suggesting that the humoral response was not responsible for the hepatocellular necrosis.

The effective lysis of virally infected cells by cytotoxic T lymphocytes requires recognition of foreign viral antigens in association with HLA self-antigens (Fig. 13–2).[30] Vallbracht and colleagues recently tested cell-mediated cytotoxicity to HAV in a microtoxicity assay employing peripheral blood lymphocytes from HAV-infected patients or nonimmune controls and autologous skin fibroblasts supporting persistent HAV infection after in vitro inoculation with virus.[31] Significant cytotoxicity was demonstrated in all seven patients with acute HAV infection but in neither of the two control subjects. Cytolytic activity was maximal in T-cell-enriched lymphocyte fractions. Limited observations in experiments with HLA mismatched lymphocytes and target cells showed diminished cytotoxicity, suggesting that a maximal cytotoxic response to HAV-infected cells is HLA-restricted.

Virally infected cells may also be lysed by non-HLA-restricted cytotoxic lymphocytes of the NK class. Mononuclear cells from healthy subjects lacking antibody to HAV showed a greater cytotoxic response to a HAV-infected continuous simian kidney cell line (BS-C-1 cells) than to uninfected cells.[32] Characterization of the effector cells revealed a Leu11$^+$, M1$^+$, T3$^-$, T4$^-$ phenotype that is widely accepted to contain cells exhibiting NK activity. The mononuclear cells exposed to BS-C-1 cells harboring virus produced high titers of α-interferon,[32] which is known to enhance NK cell activity.[33] Interferon activity is also detectable in the serum of patients with HAV infection,[34] suggesting that NK cell activity, augmented by endogenous interferon production, contributes to the immune-mediated hepatocellular necrosis in HAV infection.

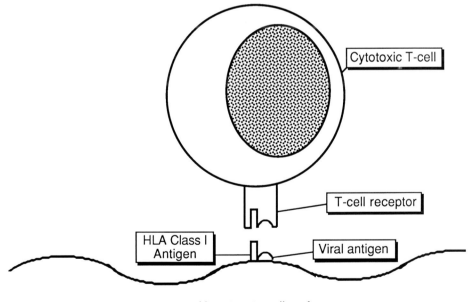

Hepatocyte cell surface

Figure 13–2 T-cell recognition. The T-cell receptor recognizes viral antigens displayed on the surface of the hepatocyte in association with HLA class I antigens. Receptor binding activates the T cell, enabling it to lyse the virus-infected cell.

HEPATITIS B VIRUS

Hepatitis B virus is an important cause of human infection, with over 200 million carriers worldwide. These carriers are at risk for the development of cirrhosis, portal hypertension, and hepatocellular carcinoma.[35,36] Furthermore, these carriers are the reservoir for the continued spread of HBV infection, and despite the availability of an effective and safe vaccine, HBV-related morbidity and mortality will continue for many years after its universal application.

Virology

HBV is among the hepadnaviruses, which display striking hepatotropism and share a tendency to cause persistent infections, resulting in chronic hepatitis and risk of hepatocellular carcinoma.[37] Hepadnaviruses produce a marked excess of their surface coat protein, which is detectable in the serum of the host as surface antigen (specific to HBV.) They possess a small, incompletely double-stranded circular DNA genome that replicates in a unique fashion by reverse transcription of an RNA template.[38]

Four different hepadnaviruses have now been identified and characterized (Table 13–2). Similar viruses affect the tree squirrel, heron, and snake, but these latter hepadnaviruses have been less well studied. Further study of these animal models could provide important clues to the immunopathogenesis of HBV-induced liver disease in man; however, these studies have been hampered by high costs and limited knowledge of the immune systems of these animals.

HBV is a 42-nm spherical particle[39] consisting of a core particle enveloped by a surface coat that contains the surface antigen (HBsAg.)[40] Treatment of the virion with detergent releases the 27-nm core particle containing the small DNA genome (3.1 kb) and DNA polymerase[41] enclosed by the core protein or core antigen (HBcAg). The complete virion (Dane particle) circulates in the blood; much more frequently found, however, are 22-nm spherical and tubular particles containing excess HBsAg. Failure to clear HBsAg from the blood after acute infection is the hallmark of chronic HBV infection. The e antigen (HBeAg), found in the serum of some patients, is a cleavage product of HBcAg and indicates ongoing viral replication.

The HBV genome has been well characterized and consists of four overlapping open reading frames designated S/pre-S, C, P, and X. Each is flanked by start and stop codons and encodes a viral polypeptide (Table 13–3).

Table 13–2 THE HEPADNAVIRUSES[a]

	HBV	WHV	GSHV	DHV
Host	Human, chimpanzee	Eastern woodchuck	Beechey ground squirrel	Peking duck
Carrier state	Yes	Yes	Yes	Yes
Hepatitis	Acute and chronic	Acute and chronic	—	Mild
HCC	Yes	Yes	Yes	Yes

[a] Abbreviations: HBV, hepatitis B virus; WHV, woodchuck hepatitis virus; GSHV, ground squirrel hepatitis virus; DHV, duck hepatitis virus; HCC, hepatocellular carcinoma.

Table 13–3   HBV POLYPEPTIDES

HBV Gene	Polypeptide
S	HBsAg (major protein)
pre-S_2 + S	pre-S_2peptide (middle protein)
pre-S_1 + pre-S_2 + S	pre-S_1 peptide (large protein)
C	HBcAg and HBeAg
P	DNA polymerase
X	X protein (?)

The S/pre-S region of the genome codes for the proteins of the viral envelope. The S gene codes for the major protein, which is related to HBsAg. The pre-S region, together with the S gene, encodes two additional translational products, pre-S_2 (middle protein) and pre-S_1 (large protein), the significance of which is discussed in the next section. Both HBcAg and HBeAg are encoded by the C gene, which includes a pre-C region. When pre-C is transcribed, the core protein is targeted to the endoplasmic reticulum, where it is subsequently cleaved and HBeAg is secreted from the cell.[42] The products of the X gene are just beginning to be studied.

Acute infection with HBV is associated with characteristic biochemical and serologic changes (Fig. 13–3). The first viral antigen to appear is HBsAg, at 1 month postinfection. The HBeAg becomes detectable but is rapidly cleared from the serum; indeed, persistence beyond 11 weeks postinfection (when exposure is identifiable) is an early indicator of risk of chronicity.[43] Typical symptoms of malaise, anorexia, right upper quadrant discomfort, dark urine, and eventually jaundice appear at approximately 2–3 months, although the incubation period may be highly variable. Clearance of the virus is signified by disappearance of HBsAg,

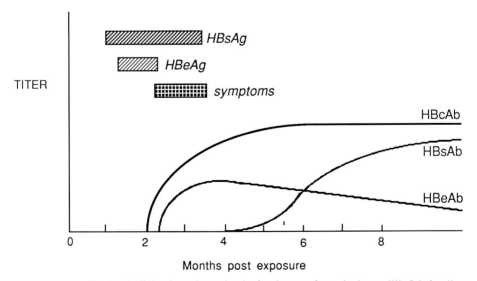

Figure 13–3   Typical clinical and serologic features of acute hepatitis B infection.

followed by the appearance of antibody to HBsAg (HBsAb), which is associated with long-term immunity to the virus and hence is the basis for immunization with HBsAg. Antibody to HBcAg (IgM-HBcAb) is the first antibody to appear, however, and may be the only serologic evidence of infection during the "window" period, when neither HBsAg nor HBsAb is present.

Individuals failing to clear HBsAg by 6 months are considered by definition to be chronically infected; most chronic carriers, however, have no history of preceding acute hepatitis,[44] suggesting an anicteric acute phase or infection at birth. The corollary also appears to be true; the vast majority of patients with acute HBV will not become chronic carriers.[45,46] Those with no evidence of inflammation have been considered as "healthy" carriers, although their disease may become active in the future.[47] Others have chronic hepatitis, which is designated chronic persistent hepatitis (CPH) if characterized by a predominantly mononuclear inflammatory infiltrate in the portal tract, as chronic active hepatitis (CAH) if associated with inflammation breaching the limiting plate of hepatocytes around the portal tract (piecemeal necrosis), or as chronic lobular hepatitis (CLH) if inflammation involves mainly the hepatic lobule. CAH is the most destructive lesion; however, CPH and CLH may progress to CAH and eventually cirrhosis.[48]

With chronicity, HBV-DNA may become integrated into the host genome.[49] Incorporation of the S gene accounts for the persistence of HBsAg in the blood of chronic carriers who are free of any markers of viral replication. More importantly, integrated HBV-DNA has been implicated in the genesis of hepatocellular carcinoma in chronic HBV carriers.[50]

Immunopathology

Although new information is accumulating from many disciplines, the precise mechanism whereby HBV selectively enters the hepatocyte and eventually causes cell death is unknown. There is indirect evidence to suggest that the immune response to viral components rather than a direct viral cytopathic effect is responsible for liver damage. Furthermore, the modulatory effects of the immune system have been implicated in the genesis of the chronic carrier state.

Mechanism of Hepatotropism

HBV-DNA has been detected in cells outside the liver, including monocytes and pancreatic cells; however, its hepatotropism is striking. Insight into the mechanism of hepatotropism occurred when a number of investigators using different techniques observed that serum from HBV-infected individuals had the capacity to bind polyalbumin, and furthermore, binding capacity appeared to correlate with infectivity.[43,51,52] Thus chronic HBV carriers with HBeAg positivity exhibited a greater propensity to bind polyalbumin. Electron microscopic studies demonstrated aggregation of Dane particles and HBsAg by polyalbumin compatible with the existence of receptors on the surface coat of the virus.[52] More recent studies have localized the putative receptor to the pre-S_2 region of the peptide.[53,54]

An attractive hypothesis, therefore, is that circulating HBV virions bind polyalbumin to their surface coat. Polyalbumin then serves as a linker molecule between HBV and hepatocyte albumin receptors.[55-57] HBV then gains access to the cell by endocytosis or by fusion with the hepatocyte membrane, with release of the core particle into the cytoplasm. Further support comes from studies in chimpanzees in which immunization with pre-S$_2$ peptide provided protection against HBV infection,[58] suggesting a role for extrahepatic virus neutralization in HBV clearance. The use of pre-S$_2$-containing vaccines has been proposed to overcome nonresponsiveness to HBsAg major protein; however, this remains controversial.[59,60] Polyalbumin receptor antibodies, first identified as anti-Dane antibodies,[61] have been demonstrated by Alberti and coworkers in 83% of patients recovering from acute HBV infection; those with HBsAg-positive CAH lacked this antibody, suggesting a failure of free virus neutralization.[62]

Very recently, however, the biologic significance of polyalbumin has been challenged[63] because it is not demonstrable in normal serum and because it must be cross linked by glutaraldehyde before binding to the viral coat protein may occur.[64]

Mechanisms of Hepatocellular Damage

The extent of hepatocellular damage in acute and chronic HBV infection will in large part determine the clinical outcome. Unfortunately, the precise mechanism(s) are still incompletely understood, partly owing to an inability to grow HBV in tissue culture. Indirect evidence implicating immune-mediated damage rather than a primary HBV cytopathic effect has now accumulated, including:

1. Lack of disease activity (hepatic inflammation) in many chronic HBV carriers despite ongoing viral replication and secretion.

2. Extensive mononuclear inflammatory infiltrates on liver biopsy are the hallmark of acute and chronic hepatitis (i.e., liver cell necrosis).

3. Lack of disease activity in subgroups of patients with impaired immunity, e.g., acquired immunodeficiency disease (AIDS), chronic renal failure, and Down's syndrome.[65,66]

4. Exacerbation of hepatic necrosis following immune stimulation, e.g., by levamisole,[67] corticosteroid withdrawal,[68,69] or interferon.[70]

5. Evidence for a hyperimmune response in HBV-infected individuals with fulminant hepatic failure.[71,72]

These observations suggest that an active immune response is an essential element in the pathogenesis of liver injury and raises the obvious question of the target of the immune response.

Target of the Immune Attack

An immune response can only be mounted against antigens that come into contact with the constituent cells of the immune system. A relevant antigen could therefore be expected to be present on the hepatocyte membrane. It could be a virally encoded protein or a normal component of the hepatocyte membrane, i.e., a virally induced autoimmune reaction. Those hepatocytes that are selectively targeted by the immune system are difficult to identify because they are rapidly being lyzed, especially in acute hepatitis. Studies performed after hepatitis is already established may therefore yield only limited information.

In order to overcome this problem, Vento and coworkers[73] screened individuals known to have had sexual exposure to patients with HBV infection (acute or chronic) and thereby identified five asymptomatic individuals with HBsAg positivity but no other markers of HBV infection. Sequential studies of humoral and cellular immune reactivity to HBV antigens were performed on the sera of these five individuals, all of whom eventually developed acute symptomatic HBV infection, providing a unique opportunity to study the temporal relationship between the development of specific immune responses and the onset of hepatocellular necrosis, as evidenced by rising serum transaminases. Cellular immunity was measured indirectly using the T-lymphocyte migration-inhibitory factor (T-LIF) assay,[74] in which T-cell sensitization to an antigen is detected by the release of factors (T-LIF) that inhibit the migration of normal T lymphocytes. The temporal development of the immune responses of the five subjects relative to the rise of transaminases were remarkably similar. Sequentially, the immune responses were: cellular response to pre-S containing HBsAg, cellular response to HBcAg, humoral (IgM) response to HBcAg, and, finally, cellular response to pre-S-negative HBsAg occurring 10 days before the serum transaminases became elevated. The number of subjects in this study was small due to obvious practical limitations; however, the results are consistent with the hypothesis that HBsAg-reactive T cells generated just prior to hepatocellular injury attack hepatocytes bearing HBsAg on their cell membrane. This is supported by another study demonstrating membranous HBsAg on the hepatocytes of six of nine patients during the first week of clinical acute hepatitis B but in none of nine patients studied after 4 weeks of illness, presumably due to immune lysis.[75] Older studies utilizing lymphocyte transformation and/or migration inhibition assays, as summarized by Edgington and Chisari,[76] have shown widely variable sensitization to HBsAg in acute HBV infection; this finding probably reflects the timing of testing and variable HBsAg sources in regard to purity and pre-S content. Most recently, HBcAg has also been implicated as a target for cytotoxic T cells in acute hepatitis B.[77]

In chronic HBV hepatitis, accumulating evidence favors HBcAg on the hepatocyte membrane as the dominant target of the immune system;[74,78–80] however, controversy remains. Whereas the predominant phenotype of the mononuclear infiltrate at the sites of liver damage has been identified as OKT8+, which defines cytotoxic/suppressor T cells and NK cells,[81–83] the question of the antigen specificity of these cells has only recently been directly addressed. Ferrari and coworkers separated lymphocytes from diagnostic liver biopsies of chronic hepatitis B patients and successfully established and characterized polyclonal HBcAg-specific CD4+ and CD8+ T cell lines; HBsAg-specific cell lines could not be identified.[78] They have subsequently cloned one of these lines to produce four CD4+ T-cell clones that undergo class II-restricted proliferation in response to HBcAg and are capable of providing antigen-specific help to autologous B cells producing HBcAb.[79] Clearly, HBcAg-specific T cells are present in the inflammatory infiltrate of the livers of patients with chronic hepatitis B.

In order to satisfy HLA restriction requirements,[30,84] Mondelli studied the cytotoxicity of peripheral T lymphocytes from patients with chronic hepatitis B toward their own hepatocytes obtained from diagnostic liver biopsy.[80] T-cell cytotoxicity toward autologous hepatocytes was increased in 61% of cases compared with HBV negative controls. Cytotoxicity was profoundly reduced if the hepatocytes were preincubated with HBcAb-containing serum; however, HBsAb or normal serum were without blocking effects, suggesting that HBcAg-bearing hepatocytes were the target of the T lymphocytes. Hepatocyte staining for HBV antigens before and after the cytotoxicity experiments showed selective deletion of core antigen-positive cells; however, other cells were also lysed, implying that other mechanisms of cytotoxicity may also be important.[85] The degree of cytotoxicity did not correlate with the amount of inflammatory activity on the liver biopsy, again supporting a role for other mechanisms.[80] Recent studies using a similar in vitro system have reaffirmed the importance of HBcAg as a target but have also implicated HBeAg.[86,87]

Studies using the T-LIF assay described earlier revealed that T cells from patients with chronic HBV-associated hepatitis showed reactivity to core antigen, but were consistently anergic to HBsAg, whereas T lymphocytes from HBV vaccinees or from patients who had recovered from acute HBV hepatitis showed strong reactivity to HBsAg.[74] Other studies using various techniques have produced both conflicting and supportive data.[76,88–90]

In summary, cytotoxic T cells sensitized to HBsAg in acute HBV infection and HBcAg in chronic infection play a major role in the induction of hepatocellular necrosis. These conclusions, however, must be tempered in consideration of the crude nature of present assays for measuring cell-mediated immunity. Assays measuring RNA transcripts of T-lymphocyte activation products (e.g., interleukin-2) will aid in a more accurate analysis of cell-mediated immunity in HBV infection.

Nonviral Targets

Non-T lymphocytes in addition to T lymphocytes were found to exhibit significant cytotoxicity toward hepatocytes from chronically infected individuals in the autologous lymphocyte-hepatocyte model system.[91] Non-T-lymphocyte but not T-lymphocyte cytotoxicity was blocked by liver-specific membrane lipoprotein (LPS), an antigenically diverse component of the normal hepatocyte cell membrane and by aggregated immunoglobulin G. The Fab$'_2$ fragment of an anti-human IgG also blocked the non-T-cell cytotoxicity. The results suggest that non-T lymphocytes participate in an antibody dependant cell-mediated cytotoxic reaction directed against a component of the LSP complex.

Antibodies to LSP were detected in 21 of 27 patients with HBV-related chronic hepatitis (CPH or CAH); furthermore, the anti-LSP titer correlated with biochemical and histologic measurements of disease activity.[92] In contrast, anti-LSP appeared only transiently in acute HBV hepatitis, and the titer did not correlate with hepatic necrosis. Although extrapolation to HBV infection in vivo must be done with caution, these observations support the hypothesis put forward by Eddleston and Williams[93] that T cells activated by persistent HBV infection trigger a humoral response against LSP determinants that subsequently contribute to the hepatocellular damage.

Immunohistochemical Techniques

Immunohistochemical staining of hepatocyte sections for HBV antigens has complemented virologic and molecular biologic techniques in defining different phases of chronic HBV infection. Many chronic HBV carriers are symptom-free despite high serum levels of HBV-DNA and the presence of HBeAg, indicating active viral replication. Their liver biopsies show little disease activity (nonspecific reactive hepatitis or CPH); however, immunohistochemical staining for HBcAg reveals intense uptake by the nuclei of many cells.[94] This constellation of findings is common in carriers in childhood or young adulthood[95] and reflects immunotolerance to the virus and its products. The duration of this first phase varies from months to decades. Indeed, this same pattern is seen in immunosuppressed individuals.[47,96] Clearly, viral replication alone does not inflict hepatic damage — a host immune response against the virus must also be present.

The second phase of chronic HBV carriage is represented by patients with ongoing liver damage (CAH or CLH), who usually display cytoplasmic and membranous/submembranous in addition to nuclear HBcAg.[94,95,97-100] These patients demonstrate falling levels of HBV-DNA and often undergo conversion from HBeAg to HBeAb. These indices of diminishing viral replication and the ongoing hepatocellular necrosis reflect immune clearance of those hepatocytes harboring replicating virus. The duration and extent of this phase will determine whether cirrhosis will develop and how much residual hepatocellular function will remain. Some patients therefore develop progressive hepatic failure despite successful clearance of replicating virus.

In the final phase of chronic HBV carriage, all indices of viral replication are absent, including stainable hepatic HBcAg; this is accompanied by diminished biochemical and histologic markers of inflammatory activity.[101,102] Some patients will have developed cirrhosis; however, it will now be inactive. The vast majority will continue to secrete HBsAg, although at lower titer, reflecting integration of HBV-DNA into the host genome. Not all phases are seen in every patient; many appear to become arrested in the replicative or immunotolerant phase and therefore never develop serious liver disease but remain as an important reservoir for viral spread.

Immunoregulatory Abnormalities

The fundamental difference between individuals who successfully clear HBV after acute infection and those who develop chronic infection is still largely unknown. Epidemiologic studies have revealed a high incidence of chronicity in males and in those infected at birth or shortly thereafter,[103] but the mechanisms remain obscure.

Recent studies have detected a lower endogenous interferon response in individuals with chronic HBV infection. Type I interferons, normally produced in response to a viral infection, will increase the display of HLA class I proteins on the cell membrane;[104,105] these are recognized by T cells in association with viral antigens, and cytotoxicity against infected cells is enhanced.[30] Reduced production and secretion of interferon in chronic hepatitis B[106,107] may thereby impede clearance of hepatocytes harboring replicating virus.[108] Chronic HBV carriage may therefore in part result from a genetic or acquired interferon deficiency.

The absence of an appropriate humoral response to HBsAg in chronic carriers, however, suggests that additional factors are important. These individuals do not lack B cells capable of HBsAb production,[109] but rather there is growing evidence for antigen-specific suppression.[74,110,111] T lymphocytes from patients with HBsAg-positive chronic hepatitis could specifically inhibit the elaboration of T-LIF by T lymphocytes from HBV vaccinees in response to HBsAg; this inhibitory effect was abolished by mitomycin-C, which is consistent with mediation by T-suppressor cells.[74] Similarly, the in vitro HBsAb response of B cells from vaccinees was markedly diminished by the addition of supernatants of T cells obtained from chronic HBV carriers.[110] The specificity of this soluble factor was shown by its failure to inhibit polyclonal immunoglobulin responses or specific antibody production in response to tetanus toxoid and by its loss of activity after passage through a column containing bound HBsAg. Non-antigen-specific T-suppressor defects have been demonstrated in chronic HBV carriers, especially those with active liver disease;[112,113] however, similar defects in various organ-specific and non-organ-specific autoimmune diseases suggest that antigen-specific T-suppressor abnormalities are more important.

In summary, these experiments implicate HBsAg-specific T-suppressor cells in the genesis and maintenance of HBsAg nonresponsiveness in chronic HBV carriers. The mode of their induction remains unknown; however, it was recently suggested that the close physical association of various pre-S and S epitopes with self-proteins such as albumin may play an important role.[109] Finally, Celis and coworkers have reported preliminary data suggesting that the T-cell response to HBsAg may be HLA class II-restricted.[114]

Fulminant Hepatitis B

In a small number of cases, acute HBV infection assumes a fulminant course, characterized by acute liver failure and encephalopathy. One might expect rampant viral replication in such patients, but in fact the converse is correct. Two large series detected serum HBV-DNA in only 9% and 0% of patients, respectively;[115,72] furthermore, HBeAg is more rapidly cleared from serum compared with nonfulminant cases.[71,72,] Fulminant hepatitis patients have lower titers of HBsAg,[71,116] and shorter periods of surface antigenemia;[116,117] antibodies to HBsAg, HBeAg, and HBcAg appear more rapidly than in nonfulminant cases.[71,116] Immunohistochemical staining reveals absence of HBsAg or HBcAg within hepatocytes in virtually all cases.[118]

Massive hepatic necrosis is demonstrable on liver biopsy or at autopsy, but there is a paucity of infiltrating inflammatory cells, and the histologic picture resembles that of ischemic necrosis.[119,120] It has been postulated that antibodies produced in the spleen and transported to the liver via the portal vein combine with viral antigens released into the hepatic sinusoids to form immune complexes. These may interfere with the hepatic microcirculation to cause ischemic necrosis. Others have suggested that a localized Shwartzman reaction leads to hypercoagulability, with formation of fibrin thrombi and ischemia.[121] Not surprisingly, therefore, treatment with antiviral agents or infusion of surface antibody has been uniformly unsuccessful in fulminant HBV hepatitis.

HEPATITIS D VIRUS

Antibodies directed against the hepatitis D virus (HDV), or delta agent, were first detected in the sera of chronic HBV carriers in 1977 by Rizzetto.[122] Further studies have shown that HDV is an incomplete virus capable of replicating and inducing infection only in the presence of HBV; once established, however, it is associated with severe and progressive liver disease.[123-127]

The epidemiology of HDV infection is unusual; it has worldwide distribution[128] but tends to cause infection in localized epidemics involving HBV carriers in affected communities, presumably following introduction of HDV from endemic regions.[123,129] Delta infection is endemic in Italy, the Middle East, and some areas of Africa and South America but is rare in Western Europe, North America, and Asia, despite the existence of susceptible HBV carriers in many of these areas.[123,130] Family clustering of cases in endemic areas suggests viral spread by close or intimate contact,[131] whereas intravenous drug use is likely to be the major source of viral spread in nonendemic regions of the Western world;[123,132,133] maternal-infant transmission does not appear to be an important cause of HDV spread.[134]

Virology

HDV is a 36-nm particle comprised of an HBsAg coat enveloping the hepatitis D antigen (HDAg) and its genome.[135] The genome is a 1.7-kb RNA strand that lacks a 3' poly-A tail, suggesting (−) polarity.[123] HDV-RNA (a sensitive indicator of delta infection) may be reliably detected in serum using cDNA transcripts of the genome.[136] HDAg may be detected within the nuclei and occasionally the cytoplasm of infected hepatocytes using immunohistochemical staining techniques;[137,138] however, ultrastructural studies have failed to visualize a discreet viral particle.[123]

Susceptibility to HDV requires either a simultaneous coinfection with HBV or superinfection of a pre-existing HBV infection; individuals with HBsAb (natural infection of postvaccination) are immune to delta infection.[139] Coinfection is characterized by a clinical illness generally indistinguishable from acute HBV infection,[140] but fulminant hepatitis occurs more frequently than in uncomplicated acute HBV infection.[124,126] Progression to chronicity is rare.[140,141]

Superinfection of a chronic HBV carrier provides the optimum conditions for HDV replication. These patients present with acute hepatitis or with deterioration of previously stable liver disease.[142,143] Delta superinfection is distinguished from acute coinfection by the absence of an IgM HBcAb response and the presence of a prominent and sustained anti-HDV response.[124,140] Although the course may be self-limited, chronicity develops in the majority of superinfections.[140,144]

Immunopathology

It is clear that HDV infection is associated with aggressive liver disease.[125] Fulminant hepatitis B is associated with HDV markers in 34–39% of cases versus only 4–19% in nonfulminant cases.[126,145] In chronic hepatitis B, hepatic HDAg and positive HDV serology are more prevalent in those with severe disease (CAH or cirrhosis) compared with those with mild (CPH) or absent liver disease.[127,146,147]

The mechanism by which HDV promotes its liver-damaging effects is unknown. The histologic appearance of delta hepatitis is considered to be compatible with a cytopathic process;[148] lobular involvement is pronounced, with eosinophilic degeneration and necrosis of hepatocytes but with less marked lymphocytic infiltrates than is common in uncomplicated HBV hepatitis.[125,148,149] Until HBV can successfully be grown in tissue culture, the cytopathic potential of HDV will remain open to speculation.

Modification of self-antigens by a viral infection is a frequently proposed mechanism of autoimmune-induced liver disease. Of interest, therefore, are recent reports of microsomal autoantibodies[150] and antibodies to the basal cell layer of rat forestomach[151] in high titer in 13% and 50%, respectively, of patients with chronic HDV infection. These antibodies appear to be a consequence rather than a cause of chronic HDV hepatitis,[152] but these reports raise support for the idea that autoimmune hepatic diseases may have an initial viral origin.

The relationship between hepatic expression of HDAg and liver damage is consistent with a direct cytopathic effect. However, much work remains to be done, particularly the elucidation of the precise mechanism of cellular injury.

NON-A, NON-B HEPATITIS

Although non-A, non-B hepatitis is still defined by excluding other hepatotrophic viruses and those systemic viral infections such as Epstein-Barr virus and cytomegalovirus that commonly affect the liver, it is clear on epidemiologic grounds that there are at least two main varieties, one spread by the fecal/oral route and the other transmitted by parenteral inoculation.

Enteric Non-A Non-B

The first major outbreak of what was later recognized as acute enteric non-A, non-B hepatitis occurred in Delhi, in 1956, when 29,300 individuals developed icteric hepatitis,[153] originally thought to be an epidemic of hepatitis A. This form was definitively excluded as a cause of the outbreak after serologic tests for HAV were developed.[154]

Epidemic non-A, non-B hepatitis is a major public health problem in Southeast Asia;[155] most outbreaks are associated with floods that have allowed sewage to enter water pipes. The incubation period is around 6 weeks. Clinically, the illness is similar to epidemic hepatitis A, although there seems to be a higher incidence and mortality (10–20%) in pregnant women. One of the unexplained epidemiologic observations is that the age range affected is 15–40 years, with young children apparently spared from infection. No long-term sequelae have been observed in careful follow-up studies in India.

Epidemic forms of non-A, non-B hepatitis are relatively easy to identify and classify, but an identical disease seems to occur between epidemics, especially in Asia.[156] This sporadic form of enteric non-A, non-B infection is also associated with a higher attack rate among young adults, higher mortality in pregnant women, and an absence of chronic sequelae. It may represent the commonest cause of acute viral hepatitis in the Far East.

Virology

In 1983, Balayan et al. reported the successful fecal-oral transmission of hepatitis to a volunteer from patients with enteric non-A, non-B hepatitis in Tashkent, USSR.[157] Since the volunteer had serologic evidence of previous hepatitis A infection, the finding of clinical illness associated with 27–30-nm virus-like particles in stools from the volunteer, together with seroconversion from antibody-negative to antibody-positive (as judged by immune electron microscopy using sera and particles from the stools), was the first direct evidence for a distinct viral agent responsible for enteric non-A, non-B hepatitis. Similar serologic responses to 27–30-nm virus-like particles in acute phase stool samples have been confirmed by others,[158–162] but a clinically useful, robust diagnostic test has not yet been developed.

Immunopathology

Because progress in the virology of enteric non-A, non-B hepatitis has only recently been achieved, there have been no studies of immune reactions to the virus or virally infected liver cells. Pathologically, there is the usual focal necrosis of hepatocytes, but there is little inflammatory infiltration and few lymphocytes.[163] These histologic findings, together with the apparent absence of a carrier state, argue in favor of a cytopathic effect of the virus rather than immune-mediated liver damage.

Parenteral Non-A Non-B

Following the development of specific serologic tests for hepatitis B infection, it has become possible to detect and eliminate most blood donations capable of transmitting this virus infection. Such screening has not, however, eliminated posttransfusion hepatitis. Experimental transmission studies in chimpanzees have shown that such transmission is due to other hepatitis viruses in some blood donations.[164] These non-A, non-B viruses transmitted by the parenteral route are different from the agent responsible for enteric non-A, non-B hepatitis. The most important clinical difference is the rather high rate of chronicity (20–50%) found after posttransfusion non-A, non-B hepatitis.[165]

Epidemiology
Parenteral non-A, non-B infection has been found in every country in which it has been sought; where hepatitis B screening of blood donations is carried out using sensitive techniques, non-A, non-B hepatitis may constitute 90% of posttransfusion hepatitis.[166] Administration of blood clotting factors VIII and IX and intravenous drug addiction have been incriminated in the transmission of non-A, non-B infection, and outbreaks have been reported from hemodialysis units. Differences in the epidemiologic pattern of hepatitis B are found in heterosexual or homosexual individuals. The incubation period is usually around 2 months, but much shorter times have been reported after administration of some clotting factor preparations. This and evidence from experimental transmission studies suggests that there may be more than one agent involved.[167]

Virology
Many attempts have been made to develop a serologic test for parenteral non-A, non-B hepatitis, but none have proved to be reproducible or specific.[166] Very recently, however, Houghton and his colleagues at the Chiron Corporation appear to have identified viral RNA in serum known to transmit non-A, non-B infection, and they have developed a test for specific antibody to a corresponding viral protein. cDNA libraries were prepared from RNA pelleted from infectious serum and screened in expression vectors for production of a protein antigen reacting with antibodies in serum from patients with non-A, non-B hepatitis. One clone was eventually found that seemed to be producing a relevant antigen, from which a serologic test for antibody to the putative non-A, non-B virus has been developed. Although rigorous testing of specificity and sensitivity has yet to be performed, the initial results are promising. The virus itself appears to contain a single RNA strand and has been tentatively assigned to the togavirus family. This most exciting development, if confirmed, is clearly of enormous potential not only for screening blood donations but also for developing detailed knowledge of the immunology and virology of this important infection.

Immunopathology
Although there is little direct evidence with which to develop hypotheses to explain the mechanism of liver damage in non-A, non-B hepatitis, the fact that apparently

healthy carriers of the virus exist in the general population might suggest that the virus is noncytopathic. This in turn would suggest that immune reactions to viral antigens might be important in promoting liver damage. Evidence to support this hypothesis includes the finding of T cells cytotoxic to isolated hepatocytes in the peripheral blood of patients with chronic non-A, non-B hepatitis[168] and the presence of CD8-positive cytotoxic/suppressor lymphocytes in liver biopsies.[169]

Therapy
The most encouraging recent development has been the finding in small pilot studies that α-interferons may be remarkably effective in small doses in reducing serum transaminases and in controlling liver inflammation in chronic hepatitis due to parenteral non-A, non-B virus infection.[170,171] Unfortunately, most patients seem to show relapse on withdrawal of therapy, at least after short courses, and prolonged treatment may be necessary.

REFERENCES

1. Krugman S, Giles JP, Hammond J: Infectious hepatitis. Evidence for two distinctive clinical, epidemiological and immunological types of infection. *JAMA* 200:365–373, 1967.

2. Feinstone SM, Kapikian AZ, Purcell RH: Hepatitis A: detection by immune electron microscopy of a virus-like antigen associated with acute illness. *Science* 182:1026–1028, 1973.

3. Kojima H, Shibayama T, Sato A, et al: Propagation of human hepatitis A virus in conventional cell lines. *J Med Virol* 7:273–286, 1981.

4. Gingrich GA, Hadler SC, Elder HA, et al: Serologic investigation of an outbreak of hepatitis A in a rural day-care center. *Am J Public Health* 73:1190–1193, 1983.

5. Lemon SM: Type A viral hepatitis. New developments in an old disease. *N Engl J Med* 313:1059–1067, 1985.

6. Mathiesen LR: The hepatitis A virus infection. *Liver* 1:81–109, 1981.

7. Hess G, Arnold W, Hopf U, et al: Etiology of hepatitis B surface antigen negative chronic hepatitis. *Digestion* 19:202–209, 1979.

8. Rakela J, Redeker AG, Edwards VM et al: Hepatitis A virus infection in fulminant hepatitis and chronic active hepatitis. *Gastroenterology* 74:879–882, 1978.

9. Papaevangelou GJ: Global epidemiology of hepatitis A. In Gerety RJ: *Hepatitis A.* London, Academic Press, 1984, p 101.

10. Ticehurst JR, Racaniello VR, Baroudy BM, et al: Molecular cloning and characterization of hepatitis A virus cDNA. *Proc Natl Acad Sci USA* 80:5885–5889, 1983.

11. Najarian R, Caput D, Gee W, et al: Primary structure and gene organization of human hepatitis A virus *Proc Natl Acad Sci USA* 82:2627–2631, 1985.

12. Shimizu YK, Mathiesen LR, Lorenz D, et al: Localisation of hepatitis A antigen in liver tissue by peroxidase-conjugated antibody method: light and electron microscopic studies. *J Immunol* 121:1671–1679, 1978.

13. Lemon SM, Brown CD, Brooks DS, et al: Specific IgM response to hepatitis A virus determined by solid-phase radioimmunoassay *Infect Immun* 28:927–936, 1980.

14. Miller HFA, Legler K, Thomssen R: Increase in IgM antibodies against gut bacteria during acute hepatitis A. *Infect Immun* 40:542–547, 1983.

15. Zhuang H, Kaldor J, Locarnini SA, et al: Serum immunoglobulin levels in acute A, B and non-A, non-B hepatitis. *Gastroenterology* 82:549–553, 1982.

16. Yoshizawa H, Itoh Y, Iwakiri S, et al: Diagnosis of type A hepatitis by fecal IgA, antibody against hepatitis A antigen. *Gastroenterology* 78:114–118, 1980.

17. Friedman LS, Dienstag JL: The disease and its pathogenesis. In Gerety RJ: *Hepatitis A*. London, Academic Press, 1984, p 55.

18. Kawanishi M: Intranuclear crystal formation in picornavirus-infected cells. *Arch Virol* 57:123–132, 1978.

19. Provost PJ, Villarejos VM, Hilleman MR: Suitability of the rufiventer marmoset as a host animal for human hepatitis A virus. *Proc Soc Exp Biol Med* 155:283–286, 1977.

20. Nasser AM, Metcalf TG: Production of cytopathology in FRhK-4 cells by BS-C-1 passaged hepatitis A virus. *Appl Environ Microbiol* 53:2967–2971, 1987.

21. Provost PJ, Hilleman MR: Propagation of human hepatitis A virus in cell culture in vitro. *Proc Soc Exp Biol Med* 160:213–221, 1979.

22. Daemer RJ, Feinstone SM, Gust ID, et al: Propagation of human hepatitis A virus in African green monkey kidney cell culture: primary isolation and serial passage. *Infect Immun* 32:388–393, 1981.

23. Binn LN, Lemon SM, Marchwicki RH, et al: Primary isolation and serial passage of hepatitis A virus strains in primate cell cultures. *J Clin Microbiol* 20:28–33, 1984.

24. Lemon SM, Binn LN: Serum neutralizing antibody response to hepatitis A virus. *J Infect Dis* 148:1033–1039, 1983.

25. Flehmig B, Zahn J, Vallbracht A: Level of neutralizing and binding antibodies to hepatitis A virus after onset of icterus: a comparison. *J Infect Dis* 150:461, 1984.

26. Gauss-Muller V, Deinhardt F: Immunoreactivity of human and rabbit antisera to hepatitis A virus. *J Med Virol* 24:219–228, 1988.

27. Mosley JW, Reisler DM, Brachott D, et al: Comparison of two lots of immune serum globulin for prophylaxis of infectious hepatitis. *Am J Epidemiol* 87:539–550, 1968.

28. Gabriel P, Vallbracht A, Flehmig B: Lack of complement-dependent cytolytic antibodies in hepatitis A virus infection. *J Med Virol* 20:23–31, 1986.

29. Slusarczyk J, Hansson BG, Nordenfelt E, et al: Etiopathogenetic aspects of hepatitis A. Specific and non-specific humoral immune response during the course of infection. *J Med Virol* 14:269–276, 1984.

30. Zinkernagel RM, Doherty PC: Restriction of in vitro T cell-mediated cytotoxicity in lymphocytic choriomeningitis within a syngeneic or semiallogeneic system. *Nature* 248:701–702, 1974.

31. Vallbracht A, Gabriel P, Maier K, et al: Cell-mediated cytotoxicity in hepatitis A virus infection. *Hepatology* 6:1308–1314, 1986.

32. Kurane I, Binn LN, Bancroft WH, et al: Human lymphocyte responses to hepatitis A virus-infected cells: interferon production and lysis of infected cells. *J Immunol* 135:2140–2144, 1985.

33. Herberman RR, Ortaldo JR, Bonnard GD: Augmentation by interferon of human natural and antibody-dependent cell mediated cytotoxicity. *Nature* 277:221–223, 1979.

34. Levin S, Hahn T: Interferon system in acute viral hepatitis. *Lancet* 1:592–594, 1982.

35. Szmuness W: Hepatocellular carcinoma and the hepatitis B virus: evidence for a causal association. *Prog Med Virol* 24:40–69, 1978.

36. Beasley RP, Hwang LY, Lin CC, et al: Hepatocellular carcinoma and hepatitis B virus. A prospective study of 22,707 men in Taiwan. *Lancet* 2:1129–1133, 1981.

37. Robinson WS, Marion PL: Biological features of hepadna viruses. In Zuckerman AJ: *Viral Hepatitis and Liver Disease*. New York, Alan R Liss, 1988. p 449.

38. Summers J, Mason WS: Replication of the genome of a hepatitis B-like virus by reverse transcription of an RNA intermediate. *Cell* 29:403–415, 1982.

39. Dane DS, Cameron CH, Briggs M: Virus-like particles in serum of patients with Australia-antigen associated hepatitis. *Lancet* 1:695–698, 1970.

40. Robinson WS, Lutwick LI: The virus of hepatitis, type B (part 1). *N Engl J Med* 295:1169–1175, 1976.

41. Robinson WS: The genome of hepatitis B virus. *Ann Rev Microbiol* 31:357–377, 1977.

42. Ou JH, Laub O, Rutter WJ: Hepatitis B virus gene function: the precore region targets the core antigen to cellular membranes and causes the secretion of the e antigen. *Proc Natl Acad Sci USA* 83:1578–1582, 1986.

43. Neurath AR, Strick N: Radioimmunoassay for albumin-binding sites associated with HBsAg: correlation of results with the presence of e antigen in serum. *Intervirology* 11:128–132, 1979.

44. Klatskin G: Subacute hepatic necrosis and postnecrotic cirrhosis due to a anicteric infections with the hepatitis virus. *Am J Med* 25:333–358, 1958.

45. Tassopoulos NC, Papaevangelou GJ, Sjogren MH, et al: Natural history of acute hepatitis B surface antigen positive hepatitis in Greek adults. *Gastroenterology* 92:1844–1850, 1987.

46. Seeff LB, Beebe CW, Norman JE, et al: Serologic followup of 1942 yellow fever vaccine associated hepatitis outbreak. *Hepatology* 5:959, 1985 (abs).

47. Hoofnagle JH, Shafritz DA, Popper H: Chronic type B hepatitis and the "healthy" HBsAg carrier state. *Hepatology* 7:758–763, 1987.

48. Aldershivile J, Dietrichson O, Skinhoj P, et al: Chronic persistent hepatitis: serological classification and meaning of the hepatitis B e system. *Hepatology* 2:243–246, 1982.

49. Shafritz DA, Shouval D, Sherman HI, et al: Integration of hepatitis B virus DNA into the genome of liver cells in chronic liver disease and hepatocellular carcinoma. *N Engl J Med* 305:1067–1073, 1981.

50. Popper H, Shafritz DA, Hoofnagle JH: Relation of the hepatitis B virus carrier state to hepatocellular carcinoma. *Hepatology* 7:764–772, 1987.

51. Hansson BG, Purcell RH: Sites that bind polymerized albumin on hepatitis B surface antigen particles: detection by radioimmunoassay. *Infect Immun* 26:125–130, 1979.

52. Imai M, Yanase Y, Nojiri T, et al: A receptor for polymerized human and chimpanzee albumins on hepatitis B virus particles co-occurring with HBeAg. *Gastroenterology* 76:242–247, 1979.

53. Machida A, Kishimoto S, Ohnuma H, et al: A hepatitis B surface antigen polypeptide (P31) with the receptor for polymerized human as well as chimpanzee albumins. *Gastroenterology* 85:268–274, 1983.

54. Machida A, Kishimoto S, Ohnuma H, et al: A polypeptide containing 55 amino acid residues coded by the pre-s region of hepatitis B virus DNA, bears the receptor for polymerized human as well as chimpanzee albumins. *Gastroenterology* 86:910–918, 1984.

55. Thung SN, Gerber MA: Polyalbumin receptors: their role in the attachment of hepatitis B virus to hepatocytes. *Semin Liver Dis* 4:69–75, 1984.

56. Thung SN, Gerber MA: Albumin binding sites of human hepatocytes. *Liver* 3:290–294, 1983.

57. Trevisan A, Gudat F, Guggenheim R, et al: Demonstration of albumin receptors on isolated human hepatocytes by light and scanning electron microscopy. *Hepatology* 2:832–835, 1982.

58. Itoh Y, Takai E, Ohnuma H, et al: A synthetic peptide vaccine involving the product of the pre-S2 region of hepatitis B virus DNA: protective efficacy in chimpanzees. *Proc Natl Acad Sci USA* 83:9174–9178, 1986.

59. Berthelot P, Neurath R, Courouce AM, et al: Hepatitis B vaccines with pre-S gene product. *Lancet* 1:1150, 1986 (letter).

60. Hellstrom U, Sylvan S, Kuhns M, et al: Absence of pre-S2 antibodies in natural hepatitis B virus infection. *Lancet* 2:889–893, 1986.

61. Alberti A, Diana S, Scullard GH, et al: Detection of a new antibody system reacting with Dane particles in hepatitis B virus infection. *Br Med J,* 2:1056–1058, 1978.

62. Pontisso P, Schiavon E, Fraiese A, et al: Antibody to the hepatitis B virus receptor for polymerized albumin in acute infection and in hepatitis B vaccine recipients. *J Hepatol* 3:393–398, 1986.

63. Heermann KH, Waldeck F, Gerlich WH: Interaction between native human serum and the pre-S2 domain of HBsAg. In Zuckerman AJ: *Viral Hepatitis and Liver Disease.* New York, Alan R Liss, 1988. p 697.

64. Yu MW, Finlayson JS, Shih JWK: Interaction between various polymerized human albumins and HBsAg. *J Virol* 55:736–743, 1985.

65. Perrillo RP, Regenstein FG, Roodman ST: Chronic hepatitis B in asymptomatic homosexual men with antibody to the human immunodeficiency virus. *Ann Intern Med* 105:382–383, 1986.

66. Briggs WA, Lazarus M, Birtch AG, et al: Hepatitis affecting haemodialysis and transplant patients. Its considerations and consequences. *Arch Intern Med* 132:21–28, 1973.

67. Thomas HC, Chadwick G, Jain S, et al: Levamisole in the treatment of HBsAg positive chronic active liver disease. *Gastroenterology* 73:1250, 1977 (abs).

68. Nair PV, Tong MJ, Stevenson D, et al: A pilot study on the effects of prednisone withdrawal on serum HBV DNA and HBeAg in chronic active hepatitis B. *Hepatology* 6:1319–1324, 1986.

69. Hoofnagel JH, Davis GL, Pappas SC, et al: A short course of prednisolone in chronic type B hepatitis. Report of a randomised double-blind placebo-controlled trial. *Ann Intern Med* 104:12–17, 1986.

70. Alexander GJM, Brahm J, Fagan EA, et al: Loss of HBsAg with interferon therapy in chronic hepatitis B virus infection. *Lancet* 2:66–69, 1987.

71. Gimson AES, Tedder RS, White YS, et al: Serological markers in fulminant hepatitis B. *Gut* 24:615–617, 1983.

72. De Cock KM, Govindarajan S, Valinluck B, et al: Hepatitis B virus DNA in fulminant hepatitis B. *Ann Intern Med* 105:546–547, 1986.

73. Vento S, Rondanelli EG, Ranieri S, et al: Prospective study of cellular immunity to hepatitis B virus antigens from the early incubation phase of acute hepatitis B. *Lancet* 2:119–122, 1987.

74. Vento S, Hegarty JE, Alberti A, et al. T lymphocyte sensitization to HBcAg and T cell mediated unresponsiveness to HBsAg in hepatitis B virus-related chronic liver disease. *Hepatology* 5:192–197, 1985.

75. Alberti A, Realdi G, Tremolada F, et al: Liver cell surface localisation of hepatitis B antigen and of immunoglobulins in acute and chronic hepatitis and in liver cirrhosis. *Clin Exp Immunol* 25:396–402, 1976.

76. Edgington TS, Chisari FV: Immune responses to hepatitis B virus coded and induced antigens in chronic active hepatitis. In Eddleston ALWF, Weber JCP, Williams R: *Immune Reactions in Liver Disease.* London, Pitman Medical, 1979. p 44.

77. Mondelli MU, Bortolotti F, Pontisso P, et al: Definition of HBV-specific target antigens recognized by cytotoxic T cells in acute HBV infection. *Clin Exp Immunol* 68:242–250, 1987.

78. Ferrari C, Penna A, Giuberti T, et al: Intrahepatic nucleocapsid antigen specific T cells in chronic active hepatitis B. *J Immunol* 139:2050–2058, 1987.

79. Ferrari C, Mondelli MU, Penna A, et al: Functional characterization of cloned intrahepatic HBV nucleoprotein specific helper T cell lines. *J Immunol* 139:539–544, 1987.

80. Mondelli M, Mieli-Vergani G, Alberti A, et al: Specificity of T lymphocyte cytotoxicity to autologous hepatocytes in chronic HBV infection: evidence that T cells are directed against HBcAg expressed on hepatocytes. *J Immunol* 129:2773–2778, 1982.

81. Eggink HF, Houthoff HJ, Huitema S, et al: Cellular and humoral immune reactions in chronic active liver disease. Lymphocyte subsets in liver biopsies of patients with untreated idiopathic auto-immune hepatitis, chronic active hepatitis B and primary biliary cirrhosis. *Clin Exp Immunol* 50:17–24, 1982.

82. Pape GR, Rieber EP, Eisenburg J, et al: Involvement of the cytotoxic/suppressor T cell subset in liver tissue injury of patients with acute and chronic liver diseases. *Gastroenterology* 85:657–662, 1983.

83. Montano L, Aranguibel F, Boffill M, et al: An analysis of the composition of the inflammatory infiltrate in autoimmune and hepatitis B virus-induced chronic liver disease. *Hepatology* 3:292–296, 1983.

84. Chu CM, Shyu WC, Kuo RW, et al: HLA class 1 antigen display on hepatocyte membrane in chronic hepatitis B virus infection: its role in the pathogenesis of chronic type B hepatitis. *Hepatology* 7:1311–1316, 1987.

85. Naumov NV, Mondelli M, Alexander GJM, et al: Relationship between expression of hepatitis B virus antigens in isolated hepatocytes and autologous lymphocyte cytotoxicity in patients with chronic hepatitis B virus infection. *Hepatology* 4:63–68, 1984.

86. Pignatelli M, Waters J, Thomas HC: Evidence that cytotoxic T cells sensitized to HBE are responsible for hepatocyte lysis in chronic hepatitis B virus infection. *Hepatology* 5:988, 1985 (abs).

87. Pignatelli M, Waters J, Lever A, et al: Cytotoxic T cell responses to the nucleocapsid proteins of HBV in chronic hepatitis. Evidence that antibody modulation may cause protracted infection. *J Hepatol* 4:15–21, 1987.

88. Lee WM, Reed WD, Mitchell CG, et al: Cellular and humoral immunity to HBsAg in active chronic hepatitis. *Br Med J* 1:705–708, 1975.

89. De Moura MC, Vernace SJ, Paronetto F: Cell-mediated immune reactivity to HBsAg in liver diseases. *Gastroenterology* 69:310–317, 1975.

90. Tong MJ, Wallace AM, Peters RL, et al: Lymphocyte stimulation in hepatitis B infections. *N Engl J Med* 283:318–322, 1975.

91. Mieli-Vergani G, Vergani D, Portmann B, et al: Lymphocyte cytotoxicity to autologous hepatocytes in HBsAg positive chronic liver disease. *Gut* 23:1029–1036, 1982.

92. Jensen DM, McFarlane IG, Portmann BS, et al: Detection of antibodies directed against a liver specific membrane lipoprotein in patients with acute and chronic active hepatitis. *N Engl J Med* 299:1–7, 1978.

93. Eddleston ALWF, Williams R: Inadequate antibody response to HBAg or suppressor T cell defect in development of active chronic hepatitis. *Lancet* 2:1543–1545, 1974.

94. Hsu HC, Su IJ, Lai MY, et al: Biologic and prognostic significance of hepatocyte hepatitis B core antigen expression in the natural course of chronic HBV infection. *J Hepatol* 5:45–50, 1987.

95. Hsu HC, Lin YH, Chang MH, et al: Pathology of chronic hepatitis B virus infection in children: with special reference to the intrahepatic expression of hepatitis B virus antigens. *Hepatology* 8:378–382, 1988.

96. Gudat F, Bianchi L, Sonnabend W, et al: Pattern of core and surface expression in liver reflects state of specific immune response in hepatitis B. *Lab Invest* 32:1–9, 1975.

97. Gudat F, Bianchi L: Evidence for phasic sequences in nuclear HBcAg formation and cell membrane directed flow of core particles in chronic hepatitis B. *Gastroenterology* 73:1194–1197, 1977.

98. Chu CM, Liaw YF: Intrahepatic distribution of hepatitis B surface and core antigens in chronic HBV infection. *Gastroenterology* 92:220–225, 1987.

99. Ramalho F, Brunetto MR, Rocca G, et al: Serum markers of HBV replication, liver histology and intrahepatic expression of HBcAg. *J Hepatol* 7:14–20, 1988.

100. Sansonna DE, Fiore G, Bufano G, et al: Cytoplasmin localization of hepatitis B core antigen in hepatitis B virus infected livers. *J Immunol Methods* 109:245–252, 1988.

101. Hoofnagle JH, Dusheiko GM, Seeff LB, et al: Seroconversion from HBeAg to HBeAb in chronic type B hepatitis. *Ann Intern Med* 94:744–748, 1981.

102. Fattovich G, Rugge M, Brollo L, et al: Clinical, virologic and histologic outcome following seroconversion from HBeAg to anti-HBe in chronic hepatitis type B. *Hepatology* 6:167–172, 1986.

103. Seeff LB, Koff RS: Evolving concepts of the clinical and serologic consequences of HBV infection. *Semin Liver Dis* 6:11–22, 1986.

104. Durandy A, Virelizier JL, Griscelli C: Enhancement by interferon of membrane HLA antigens in patients with combined immunodeficiency with defective HLA expression. *Clin Exp Immunol* 52:173–178, 1983.

105. Pignatelli M, Waters J, Brown D, et al: HLA class I antigens on the hepatocyte membrane during recovery from acute HBV infection and during interferon therapy in chronic HBV infection. *Hepatology* 6:349–353, 1986.

106. Poitrine A, Chousterman S, Chousterman M, et al: Lack of in vivo activation of the interferon system in HBsAg positive chronic active hepatitis. *Hepatology* 2:171–174, 1985.

107. Ikeda T, Lever AML, Thomas HC: Evidence for a deficiency of interferon production in patients with chronic HBV infection acquired in adult life. *Hepatology* 6:962–965, 1986.

108. Montano L, Miescher GC, Goodall AH, et al: Hepatitis B virus and HLA antigen display in the liver during chronic hepatitis B virus infection. *Hepatology* 2:557–561, 1982.

109. Sylvan SPE, Hellstrom U: Immunological mechanisms in asymptomatic carriers of HBsAg. In Zuckerman AJ: *Viral Hepatitis and Liver Disease.* New York, Alan R Liss, 1988, p 704.

110. Yamauchi K, Nakanishi T, Chiou SS, et al: Suppression of hepatitis B antibody synthesis by factor made by T cells from chronic HBV carriers. *Lancet* 1:324–326, 1988.

111. Dusheiko GM, Hoofnagle JH, Cooksley WG, et al: Synthesis of antibodies to HBV by cultured lymphocytes from chronic hepatitis B surface antigen carriers. *J Clin Invest* 71:1104–1113, 1983.

112. Kakumu S, Yata K, Kashio T: Immunoregulatory T cell function in acute and chronic liver disease. *Gastroenterology* 79:613–619, 1980.

113. Nouri-Aria KT, Hegarty JE, Alexander GJ, et al: Effect of corticosteroids on suppressor cell activity in autoimmune and viral chronic active hepatitis. *N Engl J Med* 307:1301–1304, 1982.

114. Celis E, Ou D, Otvos L: Recognition of HBsAg by human T lymphocytes. Proliferative and cytotoxic responses to a major antigenic determinant defined by synthetic peptides. *J Immunol* 140:1808–1815, 1988.

115. Brechot C, Bernuau J, Thiers V, et al: Multiplication of hepatitis B virus in fulminant hepatitis B. *Br Med J* 288:270–271, 1984.

116. Trepo CG, Robert D, Motin J, et al: HBsAg and/or antibodies (anti-HBs and anti-HBc) in fulminant hepatitis: pathogenic and prognostic significance. *Gut* 17:10–13, 1976.

117. Woolf IL, Sheikh NE, Cullens H, et al: Enhanced HBsAb production in pathogenesis of fulminant viral hepatitis type B. *Br Med J* 2:669–671, 1976.

118. Omata M, Afroudakis A, Liew CT, et al: Comparison of serum HBsAg and serum anticore with tissue HBsAg and HBcAg. *Gastroenterology* 75:1003–1009, 1978.

119. Dupuy JM, Frommel D, Alagille D: Severe viral hepatitis type B in infancy. *Lancet* 1:191–194, 1975.

120. Horney JT, Galambos JH: The liver during and after fulminant hepatitis. *Gastroenterology* 73:639–645, 1977.

121. Mori W, Shiga J, Irie H: Shwartzman reaction as a pathogenic mechanism in fulminant hepatitis. *Semin Liver Dis* 6:267–276, 1986.

122. Rizzetto M, Canese MG, Arico S, et al: Immunofluorescence detection of new antigen-antibody system (delta/anti-delta) associated with HBV in liver and serum of HBsAg carriers. *Gut* 18:997–1003, 1977.

123. Rizzetto M: The delta agent. *Hepatology* 3:729–737, 1983.

124. Shattock AG, Irwin FM, Morgan BM, et al: Increased severity and morbidity of acute hepatitis in drug abusers with simultaneously acquired hepatitis B and hepatitis D virus infections. *Br Med J* 290:1377–1380, 1985.

125. Rizzetto M, Verme G, Recchia S, et al: Chronic hepatitis in carriers of HBsAg with intrahepatic expression of the delta antigen. *Ann Intern Med* 98:437–441, 1983.

126. Govindarajan S, Chin KP, Redeker AG, et al: Fulminant B viral hepatitis: role of delta agent. *Gastroenterology* 86:1417–1420, 1984.

127. Weller IVD, Karayiannis P, Lok ASF, et al: Significance of delta agent infection in chronic hepatitis B virus infection: a study in British carriers. *Gut* 24:1061–1063, 1983.

128. Rizzetto M, Purcell RH, Gerin JL: Epidemiology of HBV-associated delta agent: geographical distribution of anti-delta and prevalence in polytransfused HBsAg carriers. *Lancet* 1:1215–1219, 1980.

129. Hadler SC, De Monzon M, Ponzetto A, et al: Delta virus infection and severe hepatitis. An epidemic in the Yucpa Indians of Venezuela. *Ann Intern Med* 100:339–344, 1984.

130. Hoofnagle JH: Type D hepatitis and the hepatitis delta virus. In Thomas HC, Jones EA: *Recent Advances in Hepatology*–II. New York, Churchill Livingstone, 1986, p 73.

131. Bonino F, Caporaso N, Dentico P, et al: Familial clustering and spreading of hepatitis delta virus infection. *J Hepatol* 1:221–226, 1985.

132. Raimondo G, Smedile A, Gallo L, et al: Multicenter study of prevalence of HBV-associated delta infection and liver disease in drug addicts. *Lancet* 1:249–251, 1982.

133. Ponzetto A, Seeff LB, Buskell-Bales Z, et al: Hepatitis B markers in United States drug addicts with special emphasis on the delta hepatitis virus. *Hepatology* 4:1111–1115, 1984.

134. Zanetti AR, Ferroni P, Magliano EM, et al: Perinatal transmission of HBV and HBV-associated delta agent from mothers to offspring in northern Italy. *J Med Virol* 9:139–148, 1982.

135. Bonino F, Hoyer B, Shih JW, et al: Delta hepatitis agent: structural and antigenic properties of the delta-associated particle. *Infect Immun* 43:1000–1005, 1984.

136. Smedile A, Rizzetto M, Denniston K, et al: Type D hepatitis: the clinical significance of hepatitis D virus RNA in serum as detected by a hybridization-based assay. *Hepatology* 6:1297–1302, 1986.

137. Stocklin E, Gudat F, Krey G, et al: Delta antigen in hepatitis B: immunohistology of frozen and paraffin-embedded liver biopsies and relation to HBV infection. *Hepatology* 1:238–242, 1981.

138. Negro F, Baldi M, Bonino F, et al: Chronic HDV hepatitis: intrahepatic expression of delta antigen, histologic activity and outcome of liver disease. *J Hepatol* 6:8–14, 1988.

139. Rizzetto M, Canese MG, Gerin JL, et al: Transmission of hepatitis B virus-associated delta antigen to chimpanzees. *J Infect Dis* 141:590–602, 1980.

140. Caredda F, Rossi E, Monforte AA, et al: Hepatitis B virus associated coinfection and superinfection with delta agent: indistinguishable disease with different outcome. *J Infect Dis* 151:925–928, 1985.

141. Caredda F, Antinori S, Re T, et al: Course and prognosis of acute HDV hepatitis. In Rizzetto M, Gerin JL, Purcell RH: *The Hepatitis Delta Virus and its Infection.* New York, Alan R Liss, 1987, p 267.

142. Farci P, Smedile A, Lavarini C, et al: Delta hepatitis in inapparent carriers of HBsAg. A disease simulating acute hepatitis B progressive to chronicity. *Gastroenterology* 85:669–673, 1983.

143. Smedile A, Dentico P, Zanetti A, et al: Infection with the delta agent in chronic HBsAg carriers. *Gastroenterology* 81:992–997, 1981.

144. De Cock KM, Govindarajan S, Chin KP, et al: Delta hepatitis in the Los Angeles Area: a report of 126 cases. *Ann Intern Med* 105:108–114, 1986.

145. Smedile A, Farci P, Verme G, et al: Influence of delta infection on severity of hepatitis B. *Lancet* 2:945–947, 1982.

146. Govindarajan S, Kanel GC, Peters RL: Prevalence of delta antibody among chronic HBV infected patients in the Los Angeles area: its correlation with liver biopsy diagnosis. *Gastroenterology* 85:160–162, 1983.

147. Colombo M, Cambieri R, Rumi MG, et al: Long term delta superinfection in HBsAg carriers and its relationship to the course of chronic hepatitis. *Gastroenterology* 85:235–239, 1983.

148. Popper H, Thung SN, Gerber MA, et al: Histologic studies of severe delta agent infection in Venezuelan Indians. *Hepatology* 3:906–912, 1983.

149. Kanal GC, Govindarajan S, Peters RL: Chronic delta infection and liver biopsy changes in chronic active hepatitis B. *Ann Intern Med* 101:51–54, 1984.

150. Crivelli O, Lavarini C, Chiaberge E, et al: Microsomal autoantibodies in chronic infection with the HBsAg associated delta agent. *Clin Exp Immunol* 54:232–238, 1983.

151. Zauli D, Fusconi M, Crespi C, et al: Close association between basal cell layer antibodies and HBV associated chronic delta infection. *Hepatology* 4:1103–1106, 1984.

152. Lavarini C, Caredda F, Ballare M, et al: Development of tissue antibodies in hepatitis delta virus infection. In Zuckerman AJ: *Viral Hepatitis and Liver Disease.* New York, Alan R Liss, 1988, p 439.

153. Viswanathan R: Infectious hepatitis in Delhi (1955–1956): a critical study; epidemiology. *Ind J Med Res* 45(Suppl):1–30, 1957.

154. Wong DC, Purcell RH, Sreenivarsan MA, et al: Epidemic and endemic hepatitis in India: evidence for a non-A non-B hepatitis virus aetiology. *Lancet* 2:882–885, 1980.

155. Purcell RH, Ticehurst JR: Enterically transmitted non-A non-B Hepatitis: Epidemiology and clinical characteristics. In Zuckerman AJ ed: *Viral Hepatitis and Liver Disease.* New York, Alan R Liss, 1988, p 131.

156. Khuroo MS, Duermeyer W, Zargar SA, et al: Acute sporadic non-A, non-B hepatitis in India. *Am J Epidemiol* 118:360–364, 1983.

157. Balayan MS, Andzhaparidze AG, Savinskaya SS, et al: Evidence for a virus in non-A, non-B hepatitis transmitted via the fecal-oral route. *Intervirology* 20:23–31, 1983.

158. Bradley DW, Maynard JE: Etiology and natural history of post-transfusion and enterically transmitted non-A, non-B hepatitis. *Semin Liver Dis* 6:56–66, 1986.

159. Favorov MO, Khukhlovich PA, Zairov GK, et al: Clinical and epidemiological features and diagnosis of viral non-A, non-B hepatitis with fecal-oral transmission mechanism. *Voprosy Virusologii* (Moskva) 31:65–69, 1986.

160. Kane MA, Bradley DW, Shrestha SM, et al: Epidemic non-A, non-B hepatitis in Nepal: recovery of a possible etiologic agent and transmission studies in marmosets. *JAMA* 252:3140–3145, 1984.

161. Sreenivasan MA, Arankalle VA, Sehgal A, et al: Non-A, non-B epidemic hepatitis: visualisation of virus-like particles in the stool by immune electron microscopy. *J Gen Virol,* 65:1005–1007, 1984.

162. Zairov GK, Stakhanova VM, Listovskaya EK, et al. Electron microscopic investigations in non-A, non-B hepatitis with fecal-oral transmission mode. *Voprosy Virusologii (Moskva)* 31:172–175, 1986.

163. Tabor E, Gerety RJ, Drucker JA, et al: Transmission of non-A, non-B hepatitis from man to chimpanzee. *Lancet* 1:463–466, 1978.

164. Dienstag JL: Non-A, non-B hepatitis. I. Recognition, epidemiology and clinical features. *Gastroenterology* 85:439–462, 1983.

165. Kiyosawa K, Akahane Y, Nagata A, et al: The significance of blood transfusion in non-A, non-B chronic liver disease in Japan. *Vox Sang* 43:45–52, 1982.

166. Gerety RJ, Tabor E, Schaff Z, et al: Non-A, non-B hepatitis agents. In Vyas GN, Dienstag JL, Hoofnagle JH: *Viral Hepatitis and Liver Diseases.* New York, Grune and Stratton, 1984, p 23.

167. Wyke RJ, Tsiquaye KN, Thornton A, et al: Transmission of non-A non-B hepatitis to chimpanzees by factor IX concentrates after fatal complications in patients with chronic liver disease. *Lancet* 1:520–524, 1979.

168. Mondelli M, Alberti A, Tremolada F, et al: In-vitro cell-mediated cytotoxicity for autologous liver cells in chronic non-A, non-B hepatitis. *Clin Exp Immunol* 63:147–155, 1986.

169. Spengler U, Kaczmarska A, Grunerbl A, et al: Involvement of immunological mechanisms in the pathogenesis of non-A, non-B hepatitis. In Zuckerman AJ: *Viral Hepatitis and Liver Disease.* New York, Alan R Liss, 1988, p 576.

170. Hoofnagle JH, Mullen K, Jones B, et al: Treatment of chronic non-A, non-B hepatitis with recombinant human alpha interferon. Gastroenterology 315:1575–1578, 1986.

171. Thomson BJ, Doran M, Lever AMI, et al: Alpha-interferon therapy for non-A, non-B hepatitis transmitted by gammaglobulin replacement therapy. *Lancet* 1:539–541, 1987.

CHAPTER 14

Chronic Active Hepatitis

IAN G. MCFARLANE

ADRIAN L.W.F. EDDLESTON

INTRODUCTION

Chronic active hepatitis (CAH) is a progressive inflammatory disorder of the liver that leads to cirrhosis if untreated. The term was first used by Saint and colleagues[1] to describe a condition that, as noted by Waldenstrom in 1950,[2] affected mainly young women and was associated with hypergammaglobulinemia. Bearn et al.[3] drew attention to the prominent systemic manifestations of the disease, which include profound lassitude, malaise, arthralgia/arthritis, swinging pyrexia, and rashes (usually acneform). The finding that a proportion of patients had circulating lupus erythematosus (LE) cells[4] and antinuclear antibodies (ANA), suggesting an autoimmune pathogenesis, led Mackay[5] to coin the term "lupoid hepatitis."

This early definition of autoimmune (lupoid) CAH was later broadened to include patients with anti-smooth muscle antibodies (SMA) in their sera, whether or not they are also seropositive for ANA. Although females still predominate (4 : 1) among patients with CAH conforming to this wider definition, it is now recognized that the disease also affects males and is biphasic with respect to age of presentation, having two peaks of onset, at 10 – 30 years of age and > 40 years (i.e., postmenopausal in women). An important additional difference is the low frequency (about 20%) of LE cells in this group.

The hypergammaglobulinemia in this disorder is due predominantly to increased IgG concentrations, which can be quite markedly elevated (two- to fourfold). The ANA give a "homogeneous" pattern of immunofluorescent staining on tissue sections similar to that seen with ANA in the sera of patients with systemic lupus erythematosus (SLE) and, as in the latter, are usually associated with serum autoantibodies against double-stranded DNA (dsDNA). These antibodies, however, react with a different antigen to that recognized by anti-dsDNA in SLE.[6] The

SMA in autoimmune CAH (AI-CAH) are specific for F-actin (which distinguishes them from autoantibodies reacting with other muscle components in some other diseases).

A subgroup of patients with particularly severe CAH who have circulating autoantibodies against a microsomal antigen in liver and kidney (LKM antibody) has been defined.[7,8] These antibodies, designated LKM-1, must be distinguished from a similar autoantibody (LKM-2), which reacts against a different antigen (see below) and which is associated with drug-induced hepatitis. CAH associated with LKM-1 antibodies can affect both sexes of any age but is most commonly seen in young females (aged 2–14 years).

Other circulating autoantibodies may be found at variable frequencies (up to about 20%) in CAH patients who are seropositive for ANA or SMA. These include antithyroid, gastric parietal cell, and even antimitochondrial (see Chapter 12) antibodies, as well as rheumatoid factor, but they seem to have little direct relevance to CAH.

The two criteria that are now regarded as perhaps the most important for a diagnosis of chronic active hepatitis (CAH) are:

1. Clinical and/or biochemical evidence of persisting liver damage. Most authorities require a minimum of 6 months' duration, to reduce the possibility that the liver damage might be due to protracted or "unresolved" acute hepatitis.
2. The histologic finding of an intense inflammatory (mainly mononuclear) cell infiltrate in the portal tracts that extends beyond the limiting plate of hepatocytes, into the periportal area, isolating and surrounding individual hepatocytes in a pattern described as "piecemeal necrosis."

Nevertheless, neither of these criteria is entirely clear-cut. Accurate documentation of duration is often difficult because the biochemical and clinical features vary between patients and tend to fluctuate. Also, the onset can be quite insidious, and it is not uncommon for the disease to present as an acute hepatic illness with an already established cirrhosis following a short prodrome. The classical histologic picture of periportal inflammation with piecemeal necrosis is generally accepted, but less certain is whether the additional finding of patches of inflammatory activity within the liver lobules should be included as part of the histologic spectrum of CAH. The current practice is to describe this latter picture as "chronic lobular hepatitis" (CLH), which has a prognosis that appears to vary with etiology.[9]

There is also the problem of how to classify "chronic persistent hepatitis" (CPH), which is defined histologically as a condition in which the inflammatory infiltrate is largely confined to the portal tracts, with little or no extension to the periportal area or piecemeal necrosis. However, distinctions must be made between CPH in the *absence* of any previous evidence of CAH, which is considered to have a good prognosis, and CPH as a *sequel* to CAH (i.e., following either spontaneous or treatment-induced remission), in which the prognosis is very variable. An additional distinction must be made between CPH and what is sometimes referred to as "mild" CAH. This last gray area highlights the fact that the histologic features of CPH and CAH really only define the two extremities of what is probably a continuous spectrum of inflammatory liver injury.

ETIOLOGIC FACTORS

After the early definitions of "autoimmune" CAH, it soon became apparent that very similar clinical, biochemical, histologic, and even serologic features can result from any one of several quite distinct etiologic stimuli. Thus CAH may be related to persistent infection with the hepatitis B (HBV),[10] hepatitis delta (HDV),[11] or non-A, non-B (NANB)[12] viruses, to α_1-antitrypsin deficiency, or to Wilson's disease,[9] or it may be drug-induced[13] (Table 14–1). The histologic features of CAH may also be seen at various stages of primary biliary cirrhosis (PBC),[14] primary sclerosing cholangitis (PSC),[15,16] and alcoholic liver disease.[9]

As mentioned above, ANA are not exclusive to AI-CAH. In addition to SLE and other autoimmune disorders, they occur in overtly healthy subjects with a frequency that increases with age (up to 25% at > 60 years)[17] as well as in PSC[18] and in some patients with HBV-CAH or PBC (although in the latter the ANA tend to be anticentromere antibodies). Similarly, SMA with antiactin specificity are found in a wide range of acute and chronic microbial infections including hepatitis A and B, cytomegalovirus, malaria, and even in patients with plantar warts.[19,20] Thus the distinction between AI-CAH and CAH of other etiologies on the basis of seropositivity for ANA and/or SMA can be very difficult, since the finding of either of these autoantibodies may be only coincidental to the underlying liver disease.

Table 14–1 SPECTRUM OF CHRONIC ACTIVE HEPATITIS

Persistent viral infection
   Hepatitis B
   Non-A, non-B
   Delta

Autoimmune
   Classical (ANA/SMA positive); also anti-LSP/anti-
      ASGP-R positive
   ANA/SMA negative
     LKM-positive
     Anti-LSP/anti-ASGP-R-positive
     Anti-SLA-positive

Drug-induced
   α-Methyldopa
   Nitrofurantoin
   Rifampicin/isoniazid
   Oxyphenisatin
   Alcohol?

Metabolic
   Wilson's disease
   α_1-Antitrypsin deficiency
   Alcoholic liver disease?

There is, in addition, a group of patients with CAH who are seronegative for ANA and SMA and in whom no etiologic factor can be identified. Some of these *idiopathic* cases have other features (e.g., concomitant autoallergic conditions) suggestive of an autoimmune diathesis. The remainder constitutes a truly idiopathic group that may include some with occult NANB infections (i.e., with no evidence to support a viral etiology) but also comprises patients whose CAH requires prolonged corticosteroid therapy to maintain remission, suggesting some underlying (possibility autoreactive) immunopathology.

In 1968, Geall et al.[21] attempted to introduce some order into the classification of these various forms of chronic hepatitis by grouping them all under a general heading of "chronic active liver disease" (CALD), but, with advances in diagnostic techniques and greater understanding of the pathogenesis of at least some of these disorders during the subsequent two decades, there is decreasing use of this term.

This chapter deals primarily with hepatocellular immunoautoreactivity in idiopathic CAH. The biliary disorders (PBC and PSC) and HBV-CAH have been considered in detail in preceding chapters and are touched on only in relation to associated immunopathology that might be involved in hepatocellular damage. The term "autoimmune" chronic active hepatitis (AI-CAH) is reserved here for those patients with idiopathic CAH who have circulating ANA and/or SMA and/or LKM antibodies.

IMMUNOGENETICS

In AI-CAH, in common with other autoimmune diseases, there is a high frequency of the HLA allotypes B8 and DR3.[22] Familial AI-CAH is comparatively rare, but healthy first-degree relatives frequently have circulating ANA, SMA, and/or other autoantibodies,[23,24] and those with the B8, DR3 allotypes tend to have a defect in concanavalin A-induced suppressor T-cell function of the same magnitude as that seen in untreated AI-CAH.[25] AI-CAH was also reported to be associated with the immunoglobulin allotype Gm a+ x+[26] but this has not been confirmed by later studies,[27,28] in which segregation and logistic regression analyses failed to find support for either autosomal or sex-linked inheritance of a disease susceptibility gene[28] — suggesting that the disease does not have a simple genetic basis. A high prevalence of HLA B8 and DR3 is also seen in PSC[29,30] but not in other liver disorders.

ANTIGENIC TARGETS OF HEPATOCELLULAR AUTOREACTIVITY

If autoimmune reactions are involved in hepatocellular damage in CAH, it is presumed that the antigenic targets of such autoreactions must be accessible to the immune system in vivo, i.e., expressed on the surfaces of the liver cells. Second, in order to account for the relative organ specificity of the tissue damage, it is further presumed that such antigens must be specific to the liver. It was obvious from the outset that the antigens with which ANA and SMA react fulfill neither of these criteria and that immune reactions against them are more likely to be a consequence than a cause of tissue damage. During the past two decades, efforts have therefore been made to define antigens that conform to one or both of these criteria. Several such components have been identified, and those that have received the most attention are considered here in chronological order.

Liver-Specific Membrane Lipoprotein

Liver-specific membrane lipoprotein (LSP) is a relatively crude but well-standardized[31] macromolecular preparation from normal liver that was first described by Meyer zum Buschenfelde and colleagues[32] and has been found to contain at least two liver-specific antigens: one that appears to be peculiar to the species from which the LSP is derived (i.e., species-specific) and one that is species cross-reactive, in that it can be demonstrated in LSP from human, rat, rabbit, mouse, or bovine liver.[33] It was subsequently shown that this preparation contains fragments of liver plasma membranes and probably also various other macromolecular constituents,[34-36] but, despite its obvious antigenic heterogeneity, use of the term liver-specific membrane lipoprotein to describe the preparation has persisted. For historical reasons, and to avoid confusion, it is retained here.

The finding that humoral and cellular immune reactions (see below) in patients with liver disease could be demonstrated against LSP prepared from different species suggested that the relevant target antigen(s) must be species cross-reactive,[33] but attempts over many years to isolate and characterize these antigens in LSP proved largely fruitless, even when hybridoma technology was applied to the problem. Of several hundred monoclonal anti-LSP antibodies produced in various laboratories,[37-42] only one was found to react with an unequivocally liver-specific epitope expressed on the surfaces of hepatocytes, but this epitope is peculiar to rabbits.[39] However, very recently, four monoclonal antibodies against human LSP have been produced[43] that react with species cross-reactive epitopes on a liver-specific component of the LSP preparation, the hepatic asialoglycoprotein receptor (see below).

Liver-Kidney Microsomal Antigen(s)

Circulating autoantibodies reacting with microsomes in kidney and liver were originally described in patients with idiopathic CAH and were first characterized by Rizetto and colleagues[44] in 1973. Subsequently, apparently similar autoantibodies were found in the sera of patients with drug-induced CAH. It was later found[45] that the antibodies in AI-CAH are distinct from those in drug-induced hepatitis, and the two autoantibodies were designated LKM-1 and LKM-2, respectively.

Recent work has shown that LKM-1 and LKM-2 are both directed at the cytochrome P-450 complex in the smooth endoplasmic reticulum but react with different P-450 isoenzymes.[46,47] Evidence that either antigen may be expressed on the surfaces of hepatocytes is inconclusive, and, since they are also not absolutely specific to the liver, it seems unlikely that they are primary targets of immune-mediated liver damage.

Liver Membrane Antigen

A liver-specific antigen that appears to be the target of the liver membrane antibody (LMA) was described by Meyer zum Buschenfelde and his colleagues[48] in

1979. The main characteristics reported were that this antigen was located on hepatocellular surfaces and was distinct from LSP. Recently, however, the same group of investigators has shown that the antigen (LMAg) can be demonstrated only on the surfaces of mechanically isolated nonviable hepatocytes and is not normally expressed on the surfaces of viable liver cells.[49] They have concluded that it is probably a submembranous component that is exposed by disruption of the plasma membrane.

Asialoglycoprotein Receptor

In 1984, studies in our laboratories revealed that the hepatic asialoglycoprotein receptor is a component of the LSP preparation.[50] This receptor (ASGP-R) is expressed on the surfaces of hepatocytes and is responsible for the endocytic removal of galactose-terminating desialylated glycoproteins, a function that is unique to hepatocytes.[51–53] From cDNA libraries encoding the receptor in human and rat liver, it has been determined that there is marked amino acid sequence homology in ASGP-R from different mammalian species.[54–56] It is thus a functionally and physicochemically, as well as immunochemically[50] liver-specific and species cross-reactive, cell surface-expressed component.

The term "hepatic lectin," originally used to describe this receptor, has now largely fallen into disuse (because of a tendency for confusion with other animal and plant lectins) and will be avoided here.

CELL-MEDIATED IMMUNITY

Early investigations of cellular immune mechanisms that might be involved in autoreactions leading to the characteristic pattern of periportal liver damage in CAH were largely concerned with studies using a variety of in vitro tests of delayed hypersensitivity to crude liver antigen preparations or cytotoxicity test systems with mixed populations of peripheral blood leukocytes as effector cells and, as targets, various heterologous isolated hepatocyte preparations or avian erythrocytes coated with LSP. The consensus opinion derived from these studies was that patients with idiopathic (including autoimmune) CAH had circulating lymphocytes that were "sensitized" to liver antigens and were able to "kill" the various target cells in vitro and that this was true also of patients with HBV-CAH and of some with PBC.[33,57]

It was recognized that these early test systems were unsuitable for investigating T-lymphocyte-mediated cytotoxic reactions, which require histocompatibility between target and effector cells for full expression.[58] This was confirmed by studies using separated T- and non-T-cell populations of peripheral blood lymphocytes from CAH patients and heterologous target cells, which showed that the effector cells are present in the non-T-cell fraction.[59] Subsequent experiments with separated lymphocyte populations established that even when *autologous* hepatocytes from liver biopsies are used as target cells (to overcome the problem of histocompatibility restriction),[60,61] the cytotoxic reactions in AI-CAH are still a function of non-T lymphocytes, i.e., T-cell cytotoxic autoreactions do not seem to occur in AI-CAH. In contrast, in HBV-CAH, both T- and non-T-cell cytotoxic reactions were demonstrable in vitro against patients' own liver cells. An important additional finding is that, whereas non-T cytotoxicity in both AI-CAH and HBV-CAH can be inhibited by preincubating the patients' lymphocytes with LSP, the T-cell cytotoxicity in HBV-CAH cannot be blocked in this way.[60,61]

These findings suggested that, both in AI-CAH and in HBV-CAH, non-T-cell cytotoxic reactions are directed against normal liver antigens in the LSP preparation and that, in HBV-CAH, there is an additional T-cell cytotoxic component that is not directed at such antigens. Further interpretation suggests that the T-cell cytotoxicity in HBV-CAH is directed at either: 1) normal hepatocellular antigens that are not present in the LSP preparation; or 2) viral antigens on the surfaces of the patients' liver cells. To test these hypotheses would require two histocompatible cell lines, one that demonstrably expresses the entire range of normal liver cell surface antigens but is not infected with HBV and the other expressing the full repertoire of HBV genomic products.

Unfortunately, no such cell lines exist. However, indirect evidence supporting the hypothesis that the T-cell reactions are directed at viral antigens was obtained by Mondelli,[62] who showed that in vitro autologous T-cell cytotoxicity in HBV-CAH could be blocked by preincubating the patients' liver cells with antisera against the HBV "core" antigen (HBcAg) but not by anti-HBs antisera. This finding was later confirmed in similar experiments showing blocking of cytotoxicity by monoclonal antibodies against HBcAg[63] or against the HBV e antigen (HBeAg, which is closely related to HBcAg)[64] but not by monoclonal anti-HBs. Additional confirmation came from the finding of T-cell cytotoxic reactions against autologous liver cells expressing HBcAg but not against cells expressing only HBsAg[65] and from the observation that increased numbers of cytotoxic/suppressor (CD8+) T cells are present at the site of tissue injury.[66,67] Other studies have shown that T cells obtained from liver biopsies from HBV-CAH patients exhibit cytotoxic properties in vitro[68] and that clonal expansion of such cells in vitro reveals both CD4+ and CD8+ T cells recognizing HBcAg.[69,70]

Attempts have also been made to elucidate the T-lymphocyte-mediated events in HBV-CAH and in AI-CAH by using an indirect agarose microdroplet assay for T-lymphocyte migratory inhibitory factor (T-LIF) production in response to HBV gene products and to liver autoantigens.[71,72] The finding that T-LIF production by T cells from HBV-CAH patients occurred in response to HBcAg but not to HBsAg[72] confirmed the above implication that HBcAg is the major target of T-cell immunity in this condition. These studies also revealed that T cells in HBV-CAH patients do not recognize LSP — in contrast to AI-CAH, in which LSP-stimulated T-LIF production is an almost universal finding.[71]

Coculture experiments with lymphocytes from patients and normal subjects have shown that, in AI-CAH, the T-LIF production in response to LSP is related to a specific defect in T-suppressor (Ts) control of this autoimmune response.[71] Thus, when normal lymphocytes are cultured with patients' T cells (in a ratio of 1:9) the former are able to "switch off" LSP-stimulated T-LIF production by the latter, but this cannot be achieved by coculturing lymphocytes from different AI-CAH patients. Almost identical results are obtained when ASGP-R is used as the antigen in place of LSP,[73] indicating that this component of LSP is a major T-cell recognition antigen on hepatocytes.

Family studies subsequently revealed that this antigen-specific Ts defect in controlling autoreactivity to ASGP-R in AI-CAH patients is a genetic trait with, possibly, an autosomal dominant mode of inheritance but that it is not HLA-linked.[74] By using different T-cell subpopulations in coculture experiments, it has been possible to show that the defect is restricted to the CD4+ suppressor/inducer

Table 14–2 SUMMARY OF EVIDENCE RELATING TO CELLULAR AND HUMORAL AUTOIMMUNE REACTIONS IN AI-CAH PATIENTS AND THEIR FIRST- AND SECOND-DEGREE RELATIVES AND SPOUSES AND IN PATIENTS WITH HBV-CAH OR PBC

Feature	Patients	Relatives 1st degree	Relatives 2nd degree	Spouses	HBV-CAH	PBC
T-cell cytotoxicity vs. *autologous* hepatocytes	No	—	—	—	Yes	—
Non-T cytotoxicity vs. *autologous* and *heterologous* hepatocytes	Yes	—	—	—	Yes	—
T cells "sensitized" to						
LSP	Yes	Some	No	Some	No	Some
ASGP-R	Yes	No	No	No	No	No
T-suppression defect related to ASGP-R	Yes	Some	Some	No	No	No
Anti-LSP antibodies	Yes	No	No	No	Yes	Yes
Anti-ASGP-R antibodies	Yes	No	No	No	Yes	Rare

subset.[75] In normal subjects, these cells seem to be activated by ASGP-R to suppress the antigen-specific autoreaction, and it is the failure to respond in this way that is a feature of AI-CAH.

About 50% of PBC patients also produce T-LIF in response to LSP but, like normal subjects, these patients' lymphocytes are able to suppress the autoreaction to LSP in AI-CAH in coculture experiments,[73] indicating that the PBC patients do not have a defect in Ts control of the response to LSP. This finding further suggests that PBC patients' lymphocytes recognize an antigen in the LSP complex different from that recognized by T cells in AI-CAH; this hypothesis was confirmed by the observation that T-LIF production in vitro cannot be stimulated by ASGP-R in PBC[73] (Table 14–2).

A very recent study in children[76] has shown that, in PSC, there is also autoreactivity to LSP but not to ASGP-R, suggesting that (as in PBC) T-cell responses to hepatocellular antigens are directed at targets different from those in AI-CAH. Similar detailed studies have not been performed in CAH of other etiologies (e.g., Wilson's disease, α_1-antitrypsin deficiency, NANB infections, or drug-induced CAH) nor with other defined antigens; whether or not analogous autoimmune responses and defects in Ts control involving antigens other than ASGP-R occur in CAH associated with other diseases is unknown at the present time.

HUMORAL IMMUNITY

ANA, SMA, and LKM

Antinuclear and smooth muscle antibodies, as noted above, are part of the diagnostic criteria of AI-CAH. These antibodies often disappear as a response to corticosteroid therapy and may not reappear even during relapses. Also, titers tend to fluctuate, and the antibodies may even disappear without treatment (which may account for some patients with idiopathic CAH). The liver-kidney microsomal (LKM-1) antibody occurs much less frequently and, apart from defining a subgroup of patients with particularly severe disease (which is not to say that severe disease is only associated with this antibody), it is not at all clear that they identify a form of AI-CAH that differs pathogenetically from that in which they are absent. In our experience, adults with LKM-1-positive CAH are usually ANA- and SMA-seronegative, and the LKM-1 antibodies tend to persist (whether or not there is a response to corticosteroid therapy), whereas children with LKM-1-positive CAH are often also positive for ANA and/or SMA, and titers of all three antibodies tend to fluctuate with response to treatment. However, a recent study of a large group of patients with LKM-1-positive CAH,[77] about one-half of whom were young females (<15 years old), found ANA in only one patient (1.5%) and SMA of antiactin specificity in none. Notwithstanding their diagnostic utility, for the reasons already given, these three autoantibodies are unlikely to be primarily related to the pathogenesis of AI-CAH.

Anti-LSP

The early evidence that non-T-lymphocyte-mediated cytotoxic reactions directed at antigens in the LSP preparation occur in AI-CAH and HBV-CAH[59] suggested that antibody-mediated cellular cytotoxic (ADCC) autoreactions might be involved in hepatocellular damage in both conditions. It was not until 1978, however, that direct evidence for circulating autoantibodies against LSP was obtained.[78] Since that time, numerous studies have shown that anti-LSP antibodies occur in almost all patients with AI-CAH who are tested before institution of immunosuppressive therapy.[79] Anti-LSP also occurs at high titers in the majority of patients with acute virus A or B (but not NANB) hepatitis at onset, but titers decline rapidly and patients become seronegative during recovery. These autoantibodies are also present in about 50% of patients with PBC, up to 90% of those with HBV-CAH, and about 20% of alcoholic liver disease patients but are very rare in Wilson's disease, hemochromatosis, NANB-CAH, and other conditions in which there does not appear to be any underlying autoreactive immunopathology.[79]

As with ANA and SMA, anti-LSP antibodies in AI-CAH decrease in titer, and patients often become seronegative when remission is induced by corticosteroids but, unlike ANA and SMA, anti-LSP almost always reappears and/or rises in titer several weeks (often months) in advance of relapses following reduction or withdrawal of corticosteroid therapy.[80] In addition, in all of the chronic liver disorders associated with a high frequency of anti-LSP seropositivity, the antibodies correlate with the presence and severity of periportal liver cell necrosis; this finding, together with the temporal relationship between anti-LSP and response to immunosuppressive therapy and relapse in AI-CAH,[80] suggests that the antibodies may be causally related to liver damage in these conditions. However, the polyantigenic composition of the LSP preparation precludes confident global conclusions of this nature.

In our experience (unpublished observations), a proportion of patients with idiopathic CAH (i.e., ANA-, SMA-, and LKM-seronegative in whom all other possible etiologies have been excluded) are found to be seropositive for anti-LSP and/or anti-ASGP-R (see below) at presentation. These patients all require continued immunosuppressive therapy to maintain remission, and the dynamics of the anti-LSP response are indistinguishable from those in AI-CAH. Whether these patients represent a separate autoimmune subgroup is uncertain, but it is unlikely that their disease is due to occult NANB infection because of the rarity of anti-LSP and anti-ASGP-R in those patients with acute or chronic hepatitis in whom there is good reason to suspect a NANB viral etiology.[79,81,85]

Anti-Anti-LSP

The possibility that control of autoreactions to LSP might be mediated by idio-type/anti-idiotype interactions involving anti-LSP antibodies has been investigated by Kakumu and colleagues[83] by using a competitive inhibition assay in which blocking of the binding of a monoclonal anti-LSP antibody to LSP determinants on the surfaces of SK-Hep-1 cells by $F(ab')_2$ of IgG obtained from anti-LSP-depleted sera of patients was taken as evidence of anti-anti-LSP activity in the sera. These investigators found anti-anti-LSP activity in sera from patients with CPH, from patients who had recovered from acute viral hepatitis, and from healthy medical staff who had had contact with hepatitis patients but found no evidence of anti-anti-LSP in patients with CAH who had active disease. By analogy with the demonstration of antiidiotypic antibodies in animal models of autoimmune thyroid disease[84] and SLE,[85] it was suggested that these anti-anti-LSP antibodies may provide a mechanism for control of autoreactivity to LSP that is complementary to the modulation by T-cell suppression.

This is an attractive hypothesis but, unfortunately, the monoclonal antibody used in these studies is not directed at a liver-specific epitope. In addition, the method employed did not absolutely exclude the possibility that inhibition in the assay might have been due to LSP/anti-LSP immune complexes in the sera, and further experimentation is required to establish whether such antiidiotypic antibodies do indeed exist.

Anti-ASGP-R

Antibodies reacting with ASGP-R have recently been demonstrated in the sera of the majority of patients with AI-CAH or HBV-CAH[82] at titers that correlate with histologic severity. These antibodies are found infrequently in PBC, even in those patients who are anti-LSP seropositive,[82] and while they occur transiently in acute virus A and B hepatitis, they are very rare in acute or chronic NANB infections[81,82] and in other conditions such as Wilson's disease and PSC (unpublished observations). Like anti-LSP, anti-ASGP-R antibodies also disappear rapidly with response to corticosteroids and reappear (but more slowly than anti-LSP) with relapse.

LMA

The liver membrane antibody detected by immunofluorescent staining of isolated hepatocytes[86] was originally thought to be found only in sera from patients with AI-CAH but was subsequently shown to occur in about 50% of patients with PBC and to a lesser extent in other liver disorders.[79] As noted above, the antigenic target of this autoantibody is now thought to be a submembranous component of the liver cell plasma membrane,[49] and there is little evidence to suggest that LMA is causally related to liver damage in CAH.

Anti-SLA

An antibody (anti-SLA) that reacts with a soluble liver antigen (SLA) has recently been detected in the sera of a small group of idiopathic CAH patients who were seronegative for ANA and LKM.[87] Thirty percent of the group had SMA (and therefore conformed to the broader definition of AI-CAH), and 45% had one or more of the following: LMA, rheumatoid factor, and antithyroid or antimitochondrial antibodies. The remaining 25% were seronegative for all of these autoantibodies, but sera were not tested for anti-LSP or anti-ASGP-R, and it is therefore not possible to say whether this group is distinct from the abovementioned patients with anti-LSP-positive idiopathic CAH. The target for anti-SLA is reportedly unrelated to LSP and appears to be a cytosolic liver protein that is also present in kidney and (at lower concentrations) in a wide range of other tissues.[87] Therefore, although it is a potentially useful marker of autoimmunity in this small group of idiopathic CAH patients, it seems unlikely that anti-SLA is primarily related to pathogenesis.

Other Antibodies

A number of other autoantibodies occur occasionally in AI-CAH. These include antimitochondrial antibodies (which make the differential diagnosis from PBC difficult) and gastric parietal cell, reticulin, thyroid microsomal, and thyroglobulin antibodies, which are not specific for liver disease but seem to be part of the overall immunopathology and may reflect concurrent underlying autoimmune disorders of other organs. In addition, antibodies that give a linear polygonal immunofluorescent plasma membrane staining outlining hepatocytes in liver sections fixed with Bouin's solution have been described.[88] The target epitopes of these hepatocyte membrane antibodies (HMA) have not been defined, but at least one appears to be present in polymerized human albumin, and others are demonstrable in LSP. HMA is found more frequently in untreated AI-CAH patients than in those receiving corticosteroids, but it also occurs frequently in HBV-CAH, PBC, acute viral hepatitis (A, B, and NANB), and in a wide range of other liver disorders including hemochromatosis, Wilson's disease, and sarcoidosis, as well as primary sclerosing cholangitis and other causes of extrahepatic biliary obstruction.[88]

In addition to the above, antibodies reacting with chemically induced haptenic alterations of host proteins have been described in certain liver disorders. These include "antihalothane" and "antialcohol" antibodies. The former are found in the sera of patients who develop severe acute hepatitis following multiple halothane anesthesia and are detected by immunofluorescence on isolated hepatocytes from rabbits that have been pretreated with halothane,[89] while the latter are associated with alcoholic liver disease and appear to react with neoantigens formed by covalent binding of acetaldehyde to various cellular macromolecules.[90] In both conditions, sera also contain antibodies that react with normal animal hepatocytes, but it is not known whether the immune reactions against haptenically altered hepatocytes trigger reactions against autoantigens or vice versa.

ANIMAL MODELS OF AI-CAH

The first attempts to induce AI-CAH in animals were made by Meyer zum Bus-chenfelde and colleagues in the late 1960s and early 1970s. These investigators found that by repeatedly immunizing normal rabbits with LSP and LSP-containing liver fractions over a period of many months they could produce a lesion with the histologic appearances of CAH.[91] Although others were unable to reproduce this rabbit model convincingly,[92] these early studies acted as a stimulus to much of the subsequent research into a disorder that, at the time, was still only tentatively considered to be an autoimmune condition.

Later attempts to reproduce this model in rabbits or in mice met with variable success.[93-95] Although the animals produced anti-LSP antibodies and showed LSP-stimulated cellular immune responses in vitro, liver damage did not always occur or was not invariably attributable to induction by LSP. However, recent studies by Mori and colleagues in Japan[96-98] have shown that, in mice, induction of CAH by immunization with LSP is partly strain-dependent (C57 BL/6 being the most susceptible strain) and is inhibited by EDTA, which is routinely used to stabilize LSP preparations[31] and which was not excluded from the immunizing preparations used in many of the earlier studies.

Very recently, in a series of elegant adoptive transfer experiments, the Japanese group has provided persuasive evidence of cellular interactions that are reminiscent of the interplay of cellular immune events that seemingly occur in patients with AI-CAH.[99] Spleen cells from mice in which a CAH-like lesion had been induced by immunization with a 100,000g liver supernatant (containing LSP) were transferred to unimmunized mice, which led to development of a similar lesion in the livers of the recipient mice. These investigators found that the liver damage induced in recipient mice by transfer of nylon wool adherent spleen cells from the hyperimmune (donor) mice is more severe if the donors are first subjected to low-dose (300-rad) irradiation to deplete suppressor T-cell function. However, if this suppressor/cytotoxic T-cell subpopulation is similarly depleted in the *recipient* mice, no liver damage occurs unless the recipients are first reconstituted with spleen cells from normal (untreated) mice — indicating that the transferred donor T cells are not the ultimate effector cells. This conclusion is supported by two additional lines of evidence:

1. [51]Cr labeling of recipient mouse lymphocytes showed that a significant proportion of the inflammatory cells invading the liver after transfer of primed donor T cells are derived from the recipient mice themselves.

2. Total lymphocyte depletion by high-dose (700-rad) irradiation of recipient mice abrogates induction of liver damage by subsequent transfer of primed cells from donor mice.

These findings suggest that the liver damage in the recipient mice is mediated by their own effector lymphocytes that have been recruited and educated by the primed donor cells and are supported by very similar results obtained from analogous studies of experimental allergic encephalomyelitis in rats.[100]

In all of the above studies, LSP or LSP-containing liver fractions have been used for induction of liver damage in the various animal models. Since LSP contains ASGP-R, this antigen must have been present in all of these preparations, but any speculation as to whether it might have been the principal target must await repetition of these experiments using purified ASGP-R as the immunogen.

MECHANISTIC ASPECTS OF IMMUNOSUPPRESSIVE THERAPY IN AI-CAH

The efficacy of corticosteroids (prednisone or prednisolone) with or without azathioprine for the treatment of AI-CAH is now well established.[101] The usual practice is to induce remission with corticosteroids and then to add azathioprine for its steroid-sparing effect. The latter drug cannot be used alone to initially control the disease but, once this has been achieved with corticosteroids, patients can be maintained in remission on lower doses of steroids with azathioprine than without it, and this drug can be used on its own to maintain remission in selected patients.[102]

These treatment regimens have been devised on a largely empirical basis, but developing knowledge of the differential modes of action of corticosteroids and azathioprine reveals that the rationale is in fact based on sound mechanistic principles. The evidence relating to the modes of action of the two drugs also supports the current hypothesis that the principal mechanism of liver damage in AI-CAH involves an ADCC reaction in which circulating autoantibodies against liver cell surface determinants cooperate with a subpopulation of non-T lymphocytes (K cells) to cause hepatocellular injury (Fig. 14–1).

Corticosteroids have rapid and profound effects on T lymphocytes. Although some studies have reported numerical changes in certain subpopulations of T cells in response to corticosteroids,[103] the rapidity of response in vivo and the fact that the effects can be demonstrated in vitro using pharmacologic concentrations of the drug[104] suggest that corticosteroids exert their effects by directly altering function rather than by causing selective depletion of specific subsets of T lymphocytes. The principal effects of corticosteroids in AI-CAH are: 1) to restore suppressor T-cell function; and 2) either by this action or by an additional effect on a separate T-lymphocyte subset, to indirectly suppress immunoglobulin production by B lymphocytes.[105] All of the evidence to date indicates that steroids do not act directly on non-T cells (including B lymphocytes and K cells).

Azathioprine, in contrast, affects killer (K) and natural killer (NK) cells.[106–109] Continuous administration of this drug leads to a gradual reduction in the numbers of these cells in the circulation, requiring 6–12 months before they reach about 5% of normal. Upon cessation of azathioprine therapy, there is a gradual reappearance of K and NK cells, but it may take several months before numbers reach the pretreatment level. If azathioprine acts directly on mature K and NK cells, it might be expected that they would disappear more rapidly. The gradual depletion from the circulation suggests rather loss during normal turnover without replenishment, and it is presumed therefore that the drug acts on K/NK stem cells in the bone marrow.

The contrasting mechanisms of action of the two drugs explains their clinical and serologic effects. The rapid action of corticosteroids on immunoglobulin (including autoantibody) production is reflected in the typical early clinical improvement and the sharp fall in autoantibody titers. The slow effect of azathioprine on the other arm of the ADCC reaction system, the K cells, means that for several months there will be sufficient numbers of these cells circulating to cooperate with

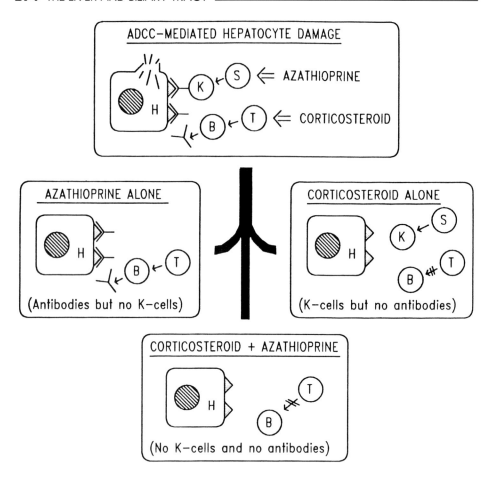

S=Stem cell   K=K-cell   T=T-lymphocyte   B=B-lymphocyte   H=Hepatocyte

▷ =Liver-specific autoantigen (AGP-R?)   ⟩—=Specific autoantibody (anti-AGP-R?)

Figure 14-1   Schematic representation of the mechanisms of action of corticosteroids and azathioprine on antibody-dependent cellular cytotoxic (ADCC) damage to hepatocytes.

autoantibodies (unless they are first reduced by corticosteroids) in ADCC-mediated hepatocellular damage; this fact explains why the drug does not induce remission when used alone. The combined action of the two drugs on the two arms of the ADCC system explains their synergistic effects (Fig. 14-1).

IMMUNOPATHOLOGIC MECHANISMS

It is presumed that control of autoreactivity operates mainly with respect to cell surface antigens, for there seems to be little need in nature to control autoimmune reactions to cryptic antigens that are not normally exposed to the immune system in vivo. The cellular and humoral immune reactions against LSP documented above are difficult to interpret in mechanistic terms because of the antigenic heterogeneity of the preparation, which very likely contains a number of immunogenic components that may be located within the plasma membrane or on intracellular structures and to which the immune system presumably does not have access in vivo. This is not the case with ASGP-R, which is purifiable to homogeneity. This receptor is synthesized in the endoplasmic reticulum and is transported to, and inserted in, the plasma membrane.[110] Structural analyses of the receptor protein indicate that it has a transmembrane disposition such that some 80% of the molecule is expressed on the outer (sinusoidal and basolateral) surface of the hepatocyte.[54–56] Although a variable proportion of the ASGP-R in the liver cell (either nascent receptor protein en route to the plasma membrane or mature ASGP-R participating in cyclical endocytic functions) is attached to various endomembranes, at steady state up to 60% of the receptor in the liver may be expressed on the hepatocyte surfaces.[111] It is thus a component that is normally exposed to the immune system in vivo and against which autoreactions could presumably therefore occur. This fact, in turn, implies that some control of autoreactivity is required to avoid tissue damage.

The available evidence suggests that ASGP-R is indeed recognized by CD4 + T cells in healthy individuals but that these cells are of the subset that normally induce suppressor cells rather than offering help for the proliferation of B- or T-cell effector populations.[75] The finding that there is apparently a defect in this control system in patients with AI-CAH could explain the persistence of autoreactions to hepatocellular antigens, but, since relatives of these patients also have the defect without the disease (or even demonstrable autoreactions), other factors are clearly involved. Either there is some (as yet undiscovered) additional control mechanism that is present in the relatives but lacking in the patients and/or, by analogy with diabetes, some triggering factor (viruses, drugs, alcohol, or other environmental agents) is required. The measles virus has been suggested as one possible triggering agent,[112] but a direct causal relationship has not been established.[113] More concrete support for the involvement of environmental agents comes from the finding that mice infected with murine cytomegalovirus develop anti-LSP responses and (from studies in athymic nude mice infected with the virus) that these autoreactions are under T-lymphocyte control.[114]

Interestingly, in the family studies,[74] while only the probands showed in vitro T-LIF production in response to ASGP-R, 24% of first-degree relatives and 27% of their spouses (but none of the second-degree relatives) did respond in this way to LSP. This response could not be suppressed by coculture with lymphocytes from unrelated normal subjects, and, since none of the relatives or spouses had any evidence of liver disease, these findings suggested that the epitopes in LSP that were recognized by the relatives' lymphocytes are probably cryptic components not normally expressed on hepatocellular surfaces. The finding that as many genetically unrelated spouses as first-degree relatives showed sensitization to these epitopes points to involvement of environmental factors. However, 15% of the healthy first-degree relatives were not only sensitized to these epitopes but also had the Ts defect, relating to control of autoreactivity to ASGP-R. These individuals differed from the probands only with respect to the fact that they did not show sensitization to ASGP-R and were seronegative for anti-LSP and anti-ASGP-R, suggesting that the disease is not precipitated by environmental factors alone.

Taken altogether, the evidence suggests that additional (possibly genetic) factors must be involved both in generating CD4+ effector cells and those capable of providing help for proliferation of B cells responding to specific autoantigens. This hypothesis underlines the immunogenetic evidence (see above), suggesting that AI-CAH does not have a simple genetic basis but is almost certainly due to polygenic interactions with environmental stimuli.

As in AI-CAH, non-T-lymphocytotoxic reactions and circulating anti-LSP and anti-ASGP-R autoantibodies are demonstrable in HBV-CAH (see above). Thus, in both diseases, liver damage could arise through ADCC reactions involving anti-ASGP-R antibodies. HBV-CAH patients do not, however, have circulating T cells that recognize ASGP-R and do not have the defect in Ts control of this autoimmune response. It must be presumed, therefore, that anti-ASGP-R production is related to a virus (HBV)-induced expansion of autoreactive B cells, possibly by recruitment of T-helper cells recognizing viral antigens that (by analogy with halothane hepatitis and alcoholic liver disease) are haptenically coupled to self-components, thereby overriding the normal control mechanism in these patients (Fig. 14–2). Alternatively, the virus might in some way generally downregulate suppression of autoreactivity, but, if this were the case, it might be expected that high titers of a wide range of other organ-specific autoantibodies would be found frequently in HBV-CAH.

In PBC and in PSC, autoimmune recognition of ASGP-R seems to be a rare occurrence but autoreactions to LSP are common. Since, at least in PBC, the patients seem to have normal Ts control of autoreactivity to LSP, it seems likely that the targets of the reactions are not components of LSP that are normally exposed to the immune system in vivo but may be sequestered antigens (possibly of biliary origin, but evidence for this is lacking) and that the immune responses are secondary reactions arising through exposure of the antigens as a consequence of hepatocellular necrosis.

Any hypothesis concerning mechanisms of liver damage in CAH must take account of the characteristic periportal pattern of hepatocellular injury. The location of these hepatocytes relative to portal blood flow may be a factor because this is the area of highest oxygen tension across the liver lobule, which would favor many metabolic events. It is also the area that presumably receives the highest concentrations of potentially tissue-damaging autoantibodies entering the liver. Periportal hepatocytes would thus be more likely to be densely coated with such autoantibodies than liver cells elsewhere in the lobule, making them particularly susceptible to damage via ADCC reactions.

Very recent studies in our laboratories have tested the latter hypothesis.[115] Rat livers were perfused in situ with polyclonal anti-rabbit ASGP-R or monoclonal anti-human ASGP-R antibodies via the portal vein (antegrade) or through the hepatic vein via the vena cava (retrograde) at 10°C (to allow binding of anti-ASGP-R to hepatocyte surfaces without internalization of the antibody). Control perfusions with hyperimmune sera raised against normal human plasma proteins were also performed. The livers were then snap-frozen and sectioned, and the distribution of anti-ASGP-R was investigated by using a sensitive avidin-biotin enzyme-immunohistochemical technique. The anti-ASGP-R was found to be prominently deposited on the surfaces of hepatocytes in the periportal areas of the lobules, with essentially no antibody found attached to midzonal or centrilobular hepatocytes. This pattern was seen in all perfusions with anti-ASGP-R, regardless

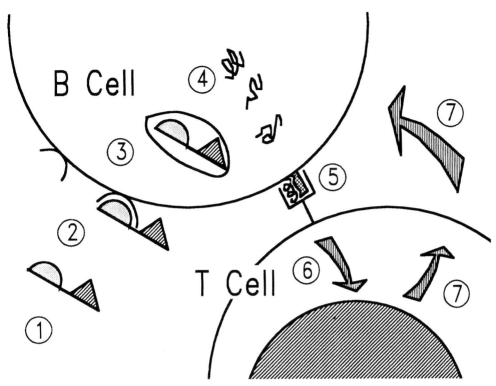

Figure 14–2 Proposed steps in the activation of autoreactive B cells by T cells responsive to foreign (viral) antigens. It is assumed that autoantigens could be linked in a carrier/hapten configuration to viral antigens (1). B cells recognizing the autoantigen would then bind the antigen complex (2) and internalize it (3). Proteolytic digestion would release peptides from the constituent auto- and foreign antigens (4), which would be presented on the B-cell surface with class II molecules (5). T cells reacting with peptide fragments from the foreign antigen would then be activated (6) and, by secreting B-cell growth factors (7), could stimulate B-cell clonal expansion and autoantibody production.

of the direction of perfusion or of the anti-ASGP-R antibody used. There was no deposition of immunoglobulins with the control perfusions. These findings suggest that periportal hepatocytes are preferentially coated by anti-ASGP-R but that this is not related to high concentrations of these antibodies entering via the afferent blood. It may rather be related to preferential expression of the receptor on the surfaces of periportal hepatocytes. If similar events occur in man in vivo, this might account for the characteristic liver lesion in AI-CAH and in HBV-CAH, which are the only chronic liver disorders of the several studied (see above) in which there is a high frequency of circulating anti-ASGP-R antibodies.

CONCLUSIONS

There is now more than ample evidence to indicate that, in AI-CAH, immunogenetic factors combine to precipitate an autoreactive condition that leads to hepatocellular destruction. It also seems likely that environmental factors play a role in triggering these autoreactive events in susceptible individuals. The challenge that now faces those with an interest in hepatology is to define the genetic defect(s) at the chromosomal level and the precise interactions between the cellular and humoral components of the immune system that lead to cell damage. The latter will require definition of the modes of communication between the various subsets of T and B lymphocytes and how they interact with target antigens on the surfaces of hepatocytes.

The earlier studies using relatively crude liver fractions, such as LSP or purified liver plasma membranes, as a source of antigens for the study of hepatocellular autoreactions, provided valuable information, but the emphasis must now be placed on defining specific targets. One such target, ASGP-R, has been identified, but others may be equally important — although theoretically a cytotoxic reaction against only one cell surface component should be sufficient to cause cell damage. It is interesting to note that in other autoimmune disorders such as Graves' disease, myasthenia gravis, and insulin-dependent diabetes, the principal target antigens have been found to be receptors (for thyroid stimulating hormone, acetylcholine, and insulin, respectively) that, like the ASGP-R, perform functions peculiar to the affected tissues.

Dissection of the ASGP-R molecule to identify submolecular domains (epitopes) that are recognized by CD4+ suppressor/inducer cells in normal subjects and to determine whether these are the same epitopes recognized by anti-ASGP-R autoantibodies (which may not be the case) is essential to elucidation of the mechanisms whereby control of autoreactivity is maintained or lost and of how the cellular and humoral interactions lead to hepatocellular damage. Such studies will also be important to determine whether anti-ASGP-R antibodies in AI-CAH and HBV-CAH recognize the same or different epitopes and to define the mechanisms by which the virus manages to override control of autoreactivity.

From a more practical clinical standpoint, identification of the target epitopes of hepatocellular autoantibodies may give rise to a new generation of laboratory tests for the diagnosis and monitoring of patients with various liver disorders. We have been routinely using anti-LSP antibodies in our unit for several years for monitoring corticosteroid therapy in AI-CAH and as part of the laboratory investigations into what is probably one of the most difficult diagnostic problems, namely, the differentiation of idiopathic (autoimmune?) CAH from NANB-CAH. The tedium of the present methods for anti-LSP determination thus far has precluded their wider application, for example, in the differentiation of HBV-CAH from HBV-CPH in the absence of a liver biopsy. Identification of specific epitopes that are targets of these autoantibodies should make the development of routine test systems, based on synthetic peptides, a much more practical proposition.

REFERENCES

1. Saint EG, King WE, Joske RA, et al: The course of infectious hepatitis with special reference to prognosis and the chronic stage. *Aust Ann Med* 2:113–127, 1956.
2. Waldenstrom J: Leber, Blutproteine und Nahrungseiweiss. *Dtsch Z Verdau Stoffwechselkr* 15:113–119, 1950.

3. Bearn AG, Kunkel HG, Slater RJ: The problem of chronic liver disease in young women. *Am J Med* 21:3–15, 1956.

4. Joske RA, King WE: The "LE cell" phenomenon in active chronic viral hepatitis. *Lancet* ii:477–479, 1955.

5. MacKay IR, Taft LI, Cowling DC: Lupoid hepatitis. *Lancet* ii:1323–1326, 1956.

6. Gurian LE, Rogoff TM, Ware AJ, et al: The immunologic diagnosis of chronic active "autoimmune" hepatitis: distinction from systemic lupus erythematosus. *Hepatology* 5:397–402, 1985.

7. Rizetto M, Bianchi FB, Doniach D: Characterization of the microsomal antigen related to a subclass of active chronic hepatitis. *Immunology* 26:589–601, 1974.

8. Odievre M, Maggiore G, Homberg JC, et al: Seroimmunologic classification of chronic hepatitis in 57 children. *Hepatology* 3:407–409, 1983.

9. Ludwig J: Morphology of chronic active hepatitis: Differential diagnosis and therapeutic implications. In Czaja AJ, Dickson ER: *Chronic Active Hepatitis: The Mayo Clinic Experience.* New York, Marcel Dekker, 1986, pp 83–104.

10. Hoofnagle JH: Chronic type B hepatitis. *Gastroenterology* 84:422–424, 1983.

11. Fagan E, Vergani D, Williams R: Delta hepatitis. *Lancet* ii:1322–1323, 1987.

12. Rakela J, Taswell HF, Ludwig J: Chronic non-A, non-B hepatitis. In Czaja AJ, Dickson ER: *Chronic Active Hepatitis: The Mayo Clinic Experience.* New York, Marcel Dekker, 1986, pp 153–170.

13. Ludwig J, Axelsen R: Drug effects on the liver: an updated tabular compilation of drugs and drug-related hepatic diseases. *Dig Dis Sci* 28:651–666, 1983.

14. MacSween RNM: Primary biliary cirrhosis. In MacSween RNM, Anthony PP, Scheuer PJ: *Pathology of the Liver.* New York, Churchill Livingstone, 1979, pp 306–314.

15. Chapman RWG, Arborgh BAM, Rhodes JM, et al: Primary sclerosing cholangitis: a review of its clinical features, cholangiography and hepatic histology. *Gut* 21:870–877, 1980.

16. Lindor KD, Wiesner RH, LaRusso NF, et al: Chronic active hepatitis: overlap with primary biliary cirrhosis and primary sclerosing cholangitis. In Czaja AJ, Dickson ER: *Chronic Active Hepatitis: The Mayo Clinic Experience.* New York, Marcel Dekker, pp 171–187, 1986.

17. Tan EM: Autoantibodies to nuclear antigens (ANA). *Adv Immunol* 33:167–240, 1982.

18. Zauli D, Schrumpf E, Crespi C, et al: An autoantibody profile in primary sclerosing cholangitis. *J Hepatol* 5:14–18, 1987.

19. Lidman K: Clinical diagnosis in patients with smooth muscle antibodies. *Acta Med Scand* 200:403–407, 1976.

20. Andersen P: Incidence and titres of smooth muscle antibodies in human sera. *Acta Pathol Microbiol Scand [c]* 87:11–16, 1979.

21. Geall MG, Schoenfield LJ, Summerskill WHJ: Classification and treatment of chronic active liver disease. *Gastroenterology* 55:724–729, 1968.

22. MacKay IR, Tait DB: HLA associations with autoimmune type chronic active hepatitis: identification of B8-DRw3 haplotype by family studies. *Gastroenterology* 79:95, 1980.

23. Galbraith RM, Smith M, Mackenzie RM, et al: High prevalence of seroimmunologic abnormalities in relatives of patients with active chronic hepatitis or primary biliary cirrhosis. *N Engl J Med* 290:63–69, 1974.

24. Salaspuro MP, Laitinen OI, Lehtola J, et al: Immunological parameters, viral antibodies, and biochemical and histological findings in relatives of patients with chronic active hepatitis and primary biliary cirrhosis. *Scand J Gastroenterol* 11:313–320, 1976.

25. Nouri-Aria KT, Donaldson PT, Hegarty JE, et al: HLA A1-B8-DR3 and suppressor cell function in first-degree relatives of patients with autoimmune chronic active hepatitis. *J Hepatol* 1:235–241, 1985.

26. Whittingham S, Mathews JD, Scanfield MS, et al: Interaction of HLA and Gm in autoimmune chronic active hepatitis. *Clin Exp Immunol* 43:80–86, 1981.

27. Walsh LJ, Cox DW: Immunoglobulin (Gm) markers and α-1 antitrypsin (pi) types in rheumatoid arthritis and early onset chronic active hepatitis. *J Immunogenet* 11:115–120, 1984.

28. Krawitt EL, Kilby AE, Albertini RJ, et al: Immunogenetic studies of autoimmune chronic active hepatitis: HLA, immunoglobulin allotypes and autoantibodies. *Hepatology* 7:1305–1310, 1987.

29. Schrumpf E, Fausa O, Forre O, et al: HLA antigens and immunoregulatory T cells in ulcerative colitis associated with hepatobiliary disease. *Scand J Gastroenterol* 17:187–191, 1982.

30. Chapman RW, Varghese Z, Gaul R, et al: Association of primary sclerosing cholangitis with HLA-B8. *Gut* 24:38–41, 1983.

31. McFarlane IG, Wojcicka BM, Zucker GM, et al: Purification and characterization of human liver-specific membrane lipoprotein (LSP). *Clin Exp Immunol* 27:381–390, 1977.

32. Meyer zum Buschenfelde KH, Miescher PA: Liver specific antigens, purification and characterization. *Clin Exp Immunol* 10:89–102, 1972.

33. McFarlane IG: Autoimmunity in liver disease. *Clin Sci* 67:569–578, 1984.

34. De Kretser TA, McFarlane IG, Eddleston ALWF, et al: A species nonspecific liver plasma membrane antigen and its involvement in chronic active hepatitis. *Biochem J* 186:679–685, 1980.

35. Lebwohl NA, Gerber MA: Characterization and demonstration of human liver-specific protein (LSP) and apo-LSP. *Clin Exp Immunol* 46:435–442, 1981.

36. Jensen DM, Hall C, Majewski T: The plasma membrane origin of liver-specific protein (LSP). *Liver* 3:213–219, 1983.

37. Lambert KJ, Major GN, Welsh CJR, et al: Production and preliminary characterization of monoclonal antibodies to human liver-specific protein (LSP). *Liver* 4:122–127, 1984.

38. Murakami H, Kuriki J, Kakumu S, et al: The specificity of human liver membrane lipoprotein: studies with monoclonal antibodies. *Hepatology* 4:192–198, 1984.

39. Poralla T, Dippold HP, Dienes M, et al: A monoclonal antibody against an organ-specific liver-cell-membrane antigen in rabbits. *J Immunol Methods* 68:341–348, 1984.

40. Kenna JG, Major GN, Lambert KJ, et al: Murine monoclonal antibodies against liver-specific lipoprotein (LSP) defining three antigenic sites which differ in tissue- and species-distribution and subcellular location. *Liver* 5:13–20, 1985.

41. Wiedmann KH, Trejdosiewicz LK, Goodall AH, et al: Analysis of the antigenic composition of liver-specific lipoprotein using murine monoclonal antibodies. *Gut* 26:510–517, 1985.

42. Poralla T, Manns M, Dienes HP, et al: Analysis of liver-specific protein (LSP) using murine monoclonal antibodies. *Eur J Clin Invest* 17:360–367, 1987.

43. McSorley CG, Isaac JE, McFarlane BM, et al: Production of murine monoclonal antibodies against a liver-specific, species cross-reactive antigen in the liver-specific lipoprotein (LSP) preparation. *J Immunol Methods* 114:161–166, 1988.

44. Rizzetto M, Swana G, Doniach D: Microsomal antibodies in active chronic hepatitis and other disorders. *Clin Exp Immunol* 15:331–344, 1973.

45. Homberg JC, Andre C, Abuaf N: A new anti-liver-kidney microsomal antibody (anti-LKM2) in tienilic acid-induced hepatitis. *Clin Exp Immunol* 55:561–570, 1984.

46. Alvarez F, Bernard O, Homberg JC, et al: Anti-liver-kidney microsome antibody recognizes a 50,000 molecular weight protein of the endoplasmic reticulum. *J Exp Med* 161:1231–1236, 1985.

47. Beaune P, Dansette PM, Mansuy D, et al: Human anti-endoplasmic reticulum autoantibodies appearing in a drug-induced hepatitis are directed against a human liver cytochrome P-450 that hydroxylates the drug. *Proc Natl Acad Sci USA* 84:551–555, 1987.

48. Meyer zum Buschenfelde KH, Manns M, Hutteroth TH, et al: LM-Ag and LSP — two different target antigens involved in the immunopathogenesis of chronic active hepatitis? *Clin Exp Immunol* 37:205–212, 1979.

49. Gerken G, Manns M, Ramadori G, et al: Liver membrane autoantibodies in chronic active hepatitis: studies on mechanically and enzymatically isolated rabbit hepatocytes. *J Hepatol* 5:65–74, 1987.

50. McFarlane IG, McFarlane BM, Major GN, et al: Identification of the hepatic asialoglycoprotein receptor (hepatic lectin) as a component of liver specific membrane lipoprotein (LSP). *Clin Exp Immunol* 55:347–354, 1984.

51. McFarlane IG: Hepatic clearance of serum glycoproteins. *Clin Sci* 64:127–135, 1983.

52. Schwartz AL: The hepatic asialoglycoprotein receptor. *CRC Crit Rev Biochem* 16:207–233, 1984.

53. Steer CJ, Ashwell G: Hepatic membrane receptors for glycoproteins. In Popper H, Schaffner F: *Progress in Liver Diseases,* Vol VIII. New York, Grune & Stratton, 1986, pp 99–123.

54. Drickamer K, Mamon JF, Binns G, et al: Primary structure of the rat liver asialoglycoprotein receptor: structural evidence for multiple polypeptide species. *J Biol Chem* 259:770–778, 1984.

55. Spiess M, Schwartz A, Lodish HF: Sequence of human asialoglycoprotein receptor cDNA. *J Biol Chem* 260:1979–1982, 1985.

56. Spiess M, Lodish HF: Sequence of a second human asialoglycoprotein receptor: conservation of two receptor genes during evolution. *Proc Natl Acad Sci USA* 82:6465–6469, 1985.

57. Vento S, Eddleston ALWF: Immunological aspects of chronic active hepatitis. *Clin Exp Immunol* 68:225–232, 1987.

58. Zinkernagel RM, Doherty PC: MHC-restricted cytotoxic T cells: studies on the biological role of polymorphic major transplantation antigens determining T-cell restriction-specificity, function and responsiveness. In Kunkel HG, Dixon FJ: *Advances in Immunology,* Vol 27. Academic Press, New York, 1979, pp 51–177.

59. Cochrane MAG, Moussouros A, Thomson AD, et al: Antibody-dependent cell-mediated (K-cell) cytotoxicity against isolated hepatocytes in chronic active hepatitis. *Lancet* 1:441–444, 1976.

60. Mieli-Vergani G, Vergani D, Jenkins PJ, et al: Lymphocyte cytotoxicity to autologous hepatocytes in HBsAg-negative chronic active hepatitis. *Clin Exp Immunol* 38:16–21, 1979.

61. Mieli-Vergani G, Vergani G, Portmann B, et al: Lymphocyte cytotoxicity to autologous hepatocytes in HBsAg-positive chronic liver disease. *Gut* 23:1029–1036, 1982.

62. Mondelli M, Mieli-Vergani G, Alberti A, et al: Specificity of T-lymphocyte cytotoxicity to autologous hepatocytes in chronic hepatitis B virus infection: evidence that T cells are directed against HBV core antigen expressed on hepatocytes. *J Immunol* 129:2773–2778, 1982.

63. Mondelli M, Eddleston ALWF: Mechanisms of liver cell injury in acute and chronic hepatitis B. *Semin Liver Dis* 4:47–58, 1984.

64. Pignatelli M, Waters J, Lever A, et al: Cytotoxic T-cell responses to the nucleocapsid

proteins of HBV in chronic hepatitis. Evidence that antibody modulation may cause protracted infection. *J Hepatol* 4:15–21, 1985.

65. Naumov NV, Mondelli M, Alexander GJM, et al: Relationship between expression of hepatitis B virus antigens in isolated hepatocytes and autologous lymphocyte cytotoxicity in patients with chronic hepatitis B virus infection. *Hepatology* 4:63–68, 1984.

66. Eggink HF, Houthoff HJ, Huitema S, et al: Cellular and humoral immune reactions in chronic active liver disease. I. Lymphocyte subsets in liver biopsies. *Clin Exp Immunol* 50:17–24, 1982.

67. Pape GR, Rieber EP, Eisenburg J, et al: Involvement of the cytotoxic/suppressor T cell subset in liver tissue injury of patients with acute and chronic liver diseases. *Gastroenterology* 85:657–662, 1983.

68. Hoffmann RM, Rieber EP, Eisenburg J, et al: Cytotoxic T lymphocyte clones derived from liver tissue of patients with chronic hepatitis B. *Hepatology* 5:980, 1985, (Abstr).

69. Ferrari C, Penna A, Giuberti T, et al: Intrahepatic nucleocapsid antigen-specific T cells in chronic active hepatitis B. *J Immunol* 139:2050–2058, 1987.

70. Ferrari C, Penna A, Degliantoni A, et al: Cellular immune response to hepatitis B virus antigens. An overview. *J Hepatol* 7:21–33, 1988.

71. Vento S, Hegarty JE, Bottazzo GF, et al: Antigen-specific suppressor cell function in autoimmune chronic active hepatitis. *Lancet* i:1200–1204, 1984.

72. Vento S, Hegarty JE, Alberti A, et al: T lymphocyte sensitisation to hepatitis BcAg and T cell-mediated unresponsiveness to hepatitis BsAg in hepatitis B virus-related chronic liver disease. *Hepatology* 5:192–197, 1985.

73. Vento S, O'Brien CJ, McFarlane BM, et al: T-lymphocyte sensitisation to hepatocyte antigens in autoimmune chronic active hepatitis and primary biliary cirrhosis: evidence for different underlying mechanisms and different antigenic determinants as targets. *Gastroenterology* 91:810–817, 1986.

74. O'Brien CJ, Vento S, Donaldson PT, et al: Cell-mediated immunity and suppressor-T-cell defects to liver-derived antigens in families of patients with autoimmune chronic active hepatitis. *Lancet* i:350–353, 1986.

75. Vento S, O'Brien CJ, McFarlane IG, et al: T-cell inducers of suppressor lymphocytes control liver-directed autoreactivity. *Lancet* i:886–887, 1987.

76. Mieli-Vergani G, Lobo-Yeo A, McFarlane BM, et al: Different immune mechanisms leading to autoimmunity in primary sclerosing cholangitis and autoimmune chronic active hepatitis of childhood. *Hepatology,* 9:198–203, 1989.

77. Homberg JC, Abuaf N, Bernard O, et al: Chronic active hepatitis associated with antiliver/kidney microsome antibody type 1: a second type of "autoimmune" hepatitis. *Hepatology* 7:1333–1339, 1987.

78. Jensen DM, McFarlane IG, Portmann B, et al: Detection of antibodies directed against a liver-specific membrane lipoprotein in patients with acute and chronic active hepatitis. *N Engl J Med* 299:1–7, 1978.

79. McFarlane IG, Williams R: Review: liver membrane antibodies. *J Hepatol* 1:313–319, 1985.

80. McFarlane IG, Hegarty JE, McSorley CG, et al: Antibodies to liver-specific protein predict outcome of treatment withdrawal in autoimmune chronic active hepatitis. *Lancet* ii:954–956, 1984.

81. Vento S, McFarlane BM, McSorley CG, et al: Liver autoreactivity in acute virus A, B and non-A, non-B hepatitis. *J Clin Lab Immunol* 25:1–7, 1988.

82. McFarlane BM, McSorley CG, Vergani D, et al: Serum autoantibodies reacting with the asialoglycoprotein receptor protein (hepatic lectin) in acute and chronic liver disorders. *J Hepatol* 3:196–205, 1986.

83. Tsubouchi A, Yoshioka K, Kakumu S: Naturally occurring serum antiidiotypic antibody against antiliver-specific membrane lipoprotein in patients with hepatitis. *Hepatology* 5:752–757, 1985.

84. Zanetti M, Bigazzi PE: Anti-idiotypic immunity and autoimmunity. I. In vitro and in vivo effects of anti-idiotypic antibodies to spontaneously occurring autoantibodies to rat thyroglobulin. *Eur J Immunol* 11:187–195, 1981.

85. Hahn BH: Suppression of autoimmune diseases with anti-idiotypic antibodies: murine lupus nephritis as a model. *Springer Semin Immunopathol* 7:25–34, 1984.

86. Hopf U, Meyer zum Buschenfelde KH, Arnold W: Detection of a liver-membrane autoantibody in HBsAg-negative chronic active hepatitis. *N Engl J Med* 294:578–582, 1976.

87. Manns M, Gerken G, Kyriatsoulis A, et al: Characterisation of a new subgroup of autoimmune chronic active hepatitis by autoantibodies against a soluble liver antigen. *Lancet* i:292–294, 1987.

88. Lee WM, Shelton LL, Galbraith RM: Antibodies to hepatocyte membrane antigens in chronic liver disease: detection by immunofluorescence after Bouin's fixation. *J Histochem Cytochem* 31:1246–1249, 1983.

89. Neuberger J, Kenna JG: Halothane hepatitis: a model of immune mediated drug hepatotoxicity. *Clin Sci,* 72:263–270, 1987.

90. Neuberger J, Williams R: Immunology of drug and alcohol-induced liver disease. In Wright R, Hodgson HJF: *Bailliere's Clinical Gastroenterology,* Vol 1, No. 3, 1987, pp 707–722.

91. Meyer zum Buschenfelde KH, Kossling FK, Miescher PA: Experimental chronic active hepatitis in rabbits following immunization with human liver proteins. *Clin Exp Immunol* 11:99–108, 1972.

92. Feighery C, McDonald GSA, Greally JF, et al: Histological and immunological investigation of liver-specific protein (LSP) immunized rabbits compared with patients with liver disease. *Clin Exp Immunol* 45:143–151, 1981.

93. Bartholomaeus WN, Reed WD, Joske RA, et al: Autoantibody responses to liver-specific lipoprotein in mice. *Immunology* 43:219–226, 1981.

94. Uibo RM, Helin KJ, Krohn KJE: Immunological reactions to liver specific membrane lipoprotein (LSP) in experimental autoimmune liver disease in rabbits. *Clin Exp Immunol* 48:505–512, 1982.

95. Kuriki J, Murakami H, Kakumu S, et al: Experimental autoimmune hepatitis in mice after immunization with syngeneic liver proteins together with the polysaccharide of *Klebsiella pneumoniae. Gastroenterology* 84:596–603, 1983.

96. Mori Y, Mori T, Yoshida H, et al: Study of cellular immunity in experimental autoimmune hepatitis in mice. *Clin Exp Immunol* 57:85–92, 1984.

97. Mori Y, Mori T, Ueda S, et al: Study of cellular immunity in experimental autoimmune hepatitis in mice: transfer of spleen cells sensitized with liver proteins. *Clin Exp Immunol* 61:577–584, 1985.

98. Mori T, Mori Y, Yoshida H, et al: Cell-mediated cytotoxicity of sensitized spleen cells against target liver cells — in vivo and in vitro study with a mouse model of experimental autoimmune hepatitis. *Hepatology* 5:770–777, 1985.

99. Ogawa M, Mori Y, Mori T, et al: Adoptive transfer of experimental autoimmune hepatitis in mice — cellular interaction between donor and recipient mice. *Clin Exp Immunol* 73:276–282, 1988.

100. Holda JH, Silberg D, Swanborg RH: Autoimmune effector cells. IV. Induction of experimental allergic encephalomyelitis in Lewis rats without adjuvant. *J Immunol* 130:732–734, 1983.

101. Czaja AJ: Treatment strategies in chronic active hepatitis. In Czaja AJ, Dickson ER: *Chronic Active Hepatitis: The Mayo Clinic Experience.* New York, Marcel Dekker, 1986, pp 247–267.

102. Stellon AJ, Keating JJ, Johnsons PJ, et al: Maintenance of remission in autoimmune chronic active hepatitis with azathioprine after corticosteroid withdrawal. *Hepatology* 8:781–784, 1988.

103. Thomas HC, Brown D, Labrooy J, et al: T cell subsets in autoimmune and HBV induced chronic liver disease: a review of the abnormalities and the effects of treatment. *J Clin Immunol* 2:575–605, 1982.

104. Nouri-Aria KT, Hegarty JE, Alexander GJM, et al: Effects of corticosteroids on suppressor cell activity in autoimmune and viral chronic active hepatitis. *N Engl J Med* 307:1310–1304, 1982.

105. Nouri-Aria KT, Hegarty JE, Alexander GJM, et al: IgG production in "autoimmune" chronic active hepatitis. Effect of prednisolone on T and B lymphocyte function. *Clin Exp Immunol* 61:290–296, 1985.

106. Campbell AC, Skinner JM, MacLennan IC, et al: Immunosuppression in the treatment of inflammatory bowel disease. II. The effects of azathioprine on lymphoid cell populations in a double blind trial in ulcerative colitis. *Clin Exp Immunol* 24:249–258, 1976.

107. Prince HE, Ettenger RB, Dorey FJ, et al: Azathioprine suppression of natural killer activity and antibody-dependent cellular cytotoxicity in renal transplant recipients. *J Clin Immunol* 4:312–318, 1984.

108. Pedersen BK, Beyer JM, Rasmussen A, et al: Azathioprine as single drug in the treatment of rheumatoid arthritis induces complete suppression of natural killer cell activity. *Acta Pathol Microbiol Immunol Scand [C]* 92:221–225, 1984.

109. Pedersen BK, Beyer JM: A longitudinal study of the influence of azathioprine on natural killer cell activity. *Allergy* 41:286–289, 1986.

110. Nakada H, Sawamura T, Tashiro Y: Biosynthesis and insertion of a hepatic binding protein specific for asialo-glycoproteins into rough endoplasmic reticulum membranes. *J Biochem (Tokyo)* 89:135–141, 1981.

111. Bischoff J, Lodish HF: Two asialo-glycoprotein receptor polypeptides in human hepatoma cells. *J Biol Chem* 262:11825–11832, 1987.

112. Robertson DAF, Zhang SL, Guy EC, et al: Persistent measles virus genome in autoimmune chronic active hepatitis. *Lancet* ii:9–11, 1987.

113. Black FL: Persistent measles virus genome in autoimmune chronic active hepatitis: cause or coincidence? *Hepatology* 8:186–187, 1988.

114. Bartholomaeus WN, O'Donoghue H, Reed WD: Thymus dependence of autoantibody responses to liver-specific lipoprotein in the mouse. *Clin Exp Immunol* 55:541–545, 1984.

115. McFarlane BM, Sipos J, Gove CD, et al: Antibodies against the hepatic asialoglycoprotein receptor preferentially coat periportal hepatocytes in the in situ perfused rat liver. *Gut.* 29:A1461–A1462, 1988 (Abstr).

CHAPTER 15

Immune-Mediated Drug Reactions

JAMES NEUBERGER

INTRODUCTION

Drug-associated liver damage is most usefully classified on the basis of the mechanism of toxicity. Type I or predictable drug reactions occur as a consequence of the intrinsic properties of the drug and are dose-dependent. The classical model of this type of hepatotoxin is acetaminophen. With very few exceptions, all xenobiotics require metabolic activation for the expression of hepatotoxicity. Acetaminophen is metabolized by the mixed function oxidase system in the liver and to a lesser extent in other organs such as the kidney and intestine, with the production of reactive metabolites. Once the normal detoxifying pathways are saturated, these metabolites (N-acetyl-p-benzoquinone imine) interact with cellular macromolecules, and cellular death ensues. Hence liver cell necrosis may occur either as a consequence of excessive ingestion (as in deliberate self-poisoning) or when the normal detoxifying pathways are reduced (as in severe disease or malnutrition). Since it is possible to study these reactions in animal models, logical strategies for treatment of toxicity can be developed.

In contrast to the predictable reactions are the idiosyncratic (type II) reactions. These reactions are dose-independent and are either attributed to metabolism of the drug through a usually minor route of metabolism or as a consequence of immune involvement. Increased metabolism of a drug through a usually minor route may arise because of a genetic defect in one of the drug-metabolizing enzymes or an alteration in drug metabolizing activity associated with one of many factors such as age, sex, concomitant drug ingestion (including alcohol and smoking), diet, and pre-existing disease. The evidence for possible involvement of the immune

I am grateful to Miss Veronica Foster for her assistance in typing this manuscript.

system in the pathogenesis of some instances of drug hepatotoxicity is the subject of this chapter.

FEATURES OF IMMUNE-MEDIATED DRUG HEPATOTOXICITY

The diagnosis of drug-related liver damage is almost always based on circumstantial evidence relating to the drug ingested, the onset and pattern of liver damage after exposure to the drug, and the exclusion of other causes of liver dysfunction. Clinically, the patient may present with an acute hepatitis, which may rarely progress to fulminant hepatic failure, when the mortality approaches 100%, or with chronic liver disease, manifest as either chronic active hepatitis or an established cirrhosis. Usually, the signs and symptoms rapidly resolve on discontinuation of the drug, although in some instances, the liver lesion may continue to progress. Involvement of the immune system in the pathogenesis of the liver damage is suggested by a number of clinical and serologic features (Table 15–1). The incidence of this type of reaction in humans is low, and the interval between first exposure to the drug and the development of liver dysfunction is variable but is usually less than 5 weeks. Thus there will either be a sensitizing period or, as in the case of anesthetic-related liver damage, a history of previous exposure to the agent. Associated clinical symptoms may include a skin rash, arthralgia, and pyrexia. Serologic features include a peripheral eosinophilia, circulating immune complexes, blood dyscrasias, and organ-nonspecific autoantibodies. Histologic examination of the liver using conventional stains rarely shows specific features, although eosinophilic infiltration may be found. Cross-reaction between drugs with a

Table 15–1 FEATURES OF IMMUNE-MEDIATED DRUG REACTIONS

Clinical
    Low incidence
    Not dose-related
    Previous exposure/sensitizing period
    Onset usually within 1–5 weeks
    Prompt response on challenge
    Arthralgia
    Fever
    Rash
    Blood dyscrasia

Serologic
    Eosinophilia
    Immune complexes
    Organ-nonspecific autoantibodies
    "Drug"-related antibodies

Histologic
    Eosinophilic infiltration
    Granulomatous infiltration

similar structure, as with the halogenated hydrocarbon volatile and enflurane or the nitrofurans furazolidine and nifuroxime,[1,2] may occur as a consequence of similar routes of metabolism rather than cross-sensitization.

Distinction between immune phenomena arising as a consequence of liver cell damage rather than through involvement in the pathogenesis of the liver damage is difficult. It will be evident that none of these features can be considered unique to immunologic involvement. Finally, it must be appreciated that immune responses to drug-related antigens may occur as a consequence of liver cell necrosis following a direct hepatotoxic reaction.[3,4]

POSSIBLE MECHANISMS OF DRUG-ASSOCIATED LIVER DAMAGE

Immune damage to the hepatocyte may occur as a consequence of one or more of a number of different mechanisms. These include direct lymphocyte-mediated cytotoxicity, antibody-dependent cell-mediated cytotoxicity antibody-dependent complement-mediated cytotoxicity, by immune complex, mediated damage or, theoretically, antibody inhibition of a compound vital to cellular function. The occurrence of immune-mediated cell damage may arise as a consequence of disturbance of the normal control mechanisms, so that the pre-existing repertoire of cell-damaging reactions may no longer be held in check. Alternatively, the drug may lead to the generation of a new antigen and thus to immune recognition and cell damage. The first mechanism outlined above involves breakdown of tolerance, so a drug that inhibits the normal lymphocyte suppressor function may result in the development of an autoimmune type of disease. Such a mechanism may operate in the case of alpha-methyl dopa toxicity. Kirtland and colleagues[5] have shown that exposure both in vivo and in vitro of normal human lymphocytes to therapeutic levels of methyl dopa is associated with a reduction in the activity of concanavalin A (con A)-induced suppressor cells. This was thought to be mediated by reduction of the intracytoplasmic cyclic AMP levels. Similar results have been shown for both ethanol and halothane.[6] A global reduction in suppressor cell activity might be expected to result in the appearance of organ-nonspecific autoantibodies, and indeed several types of presumed immune-mediated hepatitis are associated with autoantibodies. Possible drugs include iproniazid, halothane, ethanol, tienilic acid, clometacin, and chlorpromazine.[7] It is, however, unlikely that such a drug-induced reduction in suppressor cell activity plays a part in the pathogenesis of liver cell damage: the autoantibodies are directed against intracellular components (such as actin and mitochondrial and nuclear components). Such autoantibodies may also be a feature of liver damage in direct hepatotoxicity.[8] A global reduction in the control of immune regulation might be expected to result in the appearance of damage to other organs as well as the liver. Although alpha-methyl dopa may be associated with both an autoimmune hemolytic anemia and chronic active hepatitis, such an association is rare. Few drugs are associated with immune-mediated damage to more than one organ. If a drug induces liver damage because of a reduction in the control of immune regulation, then the drug effect must be at the level of the antigen-specific suppressor cell; there is as yet no evidence to support this concept.

Localization of the presumed immune response to the liver may occur because the liver is the major site of drug metabolism and therefore the site of generation of antigens. As indicated above, almost all drugs require metabolism for expression of toxicity, and this is usually with the production of reactive metabolites. The reactive metabolites may bind to and alter the immunogenicity of the normal cellular macromolecules, thereby generating neoantigens. Since there is good evidence[9] for translocation of proteins generated at the endoplasmic reticulum—the predominant site within the liver of drug metabolism—to the plasma membrane, it is conceivable that these putative altered antigens may be accessible for immune recognition, thereby initiating a cell-damaging response. Whether such cell surface antigens can initiate an immune response is not certain because it still is unclear whether the normal hepatocyte expresses the HLA antigens necessary for antigen presentation.[10]

EVIDENCE FOR A PATHOGENIC IMMUNE RESPONSE

Against this theoretical background for the development of immune-mediated drug hepatotoxicity, the evidence for immune involvement in drug hepatotoxicity can be evaluated. Many drugs are implicated as triggers in immune-mediated reactions (Table 15–2). As an example of acute hepatitis, this section concentrates on halothane hepatitis; in the author's opinion, this represents one of the best models, since the reaction occurs relatively often in hospital practice, the timing and extent of exposure is usually well documented, the routes of metabolism are well described, and the immune phenomena have been investigated widely. After halothane hepatitis, the possible role of immune mechanisms in drug-associated chronic liver disease and alcoholic liver disease will be discussed.

HALOTHANE HEPATITIS

Antibodies

There is strong circumstantial evidence that halothane hepatitis is immune-mediated. The reaction complicates less than 1 in 35,000 halothane exposures but is rarely, if ever, seen after only one exposure. There is no dose dependency. Pyrexia,

Table 15–2 DRUGS IMPLICATED IN IMMUNE-MEDIATED HEPATOTOXICITY

Phenytoin
Phenindione
Ethanol
Halothane
Chlorpromazine
Erythromycin
Alpha-methyl dopa
Nitrofurantoin
Para-amino salicylate
Sulphonamide

circulating eosinophilia, circulating immune complexes, organ-nonspecific autoantibodies are all associated, but rarely rash, blood dyscrasia, or arthralgia.[2,11,12] There may be cross-sensitization with other halogenated hydrocarbon anesthetics. The association with an increased incidence of "allergy" to other drugs and of eczema in those with halothane hepatitis is less clear.

It must be emphasized that numerous animal studies have shown that the drug may be directly hepatotoxic. Halothane is metabolized through at least two different routes — oxidative and reductive; both pathways are associated with the generation of highly reactive species. Rodents exposed to halothane, under conditions designed to stimulate the reductive pathway, develop liver cell necrosis.[2] The relevance of these models to the human situation is not clear; using a sensitive monitor of liver cell damage (serum glutathione-S-transferase activity) it was shown[13] that reductive metabolism of halothane in humans is associated with very minor degrees of liver damage. However, when humans with halothane hepatitis are studied, it is clear that there is no evidence of excessive reductive halothane metabolism; furthermore, the dose dependency and predictability of the animal models is not seen.[11]

Halothane (1-chloro,1-bromo,2,2,2-trifluoroethane) is a small molecular weight molecule and is therefore unlikely to be itself immunogenic. Indeed, early studies to show sensitization to halothane itself in patients with halothane hepatitis were conflicting and unconvincing. In order to circumvent the problems of selecting the appropriate antigens for in vitro testing, which as discussed above may not even directly involve halothane or even a metabolite, Vergani and colleagues[14] adopted a novel technique: rabbits were exposed to halothane under conditions comparable to those in humans undergoing surgery. The animals were allowed to recover for 18 hours, to allow for metabolism of halothane and generation of any putative antigens. The animal was then killed and the liver removed.

In early studies,[14] leukocyte migration tests were used to seek evidence of sensitization by patients' lymphocytes to homogenates from halothane-treated or control rabbit livers. Of the 12 patients studied, 8 showed either inhibition or enhancement of migration to the halothane homogenate only, suggesting strong or weak sensitization respectively to antigen(s) present only in the halothane-treated livers. Subsequent direct cytotoxicity experiments[15] showed that peripheral lymphocytes isolated from individuals were directly cytotoxic in vitro to collagenase-isolated hepatocytes from rabbits whether or not the rabbits had been exposed to halothane previously. Whereas cytotoxicity to control hepatocytes could be blocked by incubation with liver-specific lipoprotein (a preparation of liver membrane containing both liver-specific and -nonspecific lipoproteins), cytotoxicity to "halothane hepatocytes" was not blocked, suggesting that lymphocytes were sensitized both to normal and halothane-related antigens.

In studies to look at the humoral response, initial work used an antibody-dependent cell-mediated cytotoxicity (ADCC) technique. While the assay may not represent a specific physiologic process, it can be shown to assess clearly some antibody/antigen interactions. Using this assay, it was found that the majority, but not all, of patients with the presumed diagnosis of halothane hepatitis had circulating antibodies reacting with an antigen present on hepatocytes from halothane-pretreated rabbits.[16] Using indirect immunofluorescence, it was shown that the antigen was on the surface of the hepatocyte, since "capping" was observed. The presence of these so-called halothane antibodies (antibodies reacting with liver cell determinants associated with halothane exposure) was further confirmed using an enzyme-linked immunosorbent assay (ELISA),[17] (Fig. 15–1). None of these antibody responses to halothane-related antigens were found in patients who had been exposed to halothane without hepatitis, in those who had halothane anesthesia but developed liver cell necrosis from viral or other causes, in those with other liver diseases, or in normal subjects.

Demonstration of this humoral and cellular reaction to halothane-related antigens carries a number of implications for the possible pathogenesis of halothane hepatitis. The specificity of the reaction suggests that the presence of the antibody may be of diagnostic importance. However, the sensitivity is such that only 75–80% of patients have detectable levels of antibody.

It is not clear whether these immune reactions are involved in the pathogenesis of the hepatitis. The observation that the antibodies are of the IgG class, even in the first few days after the onset of the liver cell damage, suggests that the immune response is not merely secondary to a direct toxic reaction, although it is appreciated that switching from IgM to IgG can occur rapidly. This concept is further supported by the observation that when liver cell necrosis is seen in patients who develop viral hepatitis a few days after halothane exposure, no such antibodies are detectable.[8] That the "halothane antibodies" can induce normal lymphocytes to be

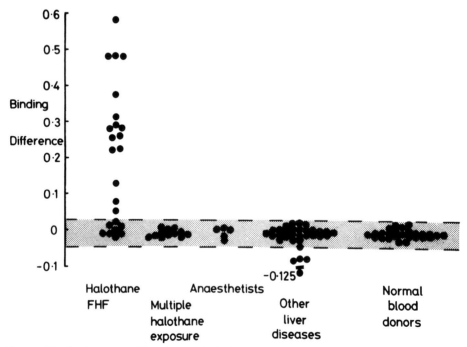

Figure 15–1 Serum antibodies to halothane-altered liver cell determinants. Sera from patients and controls more incubated with microsomes from halothane and control rabbit livers: the amount of antibody bound is determined by incubation with a second peroxidase-conjugated antibody. The shaded area indicates the normal range. Fulminant hepatic failure (FHF) . (From Kenna, et al: An enzyme linked immunosorbent assay for detection of antibodies against halothane altered hepatocyte antigens. *J Immunol Methods* 75:3–14, 1984, with permission.)

cytotoxic to the "halothane hepatocytes" in vitro and that the antigen is expressed on the cell membrane does suggest a possible mechanism whereby K lymphocytes will bind to and lyse in vivo the halothane antibody-coated hepatocytes. However, it is not clear how potent the ADCC reaction is in humans and whether this mechanism could result in a fulminant hepatic necrosis.

Antigens

The recognition by human antibodies of antigens in halothane-exposed rabbit liver cells implies that a similar, if not identical, antigen is generated in humans. Initial studies to determine the nature of the halothane antigen involved exposing the rabbits to halothane under different concentrations of oxygen preferentially to stimulate different pathways of metabolism. The presence of the antigen was detected using serum known to contain the antibody in the ADCC reaction. It was found[18] that oxidative metabolism was implicated in the generation of the antigen, contrasting with the reductive route implicated in the generation of direct toxicity. These observations were confirmed by others[19] who used both immunofluorescence and ELISA techniques to show that trifluoroacetylated (TFA) hepatocytes were stained preferentially in the centrilobular region of halothane-exposed rat hepatocytes. The fluorescence, which was concentrated in the areas of the lobule rich in the drug-metabolizing enzymes, was maximal around the periphery of the cell. The results suggest that TFA-halide, the major metabolite of oxidative halothane metabolism, reacts directly with constituents of the liver plasma membrane or with cellular components that become incorporated into the plasma membrane.

Characterization of the antigen(s) has been carried out using immunoblotting techniques. In rabbits,[20] there appear to be three polypeptide antigens that are variously recognized by serum from patients with halothane hepatitis (Fig. 15–2). These polypeptides are concentrated in the microsomal and the plasma membrane fractions of rabbit liver homogenate. Further characterization using rat liver was carried out by Kenna.[21] Rats were exposed to either halothane or deuterated halothane (which is preferentially metabolized by the reductive route) and immunoblotted with either patient serum or antibodies specific for TFA-halide. Confirmation of oxidative metabolism of halothane in generation of the antigens was again obtained; however, the demonstration that recognition of the antigens by patients' serum was only partly blocked by incubation with the hapten derivative N-e-TFA-L-lysine indicates that the patients' antibodies recognize epitopes consisting of the TFA group together with the associated structural features of the protein carriers.

Possible candidates for some of the polypeptides involved are the drug-metabolizing enzymes. It is now becoming clear that the liver-kidney microsomal antibodies observed in the sera of patients with presumed drug-associated hepatitis, as well as some other forms of hepatitis, are directed against the drug-metabolizing enzymes. In hepatitis associated with the diuretic tienilic acid, the autoantibodies react with the cytochrome P448[22] that metabolizes the drug. There is, however, no clear evidence that the cytochromes are expressed on the plasma membrane, and so these responses may occur as a consequence of direct toxicity.

Individual Susceptibility

If halothane hepatitis is immune-mediated, then the idiosyncratic nature of the syndrome must lie either in variations in generation or expression of the neoanti-

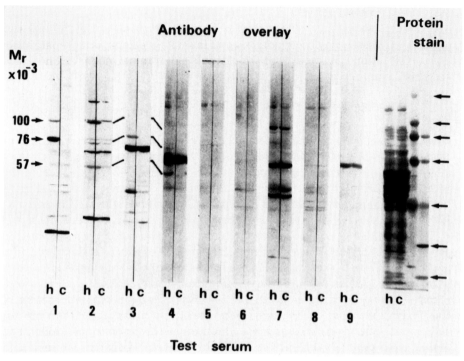

Figure 15–2 Immunoblot of sera from patients with halothane hepatitis incubated with control and halothane-treated rabbit liver microsomes. Sera recognize three polypeptides (Mr 100, 76, and 57 × 10³) in halothane-treated (h) but not control (c) rabbit livers. (From Kenna, et al: Identification by immunoblotting of three halothane induced liver microsomal antigens recognised by antibodies in sera from patient with halothane hepatitis. *J Pharm Exp Ther* 242:733–740, 1987, with permission.)

gens or in the response to those antigens. All rabbits exposed to halothane generate the neoantigen, but the data from humans are limited. Studies of immunoblotting a limited number of liver samples from humans exposed to halothane but without hepatitis suggest that generation of the antigens does occur,[23] so that the idiosyncratic nature of the response lies in the host immune system.

There are no convincing data on HLA studies in patients with halothane hepatitis: the groups studied have been either too small or too heterogenous for valid statistical analysis. The syndrome has been reported in three pairs of closely related women,[24] but no other study has reported on a family incidence. However, Farrell[25] has shown that lymphocytes from patients and some relatives are susceptible to electrophilic metabolites generated by the metabolism of phenytoin in the presence of an epoxide hydrolase inhibitor. While the immediate significance of these findings for the pathogenesis of the hepatitis is not clear, the work does provide some evidence for an abnormal lymphocyte response in susceptible individuals.

Additional factors that determine susceptibility include the effect of halothane itself as well as the stress of surgery on the immune system: both factors may be associated with reduced suppressor cell function.[26]

CHRONIC HEPATITIS

Chronic liver disease may occur as a result of immune-mediated drug hepatotoxicity in two situations: in some cases, for example chlorpromazine- or alcohol-associated liver damage, liver disease may progress despite withdrawal of the drug. Alternatively, the signs and symptoms of the liver damage may remain subclinical, so that the patient continues to take the drug and the cell-damaging reactions continue.

Chronic active hepatitis (CAH) is a syndrome described elsewhere. Estimates of the incidence of drug-induced CAH range from 3% to over 60%.[27,28] One of the first examples of drug-induced CAH was described in 1971,[29] in association with the laxative oxyphenisatin. Seven women were described, all of whom had the typical biochemical and histologic features of CAH; autoantibodies (predominantly antinuclear and antiactin) were present in all, and two had detectable lupus erythematosus cells. In all but one case, withdrawal of the drug was associated with a rapid biochemical improvement. Since the initial report of oxyphenisatin, other drugs have been implicated in the pathogenesis of CAH; these include chlorpromazine, nitrofurantoin, isoniazid, sulphonamides, dantrolene, and ethanol.

Most of the cases of drug-induced CAH that have been reported occur in women; whether this reflects a greater exposure of drugs to women rather than men or whether this reflects the greater predeliction of women to develop autoimmune diseases is not clear. As with autoimmune chronic active hepatitis, an increased prevalence of the HLA phenotype B8 has been reported.

It is tempting to deduce that drugs may initiate the immune-damaging processes, but there is little direct evidence to support this hypothesis. All the drugs that have been associated with CAH have the potential to cause a direct hepatotoxic reaction, if animal data can be extrapolated to humans. It may be that some drug-associated toxic reactions (in susceptible individuals) unmask and trigger an autoimmune process. However, the observation that the liver disease usually regresses after withdrawal of the drug may argue against this notion. Drug-related antibodies (analogous to the halothane-related antibodies described above) have been found in patients with chronic liver disease associated with alpha-methyl dopa.[30] It may be that the generation of a neoantigen on the membrane of the hepatocyte is enough to trigger the immune response and so lead to a breakdown in tolerance.

ALCOHOL LIVER INJURY

Numerous studies in both humans and animals show that alcohol may be directly hepatotoxic.[31] However, there is great individual variability in susceptibility to the hepatotoxic effects of alcohol. As outlined below, a number of factors, both clinical and serologic, suggest that immune mechanisms may be involved. Discussion of these factors is included here since the experimental observations suggest evidence for additional mechanisms whereby the immune system can be involved in the pathogenesis of liver damage.

It scarcely needs emphasis that studies of pathogenesis of alcohol-related damage in humans is difficult: assessment of the amount of alcohol consumed is not reliable, and the variability of drinking patterns and the associated diseases and malnutrition may have an effect on the immune system, so that distinguishing primary and secondary immune abnormalities is not always possible.

Evidence for immune involvement in the pathogenesis of alcohol-related liver damage is circumstantial: while population studies have shown a clear correlation between the dose of alcohol consumed and the probability of developing liver damage, the evidence is less clear-cut when the individual is assessed.[31] The observation that, dose for dose, females are more susceptible to alcoholic liver injury may relate more to the difference in body distribution, differences in xenobiotic metabolism, and variations in the activities of the isozymes of alcohol dehydrogenase and acetaldehyde dehydrogenase. The importance of the HLA phenotype in the predisposition to alcoholic liver injury is conflicting, with no clear-cut pattern emerging. Saunders et al.[32] have suggested that those with HLA B8 are more prone to the development of alcoholic cirrhosis.

Abnormalities of the humoral system are manifested by polyclonal hypergammaglobulinemia, especially of IgA. This occurs in alcoholics with and without liver disease and is probably due to increased antibody production, resulting from increased antigenic stimulation because T-cell regulation of B-cell activity is, in most studies, not markedly abnormal. The increased antigenic load probably results from either increased gut permeability or failure to sequester gut-derived antigens. There is an increased incidence of both organ-nonspecific and -specific autoantibodies. The organ-specific autoantibodies include both the liver-specific lipoprotein and the liver membrane antigen. As with halothane, studies using both immunofluorescence and antibody-dependent call-mediated cytotoxicity have shown that about one-half the patients with alcoholic liver disease have antibodies reacting with alcohol-altered liver cell components.[33,34] These antibodies are found more commonly in those with alcoholic hepatitis and cirrhosis than those with fatty liver. As with halothane, metabolism of alcohol is necessary for the generation of these antigens, and the major reactive metabolite of alcohol, acetaldehyde, is associated with the expression of the antigen.[35]

Alterations of the cellular immune system are also present in those with alcoholic liver disease. Anergy is common, and impairment of skin reactivity to common recall antigens and new antigens is also common in patients with alcoholic liver disease, but improves with improvement in the patients' clinical condition. While circulating B cells are probably normal in number, T cells are reduced, largely due to depletion of the suppressor/cytotoxic cells.[36] This depletion, which is found mainly in those with alcoholic hepatitis, is probably due to their preferential sequestration in the liver.[37] Functionally, there is in vitro reduced responsiveness to mitogens such as phytohemagglutinin (PHA), but this is likely to be due to a serum factor. In vitro, lymphocytes from patients with alcoholic hepatitis are directly cytotoxic to hepatocytes from rabbits and to autologous hepatocytes.[38] This cytotoxicity can be blocked by addition of both liver specific lipoprotein (LSP) and alcoholic hyaline (a protein probably derived from intracellular myofibrils that are common but not unique to alcoholic liver disease), suggesting that these agents may contain some of the antigens to which the lymphocytes are sensitized.

Sensitization to Acetaldehyde-Modified Proteins

In alcoholic liver disease, immune reactions may be directed against acetaldehyde-altered proteins. Acetaldehyde, the major metabolite of alcohol oxidation, is a highly reactive compound. It condenses with liver cell macromolecules by the formation of Schiff bases with free amino groups; these may be stabilized either spontaneously with ascorbic acid or by reducing agents in vitro such as cyanoborohydride.[39,40] Acetaldehyde can also react with N-terminal amino groups, forming stable imidazolidinone compounds.[41] Interaction of acetaldehyde in vitro with plasma membrane is not associated with alteration of the membrane function.[40] As with the example of halothane above, these interactions between native macromolecules and a reactive metabolite may lead to the formation of antigenic compounds either because a novel protein is produced or because the quaternary structure of the protein is sufficiently altered to become immunogenic. Israel and colleagues[42] have shown that acetaldehyde-generated epitopes are immunogenic when injected into animals. This group further showed that mice treated with ethanol chronically can generate antibodies that recognize acetaldehyde-modified proteins. Acetaldehyde forms adducts with a number of different proteins, including albumin and prothrombin. The latter two compounds are synthesized in the hepatocyte, and so it is tempting to speculate that these proteins are altered during synthesis; the demonstration of acetaldehyde-hemoglobin adducts, however, may refute this argument.[43] While several groups of compounds are more common in those with liver disease,[44] a pathogenetic role is still far from proven. It is quite possible that acetaldehyde-modified protein antibodies arise as a consequence of the release of modified proteins into the circulation on damage to the hepatocyte. It is clearly important to determine whether acetaldehyde-generated neoantigens are present on the hepatocyte surface membrane and, if so, whether they are recognized by the immune system. There are still few data on this possibility.

Another possibility is that the acetaldehyde adduct on the plasma membrane stimulates the complement cascade and attracts neutrophils (Fig. 15–3). This

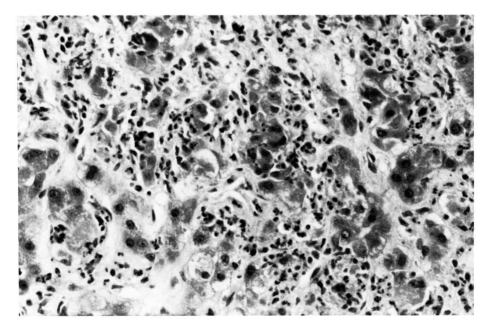

Figure 15–3 Alcoholic hepatitis showing infiltration of the liver with neutrophils. An occasional Mallory's body is seen. (Courtesy of Dr. S Hubscher).

intriguing hypothesis finds some support in work by Barry, who showed that such plasma membrane preparations can indeed stimulate complement activation and so lead to the appearance of alcoholic hepatitis.[45] This hypothesis does not explain why only a few people develop hepatitis after alcohol ingestion and why, in such patients, there is no evidence of increased complement activation.[46,47]

CONCLUSIONS

The evidence to suggest that immune mechanisms are implicated in the pathogenesis of liver damage remains circumstantial and based on the summation of clinical, histologic, and serologic features. Separation of "chicken and egg" is difficult. The lack of animal models of immune-mediated liver damage means that potential mechanisms cannot readily be studied. There remains too the paradox that all drugs that may be implicated in immune-mediated reactions can, in vitro and in vivo, generate a direct toxic effect. A good example is chlorpromazine cholestasis: clinically this falls into the category of an immune-mediated reaction (the incidence of severe damage is low, there is an associated eosinophilia and high incidence of autoantibodies, and the liver lesion may progress to cirrhosis after the drug has been stopped).[48] In vitro, however, it can be clearly demonstrated that therapeutic doses of chlorpromazine are associated reliably with features of cholestasis. Thus, at these levels why do not all patients develop cholestasis rather than less than 1 in 100? Watson[49] has shown that those with chlorpromazine jaundice are poor sulphoxidizers and so will metabolize the drug to more cholestatic metabolites: however, the incidence of poor sulphoxidizers is far greater than the incidence of chlorpromazine cholestasis. It is therefore possible that direct toxicity leading to recognition by the immune system of the drug-generated neoantigens is necessary for the occurrence of immune-mediated hepatotoxicity in humans. In susceptible individuals (by implication a tautology?), this will lead to an immune reaction and the development of severe liver damage. However, it is hard to exclude an immune involvement in such situations as an adverse reaction occurring in sensitized individuals who receive a subsequent exposure, in cases of halothane toxicity by an amount of drug from dissolved rubber in the anesthetic machine,[50] or nitrofurantoin in milk from a cow treated with the antibiotic.[51]

REFERENCES

1. Engel JJ, Vogt TR, Wilson DE: Cholestatic hepatitis after administration of furan derivative. *Arch Intern Med* 135:733–737, 1975.
2. Stock J, Strunin L: Unexplained hepatitis following halothane. *Anaesthesiology* 63:424–439, 1985.
3. Smith CI, Cooksey GE, Powell LW: Cell mediated immunity to liver antigens in toxic liver injury—I. *Clin Exp Immunol* 39:607–617, 1988.
4. Smith CI, Cooksey GE, Powell LW: Cell mediated immunity to liver antigens in toxic liver injury—II. *Clin Exp Immunol* 39:618–625, 1980.
5. Kirtland H, Daniel MD, Mohler MD, et al: Methyl dopa inhibition of suppressor lymphocyte function. *N Eng J Med* 302:825–831, 1980.
6. Neuberger J, Kenna JG: Halothane hepatitis: a model of immunoallergic disease. In Guillouzo A: *Liver Cells and Drugs*. Rouen, Inserm/John Libbey Eurotext Ltd, 1988, pp 161–173.

7. Homberg JG, Abuaf N, Helmy-Khalil H, et al: Drug induced hepatitis associated with anti-cytoplasmic auto-antibodies. *Hepatology* 5:722–725, 1985.

8. Neuberger J, Gimson AES, Davis, M et al: Specific serological markers in the diagnosis of fulminant hepatic failure associated with halothane anaesthesia. *Br J Anaesthesiol* 55:19–21, 1983.

9. Morre DJ, Kartenbeck J, Franke WW: Membrane flow and interconversions among endomembranes. *Biochem Biophys Acta* 559:71–152, 1979.

10. Franco A, Barnaba V, Natali P, et al: Expression of class I and class II major histocompatability antigens on human hepatocytes. *Hepatology* 8:449–454, 1988.

11. Neuberger J, Kenna JG: Halothane hepatitis: a model of immune mediated drug hepatotoxicity. *Clin Sci* 72:263–270, 1987.

12. National Halothane Study: Summary of the National Halothane Study. *JAMA* 197:121–134, 1966.

13. Allan LG, Hussey AJ, Howie J, et al: Hepatic glutathione-S-transferase release after halothane anaesthesia. *Lancet* 1:771–774, 1987.

14. Vergani D, Eddleston A, Tsantoulas D, et al: Sensitisation to halothane altered liver components in severe hepatic necrosis after halothane anaesthesia. *Lancet* 1:801–803, 1978.

15. Mieli Vergani G, Vergani D, Tredger J, et al: Lymphocyte cytotoxicity to halothane altered hepatocytes in patient with severe hepatic necrosis following halothane anaesthesia. *J Lab Clin Med* 4:49–51, 1980.

16. Vergani D, Mieli Vergani G, Alberti A, et al: Antibodies to the surface of halothane altered rabbit hepatocytes in patients with severe halothane associated hepatitis. *N Engl J Med* 303:66–71, 1980.

17. Kenna JG, Neuberger J, Williams R: An enzyme linked immunosorbent assay for detection of antibodies against halothane altered hepatocyte antigens. *J Immunol Methods* 75:3–14, 1984.

18. Neuberger J, Mieli Vergani G, Tredger J, et al: Oxidative metabolism of halothane in the production of altered hepatocyte antigens in acute halothane induced necrosis. *Gut* 22:669–672, 1981.

19. Satoh H, Fukada Y, Anderson DK, et al: Immunological studies on the mechanism of halothane induced hepatotoxicity. *J Pharm Exp Ther* 233:857–862, 1985.

20. Kenna JG, Neuberger JM, Williams R: Identification by immunoblotting of three halothane induced liver microsomal antigens recognised by antibodies in sera from patient with halothane hepatitis. *J Pharm Exp Ther* 242:733–740, 1987.

21. Kenna JG, Satoh H, Christ D, et al: Metabolic basis for a drug hypersensitivity. *J Pharm Exp Ther* 245:1103–1109, 1988

22. Beaune P, Dansette PM, Mansuy D, et al: Human antiendoplasmic reticulum antibodies appearing in a drug induced hepatitis are directed against a human liver cytochrome P450 that hydroxylates the drug. *Proc Natl Acad Sci USA* 84:551–555, 1987.

23. Kenna JG, Neuberger J, Williams R: Evidence for expression in human liver in halothane induced neoantigens recognised in antibodies in sera from patients with halothane hepatitis. *Hepatology* (in press)

24. Hoft RH, Bunker JP, Goodman MH, et al: Halothane hepatitis in three parts of closely related women. *N Engl J Med* 304:1023–1024, 1987.

25. Farrell S, Prendergast D, Murray M: Halothane hepatitis: detection of a constitutional susceptibility factor. *N Engl J Med* 313:1300–1314, 1985.

26. Watkins J, Salo M (eds): *Trauma, Stress and Immunity In Anaesthesia and Surgery.* London, Butterworth, 1982.

27. Hodges JR, Milward-Sadler GH, Wright R: Chronic active hepatitis: the spectrum of disease. *Lancet* i:550–552, 1982.

28. Lindberg J, Lindholm A, Lundin P, et al: Trigger factors and HLA antigens in chronic active hepatitis. *Br Med J* ii:77–79, 1975.

29. Reynolds T, Peters RL, Yamada S: Chronic active hepatitis and lupoid hepatitis caused by a laxative, oxyphenisatin. *N Engl J Med* 285:815–828, 1971.

30. Neuberger J, Kenna JG, Nouri Aria K, et al: Antibody mediated hepatocyte injury in alpha-methyl dopa induced hepatotoxicity. *Gut* 26:1233–1236, 1985.

31. Saunders J, Wodak A, Williams R: What determines susceptibility to liver damage from alcohol. *J R Soc Med* 77:204–216, 1984.

32. Saunders JB, Wodak AD, Haines A, et al: Accelerated development of alcoholic cirrhosis in patients with HLA B8. *Lancet* i:1381–1384, 1982.

33. Neuberger JM, Crossley IR, Saunders JB, et al: Antibodies to alcohol altered liver cell determinants in patient with alcoholic liver disease. *Gut* 25:300–304, 1984.

34. Anthony RS, Farquaharson N, MacSween RM: Liver membrane antibodies in alcoholic liver disease — II. *J Clin Pathol* 26:1302–1308, 1983.

35. Crossley I, Neuberger J, Davis M, et al: Ethanol metabolism in the generation of new antigenic determinants on liver cells. *Gut* 27:186–189, 1986.

36. McKeever V, O'Mahony C, Whelan C, et al: Helper and suppressor T lymphocyte function in severe alcoholic liver disease. *Clin Exp Immunol* 60:39–48, 1985.

37. Si L, Whiteside TL, Schade RR, et al: Lymphocyte subsets studied with monoclonal antibodies in liver tissue of patients with alcoholic liver disease. *Alcoholism* 7:431–435, 1985.

38. Poralla T, Hutteroth T, Meyer ZUM, et al: Cellular cytotoxicity against autologous hepatocytes in alcoholic liver disease. *Liver* 4:117–121, 1984.

39. Donohue TM, Tuma DJ, Sorrell MF: Binding of metabolically derived acetaldehyde to hepatic proteins in vitro. *Lab Invest* 49:226–229, 1983.

40. Barry RE, McGivan JD, Hayes M: Acetaldehyde binds to liver cell membranes without altering membrane function. *Gut* 25:412–416, 1984.

41. San George RC, Hoberman HD: Reaction of acetaldehyde with hemoglobin. *J Biol Chem* 26:6811–6821, 1986.

42. Israel Y, Horwitz E, Niemela O, et al: Monoclonal and polyclonal antibodies against acetaldehyde containing epitopes in acetaldehyde protein adducts. *Proc Natl Acad Sci USA* 83:7923–7927, 1986.

43. Stevens VJ, Fantl WS, Newnanco L, et al: Acetaldehyde adducts with hemoglobin. *J Clin Invest* 67:361–369, 1981.

44. Israel Y, Orrego H, Niemela O: Immune responses to alcohol metabolites: pathogenic and diagnostic implications. *Semin Liver Dis* 8:81–90, 1988.

45. Barry RE, McGivan JHD: Acetaldehyde alone may initiate hepatocellular damage in acute alcoholic liver disease. *Gut* 26:1065–1069, 1985.

46. Spinozzi F, Guercolini R, Gelri R, et al: Immunological studies in patients with alcoholic liver disease. *Int Arch Allergy Appl Immunol* 80:361–386, 1986.

47. Munoz LE, De Villiers D, Markham D, et al: Complement activation in chronic liver disease. *Clin Exp Immunol* 47:548–554, 1982.

48. Zimmerman H, Lewis J: Drug induced cholestasis. *Med Toxicol* 2:112–160, 1987.

49. Watson LGP, Olonu A, Clements D, et al: A proposed mechanism for chlorpromazine jaundice. *J Hepatol* 7:79–84, 1988.

50. Varma RR, Whitesell RC, Iskandarani M: Halothane hepatitis without halothane. *Hepatology* 5:904–906, 1985.

51. Berry WR, Warren GH, Reichen J: Nitrofurantoin-induced cholestatic hepatitis from cow's milk in a teenage boy. *World J Med* 140:278–280, 1984.

CHAPTER 16

Immunology of Liver Transplantation

JOHN G. O'GRADY

ROGER WILLIAMS

INTRODUCTION

Orthotopic liver transplantation (OLT) is now established as a feasible therapeutic option for almost the entire range of end-stage liver disorders not amenable to other forms of therapy.[1,2] At the time of writing (August 1988), the estimated total number of liver transplants performed worldwide exceeds 5,000, and the observed rate of growth persists on an upward trend with more and more programs being developed. One-year survival rates in excess of 70% are widely reported (currently in excess of 90% for elective cases in at least one major institution), while 5-year survival rates in excess of 60% are anticipated.[3] The indications for, and the contraindications to, OLT are constantly being revised in the light of greater clinical experience with transplantation and the results obtained. OLT appears to be beneficial in acute liver failure, metabolic disorders, and in most patients with end-stage chronic liver disease, but controversy surrounds hepatitis B-related chronic liver disease and malignant disorders because the benefits of transplantation are perceived by some to be attenuated to varying degrees by disease recurrence. Nevertheless, it is safe to assume that OLT will continue to expand its overall role in the management of liver disease.

This review will concentrate on the immunologic aspects of clinical liver transplantation, with particular emphasis on "acute" and "chronic" graft rejection, graft-versus-host disease, graft tolerance, and strategies of immunosuppression. A knowledge of principles of transplantation immunology is largely presumed.

We are grateful to Dr. Graeme J.M. Alexander for advice during the preparation of this manuscript and to Dr. Bernard Portmann for providing the photomicrographs.

ACUTE REJECTION

The clinical features of acute liver graft rejection are nonspecific and include fever and a reduction in both the quality and quantity of bile produced. Laboratory tests show an increase in serum transaminases and bilirubin, peripheral eosinophilia,[4] and a prolongation in prothrombin time in severe cases. Such is the degree of overlap with other causes of graft dysfunction that histologic examination of the liver is almost mandatory to diagnose acute rejection. The prominent features of severe acute rejection are a mixed portal inflammatory infiltrate (including lymphocytes, neutrophils, and eosinophils), bile duct damage with lymphocytic infiltration, and venous endothelialitis (Fig. 16–1). This complete triad was present in 86% of the initial diagnostic biopsies in one series of 36 patients with acute rejection.[5] In the absence of an endothelialitis, a portal infiltrate with >50% bile duct damage is said to be diagnostic of acute rejection.[5] Centrilobular ballooning and cell dropout are found in more severe cases and are probably secondary to ischemia. Hepatic arteriography in cases of severe acute rejection may show a marked slowing in blood flow with generalized pruning of the peripheral arterial system, a feature also seen in chronic rejection.[6,7] In some instances the blood flow rate is so decreased that secondary arterial thrombosis develops at the site of the arterial anastamosis.[7]

No functional assays have been developed to study the immunokinetics of acute rejection, but the histologic pattern suggests that bile duct epithelium and endothelial cells, the main major histocompatibility complex (MHC) antigen-expressing

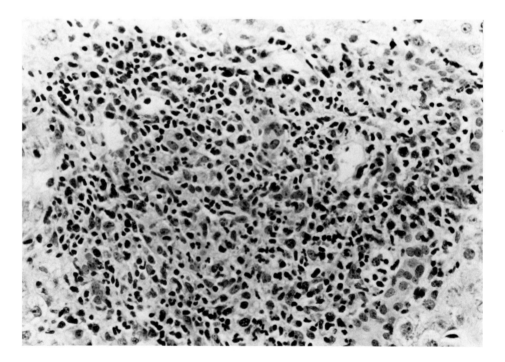

Figure 16–1 Expanded portal tract with mixed inflammatory cell infiltrate, bile duct damage, and endotheliitis in a patient with acute rejection.

cells, are the primary target cells. The pattern of MHC antigen expression in well-functioning liver grafts shows that hepatocytes express no antigens or only weak staining for class I antigens, bile ducts usually express class I antigens alone, while both class I and II antigens are expressed on Kupffer and endothelial cells, a pattern similar to the normal liver.[8] Class I antigens may be the target antigen; expression on hepatocytes is increased in acute rejection[8-10] and has been shown to decrease again after histologic resolution of the rejection episode.[10] However, increased hepatocyte class I expression has also been documented in cytomegalovirus (CMV) hepatitis, apparently uncomplicated by rejection[8] and possibly in association with other complications, e.g., cholangitis. Focal and transient expression of DR antigen (but not DP and DQ antigens) on hepatocytes related to lymphocytic infiltrates has also been demonstrated in acute rejection.[8] While there is increased expression of DR antigens (and in some cases DP antigens, but rarely DQ antigens) on bile duct epithelial cells in episodes of acute rejection, these changes were found to be relatively nonspecific and only correlated with acute rejection when there was coexisting DR expression by hepatocytes.[8] The extent to which these changes are epiphenomena associated with local production of cytokines, or truly important processes in the pathogenesis of acute rejection is currently uncertain.

The profile of inflammatory cells in the liver graft during episodes of acute rejection indicates an overall predominance of T lymphocytes, with only a modest increase in the B-cell population.[4] Among the T lymphocytes, there is an initial predominance of CD4 (helper) cells, followed by a rapid increase of CD8 (suppressor and cytotoxic) cells, restoring the CD4/CD8 ratio to prerejection levels.[4] However, acute rejection has been documented in patients having CD4 but no CD8 cells in the portal tracts,[11] and it has been shown that some CD4 cells expressing T-cell receptor (TCR) are capable of cell lysis. The portal tract T lymphocytes have been shown to express DR antigen, indicating an active state and probable involvement in the rejection process.[12] This pattern of events supports the concept that initiation of rejection is mediated by the CD4 cells and that the CD8 cells are subsequently recruited through interleukin-2 production by CD4 cells to complete the process. The presence of CD8 cells in liver tissue only correlated with rejection when they were situated in the portal tracts, and their presence in the lobule was found to be of no significance.[11] Furthermore, CD4 cells have been demonstrated in the portal tracts in patients with CMV hepatitis, so that the immunohistologic patterns of cellular infiltrates are not pathognomic.[11] In peripheral blood, a fall in CD3 and CD4 cells has been documented in patients with acute rejection, while CD8 and B cells remain unchanged.[13] The reduction in CD4 cells was noted to persist for 1 year, but this may be a function of more aggressive immunosuppression in patients who had had rejection episodes.

The role of humoral factors (including antibodies against ABO and other blood groups, lymphocytes, and HLA antigens) in the pathogenesis of acute rejection is uncertain. While hyperacute rejection appears to be inducible by presensitization to donor in the animal model,[14] and probable cases of hyperacute or accelerated rejection have been documented in patients with positive cross-matches,[15,16] this scenario is highly unusual when compared with renal graft recipients. One patient with preformed lymphocytotoxic antibodies [100% panel-reactive antibody (PRA)] in the Cambridge/King's College Hospital program had evidence of progressive graft failure from 8 hours after transplantation, and the explanted graft showed eosinophilic necrosis at 44 hours.[15] Nonetheless, successful liver transplants have been performed in the presence of preformed lymphocytotoxic antibody. In one series of 62 patients, 18% had preformed lymphocytotoxic antibody, and all developed acute rejection, compared with 70% of those without antibody.[13] All but three of the latter seroconverted after the rejection episode, peaking at 1 month and returning to normal at 1 year, a pattern that was interpreted as evidence of the development of antiidiotypic antibodies. One patient transplanted across a strong antilymphocyte cross-match who developed severe rejection failed to develop antiidiotypic antibodies to anti-HLA.[17] In another study of 505 grafts, the graft survival rates did not differ with the percent of pretransplant PRA; 48.9% of 67 with PRA >30% and 51.4% of 438 with PRA <30% survived for 2 years.[18] Transplantation across the ABO barrier is also feasible, although apparently associated with a modest decrease in graft survival. In a series of 745 patients having a primary liver transplant, 664 were given identical matches with 59.4% graft survival, compared with 40.3% and 42.1% of 62 and 19 patients given compatible and incompatible grafts, respectively.[19]

The incidence and clinical consequences of acute rejection episodes after OLT have been reasonably well defined. In one carefully studied series of 104 patients maintained on cyclosporine and prednisolone, acute rejection was diagnosed in 60.6% at a median of 8 days post-OLT (95.2% of these occurred between days 4 and 21) and was recurrent in 17.3%.[20] The frequency of acute rejection was of the order of 60% in a number of other studies, although two series put the rate as high as 80–81.5%.[21,22] The response to supplemental corticosteroid therapy is 48–60%, while an additional 19–44% respond to OKT3 or other antibodies directed against lymphocytes (as discussed later).[20,22] About 8–9% of cases fail to respond to all therapies, and urgent retransplantation is indicated.

CHRONIC REJECTION

Chronic rejection means irreversible loss of the liver graft through immunologic processes directed principally at the bile duct epithelial cell and/or the arterial endothelial cell. The prominence of the former feature on liver biopsy specimens from these patients has led to the synonymous term vanishing bile duct syndrome (VBDS). Serial liver biopsies demonstrate a progressive nonsuppurative destruction of interlobular bile ducts; VBDS is diagnosed when 50–80% of such ducts have disappeared.[23,24] In the early stages there is a mixed inflammatory cell infiltrate in the portal tracts, but subsequently these become relatively acellular (Fig. 16–2). The cells infiltrating the bile ducts appear to be mainly T lymphocytes, together with some natural killer (NK) cells and neutrophils.[25] Arterial changes may be seen in percutaneous liver biopsy specimens, but in many instances examination of the explanted graft is necessary to establish the presence of this feature. The intima is infiltrated by foamy macrophages, leading to occlusion of the arterial lumen and centrilobular ischemic change including ballooning and cell loss. Additional histologic features include cellular and canalicular cholestasis and, in the later stages, lobular fibrosis with an increase in copper-associated protein deposition.[23]

Studies from our unit have shown that susceptibility to developing VBDS appeared to be conferred by a specific pattern of donor/recipient HLA antigen matching.[26,27] In a group of 101 patients including 16 with VBDS, the stronger association was found for a match for HLA-DR antigens, which carried a relative

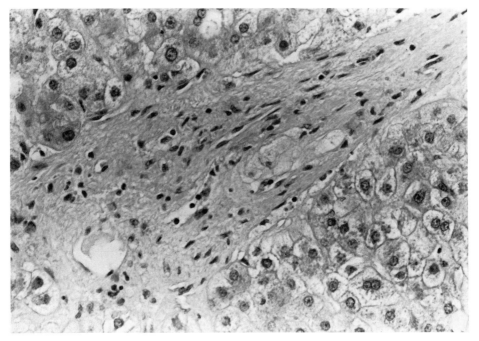

Figure 16-2 A portal tract with a sparse inflammatory cell infiltrate, absence of interlobular bile ducts, and arterial foamy cell infiltration in a patient with the vanishing bile duct syndrome.

risk of 9.4 for developing VBDS.[27] A weaker association was found for a complete mismatch for HLA-A/B antigens (relative risk 3.1), but the combination of the latter with a match for HLA-DR antigens did not have a cumulative effect in increasing susceptibility (relative risk 6.9). However, susceptibility to VBDS was increased when CMV infection developed in recipients sharing a donor HLA-DR antigen (relative risk 10.1). When either an HLA-DR antigen match or CMV infection occurred in the absence of the other factor, the relative risk of developing VBDS was reduced (both <0.5), and no case of VBDS developed in the absence of both factors. This pattern suggests that CMV infection and donor/recipient HLA antigens are interdependent cofactors in the pathogenesis of VBDS. The role of CMV infection is probably to induce cellular expression of HLA antigens as a consequence of gamma-interferon production. This effect may not be specific to CMV, which is the commonest infection after liver transplantation, but could also be caused by other viral and bacterial infections, e.g., non-A, non-B viral hepatitis or cholangitis. Alternatively, the importance of CMV may lie in its genes, which code for class I- and DR-like protein sequences.[28,29] The class I-like protein may promote binding of CMV to donor class I antigens, leading to the formation of novel antigens or the unmasking of concealed epitopes. An immediate early gene of CMV codes for a quinpeptide shared with HLA-DR protein. Hydrophilicity experiments and beta-turn potential suggest it should be externalized; it has been shown to be antigenic and to cross react with HLA-DR.[29] However, it is still unclear whether the target antigen is class I or II (or indeed either) antigen. The effector cell appears to be the T lymphocyte, and the findings described above suggest it may be class II-restrictive. However, the correlation between HLA-DR matching and VBDS was not confirmed in another study of 52 patients with six cases of VBDS, although an association with HLA-DQ mismatching was observed.[30]

The role of humoral factors in the pathogenesis of VBDS is also controversial. The frequency of retransplantation for chronic rejection was not increased in patients with positive lymphocyte cross-matches in the Pittsburg program,[18] but a significantly increased risk was found in two other smaller studies specifically studying VBDS.[26,30] Positive lymphocyte cross-matches were found in five of six patients (83%) with VBDS in the Mayo Clinic program, compared with 24% of the remaining patients.[30] In our series, high-titer, donor-specific antibodies to class I antigen were only found in association with VBDS, occurred in 43% of such patients, and developed after transplantation in all but one instance.[26]

In our experience, VBDS may develop as early as the third week after transplantation, and about 75% of cases are diagnosed within 3 months. Analysis of serial liver function tests in recipients developing VBDS, CMV infection, and neither complication shows that aspartate aminotransferase (AST) is the earliest parameter to change; AST is significantly higher in the VBDS patients than in the other two subgroups at the end of the fourth week (Fig. 16–3). The increases in alkaline phosphatase and serum bilirubin reach significance in the fifth week (Figs. 16–4 and 16–5). The predominant clinical feature is progressive cholestasis and pruritus. The bile becomes pale, while feces and urine show the characteristic color changes of cholestasis. Hepatocyte function is relatively well preserved until the later stages, so that abnormalities of synthetic function (serum albumin and pro-

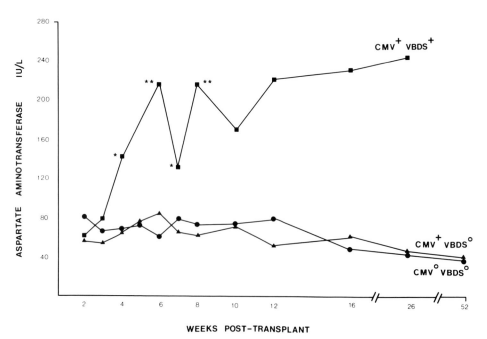

Figure 16–3 Serial median aspartate aminotransferase (AST) levels in patients with the vanishing bile duct syndrome (VBDS) and CMV, uncomplicated CMV, and those with neither complication.

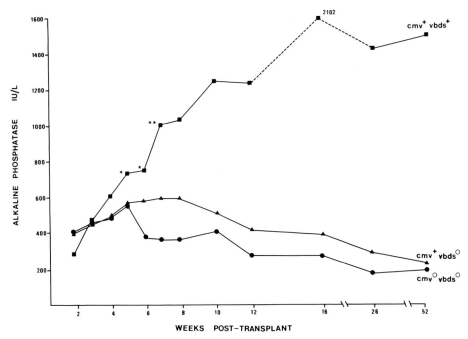

Figure 16–4 Serial median alkaline phosphatase levels in patients with VBDS and CMV, CMV alone, and neither complication.

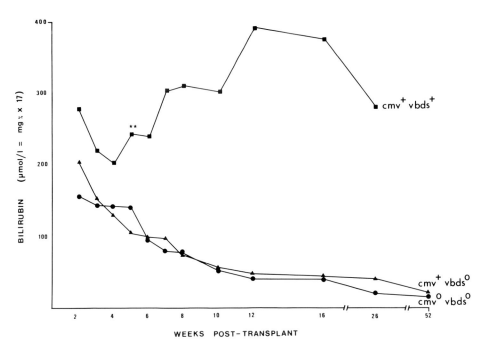

Figure 16–5 Serial median serum bilirubin levels in patients with VBDS and CMV, CMV alone, and neither complication.

thrombin time), encephalopathy, and ascites are only seen in the preterminal phase. Patients with VBDS often succumb to sepsis before progressing to this stage. Although the diagnosis is made on histologic criteria, hepatic arteriography and cholangiography may reveal the associated changes of arterial pruning or occlusion and biliary stricturing, respectively.[6]

The only effective treatment for VBDS is retransplantation, which should be performed as early as possible to minimize surgical difficulties caused by the formation of adhesions. There is no evidence that the course of VBDS can be modified by any of the immunosuppressive agents currently available, and excessive immunosuppression increases the risk of infection and might thus prejudice the eventual outcome. It is not possible on available data to determine if the risk of developing VBDS is increased after a second transplant.

GRAFT-VERSUS-HOST DISEASE

Mild graft-versus-host (GVH) disease resulting in self-limiting hemolytic anemia may be relatively common after liver transplantation when carried out across the blood group barrier.[31] Severe GVH disease has recently been reported in a single patient, with the demonstration of HLA chimerism on bone marrow cells.[32] The clinical features observed were fever, diarrhea, pancytopenia, and a skin rash. The outcome was favorable after treatment with high-dose steroids. The source of the donor-immunocompetent cells was uncertain, but may possibly have originated from transplanted lymph nodes. It has been suggested that patients immunosuppressed mainly with cyclosporine may have an increased risk of developing GVH disease because of the relative uncontrolled activity of B-lymphocyte populations.[33]

TOLERANCE

Rejection episodes are less severe and immunosuppression requirements appear lower in human patients receiving liver grafts, compared with other solid organs, e.g., kidney. This is especially true more than 6 months after transplantation, and some long-term survivors in our program maintain normal graft function on as little as 100 mg of cyclosporine daily. Animal experiments suggest that clonal deletion of alloreactive T lymphocytes, and the presence in serum of a soluble factor (possibly circulating class I antigen) explain the development of tolerance after liver grafting.[34] In humans, one contributing factor may be that donor Kupffer cells, which strongly express both class I and II MHC antigens and which function as antigen-presenting cells, are replaced by recipient cells within 8 days to 1 month of transplantation, thus removing one of the stronger immunogenic components from the transplanted graft.[9] In addition, dendritic cells that are antigen-presenting are sparse in the liver.

Two separate studies have suggested that antiidiotypic antibodies to anti-MHC develop within 2 weeks of transplantation, and that they may be important in determining graft survival.[12,17] As mentioned previously, the down-regulation of PRA with time after transplantation was interpreted as evidence of a humoral response leading to the production of antiidiotypic antibodies.[12] Another group demonstrated that inhibition of microcytotoxicity was present in the immunoglobulin fraction of serum and was specific for donor anti-HLA alloantisera,[17] but this could also be due to the presence of non-complement-fixing (nonidiotypic) antibodies. All patients losing their graft through rejection showed poor and transient antiidiotype production when compared with successful transplants.

A role for antigen-specific suppressor T cells in the facilitation of long-term graft survival has been proposed,[35] based on an increase in specific subsets of CD8 cells in patients with normal graft function 10–43 months posttransplantation. While CD8 cells are present in greater numbers, the CD11-negative and CD16-positive subsets are not, and the increase is due to CD8/CD11-positive and CD8/Leu7-positive cells. In addition, these subsets were also found to have increased expression of the CD3/TCR complex; they were interpreted to be antigen-specific cells associated with suppressive activity.[35] Animal studies suggest that both humoral and cellular factors may be important in promoting tolerance after liver transplantation. Tolerant animals were found to have strong antidonor class II MHC activity,[36] as well as a depletion of alloreactive host cytotoxic cells.[37]

IMMUNOSUPPRESSION

Immunosuppressive therapy after OLT can be considered in relation to maintenance therapy and to supplemental treatment in response to an immunologic "crisis." Prior to the introduction of cyclosporine into clinical practice, the combination of prednisolone and azathioprine was the mainstay of maintenance immunosuppression, but was associated with a high incidence of sepsis and impaired healing, which was largely attributed to the steroid component. Cyclosporine was introduced into clinical liver transplantation by Calne et al. in 1979 and was proclaimed by Starzl to be one of the most important advances in the history of OLT; he attributed a doubling in 1-year survival rates in his program to cyclosporine.[38] In retrospect, such an interpretation appears overgenerous, as a similar improvement in survival rate was observed in the Cambridge/King's College Hospital joint program 5 years after the introduction of cyclosporine and was probably secondary to a number of parallel advances in medical, anesthiologic, and surgical practices.[39] Furthermore, a 60% 1-year survival has been obtained in the Groningen program without the use of cyclosporine.[40] The mechanisms of action of cyclosporine are relatively selective; it appears to function by inhibiting transcription of lymphokine genes, thus interfering with interleukin-2 (IL-2) production. Cyclophilin, a small ubiquitous protein, has been proposed as the active cytoplasmic binding protein for cyclosporine.[41] IL-2-producing clones of helper T lymphocytes are thought to be the main target in cyclosporine-induced immunosuppression, but the recently demonstrated inhibition of antigen-presenting cells may prove to be relevant.[42]

Cyclosporine is almost universally used in the initial maintenance regimen after OLT. While in earlier years doses as high as 17.5 mg/kg/day were administered, starting doses of 3–10 mg/kg/day are now usual. Some centers commence cyclosporine before OLT, while others postpone the introduction for 48 hours or longer after surgery, until renal function has normalized. Thereafter, the drug dose is normally titrated to maintain blood levels, which vary not only from center to center, but also with the method of assay [radioimmunoassay (RIA) with polyclonal or monoclonal antibodies, high performance liquid chromatography] and the type of blood sample used (whole blood, plasma-separated at different temperatures). In our program we currently aim for levels of 100–150 ng/ml as measured by monoclonal RIA in whole blood during the first 6 months after OLT (falling to 80–120 ng/ml in stable patients after 6 months), while in the Pittsburg series levels are maintained between 600 and 1,000 ng/ml, as measured by polyclonal RIA in whole blood.[43] Cyclosporine is initially given intravenously, since adsorption is highly unpredictable while bile is draining percutaneously and graft function is abnormal. In our practice, conversion to oral cyclosporine is usually achieved 3–5 weeks after transplantation.

A corticosteroid is almost invariably used in conjunction with cyclosporine, particularly in the initial posttransplant phase. Corticosteroids impair interleukin-1 production by macrophages and as a consequence also suppress IL-2 release from activated T cells. The type, dose, and duration of therapy varies considerably from center to center. In our program, 15 mg/kg of methylprednisolone is given intravenously during the anhepatic phase of the transplant operation, and subsequently prednisolone 1 mg/kg/day is administered. The latter is decreased by weekly increments of 0.05 mg/kg until a target dose of 0.15–0.2 mg/kg/day is reached. In the Pittsburg program, 200 mg of methylprednisolone is given on the first posttransplant day, and the dose is gradually decreased to 20 mg by the sixth postoperative day.[2] At the Mayo Clinic, the initial corticosteroid doses are higher, at prednisolone 100 mg/day, but are tapered to 20 mg/day by 8 weeks.[11,30] Long-term treatment with corticosteroids is the norm, although between 1979 and 1986 in our program, 55% of patients surviving for 3–4 years after OLT were maintained on cyclosporine alone.[44]

Azathioprine, a less selective immunosuppressive agent, is again being used in immunosuppressive regimens after OLT. As a "steroid-sparing" agent, the advantage of cyclosporine over azathioprine appears to be confined to the first posttransplant year,[44] and azathioprine is often used in doses of 1.5–2.0 mg/kg/day as an alternative to cyclosporine in patients with toxicity related to the latter drug. Since January, 1987, we have incorporated azathioprine 1 mg/kg/day into the long-term immunosuppression regimen with cyclosporine and prednisolone, in an attempt to gain greater flexibility and to minimize the side effects encountered by using relatively low doses of each drug.

Supplemental immunosuppression is given to patients with evidence of acute or reversible graft rejection. High-dose corticosteroids, usually methylprednisolone (up to 1,000 mg/day) or hydrocortisone (up to 2,000 mg/day), are usually given for 3–6 days. The principal alternative approach is the use of polyclonal or monoclonal antibodies of varying specificity, including antilymphocyte globulin (ALG), antithymocyte globulin (ATG), OKT3, and six generations of Campath monoclonal antibodies. The greatest clinical experience has been gained with OKT3, a mouse antihuman pan-T-cell antibody directed against the CD3 antigen. In an uncontrolled study, the response rate to OKT3 among 250 patients in the Pittsburg series was 76% when used within 10 days of transplantation, 94% at days 10–90, and 69% after 90 days.[45] However, 25.2% of these patients were retransplanted, compared with 24.9% of 362 patients not receiving OKT3 over the same period, and the respective 1-year graft survival rates were 62.0 and 53.3%. Other smaller studies quote response rates of 25–83%, when OKT3 is used as primary therapy for rejection episodes, and 44–76% when it is used as rescue therapy for patients in whom other treatment regimens have failed.[22,46-49] However, the use of OKT3 may be associated with a higher frequency of subsequent infections, particularly due to CMV and other viruses.

REFERENCES

1. Bismuth H, Castaing D, Ericzon BG, et al: Hepatic transplantation in Europe. *Lancet* ii:674–675, 1987.
2. Maddrey WC, Van Thiel DH: Liver transplantation: an overview. *Hepatology* 8:948–959, 1988.
3. Starzl TE, Iwatsuki S, Shaw BW, et al: Immunosuppression and other nonsurgical factors in the improved results of liver transplantation. *Semin Liver Dis* 5:334–343, 1985.
4. Lautenschlager I, Hockerstedt K, Ahonen J, et al: Fine-needle aspiration biopsy in the monitoring of liver allografts. *Transplantation* 46:47–52, 1988.
5. Snover DC, Freese DK, Sharp HL, et al: Liver allograft rejection: an analysis of the use of biopsy in determining outcome of rejection. *Am J Surg Pathol* 11:1–10, 1987.
6. O'Grady J, Williams R: Long-term management, complications and disease recurrence. In Maddrey WC: *Transplantation of the Liver.* New York, Elsevier, 1988 pp 143–165.
7. White RM, Zajko AB, Demetris AJ, et al: Liver transplant rejection: angiographic findings in 35 patients. *Am J Radiol* 148:1095–1098, 1987.
8. Steinhoff G, Wonigeit K, Pichlmayr R: Analysis of sequential changes in major histocompatibility complex expression in human liver grafts after transplantation. *Transplantation* 45:394–401, 1988.
9. Gouw ASH, Houthoff HJ, Huitema S, et al: Expression of major histocompatibility complex antigens and replacement of donor cells by recipient ones in human liver grafts. *Transplantation* 43:291–296, 1987.
10. So SKS, Platt JL, Ascher NL, et al: Increased expression of class I major histocompatibility complex antigens on hepatocytes in rejecting human liver allografts. *Transplantation* 43:79–84, 1987.
11. Perkins JD, Wiesner RH, Banks PM, et al: Immunohistologic labeling as an indicator of liver allograft rejection. *Transplantation* 43:105–107, 1987.
12. Markus BH, Fung JJ, Zeevi A, et al: Analysis of T lymphocytes infiltrating human hepatic allografts. *Transplant Proc* 19:2470–2473, 1987.
13. Bryan CF, Newman JT, Nery J, et al: Quantitative and functional profile of the immune system after liver transplantation. *Transplant Proc* 19:4340–4344, 1987.
14. Gubernatis G, Lauchart W, Jonker M, et al: Signs of hyperacute rejection of liver grafts in rhesus monkeys after donor-specific presensitization. *Transplant Proc* 19:1082–1083, 1987.
15. Bird G, Friend P, Donaldson P, et al: Hyperacute rejection in liver transplantation: a case report. *Transplant Proc* (in press).
16. Rego J, Prevost F, Rumeau JL, et al: Hyperacute rejection after ABO-incompatible orthotopic liver transplant. *Transplant Proc* 19:4589–4590, 1987.
17. Mohanakumar T, Rhodes C, Mendez-Picon G, et al: Antiidiotypic antibodies to major histocompatibility complex class I and II antibodies in hepatic transplantation and their role in allograft survival. *Transplantation* 44:54–58, 1987.
18. Gordon RD, Fung JJ, Markus B: The antibody crossmatch in liver transplantation. *Surgery* 100:705–715, 1986.

19. Gordon RD, Iwatsuki S, Esquivel CO, et al: Experience with liver transplantation across ABO blood groups. *Transplant Proc* 19:4575–4579, 1987.

20. Nery J, Klintmalm G, Olson L, et al: Incidence and outcome of acute rejection in liver transplantation. *Transplant Proc* 20:375–377, 1988.

21. Gugenheim J, Samuel D, Saliba F, et al: Use of flexible triple-drug immunosuppressive therapy in liver transplantation. *Transplant Proc* 19:3805–3807, 1987.

22. Wood RP, Shaw BW, Williams L: The use of OKT3 rescue therapy after orthotopic liver transplantation—the University of Nebraska Medical Center experience. *Transplant Proc* 20:254–259, 1988.

23. Portmann B, Neuberger JM, Williams R: Intrahepatic bile duct lesions. In Calne RY: *Liver Transplantation* ed 1. New York, Grune and Stratton, 1983, pp 279–287.

24. Vierling JM, Fennel RH: Histopathology of early and late human hepatic allograft rejection: evidence of progressive destruction of interlobular bile ducts. *Hepatology* 5:1076–1082, 1985.

25. Ludwig J, Wiesner RH, Batts KP, et al: The acute vanishing bile duct syndrome (acute irreversible rejection) after orthotopic liver transplantation. *Hepatology* 7:476–483, 1987.

26. Donaldson PT, Alexander GJM, O'Grady J, et al: Evidence of an immune response to HLA class I antigens in the vanishing bile duct syndrome after liver transplantation. *Lancet* i:945–948, 1987.

27. O'Grady JG, Alexander GJM, Sutherland S, et al: Cytomegalovirus infection and donor/recipient HLA antigens: interdependent co-factors in pathogenesis of vanishing bileduct syndrome after liver transplantation. *Lancet* ii:302–305, 1988.

28. Beck S, Barrell BG: Human cytomegalovirus encodes a glycoprotein homologous to MHC class I antigens. *Nature* 331:269–272, 1988.

29. Fuginami RS, Nelson JA, Walker L, et al: Sequence homology and immunologic cross-reactivity of human cytomegalovirus with HLA-DR beta chain: a means for graft rejection and immunosuppression. *J Virol* 62:100–109, 1988.

30. Batts KP, Moore SB, Perkins JD, et al: Influence of positive lymphocyte crossmatch and HLA mismatching on vanishing bile duct syndrome in human liver allografts. *Transplantation* 45:376–379, 1988.

31. Ramsey G, Nusbacher J, Starzl TE, et al: Isohemagglutinins of graft origin after ABO-unmatched liver transplantation. *N Engl J Med* 311:1167–1170, 1988.

32. Burdick JF, Vogelsang GB, Smith WJ, et al: Severe graft-versus-host disease in a liver-transplant recipient. *N Engl J Med* 318:689–691, 1988.

33. Badosa F, de Oca J, Figueras J, et al: Is there a graft-versus-host reaction in liver transplantation? *Transplant Proc* 19:3822–3824, 1987.

34. Roser BJ, Kamada N, Zimmerman F, Davies HS: Immunosuppressive effect of experimental liver allografts. In Calne RY: *Liver Transplantation,* ed 2. London, Grune and Stratton, 1987, pp 35–56.

35. Schwinzer R, Wonigeit K, Nashan B, et al: Selective increase of CD8+ CD11+ cells in long-term liver allograft recipients. *Transplant Proc* 19:3812–3814, 1987.

36. Kamada N, Shinomiya T: Serology of liver transplantation in the rat. I: Alloantibody responses and evidence for tolerance in a nonrejector combination. *Transplantation* 42;7–13, 1986.

37. Davies HffS, Kamada N, Roser BJ: Mechanisms of donor-specific unresponsiveness induced by liver grafting. *Transplant Proc* 15:831–835, 1983.

38. Starzl TE, Iwatsuki S, Van Thiel DH, et al; Evolution of liver transplantation. *Hepatology* 2:614–636, 1982.

39. O'Grady JG, Williams R: Present position of liver transplantation and its impact on hepatological practice. *Gut* 29:566–570, 1988.
40. Krom RAF, Wiesner RH, Haagsma EB, et al: A comparison of azathioprine and cyclosporine in liver transplantation: a study of two personal series. In Sloof MJH, Houthoff HJ, eds: *Cyclosporine in Liver Transplantation,* Uden, Actua Sandoz, 1987, pp 49–54.
41. Harding MW, Handschumacher RE: Cyclophilin, a primary molecular target for cyclosporine. *Transplantation* 46:29S–35S, 1988.
42. Manca F, Fenoglio D, Kunkl A, et al: Effect of cyclosporine on the antigen-presenting function of human and murine accessory cells. *Transplantation.* 46:40S–43S, 1988.
43. Starzl TE, Iwatsuki S, Shaw BW, et al: Orthotopic liver transplantation in 1984. *Transplant Proc* 17:250–258, 1985.
44. O'Grady JG, Forbes A, Rolles K, et al: An analysis of cyclosporine efficacy and toxicity after liver transplantation. *Transplantation* 45:575–579, 1988.
45. Esquivel CO, Fung JJ, Markus B, et al: OKT3 in the reversal of acute hepatic allograft rejection. *Transplant Proc* 19:2443–2446, 1987.
46. Yandza T, de Ville de Goyet J, Salizzoni M, et al: Orthoclone OKT3 in liver transplantation: experience in 21 patients. *Transplant Proc* 19:3987–3990, 1987.
47. Cosimi AB, Cho SI, Delmonico FL, et al: A randomised clinical trial comparing OKT3 and steroids for treatment of hepatic allograft rejection. *Transplantation* 43:91–95, 1987.
48. Goldstein G, Kremer AB, Barnes L, et al: OKT3 monoclonal antibody reversal of renal and hepatic rejection in pediatric patients. *J Pediatr* 111:1046–1050, 1987.
49. Colonna JO, Goldstein LI, Brems JJ, et al: A prospective study of the use of monoclonal anti-T3-cell antibody (OKT3) to treat steroid resistant liver transplant rejection. *Arch Surg* 122:1120–1123, 1987.

PART **SIX**

THE GASTROINTESTINAL TRACT

Gastrointestinal Manifestations of Immunodeficiency Diseases in Infants, Children, and Adults

MARVIN E. AMENT

INTRODUCTION

This chapter clarifies the unique and specific abnormalities seen in immune-deficient states and stresses the newest recognized abnormalities. It highlights the fact that the most frequent and severe abnormalities occur in those with combined immune-deficient states.

SYNDROME OF X-LINKED INFANTILE AGAMMAGLOBULINEMIA (BRUTON'S AGAMMAGLOBULINEMIA, CONGENITAL AGAMMAGLOBULINEMIA)

This condition is the prototype for discussion of primary humoral immunodeficiency and was the first described and best characterized. It is known by many synonyms: "Bruton's," "congenital," "infantile," "X-linked agammaglobulinemia," and "hypogammaglobulinemia."[1-3]

Patients with this syndrome have serious, recurrent pyogenic infections commencing in infancy or early childhood because of markedly decreased levels of serum immunoglobulins of all classes. These patients have low or totally absent serum immunoglobulins of all classes, a lack of circulating immunoglobulin-bearing B cells, and an inability to make functional antibody and clear antigens. These patients have normal numbers of T lymphocytes, and they function normally. Plasma cells are absent from lymph nodes, and they do not have germinal centers and follicle formation.

In X-linked agammaglobulinemia, the primary immunologic defect is lack of development of immunoglobulin-bearing B lymphocytes. It is a block in maturation of cytoplasmic immunoglobulin-positive pre-B cells to rearrange light chain genes and thereby express functional IgM molecules on the cell surface, the hallmark of mature B lymphocytes. Cell-mediated immunity is intact, and circulating T cells and T-cell subsets are normal in number, proportion, and function.

Clinical Features

Patients with X-linked agammaglobulinemia typically begin to develop recurrent bacterial infections between 6 and 9 months of age when maternal antibody is no longer present to prevent it. Typically, they develop pyogenic infections such as recurrent pneumonia, acute and chronic sinusitis, otitis, pyoderma, osteomyelitis, meningitis, and sepsis. If diagnosis is not established early on, bronchiectasis may develop because of repeated pulmonary infections. The most typical organisms to cause infection are: *Hemophilus influenzae,* streptococci, pneumococci, and *Pseudomonas aeruginosa.*

Although immunity to viral infections appears to be intact, these patients are particularly susceptible to chronic enteroviral infections of the central nervous system (CNS). The most common pathogens to cause this infection are the echoviruses, type II in particular. Rare cases have had simultaneous infections with a second serotype. The disease is characterized by weakness, lethargy or coma, headaches, hearing loss, seizures, ataxia, and paresthesias. Some patients have neurologic manifestations of chronic enteroviral infection including fever, dermatomytositis-like syndrome, edema, rashes, and hepatitis. Patients with CNS disease may best be treated with intraventricular immunoglobulin.[5] Hepatitis has also been reported to be fatal in occasional cases.[6] Recurrent gastrointestinal infections with enteric gram-negative organisms are not typical of this group. This suggests that resistance to these infections may in part be secondary to cellular immunity or other host-resistant factors. Giardiasis has been reported to cause chronic diarrhea, steatorrhea, secondary lactase deficiency, and severe damage to the intestinal mucosa; however, it is susceptible to eradication with treatment and reversal of all abnormalities in structure and function. This infection, however, is rare in those with X-linked agammaglobulinemia.[7]

In eight cases of X-linked immunodeficiency syndrome followed for 1½ decades, giardiasis was recognized as the cause of chronic diarrhea only once and in a prospective study of the incidence of giardia in asymptomatic subjects with X-linked agammaglobulinemia, was not found in any individual.[8]

Campylobacter fetus jejuni is one of the most common causes of bacterial gastroenteritis. In a retrospective study of 51 cases of diarrhea, two patients with X-linked agammaglobulinemia and three other immune-deficient patients were infected. They represented 20% of the cases and, compared with nonimmune-deficient patients, they had fever and diarrhea for a substantially longer interval of time, i.e., 15 and 23 days, respectively. Four of the five patients excreted the bacteria in their stool for 20–27 days, and the fifth patient for 1 year. The investigators claimed the infections were not affected by treatment with erythromycin ethylsuccinate.[9] Subsequent cases have shown that *C. jejuni* can cause bacteremia as well as enteritis and that antibiotic therapy may not be sufficient to eradicate it. Death may occur because antibiotics may be insufficient.[10]

Late-onset lactase deficiency has been described in X-linked agammaglobulinemia, but there is no evidence that it is typical of this condition.[11] Idiopathic malabsorption and protein-losing enteropathy have also been reported in one case.[12]

Cases of ulcerative colitis are not well documented in X-linked agammaglobulinemia. Many in the past may have been antibiotic-induced. Acute and chronic colitis secondary to *Clostridium difficile* should be considered as the cause of bloody or blood-tinged diarrhea in these patients, especially if antibiotics have been used within 3 months of its onset. Only if this and other bacteria recognized to cause colitis have been excluded, can ulcerative colitis be diagnosed. All such patients should have stool cultured for *C. difficile* and a toxin titer determined in the stool. Crohn's disease has not been reported in any patient with X-linked agammaglobulinemia.

The total absence of plasma cells in the rectal mucosa of patients with agammaglobulinemia is characteristic, although some patients with variable immune deficiency syndrome may have a similar finding. Similarly, most asymptomatic patients with X-linked agammaglobulinemia will show early crypt abscesses in their rectal mucosa and polymorphonuclear leukocytes in the lamina propria.[8]

Recently, a case of malakoplakia of the colon with recurrent strictures has been reported. Microscopically, the disease is characterized by chronic granulomatous infiltration consisting primarily of large histiocytes and intracellular and extracellular inclusion bodies scattered in a scant fibrous stroma, infiltrated with lymphoid cells. The symptoms of malakoplakia are not specific and typically consist of abdominal pain and diarrhea. Its etiology is unknown but is suspected of being infectious in origin. It may involve one or multiple areas or the entire colon.[13] Treatment of the malakoplakia with bethanecol may be useful to treat the inflammatory lesions.[14] Its mode of action is by stabilizing lysozymal enzymes.

A rare case of recurrent purulent triaditis was reported in a patient with X-linked agammaglobulinemia, who had no anatomic obstruction of the biliary tree. In patients with X-linked agammaglobulinemia and fever of unknown origin, this condition should be considered. Patients such as this frequently have negative blood cultures and require liver biopsy with culture to diagnose the specific organism, in order to establish appropriate treatment.[15] Primary sclerosing cholangitis has also been reported in X-linked agammaglobulinemia.[16]

X-LINKED IMMUNODEFICIENCY WITH HYPER IgM (DYSGAMMAGLOBULINEMIA TYPE 1)

This syndrome is characterized by *X-linked recessive* inheritance, recurrent bacterial infections, and decreased or absent serum levels of IgG, IgA, and IgE, but elevated or normal IgM. Neutropenia and lymphoid hyperplasia (lymphadenopathy, hypertrophic tonsils, and splenomegaly) are part of this syndrome.

Although the condition has occurred predominantly in males, a few female cases have been reported. It may occur as a complication of congenital rubella. Patients with this condition may have a defect in the switch mechanism preventing the generation of IgG and IgA, a lack of "feedback inhibition" by serum IgG, further increasing the level of IgM, and, in some, a lack of helper T lymphocytes.[17] A stem cell defect may exist in some to account for the neutropenia.

Clinical Manifestations

Recurrent bacterial infections, including otitis media, pneumonia, and tonsillitis begin during the first 2 years of life. If neutropenia is present, stomatitis and mouth ulcers may develop. Esophageal ulcers with stricture formation, possibly secondary to *Candida tropicalis,* developed in one patient who had neutropenia. This was treated with antifungal and antibiotic medications. The ulcers healed, but resulted in midesophageal stricture.[18] This was treated with bougienage.

Several years later, this patient developed chronic diarrhea and malabsorption, Cryptosporidium were found in his small bowel biopsies. Treatment with sporicidin resulted in reversal of diarrhea but persistence of malabsorption. Although successful treatment of cryptosporidium with hyperimmune bovine colostrum has been documented,[19] other recent reports clearly contradict these findings.[20,21]

X-linked hypogammaglobulinemia with growth hormone deficiency
This manifestation has been described in one family, but there was no associated gastrointestinal disease.[22] This individual developed chronic enteroviral meningoencephalitis with edema and rash. The virus was isolated from his stool and pharynx.

Autosomal recessive agammaglobulinemia
This manifestation has been reported in female patients. It is indistinguishable from the X-linked type. Chronic gastrointestinal disease has not been reported in these patients,[23] but they too are susceptible to chronic enteroviral meningoencephalitis.[5]

IMMUNODEFICIENCY WITH NORMAL OR HYPERIMMUNOGLOBULINEMIA

This syndrome is characterized by recurrent bacterial infections, onset during infancy, normal or elevated serum immunoglobulins, and defective antibody responses to certain antigens.

This extremely rare syndrome may really represent a variety of immunodeficiencies. In some instances, a T-cell defect (T4 inducer cell) may account for the immune aberrations.[24]

Two patients with this condition had chronic diarrhea and malabsorption. Their biopsies showed moderate-to-severe mucosal injury without any recognizable causes and proliferation of plasma cells in the lamina propria. It is possibly due to chronic viral infection with rotavirus, since in both involvement was confined to the small intestine. One of these patients had normal immunoglobulin levels but failed to produce neutralizing antibodies to coxsackievirus B2 despite several months of infection by the virus.[5]

ATAXIA TELANGIECTASIA (AT) WITH IMMUNODEFICIENCY

This *autosomal recessive* disorder is typified by telangiectasia, progressive ataxia with degeneration of Purkinje cells, sinupulmonary infections, increased sensitivity of fibroblasts and lymphocytes to ionizing radiation, lymphocyte chromosome changes, and thymic hypoplasia with IgA and IgG2 immunodeficiencies.[25-27] Cancer risk is greatly elevated in these patients. Premature aging and increased incidence of endocrine disorders, such as diabetes mellitus, is also associated with this disorder. These patients have increased autoantibodies against endocrine organs, liver, and parietal cells of the stomach and muscle. The CNS lesions in the condition are both demyelinating and degenerative, which is also suggestive of an autoimmune process. An excess of a DNA processing or repair protein is common among patients with ataxia-telangiectasia.[27]

The elevated alpha-fetoprotein levels in patients with ataxia telangiectasia has been said to be evidence for a basic defect in organ differentiation and maturation.[28] Furthermore, their cells are extremely sensitive to radiation. With time these patients have progressive deterioration of the immune system.

Clinical Features

Symptoms of ataxia usually develop during infancy but may be delayed until age 5 years. Ataxia is cerebellar, initially involving posture and gait, ultimately involving movements of intention. The speech of these patients becomes slurred, and variable choreoathetoid movements are present. They have typical mask-like facies.

Telangiectasia occurs on the bulbar conjuntivae initially, and as early as 1 year of age. They eventually become more prominent and appear in other areas, such as the lateral aspect of the nose, the ears, the antecubital and popliteal areas, and the dorsa of the hands and feet. Recurrent sinopulmonary infections leading to bronchiectasis rarely present before the ataxia and telangiectasia.[25,29]

Gastrointestinal disease is not a major factor in patients with ataxia telangiectasia. However, death in patients with ataxia telangiectasia has been attributed to adenocarcinoma of the stomach and small intestine and lymphoma in the stomach, small intestine, and colon.[30,31] Hepatocellular carcinoma has also been described in four cases. Two were siblings.[32] The risk of dying of cancer in these children is 61-fold greater for white probands and 184-fold for black probands. The cancer excess was most pronounced for lymphoma, with 252- and 750-fold excesses observed for whites and blacks, respectively.[33]

Abnormal liver function has been described, but biopsies were not taken to assess the degree of liver damage and to determine its characteristics. Elevations of anti-smooth muscle and antimitochondrial antibodies have been described in ataxia telangiectasia; however, this finding has not been correlated histologically. Small intestinal and rectal biopsies from patients with AT show increased numbers of plasma cells without destruction of crypts, villi, or glands.[8] Patients with AT who have malignancy are very radiosensitive. Radiation therapy must be managed with lower dosage in this group of patients.

TRANSIENT HYPOGAMMAGLOBULINEMIA OF INFANCY (THI) (HYPOGAMMAGLOBULINEMIA OF EARLY CHILDGOOD "WITH RECOVERY" OR WITH DEVELOPMENT OF OTHER GYSGAMMAGLOBULINEMIA)

This syndrome is characterized by being self-limited with onset between 3–6 months of age, usually lasting 6–18 months, but extending up to 60 months. It is usually associated with increased susceptibility to infection as a result of abnormal delay in the onset of immunoglobulin synthesis.[34] Some believe the name is a misnomer because many of these patients do not develop normal immunoglobulin levels until after infancy and, in a few, dysgammaglobulinemia persists. In some, the diminished immunoglobulin levels are a prodrome of selective IgA deficiency.[35] A better name for the syndrome is hypogammaglobulinemia of early childhood, to which can be added, "with recovery" or with development of other dysgammaglobulinemia depending upon the eventual phenotype observed.[36]

Clinical Features

THI typically presents with frequent bacterial infections of the skin, lungs, meninges, and respiratory tract caused by gram-positive organisms.

Some, but not all, have a decreased number of peripheral lymph nodes and a decrease in volume of tonsillar tissue. Some may fail to thrive because of their frequent infections, while others grow and gain weight normally. Unlike those with combined immunodeficiency syndrome, who frequently have thrush, these patients do not.

Immunological Defect

THI patients have a decline in placentally transferred immunoglobulins, as all infants do, during the first months of life. They fail to synthesize their own immunoglobulins until much later than normal. Spontaneous recovery usually begins by 9–15 months of age, and they may become normal by 2–4 years of age.

They have normal or near normal numbers of circulating B cells, which distinguishes them from children with X-linked agammaglobulinemia. It has been shown that their B cells can function normally but that there is delayed maturation of T-helper-cell function for immunoglobulin production.[37] They have a thymus on chest x-ray films. Their bone marrows have a paucity of normal plasma cells.

Gastrointestinal Manifestations

Patients with transient hypogammaglobulinemia of infancy have an increased incidence of chronic diarrhea.[35] They constitute 10–15% of all such patients. Therefore, in all infants with chronic diarrhea, immunoglobulins should be measured. The etiology of diarrhea in such patients is not unique — giardiasis, *C. jejuni, Shigella, Salmonella,* rotoviruses, and *C. difficile.* However, these infections are found in a greater proportion of patients with transient hypogammaglobulinemia than in those with chronic diarrhea and normal immunoglobulins.[35] The unique factor is the chronicity of the infections.[9] Protozoan and bacterial gastrointestinal infections should be treated in this condition in the same way as in others who are not immunodeficient.

Immunotherapy

Although this is controversial, gammaglobulin therapy is generally given to such patients with THL.

SELECTIVE IgA DEFICIENCY

One in 700 in the general population has an absence of, or a marked reduction of, serum IgA. IgA deficiency may be associated with other immunologic abnormalities.[38] Studies have shown that selective IgA deficiency may be associated with IgG2 and IgG4 deficiency, and it is this subgroup that may have more symptomatic infections.[39,40] One report indicated that half of all patients with IgA deficiency were also deficient in IgE.[41] Those patients with normal or elevated IgE often suffer from allergic disorders that may mimic respiratory infection. T-cell function is generally normal in these patients. Patients with symptomatic IgA deficiency may require additional evaluation to determine the immune nature of their problem, i.e., if it is truly selective IgA deficiency. The evaluation should include quantitation of IgG subclasses, as well as studies of B- and T-cell function. Some also recommend an evaluation of IgE levels and IgA in secretions and the associated secretory component.

Patients with selective IgA deficiency may present with recurrent sinusitis, otitis media, bronchitis, and pneumonia. Chronic diarrhea and malabsorption secondary to giardiasis and/or celiac sprue as the only manifestation of IgA deficiency occur in 10% of patients with this immune defect.[42-45] It has been well documented that giardiasis is more likely to persist in patients who are IgA-deficient than in those who are not. However, there appears to be no difference in T- and B-lymphocyte subpopulations between those with and without persistent giardiasis.[46]

Ulcerative colitis and Crohn's disease have been reported in selective IgA deficiency. Their presentation and clinical course do not differ from those who are not immune deficient. Diabetes mellitus, pancreatitis, and malabsorption have been reported in one child with this deficiency.[47]

Intestinal Biopsy

The intestinal biopsy in patients with selecting IgA deficiency and celiac disease is similar to that seen in patients with celiac disease and normal IgA levels. Significant differences are found in the number of IgM-staining cells in the intestinal mucosa. In patients with selective IgA deficiency and celiac disease, almost all of the plasma cells stain for IgM.

In patients who are not immunoglobulin deficient, the plasma cells in the lamina propria stain for an increased number with IgA. Patients with IgA deficiency and celiac sprue have increased levels of IgM in their blood, whereas non-immunoglobulin-deficient individuals have increased IgA levels.

SELECTIVE IgE DEFICIENCY

No syndrome has been described in which IgE deficiency alone has been linked to gastrointestinal disease.

IgG SUBCLASS DEFICIENCIES AND ABNORMALITIES

There are four types of IgG subclasses. In normal serum the percentage of sub-classes are: IgG1 – 66%; IgG2 — 23%; IgG3 — 7%; and IgG4 — 4%. Unfortunately, the measurement of IgG subclasses is technically very difficult, and results reported from many commercial laboratories are simply not reliable or reproducible.

Patients with common variable immunoglobulin deficiency syndromes have a 20 – 25% chance of having an imbalance of IgG subclasses. There is no correlation of IgG subclass concentrations with type of immunodeficiency and/or with gastro-intestinal disease.[39]

COMMON VARIABLE IMMUNODEFICIENCY (ACQUIRED AGAMMAGLOBULINEMIA, ADULT AGAMMAGLOBULINEMIA, LATE ONSET AGAMMAGLOBULINEMIA)

This is a heterogeneous group of patients that present sometime after infancy, usually in the second or third decades. They are characterized by recurrent bacte-rial infections, decreased serum immunoglobulins, impaired antibody responses, and either normal or partially defective cellular immunity.[48–50] The majority of this group of patients has a significant amount of gastrointestinal disease. A few have chronic enteroviral meningencephalitis.[5]

Most of the cases are sporadic and cannot be attributed to genetic factors. In a select few, immunologic abnormalities in multiple family members may be de-tected. Circulating B lymphocytes are generally present, although the percentage and absolute numbers may be below the normal range. Absence of B cells suggests either acquired hypogammaglobulinemia associated with thymoma or congenital hypergammaglobulinemia.[51]

Clinical Features

The most common presenting feature in patients with common variable immuno-deficiency is recurrent sinopulmonary nfections. Pneumococci, staphylococci, and *H. influenzae* are the three organisms most commonly implicated in the respiratory tract infections early on but are later replaced by gram-negative-rods, as the pa-tient's flora becomes altered by exposure to an increasingly wide variety of antibi-otics. Most patients with common variable immunodeficiency syndrome have ton-sillar tissue and lymph nodes. A rare number will have hepatomegaly. Lymphoid hyperplasia with splenomegaly and lymphadenopathy, particularly of the GI tract, occur in about one-third of patients. Rales, clubbing of fingertips and toes, and altered chest configuration are characteristic findings in those with chronic lung disease. Gastrointestinal abnormalities and disease are frequent occurrences in common variable immunodeficiency syndrome.[8]

A generalized malabsorption syndrome characterized by steatorrhea, lactose intolerance, protein-losing enteropathy, generalized dissacharidase deficiency, and malabsorption of vitamin B_{12} and folic acid has been frequently described.[8,11] It is typically associated with varying degrees of damage to the villous architecture.

The etiology of the lesion has been described as secondary to giardiasis, cryptosporidium, and stronglyloidiasis.[52-54] In most instances, treatment of *Giardia lamblia* with metronidazole or other antiprotozoan medications, and cryptosporidium with sporicidin, has resulted in eradication of the parasite and reversal of malabsorption and of the mucosal lesions.[7,8,52-54] *Giardia lamblia* infections may be difficult to diagnose and may require aspiration of duodenal contents or examination of multiple small bowel biopsies. Cryptosporidia may be diagnosed most easily by multiple stool examinations and small intestinal biopsies.[53] This is also true of strongyloidiasis.[54] Bacterial infections of the small bowel and colon occur more frequently and are prolonged in this group of patients. *Campylobacter jejuni* has been recognized as causing a chronic diarrheal syndrome in this group of patients, which may respond to treatment with erythromycin.[55,56] Similarly, *Salmonella* infections may be frequent and severe in these patients, especially if pernicious anemia is present, with its decreased gastric acid production and defect in cellular immunity.[57] It would not be surprising to find chronic enteroviral infections in this group of patients, and a few such cases have been documented.[5]

Nodular lymphoid hyperplasia (NLH) of the small intestine has been described in acquired immunodeficiency syndrome. Microscopic examination shows large lymphoid follicles with germinal centers with the lamina propria. This causes protrusion of the overlying mucosa and a nodular or polypoid appearance. Plasma cells are either absent or diminished in the lamina propria.[58,59] The follicular lymphoid cells contain no detectable immunoglobulin by immunofluorescence. Studies have shown that these patients are unable to switch from IgM to IgG antibody production.[60,61]

The nodules seen in NLH are widespread in the large and small bowel, but they are predominantly distal in the small bowel. Small bowel enteroclysis may be necessary along with the double-contrast barium enema to demonstrate them. The lesions of NLH are said to be specific if they are umbilicated. Typically, the colonic lesions are larger than those in the small bowel. NLH is not typically seen with selective IgA deficiency but with common variable hypogammaglobulinemia.[62]

Colitis occurs in patients with common variable immunodeficiency syndrome and clinically is not different from that in the nonimmune-deficient. The lesions may be typical of ulcerative colitis but may not have as many plasma cells. Recently, a case of colitis was described confined to the rectosigmoid in which the lesions were not typical for ulcerative colitis or Crohn's disease. Radiographically, the patient had thumb printing confined to the rectosigmoid, and large elongated masses of hard, friable tissue were seen during sigmoidoscopy. Biopsies showed that glandular elements were denuded, and the lamina propria was filled with macrophages, which accounted for 80–90% of the cells in the lamina propria. The patient responded to 2 g azulfidine, 40 mg prednisone orally, and 100 mg hydrocortisone enema daily.[63,64] Two patients have been described who initially developed Crohn's disease followed by hypogammaglobulinemia. The immunologic profile of both was typical of acquired common variable hypogammaglobulinemia. They were believed to represent instances in which the "covert" suppressor T cell of Crohn's disease has become overtly active in the systemic circulation and has resulted in hypogammaglobulinemia.[65]

Some patients with common variable immunodeficiency syndrome have no recognizable cause of the malabsorption syndrome and small intestinal mucosal lesions. They do not respond to a gluten-free diet and fail to respond to antibiotic therapy for bacterial overgrowth.

Patients with common variable immunodeficiency have an increased incidence of pernicious anemia (PA). It is characterized by its earlier time of onset (in the third to fifth decades) and either presence or absence of antiparietal antibodies.[62-68] It differs from classic pernicious anemia in that both the gastric antrum and fundus are involved in the atrophic process. In classic PA only the fundus is involved. Furthermore, gastrin levels are either not elevated or only mildly in those with PA and common variable hypogammaglobulinemia, whereas they are very elevated in classic PA. Nearly one-third of adults with common variable immune deficiency syndrome and gastrointestinal disease develop adenocarcinoma or lymphoma of the stomach, small intestine, and/or colon.[68,69] In one series of 98 patients followed for up to 13 years, 11 developed cancer and 2 had had two cancers. Nine of the 11 were female, and cancer developed in the fifth or sixth decade of life for 10 of 11 patients. Seven of the 13 cancers were non-Hodgkin's lymphoma, and one had Waldenstrom's macroglobulinemia. These data show an 8- to 13-fold increase in cancer in general for patients who have this immunodeficiency and a 438-fold increase in lymphoma for females.[70]

Non-A, non-B hepatitis developed in a patient with common variable hypogammaglobulinemia while receiving fresh-frozen plasma transfusions. After the onset of hepatitis, the patient's T4/T8 cell ratio increased to nearly normal levels. The patient's serum IgG concentration stabilized at a satisfactory level in the absence of maintenance therapy, and simultaneous clinical improvement of a pre-existing condition of chronic sinusitis was noted. However, the patient was unable to produce specific antibody after immunization with a number of defined antigens. The mechanism for the increased IgG production is believed secondary to diminished suppressor T-cell activity.[71] Chronic active hepatitis that responds to corticosteroid therapy has also been reported in patients with common variable hypogammaglobulinemia.[72]

ANTIBODY DEFICIENCY WITH TRANSCOBALAMIN II DEFICIENCY

This is a very rare syndrome that was first described in an infant whose parents were first cousins. It was characterized by intractable diarrhea and megaloblastic anemia at 4 months of age. Serum immunoglobulins were low, and there was no antibody response to several antigens during the B_{12}-deficient phase. T-cell function was reportedly normal. The diarrhea was most likely due to malfunction or immaturity of the intestinal absorptive cells, which are dependent on a continuous supply of vitamin B_{12}.[73]

IMMUNODEFICIENCY WITH GENERALIZED HEMATOPOIETIC HYPOPLASIA (RETICULAR DYSGENESIS)

This is an exceedingly rare syndrome characterized by severe, congenital cellular and antibody deficiency associated with agenesis of the granulocytic precursors of the bone marrow. It presents within the first days of life with failure to thrive, vomiting, diarrhea, or localized infection. Two-thirds of cases died before 2 weeks of age. All had marked-to-mild leukopenia. Total gammaglobulin level reflects maternal transport of transplacental maternal IgG and IgA. The autopsy findings are similar to those of severe combined immunodeficiency. In addition, an absence or marked deficiency of granulocytic precursors is noted in the bone marrow. Bone marrow transplant is the only possible treatment. The etiology of the diarrhea is unknown.[74]

THYMIC HYPOPLASIA (DIGEORGE SYNDROME, CELLULAR IMMUNODEFICIENCY WITH HYPERPARATHYROIDISM)

Clinical Features

Thymic hypoplasia is a congenital immunodeficiency syndrome characterized clinically by hypocalcemic tetany, congenital heart disease, unusual facies, and increased susceptibility to infection. These patients are typically recognized by their characteristic external features. These include hypertelorism, antimongoloid slant of the eyes, low-set prominent ears with notched pinnae, reduced helix, and micrognathia. Rarely, esophageal atresia and imperforate anus may be found.[75]

If the infants survive the neonatal period, increased susceptibility to infection occurs, manifested by chronic rhinitis, recurrent pneumonia, oral candidiasis, and diarrhea. The etiology of the diarrhea is undetermined but may be linked to hyperparathyroidism.[76] Pathologically, it is characterized by absence or hypoplasia of the thymus and parathyroid glands. Immunologically, it is characterized by partial or complete T-cell immunodeficiency and normal or near-normal B-cell immunity. After the hypoparathyroidism is treated with intravenous calcium-gluconate, low phosphorous diet, calcium supplements, and large doses of vitamin D, fetal thymus transplant is the recommended therapy. Heart disease may be severe and affect survival. Correction of the cardiac anomaly may ultimately affect survival.

COMBINED IMMUNODEFICIENCY DISEASES (SEVERE COMBINED IMMUNODEFICIENCY, SWISS-TYPE AGAMMAGLOBULINEMIA, LYMPHOPENIC AGAMMAGLOBULINEMIA, THYMIC ALYMPHOPLASIA, HEREDITARY THYMIC DYSPLASIA, CELLULAR IMMUNODEFICIENCY WITH ABNORMAL IMMUNOGLOBULIN SYNTHESIS)

Combined immunodeficiency disease (CID) is congenital and usually hereditary. It includes deficiencies of both T- and B-cell systems and is associated with lymphoid aplasia and thymic dysplasia. Some have suggested that the basic defect in this condition is, in most instances, secondary to a stem cell defect, or that there is a thymic helper defect or an intrathymic defect.[76] Others maintain that CID is a group of disorders characterized by T- and B-cell dysfunction.

Clinical Features

The typical presenting symptoms are recurrent septic episodes and severe bacterial pneumonia, followed by chronic oral candidiasis that proves refractory to all forms of oral or local therapy. It has been reported to present as the Letterer-Siwe syndrome.[77] Systemic candidiasis in these patients is unusual, but they may develop esophagitis. Pulmonary symptoms are common. They may develop overwhelming infections with *Pneumocystis carinii,* cytomegalovirus, or rubeola.

Gastrointestinal Disease

Gastrointestinal manifestations can be severe and occur in 90% of these patients. They may first develop lactase deficiency and steatorrhea and ultimately a generalized malabsorption syndrome. The etiology of the mucosal injury can be idiopathic or secondary to a variety of agents. Prolonged excretion of rotavirus is a recently described phenomena and could account for the intractability of the diarrhea.[78] Quite often the agent or agents responsible for the damage cannot be isolated. Coccidiosis and cryptosporidiosis have been described in such patients.[79,80]

Fatal progressive adenovirus hepatic necrosis has been described in one patient with subacute immunodeficiency[81] and venoocclusive disease of the liver in two other siblings.[82] Survival may require total parenteral nutrition through a central venous catheter until either thymus or bone marrow transplantation may be done.[83]

SHORT-LIMBED DWARFISM WITH IMMUNODEFICIENCY CARTILAGE-HAIR HYPOPLASIA

This autosomal recessive, predominantly T-cell immunodeficiency syndrome is associated with metaphyseal or spondyloepiphyseal dysplasia. It is a variant of short-limbed dwarfism in which fine, sparse hair is present. The short stature is a result of disproportionate shortening of the extremities. Immunologically, these patients either have a T-cell defect, a B-cell defect, or a combined defect. The gastrointestinal manifestations of this syndrome include: celiac sprue, malabsorption of unknown etiology, and Hirschprung's disease.[84] The susceptibility to infection in this condition is directly related to the extent of the immunologic deficiency. Varicella has been the most common severe infection to cause death in these patients. Vaccina and poliovirus vaccine are potentially lethal pathogens. Bone marrow transplant in one child was reported to reverse malabsorption, chronic diarrhea, agenerative anemia, and growth failure.

WISKOTT-ALDRICH SYNDROME (IMMUNODEFICIENCY WITH ECZEMA AND THROMBOCYTOPENIA)

Wiskott-Aldrich syndrome is an X-linked recessive immunodeficiency syndrome characterized by thrombocytopenia, eczema, and recurrent infection. Immunologically, such patients have very elevated levels of IgA and IgE and low levels of

IgM.[85,86] They have defective T-cell function and respond poorly to stimulation with polysaccharide antigens.[87] These patients have a progressive degeneration in their ability to form specific antibody to antigen.[88] The thrombocytopenia in Wiskott-Aldrich syndrome is secondary to a metabolic defect in the platelets leading to a decreased platelet survival.

The gastrointestinal manifestations of Wiskott-Aldrich syndrome include hematemesis, melena, and chronic diarrhea. These patients often have difficulty tolerating standard infant feedings, made with intact protein. They develop malabsorption syndromes but respond to elemental formulas such as Pregestimil, Vivonex, and Nutramigen. They often have difficulty throughout infancy and beyond tolerating intact protein. Frequently, they have diets limited to fruits, vegetables, and a select group of proteins. Recently, a 19-year-old boy with this syndrome was reported to have watery, bloody diarrhea and colonoscopic findings compatible with ulcerative colitis including friability and pseudopolyposis. He responded to the use of vancomycin and corticosteroids.[89]

Patients with Wiskott-Aldrich syndrome die from bleeding or malignancy unless transplanted.[90] Bone marrow transplantation to reconstitute these individuals has been successful. Malignancies in most instances are lymphomas.[87,88]

CHRONIC MUCOCUTANEOUS CANDIDIASIS

Chronic mucocutaneous candidiasis (CMC) is a celleular immunodeficiency that manifests in five distinct clinical syndromes similar in their susceptibility to chronic *Candida* infections of the mucosa, skin, and nails. These include: 1) early-onset chronic mucocutaneous candidiasis; 2) late-onset chronic mucocutaneous candidiasis; 3) familial mucocutaneous candidiasis; 4) juvenile familial polyendocrinopathy with candidiasis; and 5) biotin-dependent carboxylase deficiency with candidiasis.[91] It has not been determined whether these five clinical syndromes are forms of a single disease or represent distinct disease processes. CMC appears to involve a defect of the T-cell response to *Candida* antigen(s). The mode of inheritance is variable among these syndromes.

CMC is characterized by persistent *Candida* infection of the mucous membranes, scalp, skin, and nails. The most common *Candida* infections are present on the oral mucous membranes. Fingernails and toenails are frequently involved. Infections of skin of the face, hands, and feet occur less commonly. CMC is frequently associated with an endocrinopathy, such as Addison's disease, hypoparathyroidism, thyroiditis, and diabetes mellitus.[92,93] The clinical manifestations differ among the syndromes and are related to the presence of endocrinopathy.[91] These manifestations include increased pigmentation, tetany, seizures, steatorrhea, alopecia, and tooth hypoplasia. Gastrointestinal manifestations include dysphagia, which can occur in patients with candidial involvement of the mouth, pharynx, or esophagus. This can be successfully treated with ketoconazole and in some instances, when this fails, with intravenous amphotericin. In some patients with CMC, acute or chronic hepatitis and cirrhosis may occur.[91]

Treatment regimens for CMC vary due to the spectrum of clinical manifestations.[94-97] Antifungals, such as topical nystatin, clotrimazole, and mycostatin, are commonly prescribed. In severe cases, treatment with ketoconazole or intravenous antifungal therapy may be indicated. In the event of total treatment failure, in the presence of confirmed immunologic deficit, immunotherapy may be attempted. Death in these patients may occur secondary to immune defects and the infections to which this makes them susceptible.

GASTROINTESTINAL INVOLVEMENT IN CHILDREN WITH ACQUIRED IMMUNODEFICIENCY SYNDROME (AIDS)

Children at high risk for developing AIDS include hemophiliacs, transfusion recipients, and infants born to high-risk parents. Most children present with fever, lymphadenopathy, hepatomegaly, splenomegaly, chronic interstital lung disease, and failure to gain weight and grow. Although gastrointestinal disease is not a major characteristic of all patients, it is still of major importance.[98]

Infants and children with AIDS are highly susceptible to life-threatening and recurrent infection with common pyogenic bacteria.[99] These include *H. influenzae, Streptococcus pneumonia,* and *Staphylococcus* species. In addition, they are highly susceptible to a variety of common enteric organisms, as well as some unique ones. These include *Shigella, Salmonella, Yersinia, Mycobacterium avium intracellulare,* cytomegalovirus, herpes simplex virus, *G. lamblia, Isospora belli,* cryptosporidium, *Candida albicans,* and *Torulopsis globrata.*

In 10% of cases, the gastrointestinal manifestations are the initial presenting complaints of AIDS. Abdominal distention, diarrhea, malabsorption, and malnutrition may be the initial symptoms. Severe jejunal atrophy may be found, but it is not secondary to gluten sensitivity.[100]

In others, the mucosa may be infiltrated with acid-fast bacilli-laden macrophages secondary to *M. intracellulare.* Pseudomembranous necrotizing jejunitis secondary to bacterial overgrowth with *Klebsiella pneumoniae* has been described in one child, and abdominal pain, diarrhea and severe gastrointestinal hemorrhage secondary to cytomegalovirus in another.

Hepatitis and pancreatitis separately and together have been recognized in some children with AIDS. The pancreatitis is typically chronic and severe, with intractable abdominal pain as a typical symptom. Although papillary stenosis and sclerosing cholangitis have not been described in children with AIDS, they have been described in adults.[101] Etiology of the hepatitis and pancreatitis is not clear, but in some may be secondary to a variety of viruses. Cytomegalovirus and cryptosporidium associated acalculous gangrenous cholecystitis has been described.[102]

Some pediatric patients with AIDS and chronic diarrhea have no demonstrable enteric pathogens to explain their symptoms or to explain the damage to the intestinal mucosa. Kaposi's sarcoma of the intestinal tract, a not infrequent complication in adults with AIDS, has not been described in pediatric patients. It has been hypothesized that in some patients with AIDS, the mucosal injury is mediated by immune complex-mediated mechanisms.

Diagnostic evaluation of pediatric patients with AIDS for gastrointestinal signs and symptoms is no different than for children free of AIDS but with similar complaints. Appropriate cultures and examination of body fluids and secretions should be done as indicated. When specific pathogenic organisms are isolated and/or parasites identified, specific treatment is possible. In many instances, treatment has to be supportive since specific therapy is not possible.

We have found parenteral nutrition both in the hospital and at home a worthwhile therapy because it allows patients to survive until specific therapy can be instituted. In some, diarrhea and malabsorption ceased without specific therapy, and total parenteral nutrition could be discontinued.

STRUCTURAL INTESTINAL DEFECTS AND SECONDARY IMMUNODEFICIENCY

Until recently, intestinal lymphangiectasia was the primary anatomic defect recognized to be associated with secondary immunodeficiency. These patients typically have protein-losing enteropathy and a cellular immune defect. The latter is secondary to loss of long-lived lymphocytes across the mucosa. Recently, two other abnormalities have been discovered to have significant defects in both humoral and cellular immunity: midgut volulus in one child and a cavernous hemanginoma of the midjejunum in another. Both of these children had reversal of their immune deficit once the anatomic abnormality was corrected surgically.[103]

REFERENCES

1. Bruton OC: Agammaglobulinemia. *Pediatrics* 9:722–728, 1952.
2. Allen GE, Hadden DR: Congenital hypogammaglobulinemia with steatorrhea in two adult brothers. *Br Med J* 2:486–490, 1964.
3. Gabrielson AE, Cooper MD, Peterson RDA, et al: The primary immunologic deficiency diseases. In Miescher PA, Muller-Eberhard HJ: *Textbook of Immunopathology,* Vol II. New York, Grune & Stratton, 1969, pp 385–405.
4. Chandra RK: *Primary and Secondary Immunodeficiency.* New York, Churchill-Livingstone, pp 1–24.
5. McKinney RE, Katz SL, Wilfert CM: Chronic enteroviral meningoencephalitis in agammaglobulinemic patients. *Rev Infect* 9:334–356, 1987.
6. Good RA, Page AR: Fatal complications of virus hepatitis in two patients with agammaglobulinemia. *Am J Med* 29:804–810, 1960.
7. Ochs HD, Ament ME, Davis SD: Giardiasis with malabsorption in X-linked agammaglobulinemia. *N Engl J Med* 287:341–342, 1972.
8. Ament ME, Ochs HD, Davis SD: Structure and function of the gastrointestinal tract in primary immunodeficiency syndromes: a study of 39 patients. *Medicine* 52:227–248, 1973.
9. Melamed I, Bujanover Y, Siegman Y, et al: *Campylobacter* enteritis in normal and immunodeficient children. *Am J Dis Child* 137:752, 1983.
10. LeBar WD, Menard RR, Check FE: Hypogammaglobulinemia and recurrent *Campylobacter jejuni* infection. *J Infect Dis* 152:1099–1100, 1985.
11. Dubois RS, Roy CC, Fulginiti VA, et al: Disaccharidase deficiency in children with immunologic deficits. *J Pediatr* 76:377–385, 1970.
12. Norman ME, Hansell JR, Holtzapple DG, et al: Malabsorption and protein-losing enteropathy in a child with X-linked agammaglobulinemia. *Clin Immunol Immunopathol* 4:157–164, 1975.
13. Mir-Madjlessi SH, Tauassolie H, Kamalian NL: Malakoplakia of the colon and recurrent colonic strictures in a patient with primary hypogammaglobulinemia. *Am J Dis Colon Rectum* 25:723–726, 1982.

14. Webb M, Pincott JR, Marshall WC, et al: Hypogammaglobulinemia and malakoplakia: response to bethanechol. *J Pediatr Pathol:* 297–302, 1986.

15. Wray B, Middleton HM, Mulls LR, et al: Recurrent purulent triaditis in a patient with congenital X-linked agammaglobulinemia. *Am J Gastroenterol* 75:140–143, 1983.

16. Naveh Y, Medelsohn H, Spirag-Auslaender L, et al: Primary sclerosing cholangitis associated with immunodeficiency. *Am J Dis Child* 137:114–117, 1983.

17. Geha RS, Hyslop N, Alami S, et al: Hyperimmunoglobulin M immunodeficiency (dysgammaglobulinemia). *J Clin Invest* 64:385–391, 1979.

18. Vanderhoof JA, Rich KC, Stiehm ER, et al: Esophageal ulcers in immunodeficiency with elevated levels of IgM and neutropenia. *Am J Dis Child* 131:551–552, 1977.

19. Tzipori S, Roberton D, Chapman C: Hyperimmune bovine colostrum treatment of cryptosporidiosis in congenital hypogammaglobulinemia. *Br Med J* 293:1276–1277, 1986.

20. Ching HH, Shaw D, Klesius P, et al: Inability of oral bovine transfer factor to eradicate cryptosporidial infection in a patient with congenital dysgammaglobulinemia. *Clin Immunol Immunopathol* 50:402–406, 1989.

21. Saxon A, Weinstein W: Oral administration of bovine colostrum anti-cryptosporidia antibody fails to alter the course of human cryptosporidiosis. *J Parasitol* 73:413–415, 1987.

22. Fleisher TA, White RM, Broder S, et al: X-linked hypogammaglobulinemia and isolated growth hormone deficiency. *N Engl J Med* 302:1429–1434, 1980.

23. Matthews WJ Jr, Williams M, Oliphant B, et al: Hypogammaglobulinemia in patients with cystic fibrosis. *N Engl J Med* 302:245–249, 1980.

24. Reinherz EL, Geha R, Wohl ME, et al: Immunodeficiency associated with loss of T4-inducer T-cell function. *N Engl J Med* 304:811–816, 1981.

25. Boder E, Sedgwick RP: Ataxia-telangiectasia: a familial syndrome of progressive cerebellar ataxia, oculocutaneous telangiectasia and frequent pulmonary infections. *Univ S Calif Med Bull* 9:15–27, 1957.

26. Ammann AF, Cain WA, Ishizaka K, et al: Immunoglobulin E deficiency in ataxia-telangiectasia. *N Engl J Med* 281:469–472, 1969.

27. Gatti RA, Izzet B, Boder E, et al: Localization of an ataxia-telangiectasia gene to chromosome 11q22-23. *Nature* 336:557–580, 1988.

28. Waldmann TA, McIntire KR: Serum alpha-fetoprotein levels in patients with ataxia-telangiectasia. *Lancet* 2:1112–1115, 1972.

29. Dunn HG, Mirwissen H, Livingstone CS, et al: Ataxia-telangiectasia. *N Engl J Med* 281:469–472, 1969.

30. Haerer AF, Jackson JF, Evers CG: Ataxia-telangiectasia with gastric adenocarcinoma. *JAMA* 210:1884–1887, 1969.

31. Swift M, Sholman L, Perry M, et al: Malignant neoplasms in the families of patients with ataxia-telangiectasia. *Cancer Res* 36:209–215, 1976.

32. Weinstein S, Scottolini AF, Loo SYT, et al: Ataxia telangiectasia with hepatocellular carcinoma in a 15-year-old girl and studies of her kindred. *Arch Pathol Lab Med* 109:1000–1004, 1985.

33. Morrell D, Cromartie E, Swift M: Mortality and cancer: incidence in 263 patients with ataxia telangiectasia. *JNCI* 77:89–92, 1986.

34. Tiller TL Jr, Buckley RH: Transient hypogammaglobulinemia of infancy; review of the literature, clinical and immunologic features of 11 cases and long term follow-up. *J Pediatr* 92:347–453, 1978.

35. Perlmutter D, Leichtner AM, Goldman H, et al: Chronic diarrhea associated with hypogammaglobulinemia and enteropathy in infants and children. *Dig Dis Sci* 30:1149–1155, 1985.

36. McGeady SJ: Transient hypogammaglobulinemia of infancy: need to reconsider name and definition. *J Pediatr* 110:47–50, 1987.

37. Geha RS, Schneeberger E, Merler E, et al: Heterogeneity of "acquired" or common variable agammaglobulinemia. *N Engl J Med* 291:1–6, 1974.

38. Ochs HD, Wedgewood RJ: Disorders of the B-cell system. In: Stiehm ER, Fulginiti AV: *Immunologic Disorders in Infants and Children,* Philadelphia, Saunders, 1980, pp 239–259.

39. Oxelius VA, Laurell AB, Lindquist B, et al: IgG subclasses in selective IgA deficiency. Importance of IgG2-IgA deficiency. *N Engl J Med* 304:1476–1477, 1981.

40. Lane P, McLennan I, deGracia J, et al: Correspondence: impaired lung function in patients with IgA deficiency and low levels of IgG2 or IgG3. *N Engl J Med* 314:924–926, 1986.

41. Buckely RH, Fiscus SA: Serum IgD and IgE concentrations in immunodeficiency states. *J Clin Invest* 55:157–165, 1975.

42. Crabbe PA, Heremans JF: Selective IgA deficiency with steatorrhea: a new syndrome. *Am J Med* 42:319–326, 1967.

43. Crabbe PA, Heremans JF: Lack of gamma-A immunoglobulin in serum of patients with steatorrhea. *Gut* 7:119–127, 1968.

44. Mann JG, Brown WR, Kern F: The subtle and variable clinical expressions of gluten-induced enteropathy (adult celiac disease, non-tropical sprue): an analysis of 21 consecutive cases. *Am J Med* 48:357–366, 1970.

45. Ammann AJ, Hong R: Selective IgA deficiency: presentation of 30 cases and a review of the literature. *Medicine* 50:223–226, 1971.

46. Vinayak VK, Fical KK, Venkateswarlu K, et al: Hypogammaglobulinemia in children with persistent giardiasis. *J Trop Pediatr* 33:140–142, 1987.

47. Penny R, Thompson RG, Palmar SH, et al: Pancreatitis malabsorption and IgA deficiency in a child with diabetes. *J Pediatr* 78:512–516, 1971.

48. Geha RS, Schneeberger E, Merler E, et al: Heterogeneity of "acquired" or common variable agammaglobulinemia. *N Engl J Med* 291:1–6, 1974.

49. Hausser C, Virelizier JL, Buriot D, et al: Common variable hypogammaglobulinemia in children. *Am J Dis Child* 137:833–837, 1983.

50. Waldman TA, Broder S, Baese RM, et al: Role of suppressor T cells in pathogenesis of common variable hypogammaglobulinemia. *Lancet* 2:609–614, 1974.

51. Saxon A, Giorgi J, Sherr EH, et al: Failure of B cells in common variable immunodeficiency to transit from proliferation to differentiation is associated with altered B cell surface molecule display. *J Clin Immunol Allergy.* In Press, 1989.

52. Nime FA, Burek JD, Page DL, et al: Acute enterocolitis in a human being infected with the protozoan cryptosporidium. *Gastroenterology* 70:592–598, 1976.

53. Portnoy D, Whiteside ME, Buckley E, et al: Treatment of intestinal cryptosporidiosis with Spiramycin. *Ann Intern Med* 101:202–204, 1984.

54. Shelhamer JH, Neva FA, Finn DR: Persistent strongyloidiasis in an immunodeficient patient. *Am J Trop Med Hyg* 31:746–752, 1982.

55. Ahnen DF, Brown WR: *Campylobacter* enteritis in immune-deficient patients. *Ann Intern Med* 96:187–188, 1982.

56. Ponka A, Tilvis R, Kosunen TU: Prolonged *Campylobacter* gastroenteritis in a patient with hypogammaglobulinemia. *Act Med Scand* 213:159–160, 1983.

57. Leen CLS, Birch ADJ, Brettle RP, et al: Case reports: salmonellosis in patients with primary hypogammaglobulinemia. *J Infect* 12:241–245, 1986.

58. Hermans PE, Huizenga KA, Hoffman HN, et al: Dysgammaglobulinemia associated with nodular lymphoid hyperplasia of the small intestine. *Am J Med* 40:78–79, 1966.

59. Crooks DJM, Brown WR: The distribution of intestinal nodular lymphoid hyperplasia of the small intestine. *Am J Med* 40:78–79, 1966.

60. Johnson VL, Goldberg LS, Pops MA, et al: Clinical and immunological studies in a case of nodular lymphoid hyperplasia of the small intestine. *Gastroenterology* 61:369–374, 1971.

61. Kohler PF, Cook RD, Brown WR, et al: Common variable hypogammaglobulinemia and T-cell nodular lymphoid hyperplasia: different lymphocyte populations with a similar response to prednisone therapy. *J Allergy Clin Immunol* 70:299–305, 1979.

62. Hermans PE, Huizenga KA, Haffman HN, et al: Dysgammaglobulinemia associated with nodular lymphoid hyperplasia of the small intestine. *Am J Med* 40:78–79, 1966.

63. Strauss RG, Ghisan F, Mitros F, et al: Rectosigmoid colitis in common variable immunodeficiency disease. *Dig Dis Sci* 25:798–801, 1980.

64. Kirk BW, Freedman SO: Hypogammaglobulinemia, thymoma and ulcerative colitis. *Can Med Assoc J* 96:1272–1277, 1967.

65. Elson CO, James SP, Graeff AS, et al: Hypogammaglobulinemia due to abnormal suppressor T-cell activity in Crohn's disease. *Gastroenterology* 86:569–576, 1984.

66. Keczkes K, Bilimoria S, Peircy DM: Pernicious anemia and granulomatous skin lesions in a case of common variable hypogammaglobulinemia. *Br J Dermatol* 101:211–217, 1979.

67. Hippe E, Jensen KB: Hereditary factors in pernicious anemia and their relation to serum immunoglobulin levels and age at diagnosis. *Lancet* 2:721–722, 1969.

68. Wright PE, Sears DA: Hypogammaglobulinemia and pernicious anemia. *South Med J* 80:243–246, 1987.

69. Hermans PE, Diaz-Buxoja, Stobo JD: Idiopathic late-onset immunoglobulin deficiency: clinical observation in 50 patients. *Am J Med* 62:221–237, 1976.

70. Cunningham-Rundles C, Siegal FP, Cunningham-Rundles S, et al: Incidence of cancer in 98 patients with common varied immunodeficiency. *J Clin Immunol* 7:294–299, 1987.

71. Osur SL, Lillie MA, Chen PB, et al: Elevation of serum IgG levels and normalization of T4/T8 ratio after hepatitis in a patient with common variable hypogammaglobulinemia. *J Allergy Clin Immunol* 79:969–975, 1987.

72. Maggiore G, DeGiacomo C, Rascio N, et al: Severe hepatitis B-negative chronic hepatitis responsive to steroids in a child with common variable hypogammaglobulinemia. *Am J Dis Child* 138:796, 1984.

73. Hitzig WH, Dohman WU, Pluss HJ, et al: Hereditary transcobalamin II deficiency: clinical findings in a new family. *J Pediatr* 85:622–628, 1974.

74. DeVaal OM, Seynhaeve V: Reticular dysgenesis. *Lancet* 2:1123–1125, 1959.

75. Ammann AJ, Hong R: Disorders of the T-cell system. In Stiehm ER, Fulginiti VA: *Immunologic Disorders in Infants and Children*. Phildelphia, Saunders, 1980, pp 287–291.

76. Ammann AJ, Hong R: Disorders of the T-cell system. In Stiehm ER, Fulginiti VA: *Immunologic Disorders in Infants and Children*. Philadelphia, Saunders, 1980, pp 291–293.

77. Cederbaum SD, Niwayama G, Stiehm ER, et al: Combined immunodeficiency presenting as the Leterr-Sive syndrome. *J Pediatr* 85:466–471, 1974.

78. Cannon RA, Blum PM, Ament ME, et al: Reversal of enterocolitis-associated combined immunodeficiency by plasma therapy. *J Pediatr* 101:711–717, 1982.

79. Hallak A, Yust I, Ratan Y, et al: Malabsorption syndrome coccidiosis, combined immune deficiency and fulminant lymphoproliferative disease. *Arch Intern Med* 142:196–197, 1983.

80. Current WL, Reese NC, Ernst JV, et al: Human cryptosporidiosis in immunocompetent and immunodeficient persons. *N Engl J Med* 308:1252–1257, 1983.

81. South MA, Dolen J, Beach DK, et al: Fatal adenovirus hepatic necrosis in severe combined immune deficiency. *Pediatr Infect Dis* 1:416–419, 1982.

82. Etzioni A, Benderly A, Rosenthal E, et al: Defective humoral and cellular immune functions associated with veno-occlusive disease of the liver. *J Pediatr* 110:54, 1987.

83. Ammann AJ, Ward D, Salmon S, et al: Thymus transplantation: permanent reconstitution of cellular immunity in a patient with sex-linked combined immunodeficiency. *N Engl J Med* 289:5–9, 1973.

84. Ammann AJ, Sutliff W, Millinchick E: Antibody mediated immunodeficiency in short-limbed dwarfism. *J Pediatr* 84:200–203, 1974.

85. Aldrich RA, Steinberg AG, Cambell DC: Pedigree demonstrating a sex-linked recessive condition characterized by draining ears, eczematoid dermatitis and bloody diarrhea. *Pediatrics* 13:133–139, 1954.

86. Wolff JA, Bertucio M: A sex-linked genetic syndrome in a negro family manifested by thrombocytopenia, eczema, bloody diarrhea, recurrent infection, anemia and epistaxis. *Am J Dis Child* 93:74, 1957.

87. Berglund G, Finnstrom O, Johansson SGO, et al: Wiskott-Aldrich syndrome: a study of six cases with determination of the immunoglobulins A, D, G, M, and ND. *Acta Paediatr Scand* 57:89–97, 1968.

88. Wolff JA: Wiskott-Aldrich syndrome: clinical, immunologic and pathologic observations. *J Pediatr* 70:221–232, 1967.

89. Hsieh KH, Chang MH, Lee CY, et al: Wiskott-Aldrich syndrome and inflammatory bowel disease. *Ann Allergy* 60:429–431, 1988.

90. Ten Bensel RW, Stadlaw EM, Krivit W: The development of malignancy in the course of Aldrich syndrome. *J Pediatr* 68:761–767, 1966.

91. Ammann AJ, Hong R: Disorders of the T cell system. In Stiehm ER: *Immunologic Disorders in Infants and Children*. Philadelphia, Saunders, 1989, pp 286–290.

92. Cahill LT, Ainbender E, Glade PR: Chronic mucocutaneous candidiasis: T-cell deficiency associated with B cell dysfunction in man. *Cell Immunol* 14:215–225, 1974.

93. Kunin AS, MacKay BR, Burns SL, et al: The syndrome of hypoparathyroidism and adrenocorticoinsufficiency: a possible sequel of hepatitis: case report and review of the literature. *Am J Med*

94. Kirkpatrick CH, Smith TK: Chronic mucocutaneous candidiasis; immunologic and antibody therapy. *Ann Intern Med* 80:310–320, 1974.

95. Leikin S, Parrott R, Randolph J: Clotrimazole: treatment of chronic mucocutaneous candidiasis. *J Pediatr* 88:864–866, 1976.

96. Meade RH: Treatment of chronic mucocutaneous candidiasis. *Ann Intern Med* 86:314–315, 1979.

97. Rosenblatt HM, Byrne WJ, Ament ME, et al: Successful treatment of chronic mucocutaneous candidiasis with ketokonazole. *J Pediatr* 97:657–660, 1980.

98. McLoughlin LC, Nord KS, Josh VV, et al: Gastrointestinal involvement in acquired immunodeficiency syndrome. *J Pediatr Gastroenterol Nutr* 6:517–524, 1987.

99. Shannon KM, Ammann AJ: Acquired immunodeficiency syndrome in childhood. *J Pediatr* 106:332–342, 1985.

100. Gottlieb MS, Groopman JE, Weinstein WM, et al: The acquired immunodeficiency syndrome. *Ann Intern Med* 99:208–220, 1983.

101. Schneiderman DJ, Cello JP, Laing FC: Papillary stenosis and sclerosing cholangitis in the acquired immunodeficiency syndrome. *Ann Intern Med* 206:546–549, 1987.

102. Blumberg RS, Kelsey P, Perrone T, et al: Cytomegalovirus and cryptosporidium-associated acalculous gangrenous cholecystitis. *Am J Med* 76:1118–1123, 1984.

103. Fawcett WA, Ferry GD, Gorin LJ, et al: Immunodeficiency secondary to structural intestinal defects. *Am J Dis Child* 140:169–172, 1986.

CHAPTER 18

The Acquired Immunodeficiency Syndrome

STEVEN M. HOLLAND

THOMAS C. QUINN

INTRODUCTION

The acquired immunodeficiency syndrome (AIDS) is an immunologic disease caused by the human immunodeficiency virus (HIV). Since its description in 1981,[1-3] AIDS has become a global epidemic with estimates of over 250,000 cases of AIDS, over 500,000 cases of symptomatic HIV infection (AIDS-related complex; ARC), and up to 10,000,000 asymptomatic carriers worldwide. It is estimated that over the next two years 1,000,000 people in 140 countries will develop AIDS. In the United States, it is estimated that 1.5 million people are currently infected with HIV and that by 1992 there will be 365,000 cumulative cases of AIDS with over 260,000 total deaths.[4] The clinical spectrum of HIV infection includes an initial "mononucleosis-like" syndrome within several weeks of exposure, characterized by fevers, sweats, lethargy, myalgias, arthralgias, headaches, photophobia, lymphadenopathy, sore throat, truncal maculopapular rash, and diarrhea.[5] This acute syndrome typically resolves over several weeks with the development of specific antibodies to HIV.[6] Patients remain asymptomatic but infectious for a prolonged period of time, and may develop immunologic abnormalities such as immune thrombocytopenic purpura, anemia, or lymphadenopathy. After a mean incubation of 8–10 years, and with further immunologic impairment, about 50% of infected individuals develop AIDS, characterized by disseminated opportunistic infections and neoplasms. It is estimated that almost all infected individuals will eventually progress to AIDS after 10–15 years of infection if no effective therapy is found.[7]

MOLECULAR PATHOGENESIS

The AIDS virus has been previously referred to as the lymphadenopathy-associated virus (LAV),[8] the human T-lymphotropic virus-3 (HTLV-III),[9] and the AIDS-related virus (ARV).[10] In May, 1986, an international committee on viral nomenclature renamed the virus the human immunodeficiency virus (HIV), since the above viruses have been shown to be essentially the same.[11] A closely related but genetically distinct human retrovirus, HIV-2, has recently been recovered from West African AIDS patients.[12-15]

HIV is a retrovirus of the lentivirus family and is composed of an mRNA and protein core surrounded by a cell-derived lipid membrane.[16] The HIV genome is about 10 kb long and contains a group antigen *(gag)* gene encoding a 55 kD precursor peptide that is processed into three smaller core proteins, p15, p18, and p24; a polymerase *(pol)* gene encoding a precursor peptide that is cleaved into p66 and p51 reverse transcriptases and the endonuclease/integrase p34; an envelope *(env)* gene encoding a precursor glycoprotein, gp160, which is cleaved into two noncovalently associated glycoproteins, gp120 and gp41; and two long terminal repeats (LTR) that contain specific DNA sequences for the binding of viral and cellular regulators.[17] In addition to the above basic retroviral genes, HIV has at least four other unique genes that are crucial to its expression and pathogenicity. The *trans*-acting *(tat)* gene product up-regulates the expression of genes linked to the LTR and is necessary for viral replication.[18,19] The regulator of viral transcription (*rev*, previously known as *art/trs*) gene product is required for viral structural gene processing and is also necessary for viral replication.[20] The negative regulatory factor (*nef*, previously known as *3′orf, f,* and *B*) gene product down-regulates viral transcription from the LTR, has GTP binding and GTPase activity, and is involved in the maintenance of viral latency.[21,22] The viral infectivity factor (*vif*, previously known as *sor* and *A*) gene product is required for efficient cell-free or cell-cell virus transmission.[23] Other open reading frames have been described, but distinct functions have not been ascribed to their products.

The pathogenic action of HIV lies in its ability to induce susceptibility to opportunistic pathogens and neoplasms by progressive destruction of the immune system. The viral envelope glycoprotein, gp120, displayed on the surface of the virus and on infected cells, binds to the CD4 receptor.[24-26] CD4 (also known as T4) is the phenotypic marker of helper T lymphocytes and serves as a ligand for the major histocompatibility complex (MHC) class II molecule.[27] CD4 is also found on monocyte/macrophage-derived cells[28] and in the brain.[29] HIV gp120 binds to CD4 with an affinity of 10^{-9} M,[30] and monoclonal antibodies against specific CD4 epitopes block the binding of HIV.[31] Recently it has been shown that cell-free CD4 binds to gp120 independent of other cellular or viral components.[32,33] Maddon et al.[29] showed that transfection and expression of the CD4 gene into CD4-negative HeLa cells conferred HIV binding capability and infectability on those cells. However, transfection of the CD4 gene into a variety of CD4-negative murine cells permitted HIV binding but not infection. The failure of CD4-transfected murine cells to permit HIV infection is not due to inability of these cells to support HIV replication, as shown by transfection and expression of an HIV plasmid into murine fibroblasts.[34] Therefore, the presence of the CD4 receptor alone is not sufficient for HIV infection. Conversely, HIV has been shown to infect colon carcinoma-derived cell lines that lack detectable surface CD4 but do produce CD4 mRNA. Normal bowel epithelium is also CD4 message-positive but has undetectable surface CD4.[35] Using in situ hybridization and immunohistochemical techniques, Nelson et al.[36] have demonstrated HIV RNA and proteins in rectal epithelium. One group has reported infection of cultured astrocytes that are negative for both CD4 mRNA and protein.[37] These data taken together suggest that CD4 is an important factor in HIV infection but that other factors are necessary and in some cases may be sufficient for HIV infection.

Site-directed, linker insertion, and deletion mutational analysis have delineated separate regions of gp120 responsible for CD4 association and gp41 association. Discrete regions of gp41 have been identified that are responsible for membrane anchoring, posttranslational processing, and virus-cell fusion.[38] In this model, the binding of gp120 to CD4 allows alignment of gp41 with a separate cell surface protein, which is directly responsible for fusion of viral and cellular membranes. This view is strengthened by the finding of highly conserved sequences within the amino terminus of gp41 that are closely related to the fusion-inducing sequences of paramyxoviruses.[39]

Controversy still exists over whether viral fusion with the cell membrane and penetration occurs at the plasma membrane[40] or in an endosome,[29,41] whether fusion is pH-dependent, and whether internalization of the CD4 receptor is required for infection.[42]

Monocyte-derived cells and cell lines are infectable by HIV in vivo and in vitro. They may be able to ingest and destroy virus through a phagocytic pathway and yet remain infectable through a CD4 pathway.[41] Infection of macrophages by certain viruses (e.g., yellow fever and dengue) is enhanced by low concentrations of antibody.[43] Takeda et al.[44] have shown that the same antiserum that has HIV neutralizing activity at high concentrations enhances infection at low concentrations. They have convincingly demonstrated that the enhancing activity is antibody and that the relevant cellular receptor is the Fc receptor. Because of the dramatic in vivo variation of HIV over time,[45,46] this mechanism may permit enhancement of infection in macrophages by the same antibody that neutralized a previous variant. Robinson et al.[47] have suggested infection enhancement by complement and complement receptors as well as antibody. Antibody and complement enhancement will need to be considered in future vaccine development.

Following cellular penetration, viral RNA is uncoated and transcribed to DNA by viral reverse transcriptase. Proviral DNA can integrate into the host genome by a mechanism dependent on the *pol* gene endonuclease. There it can persist in a double-stranded linear form, or it can assume a double-stranded closed circular form. Accumulation of unintegrated linear DNA is associated with cytopathicity in some animal retroviruses and is also seen with HIV.[48] After integration, the provirus remains clinically silent for a prolonged period, perhaps under the influence of viral or cellular negative regulatory factors. Viral transcription and replication can be induced by a number of factors, including allogeneic stimulation,[49] mitogenic or antigenic stimulation,[50] or coinfection with some DNA viruses, notably herpesviruses.[51,52] In a chronically infected promonocyte line, HIV expression and replication were induced by exposure to cytokines.[53] Chronic immune stimulation, as is found in African heterosexuals and U.S. homosexual men, may also predispose to HIV infection and disease progression.[54] Therefore, immune activation by intercurrent infection, antigenic stimulation (e.g., semen or blood), or cytokines may trigger HIV replication, cytolysis, spread, and progression.

Despite finding very few CD4 lymphocytes infected,[55] the hallmark of advanced AIDS is CD4 lymphocyte depletion. Viral replication in CD4-positive T cells usually leads to cell death. HIV-mediated cell death in vitro is caused by fusion-dependent and fusion-independent mechanisms. Lifson et al.[56] noted that HIV-infected lymphocytes formed syncytia with CD4-positive cells and thereby caused cell death. Syncytia did not form with CD4-negative cells. These findings were extended by Sodroski et al.[57] and Lifson et al.,[58] by showing that the HIV envelope was the only viral factor required for CD4-mediated cell fusion and death. Syncytium formation does not require antigenic stimulation of either the HIV-infected or the CD4-bearing uninfected cell and therefore suggests a plausible mechanism of in vivo CD4 lymphocyte depletion.[59] Disruption of proper glycosylation of the HIV envelope by castanospermine or other glucosidase inhibitors reduced or prevented syncytium formation.[60] This suggests that glycosylation is important in recognition of the fusogenic epitope. Despite firm in vitro evidence of cytotoxic syncytium formation, its importance in vivo is debated.

Fusion-independent HIV-related cell death is well described.[61] Stevenson et al.[62] propose that HIV persistence in infected cells is due to intracellular complexing of gp120 to CD4 with resultant down-regulation of HIV binding sites and prevention of superinfection. Lack of surface CD4 or gp120 secondary to intracellular complexing makes these cells refractory to syncytium formation. However, following exposure of these cells to the tumor promoter phorbol 12-myristate 13-acetate (TPA), reverse transcriptase and viral RNA increase fourfold. This is accompanied by the death of the majority of cells in the absence of syncytia or multinucleated giant cells.[62] This work suggests mechanisms of viral persistence and viral activation leading to cell death that are fusion-independent. Other groups have noted direct viral down-regulation of CD4 mRNA, which may contribute to cytolysis resistance.[21,63]

HIV may cause the death of CD4 cells indirectly through autoimmune mechanisms. Siliciano et al.[64] demonstrated gp120-specific MHC class II-restricted cytotoxic lymphocytes (CTL) and showed that these cells specifically lysed gp120-bearing class II-displaying antigen-presenting cells. This CTL effect could also be directed against CD4+ cells that bound free gp120 from the medium. This "innocent bystander" effect would lead to the destruction of activated CD4+ cells. Therefore, this autologous cytolytic effect provides a mechanism of CD4+ cell depletion that depends on T-cell stimulation to display MHC class II in response to infection [e.g., cytomegalovirus (CMV), herpes simplex virus (HSV), Epstein-Barr virus (EBV)] or foreign antigens. Circulating gp120 may also reach the thymus, where it could bind to nascent CD4+ T cells and cause their destruction. This mechanism might explain the gradual depletion of CD4+ cells seen with progressive HIV disease.[65] However, in a study of HIV-infected patients, Wahren et al.[66] were unable to find HIV-specific T-cell proliferative responses in most patients, despite preserved proliferative responses to other viruses.

Antibody-dependent cell-mediated cytotoxicity and the formation of cytotoxic autoantibodies have also been described in HIV infection.[67,68] The issue of cytopathicity of HIV for CD4 cells remains a crucial one to resolve, in so far as CD4 depletion is a cardinal feature of AIDS. The ability to detect HIV RNA in <0.01% of circulating lymphocytes indicates that these other mechanisms, or mechanisms yet to be described, are important.[55]

IMMUNOLOGIC PATHOGENESIS

Not only does HIV lead to depletion of CD4+ T-cell numbers, it induces profound functional abnormalities in immune function as well. Virtually all T-cell functions examined so far in patients with AIDS have been severely diminished or nearly absent when studied in vivo or in vitro using peripheral blood mononuclear cells.[69] With progression from asymptomatic infection to ARC to AIDS, there is progressive immune deterioration. Lane et al.[70] showed that homosexual patients with AIDS and opportunistic infection had much lower mean CD4+ cell counts and in vitro phytohemagglutinin (PHA) proliferative responses than patients with AIDS and Kaposi's sarcoma, chronic lymphadenopathy, or healthy controls. Zolla-Pazner et al.[71] have shown progressive decline in CD4/CD8 ratio, CD4 number, and total lymphocyte count in intravenous drug users (IVDU) and homosexual men with progression from seronegative to asymptomatic seropositive to AIDS. They also noted elevations of IgG, IgA, and β_2-microglobulin in infected patients. Delayed-type hypersensitivity reactions (DTH) were reduced or absent in a group of seropositive hemophiliacs.[72] However, over 40% of seropositive hemophiliac patients had one or more DTH tests positive out of a panel of seven antigens. Therefore, DTH testing for certain exposures (e.g., tuberculosis) is still of value in seropositive patients, but negative responses are difficult to interpret without appropriate controls.

Murray et al.[73] showed deficient in vitro mitogen-induced lymphokine and gamma-interferon production by T cells taken from AIDS patients with opportunistic infections. More profound deficits were noted on stimulation with specific microbial antigens. However, these investigators found monocyte killing was intact if stimulated with normal amounts of lymphokines or gamma-interferon. Examining a group of homosexual AIDS patients with Kaposi's sarcoma, Lane et al.[74] showed normal pokeweed mitogen (PWM) proliferative responses in purified T-cell subsets, absent proliferation to tetanus toxoid, diminished alloreactivity of unfractionated and purified cells, and high levels of spontaneous DNA synthesis in unstimulated circulating cells. These results suggest a profound, intrinsic defect in antigen-reactive T cells. Lane et al.[74] did not confirm significant defects of interleukin-2 (IL-2), IL-2 receptor, or gamma-interferon production in these patient cells. This may reflect differences between patients with Kaposi's sarcoma and those with opportunistic infections as their AIDS-defining illnesses.

Linnette et al.[75] have shown a specific defect in signal transduction and proliferation following CD3 stimulation that is not apparent following CD2 or IL-2 stimulation. As CD3 stimulation responses are thought to mimic antigen stimulation responses in T cells, this points to specific antigen-dependent response defects in HIV-infected cells.

Lane et al.[76] demonstrated intrinsic B-cell abnormalities in homosexual AIDS patients. These included elevated numbers of IgG-secreting B cells, deficient PWM (T-cell-dependent) responses, and deficient *Staphylococcus aureus* Cowan strain 1 (SAC) (T cell-independent) proliferation. Both humoral and cellular responses to immunization with keyhole limpet hemocyanin (KLH) were profoundly depressed in patients with AIDS, suggesting an inability to respond to new antigens. Asymptomatic homosexual men (who may have been HIV-infected) had immune responses to PWM, SAC, and KLH that were intermediate between AIDS patients and heterosexual controls. Elevations of IgG and IgA were noted.

Polyclonal activation of B cells occurs following direct exposure to HIV.[77] The mechanism of this stimulation is unproved, but may be related to the homology of gp120 to neuroleukin, a lymphokine product of lectin-stimulated T cells that induces B-cell secretion of immunoglobulin.[78,79] Neuroleukin has been shown recently to be identical to glucophosphoisomerase. However, the findings of gp120 homology and the described phenomenology are not disputed.[80,81] This homology may therefore be of importance in explaining the direct noninfectious effects of HIV and its products on B cells.

Since many of the microorganisms causing infections in AIDS are intracellular pathogens normally controlled by the reticuloendothelial system, it is likely that defective monocyte/macrophage function contributes to the occurrence and severity of infections in AIDS. Monocytes and macrophages are infectable by HIV[82–84] and are thought to be an important mode of transport of HIV into the central nervous system.[85,86] Folks et al.[87] have shown that CD4− CD34+ bone marrow precursor cells are infectable by HIV. On differentiation, these cells become CD4+ monocytes, providing a reservoir and possible source for viral dissemination. Monocytes and macrophages produce smaller quantities of virus than lymphocytes and are less often killed by infection. Smith et al.[88] showed defective in vitro chemotaxis in monocytes from AIDS patients, worse in those with opportunistic infections than in those with Kaposi's sarcoma. Bender et al.[89] showed defective antibody-dependent cellular cytotoxicity and defective clearance of IgG-sensitized erythrocytes, but no defect in nonspecific phagocytosis. HIV has also been shown to infect pulmonary alveolar macrophages, which may in part account for the high incidence of pulmonary infections in adults.[90] Muller et al.[91] have shown a diminished macrophage oxidative burst in response to antigen or mitogen stimulation in asymptomatic seropositive and AIDS patients compared with blood donors and seronegative controls. This defect of intracellular killing may further explain the propensity of HIV-infected patients to experience severe and persistent infections with intracellular pathogens.

Specific macrophage-secreted factors may influence cellular responses as well as metabolic condition. IL-1 is a macrophage-produced peptide that activates T cells, B cells, neutrophils, and fibroblasts as well as causing fever, synthesis of acute phase reactants, and proteolysis in muscle.[92] Although no overt pathologic role has been demonstrated so far in AIDS, IL-1 may be a potent mediator of the fevers and wasting seen in AIDS. Tumor necrosis factor (TNF, cachectin) is another macrophage-synthesized cytokine with potent activities including fever, inhibition of lipoprotein lipase synthesis, depletion of adipocyte stores, septic shock, and disseminated intravascular coagulation.[93] One study has noted elevated serum levels of TNF in ARC and AIDS, compared with asymptomatic seropositives.[94] Conversely, defects in the generation or secretion of these factors could lead to failure to mount an appropriate immune response and thereby predispose to infection. The importance of these mediators in AIDS is under active investigation.

Fatal consequences follow on the immunologic dysfunction caused by HIV. Gastrointestinal manifestations are discussed below. In this country the majority of cases of AIDS are diagnosed by the occurrence of pulmonary infection with the parasite *Pneumocystis carinii*. Other pulmonary pathogens include *Mycobacterium tuberculosis, M. avium-intracellulare*, cytomegalovirus, and bacteria. Although treatable, these infections frequently persist or recur. The central nervous system is the target of infection with *Cryptococcus neoformans, Toxoplasma gondii*, and papovaviruses. Dementia in patients infected with HIV may occur as a direct result of the virus. B cell derived lymphomas occur systemically and in the central nervous system. An aggressive form of Kaposi's sarcoma affecting primarily the skin, gastrointestinal tract, and lung is seen among homosexual men with AIDS.

GASTROINTESTINAL MANIFESTATIONS

The gastrointestinal manifestations of HIV are divided into primary and secondary. Primary manifestations of HIV infection are those for which no pathogen other than HIV has been identified. Secondary manifestations of HIV infection are those seen in association with known pathogens or opportunistic infections. It is possible, and in some cases likely, that certain features currently considered in one category will turn out to belong in the other.

Primary Gastrointestinal Features

Acute HIV infection can cause an acute mononucleosis-like syndrome. This may be accompanied by an acute ulcerative esophagitis with dysphagia, odynophagia, and retrosternal pain. These symptoms last up to 2 weeks and resolve with the resolution of the acute HIV infection syndrome.[95] Pharyngitis was seen in 75% and diarrhea in 33% of the cases described by Cooper et al.[5] These manifestations resolved without specific therapy, and their immediate cause is unknown. Peripheral blood may show a brisk atypical lymphocytosis, raising the possibility that these "mononucleosis-like" findings are secondary to immune response to viral infection. Whatever the immediate cause of these systemic signs and symptoms, acute HIV infection is the underlying one.

With the slow but inexorable decline in immune function, gastrointestinal complications of HIV infection emerge. In developed countries, homosexual men appear to present most commonly with gastrointestinal symptoms and signs. Approximately 40–50% of homosexual men with AIDS have a history of a clinical prodrome characterized by progressive weight loss of more than 10% of body weight and diarrhea for which no specific pathogen can be isolated.[96,97] Colebunders et al.[98] found that Zairian patients presenting with a history of persistent diarrhea for more than 1 month were likely to be HIV-positive and have weight loss >10%. Extensive evaluation of stool showed no specific pathogens in about 40%. Serwadda et al.[99] reported a disease in rural Uganda and Tanzania characterized by weight loss and diarrhea. Stool exams were reportedly negative for enteric pathogens including cryptosporidia. However, the clinical, serologic, virologic, immunologic, and epidemiologic features of "slim disease" and enteropathic AIDS are essentially identical, and they are now considered to be the same disease.

The frequency of gastrointestinal symptoms in AIDS, on the one hand, and the relative paucity of specific diarrhea-causing pathogens identified on the other, suggest a possible role for HIV per se. This role could be due to direct effects of viral infection, to viral products influencing local or distant functions, or to specific cellular responses to viral infection that might have deleterious effects. Nelson et al.[36] performed rectal, colonic, and duodenal biopsies on homosexual HIV-infected patients with advanced disease and gastrointestinal symptoms. In situ hybridization and immunohistochemistry showed HIV RNA in the bowel epithelium at the base of the crypts and in the enterochromaffin cells. In duodenal biopsies HIV RNA was demonstrated in the lamina propria. Since the enterochromaffin cell is derived from the neural crest and has gastrointestinal function, its infection by HIV may be important in the gastrointestinal dysfunction seen in HIV disease. Rene et al.[100] performed rectal and duodenal biopsies on AIDS patients with pathogen-associated diarrhea, pathogen-unassociated diarrhea, and without diarrhea. Immunohistochemistry showed reduced CD4 lymphocyte number and HIV-positive lymphocytes and macrophages in the lamina propria, but no epithelial staining for HIV. The presence of HIV-positive cells in the lamina propria did not correlate with the presence of diarrhea or gastrointestinal infection. The absence of HIV-staining bowel epithelial cells in this study may be due to methodological differences, such as not using in situ hybridization. However, both Nelson et al.[36] and Rene et al.[100] found HIV-infected lymphocytes and macrophages in the lamina propria, which thus may provide a mechanism for local HIV effects on the gut. The failure of these histologic findings to correlate well to clinical status suggests that other factors or mechanisms must be involved.

Using the feline leukemia virus, one group has isolated strains that produce an AIDS-like illness in cats.[101,102] They have found that replication-defective viruses can be complemented by replication-competent viruses, and that onset of immunodeficiency is preceded by loss of colony-forming T cells and amplification of viral DNA in target tissues. They have also shown these viruses to be cytopathic for intestinal epithelium and to cause an enteropathy with persistent diarrhea and progressive wasting. These findings have not been paralleled for HIV, but raise questions about the possibility of complementation of viruses causing cytopathic effects in vivo that can not be reproduced in vitro with standard culture techniques.

Rodgers et al.[103] examined peripheral blood and small intestinal mucosae of healthy heterosexual men, healthy homosexual men, homosexual men with the lymphadenopathy syndrome (LAS), and homosexual men with AIDS. In the gut they found an increase in the number of mononuclear cells per unit area of intestinal mucosa, a decrease in total T cells with a low CD4/CD8 ratio, and an increase in the relative number of T cells bearing an activation marker. A fall in the peripheral blood CD4/CD8 ratio seemed to precede changes in the gut ratio. These findings indicate some derangement of cellular composition at the mucosal level. The presence of activated T cells and the relative excess of CD8 cells in the intestinal mucosa suggests a state of gastrointestinal immune stimulation.

Neurologic involvement is one of the most common and devastating complications of AIDS. Dementia, vacuolar myelopathy, sensory neuropathy, and inflammatory demyelinating polyneuropathy have all been described during HIV infection.[104] Craddock et al.[105] described AIDS patients undergoing percutaneous lung aspiration who experienced hypotension or syncope. Further study of these men, using cardiovascular parameters, showed evidence of autonomic neuropathy. Gastrointestinal neuropathy was not studied. Autonomic neuropathy may play a role in the diarrhea seen in AIDS. By causing pathologic motility, HIV could be a primary gastrointestinal pathogen. By exacerbating responses to known pathogens, HIV may contribute to the severity of infectious diarrhea seen in AIDS. Further studies of these phenomena are needed to determine the role of the autonomic nervous system in AIDS.

In a prospective study of gastric secretory activity and gastric juice composition in AIDS patients, Lake-Bakaar et al.[106] found higher mean gastric pH, lower maximal acid output, lower gastric juice volume, lower mucus output and concentration, and lower pepsin output and concentration compared with controls. Cultures of gastric juice were typically positive for bacterial organisms and herpesviruses in patients but sterile in controls. Patients had elevated mean serum gastrin levels compared with controls. Antiparietal cell antibodies were found in 53% of patients compared with a 2–4% prevalence in the general population of the same age group. Biopsies of gastric and duodenal mucosa showed mild-to-moderate chronic inflammation. Whether this gastropathy is due to direct HIV infection, secondary to infection with another pathogen (e.g., *Campylobacter pylori*), neuropathy, or viral blockade of neuroendocrine signaling is unknown.

Malabsorption is another mechanism by which HIV may induce diarrhea and weight loss. It could result from defects in luminal digestion, mucosal transport, local immunity, or submucosal infiltration. Kotler et al.[107] studied homosexual AIDS patients with the diarrhea-wasting syndrome and homosexual patients with diarrhea but without AIDS. They found malabsorption with a mixed type of malnutrition, with features of both marasmus and kwashiorkor, in all AIDS patients. Jejunal biopsies showed partial villous atrophy, crypt hyperplasia, and increased numbers of intraepithelial lymphocytes. Rectal biopsies showed intranuclear viral inclusions, abundant mast cells near the base of the rectal crypt, and apoptosis, a focal degeneration of crypt epithelial cells. Gillin et al.[108] studied AIDS patients with and without the diarrhea-wasting syndrome. Mild-to-moderate chronic inflammation was found on duodenal biopsy in patients with and without gastrointestinal symptoms. All symptomatic patients tested had abnormal D-xylose absorption and all but one had abnormal ^{14}C-glycerol-tripalmitin absorption. These patients had no specific gastrointestinal pathogen identified, but cultures for CMV and *Mycobacterium avium-intracellulare* (MAI) were not performed. However, a subset of these patients did have acid-fast bacilli-laden histiocytes in duodenal biopsy specimens, and therefore probably represent disseminated mycobacterial infection. These studies confirm the importance of malabsorption in AIDS and point to local immune derangement and submucosal infiltration as possible etiologies.

Immune responses to gastrointestinal pathogens are diminished in AIDS, which may allow for persistence of some organisms. Janoff et al.[109] found homosexual AIDS patients infected with *Giardia lamblia* unable to mount de novo antibody responses despite pre-existing titers. Patients infected with *Shigella flexneri* or *Campylobacter jejuni* who failed to generate appropriate antibody responses had recurrent infection despite antibiotic therapy. The one patient who recovered developed appropriate antibody responses in all three classes.[110] Perillo et al.[111] examined 12 HIV-infected homosexual men who were asymptomatic hepatitis B virus (HBV) carriers. HIV-seropositive carriers had milder histology, lower alanine aminotransferase levels, higher HBV DNA polymerase levels, and lower CD4/CD8 ratios than homosexual HIV-seronegative carriers or heterosexual carriers. These studies show impaired immune responses to gastrointestinal parasites, bacterial pathogens, and hepatitis B. These defects cause no change in disease caused by *Giardia,* more severe disease caused by bacteria, and less severe disease caused by hepatitis B. In contrast to the milder disease due to hepatitis B, the cytopathic viruses are more virulent in AIDS (see below).

Primary manifestations of HIV may include direct infection, local immune dysregulation, neuropathic complications, gastric secretory failure, or malabsorption. Proof for any one of these mechanisms is lacking and will be difficult to obtain without good animal or in vitro models. However, these findings show that primary

HIV effects are plausible and in some cases probable. Further effort to understand basic pathophysiologic mechanisms is required.

Secondary Infections in HIV

Over the past 15 years, the sexual transmission of enteric pathogens among homosexual men has been recognized. With the advent of AIDS, new pathogens have been identified in patients with gastrointestinal symptoms. These include cryptosporidia, isospora, microsporidia, *M. avium-intracellulare,* and cytomegalovirus. These pathogens, when added to previously recognized sexually transmitted pathogens such as gonorrhea, syphilis, chlamydia, herpes simplex, and papillomavirus, demonstrate the microbial complexity of intestinal infections in homosexual men at risk for HIV infection.[96,112,113] When coupled with trauma-induced rectal lesions and gastrointestinal neoplasms such as Kaposi's sarcoma and lymphoma, these diseases span a broad spectrum of gastrointestinal problems in homosexual men. Therefore, a homosexual man with gastrointestinal symptoms must be thoroughly investigated, including microbiologic and, in some cases, histologic evaluation of the gastrointestinal tract and assessment of HIV status.

Factors contributing to the high prevalence of enteric pathogens in this population include anorectal intercourse, oral-anal contact, promiscuity, anonymity of sexual contacts, asymptomatic infections, and possibly fomite transmission via unsterile enema devices. Quinn et al.[113] recovered one or more intestinal pathogens from 80% of symptomatic homosexual men attending a sexually transmitted disease clinic, as opposed to 39% of asymptomatic homosexual men attending the same clinic. Nearly 25% of the symptomatic patients had two or more pathogens. Pathogens that are infectious at low inoculum size, such as *Shigella, Giardia, Entanoeba histolytica,* and *Campylobacter,* appeared to be transmitted by oral-anal sex and commonly caused enteritis or proctocolitis. The traditional venereal pathogens such as gonorrhea, syphilis, chlamydia, herpes, and papillomaviruses were transmitted primarily by anal intercourse and tended to cause proctitis and perianal disease.

With the immunocompromise accompanying HIV infection, pre-existing subclinical infections may emerge. Gastrointestinal disease may become severe with oroesophageal candidiasis, severe mucocutaneous herpes simplex infections of the mouth, esophagus, rectum, and perirectal skin, or dissemination of cytomegalovirus.[1,3,114-116] Infections with cryptosporidia, isospora, or other pathogens that are usually asymptomatic or readily cleared in immunocompetent hosts may become debilitating or fatal in HIV-infected patients.[117-120] Other patients may develop enteropathy in the absence of defined pathogens, as discussed above.

In tropical areas such as Central Africa, Haiti, and other developing countries, diarrhea and weight loss are present in over 80% of AIDS patients. This may indicate greater susceptibility to gastrointestinal pathogens common to a specific region.[121,122] Malebranche et al.[123] showed that greater than 90% of AIDS patients in Haiti presented with unexplained chronic diarrhea, persistent fever, weight loss, anorexia, and opportunistic infections. Infections included mucosal candidiasis in 93%, cryptosporidiosis in 38%, *Mycobacterium tuberculosis* in 24%, cytomegalovirus in 14%, and mucocutaneous herpes simplex in 10%. In contrast to the 60% of Americans who present with *Pneumocystis carinii* pneumonia, only 7% of the

Haitians had pneumocystis diagnosed. Other groups have confirmed these findings in African patients diagnosed in Europe and in Central Africa.[98,99,121,124-126]

Opportunistic Infections and Malignancies

Oroesophageal Candidiasis

Oral candidiasis (thrush) is one of the most common signs of AIDS. It appears early in the symptomatic prodrome of AIDS and is part of ARC. The occurrence of thrush in a patient at risk for HIV infection or in association with a diarrhea-wasting syndrome is suggestive of HIV infection. Klein et al.[127] found that thrush in homosexual men was a significant predictor of underlying immunosuppression and development of AIDS. Tavitian et al.[128] endoscoped ten patients with pre-existing AIDS and oral candidiasis, three without and seven with esophageal complaints. All ten had esophageal candidiasis. Symptoms did not correlate with degree of involvement seen endoscopically or histologically. Therefore, in this small study, oral candidiasis was a strong predictor of esophageal involvement in patients with AIDS. Diagnosis can be made by barium swallow or endoscopy, which shows "cottage cheese" exudates with esophageal ulceration.[114,115] Biopsies show hyphae extending into the mucosa and submucosa. Since esophageal ulceration can also be due to cytomegalovirus or herpes simplex, viral cultures are necessary.

Therapy of oral candidiasis is with either nystatin or clotrimazole. Persistent oral candidiasis or esophageal candidiasis should be treated with ketoconazole. Severe cases require intravenous amphotericin B. Long-term suppressive therapy is required due to frequent recurrence. Without aggressive therapy of esophageal disease, intractable ulceration may develop.

Cytomegalovirus

Autopsy series have shown active cytomegalovirus infection in nearly 90% of AIDS cases.[114,116,129] Serologic evidence of the virus is common, and it is readily cultured from blood, saliva, semen, and intestinal biopsy specimens of most AIDS patients.[114,116,130,131] Cytomegalovirus can infect any portion of the gastrointestinal tract, but most often presents as a diffuse colitis with abdominal pain and watery or bloody diarrhea.[132-135]

Cytomegalovirus intestinal infection may present as a solitary ulcer, toxic dilatation, or, rarely, perforation.[136,137] Lower endoscopy may show ulceration or violaceous lesions resembling Kaposi's sarcoma. Biopsies show cytomegalovirus inclusions and vasculitis with acute hemorrhage and inflammation in the lamina propria. Cytomegalovirus is associated with the acalculous cholecystitis,[138] and the biliary stenosis and sclerosis that are seen in AIDS patients.[139]

Diagnosis of cytomegalovirus infection is confirmed by biopsy showing characteristic intranuclear inclusions, viral culture of specimens, in situ hybridization, or monoclonal antibody staining.[140]

Therapy of cytomegalovirus consists of 9-(1,3-dihydroxy-2-propoxymethyl) guanine (DHPG, ganciclovir), which is effective in the therapy of gastrointestinal infection but is toxic.[141] Life-long suppressive maintenance is required. Patients presenting with cytomegalovirus gastrointestinal disease and other concurrent opportunistic infections had shorter survival times compared with those with cytomegalovirus alone.[141]

Herpes Simplex

Oral, esophageal, and anorectal herpes simplex infections are common in homosexual men with HIV infection.[3,142,143] Gastrointestinal herpes becomes progressive and chronic in the setting of the progressive immunosuppression due to HIV.[3] These lesions are usually painful and debilitating and may involve the entire gastrointestinal tract if left untreated. Perianal herpes can cause ulcers greater than 10 cm in diameter.[3] Without therapy, herpes ulcers may persist for months. Diagnosis is strongly suggested by history and inspection and confirmed by biopsy, Tzanck preparation, or viral culture. Treatment with oral or intravenous acyclovir leads to healing of the lesions, but prolonged maintenance therapy is required.

Protozoal Infections

Infections with *E. histolytica* or *G. lamblia* do not predict HIV infection nor do they pose any unusual clinical or therapeutic problems in AIDS patients.[113] This is of note in view of the failure of AIDS patients to synthesize antibody de novo in response to *G. lamblia* infection.[109] A high proportion responds to therapy with metronidazole.

Other pathogenic protozoa in HIV-infected patients include cryptosporidia, isospora, and microsporidia. Transmission appears to be fecal-oral among homosexual men and is associated with poor sanitary conditions in developing countries.[117,144,145] Although cryptosporidiosis is a zoonosis in immunocompetent hosts, no animal reservoir has been described for isospora or microsporidia.[146] One of these three parasites is identified in up to 25% of AIDS patients and causes marked morbidity and mortality.

Cryptosporidia primarily infect the lower small intestine, but can involve the entire gut, the hepatobiliary system, and the bronchi.[147-150] Ingestion of oocysts leads to hatching out of sporozoites, which invade the microvilli. There they replicate, reinvade neighboring cells, and undergo sexual division (sporogony).[151] Oocysts are released into the lumen where they can reinfect or be passed in the stool. The pathogenic features of cryptosporidia are unknown. Although a transient diarrhea occurs in immunocompetent hosts, cryptosporidiosis can be a severe, debilitating infection with maldigestion and malabsorption in AIDS patients. Complications ascribed to cryptosporidial infection include cholecystitis, sclerosis of the biliary tree, and extrahepatic biliary stenosis.[139] However, a lack of understanding of the pathogenic mechanism of cryptosporidium and coinfection of these patients with HIV and other pathogens makes determination of a clear role for cryptosporidium in these extraintestinal complications difficult.

Diagnosis is made by demonstration of oocysts in stool or by visualizing the characteristic $2-4\ \mu m$ organism along the villus border. Small intestinal histology may show partial atrophy and distortion of villi, and cellular infiltration of the lamina propria of the ileum and jejunum.[152]

Therapy for cryptosporidiosis has been disappointing.[153,154] Recent reports have shown dramatic results using the long-acting somatostatin analog SMS-201-995 (Sandoz Pharmaceutical).[155,156] Subcutaneous administration led to control of refractory diarrhea in an AIDS patient with cryptosporidia-related diarrhea and in AIDS patients with pathogen-unassociated diarrhea.

Isospora belli is another coccidian parasite infecting the microvilli of the small intestine in man. The life cycle is similar to that of cryptosporidia. In the immunocompromised host, despite the watery diarrhea, weight loss, and abdominal cramps, little if any local inflammatory response is generated.[157,158] Diagnosis is made as described for cryptosporidiosis. Therapy with trimethoprim-sulfamethoxazole is effective for isospora but must be given over a prolonged period to prevent relapses.[159,160]

Microsporidia are ubiquitous spore-forming protozoa that have been identified by electron microscopy in the cytoplasm of villous enterocytes,[118,161,162] in muscle,[163] and in the liver[164] in a small number of patients with AIDS. This organism seems to be associated with dysfunction of the respective organ system and systemic signs, but its exact role is unclear. Diagnosis is demanding, as it requires electron microscopy, and therapy is supportive.

Mycobacteria

Mycobacterium avium-intracellulare is ubiquitous in the environment and is an uncommon cause of pulmonary disease in immunocompetent hosts. However, in AIDS patients it can cause disseminated disease and is associated with fever, weight loss, abdominal pain, malabsorption, and diarrhea.[165,166] The effect of *M. avium-intracellulare* on mortality is still unclear. Although clinical, gastrointestinal, and histopathologic presentations of intestinal involvement with *M. avium-intracellulare* mimic aspects of Whipple's disease, the bacteria seen in small intestinal macrophages in the two syndromes are distinct. *Mycobacterium avium-intracellulare* is periodic-acid Schiff (PAS)-positive and acid-fast whereas the Whipple's agent is PAS-positive, non-acid-fast.[167,168] Diarrhea and malabsorption may result from local accumulation of *M. avium-intracellulare* engorged macrophages. *Mycobacterium avium-intracellulare* can also cause extrahepatic biliary obstruction from parapancreatic and portahepatic adenopathy.[165]

Diagnosis is based on acid-fast staining and culture of stool and histopathologic examination and culture of biopsy specimens. Blood cultures are almost always positive in disseminated *M. avium-intracellulare* infection.[165] Therapy has been disappointing, requiring multiple agents with poor results. Approaches using macrophage activators such as TNF along with other agents have been successful in animal models[169] and cultured human macrophages.[170] *Mycobacterium tuberculosis,* with pulmonary, extrapulmonary, and disseminated presentations is being seen with increasing frequency in patients with HIV infection.[171,172] Gastrointestinal involvement is likely to be seen more frequently with the increasing number of cases of disseminated disease. Unlike the case with *M. avium-intracellulare,* antituberculous therapy is effective against *M. tuberculosis* in HIV-infected patients, but prolonged courses of therapy may be required.[173]

Histoplasmosis

Although disseminated infection with *Histoplasma capsulatum* has been reported in <0.5% of AIDS cases so far, the number of cases in the future is certain to increase. Gastrointestinal involvement seems to occur in a small percentage of disseminated cases.[174,175] Manifestations have not been well characterized, but have included small bowel obstruction due to transmural inflammation,[176] fever of unknown origin with subsequent intestinal perforation (Bartlett JG, unpublished data), jejunal bleeding,[177] and cecal mass.[178] Johnson et al.[175] reported two cases of AIDS with positive intestinal biopsy cultures who did not have diarrhea. Diagnosis of disseminated disease can be made by careful inspection of the peripheral blood, staining and culture of bone marrow aspirates, blood or other fluid culture, or staining and culture of biopsy specimens.

Salmonella and Campylobacter

Recurrent bacteremia due to *Salmonella* has been reported in HIV-infected patients.[179-182] These infections respond to acute therapy but often recur after cessation of antibiotics. The organism's ability to survive intracellularly in macrophages for long periods and the importance of T-cell functions for the clearance of *Salmonella* infections give some explanation for these problems in AIDS patients. Therapy should be based on in vitro sensitivities and continued indefinitely.

Persistent, refractory *C. jejuni* and *C. coli* infections have been encountered in HIV-infected patients. Perlman et al.[110] reported three AIDS patients with diarrhea who grew *C. jejuni* or *C. coli* from stool, blood, or biopsy specimens and failed to clear the organism after appropriate therapy. Another HIV-infected patient with generalized lymphadenopathy responded well to one course of antibiotics. Failure to clear infection correlated with failure to mount an appropriate antibody response.

Kaposi's Sarcoma

Kaposi's sarcoma is a neoplastic proliferation of vascular endothelial cells that can occur throughout the body. Cutaneous dissemination is the most common form, but over 50% have gastrointestinal involvement as well.[183] Gastric, small intestinal, and colonic lesions are more common than esophageal lesions,[183] but oral involvement is frequent.[184] Gastrointestinal Kaposi's sarcoma is usually detected on routine endoscopy as raised sessile red nodules of 1–2 cm. Histologic confirmation may be complicated by the submucosal location of the lesion, making biopsy difficult. Histology shows typical spindle cells with slits and hemorrhage. Kaposi's sarcoma lesions rarely cause significant blood loss, although they may cause mechanical obstruction if large. Therapy is local if necessary, but may involve radiation or chemotherapy in more advanced cases.[185]

Small Bowel Lymphoma

Non-Hodgkin's lymphomas of B-cell origin and Hodgkin's disease occur with a higher than expected frequency in HIV-infected and AIDS patients.[186] Therapy with standard protocols is disappointing, and survival time from diagnosis is short. Involvement of the gastrointestinal tract seems to be more common in this population than in HIV-negative patients.[187]

Oral Hairy Leukoplakia

Oral hairy leukoplakia seems to be due to EBV-induced benign epithelial hyperplasia seen in the oral mucosa in patients infected with HIV.[188] Clinically, the lesion is a white thickening of the oral mucosa with corrugations. Biopsy shows epithelial hyperplasia, thickening of the parakeratin layer with an irregular surface, projections ("hairs"), and vacuolated prickle cells, but little inflammation.[189,190] EBV can be demonstrated in the lesions, and acyclovir is somewhat effective.[191]

Anal Warts and Anal Cancer

In 1982, Daling et al. suggested an increased rate of anal cancer in homosexual men.[192] Subsequent studies by this group compared 148 anal cancer patients with

166 colon cancer patients.[193] They found that in men the relative risk of developing anal cancer was increased by a history of anal intercourse, genital warts, gonorrhea, number of sexual partners, or presence of antibodies to herpes simplex type 2 or *Chlamydia trachomatis*. In women, relative risk was increased by a history of genital warts or presence of antibodies to herpes simplex type 2 or *C. trachomatis*. Current smokers of either sex were also at higher risk. In view of the proposed role of human papillomavirus in genital warts and cervical cancer, it seems likely that papillomavirus is involved in anal cancer. However, the effect of HIV infection on clinical presentation is still unclear.

CONCLUSIONS

Despite the fact that the gastrointestinal manifestations of HIV infection are among the most common and most debilitating encountered, enteropathy in AIDS remains rather poorly understood. A large fraction of the diarrhea in AIDS still has no clear etiology other than HIV, but clear pathophysiologic mechanisms are lacking. The spectrum of known pathogens demonstrated in gastrointestinal disease in AIDS is distinct from that seen in the normal population and is probably due, at least in part, to the disruption of local as well as systemic immunity.

Further understanding of the enteropathy found in AIDS patients that is not associated with known gastrointestinal pathogens may help shed light on the reasons for the severity of AIDS gastrointestinal disease that is associated with known pathogens.

REFERENCES

1. Gottlieb MS, Schroff R, Schanker HM, et al: *Pneumocystis carinii* pneumonia and mucosal candidiasis in previously healthy homosexual men: Evidence of a new acquired cellular immunodeficiency. *N Engl J Med* 305:1425–1431, 1981.
2. Masur H, Michelis MA, Greene JB, et al: An outbreak of community-acquired *Pneumocystis carinii* pneumonia: initial manifestation of cellular immune dysfunction. *N Engl J Med* 305:1431–1438, 1981.
3. Siegal FP, Lopez C, Hammer GS, et al: Severe acquired immunodeficiency in male homosexuals, manifested by chronic perianal ulcerative herpes simplex lesions. *N Engl J Med* 305:1939–1944, 1981.
4. Centers for Disease Control. Quarterly report to the domestic policy council on the prevalence and rate of spread of HIV and AIDS — United States. *MMWR* 37:551, 1988.
5. Cooper DA, Maclean P, Finlayson R, et al: Acute AIDS retrovirus infection: definition of a clinical illness associated with seroconversion. *Lancet* 1:537–540, 1985.
6. Tindall B, Cooper DA, Donovan B, et al: Primary human immunodeficiency virus infection. Clinical and serologic aspects. *Infect Dis Clin N Am* 2:329–351, 1988.
7. Lui KJ, Darrow WW, Rutherford GW III: A model-based estimate of the mean incubation period for AIDS in homosexual men. *Science* 240:1333–1335, 1988.
8. Barre-Sinoussi F, Chermann JC, Rey F, et al: Isolation of a T-lymphotropic retrovirus from a patient at risk for acquired immune deficiency syndrome (AIDS). *Science* 220:868–871, 1983.
9. Gallo RC, Salahuddin SZ, Popovic M, et al: Frequency, detection and isolation of cytopathic retroviruses (HTLV-III) from patients with AIDS and at risk for AIDS. *Science* 224:500–503, 1984.

10. Levy JA, Hoffman AD, Kramer SM, et al: Isolation of lymphocytopathic retroviruses from San Francisco patients with AIDS. *Science* 225:840–842, 1984.

11. Coffin J, Haase A, Levy JA, et al: What to call the AIDS virus. *Nature* 321:10, 1986.

12. Kanki PJ, Barin F, M'Boup S, et al: New human T-lymphotropic retrovirus related to simian T-lymphotropic virus type III (STLV-III agm). *Science* 232:238–243, 1986.

13. Clavel F, Guetard F, Brun-Vezinet F, et al: Isolation of a new human retrovirus from West Africa patients with AIDS. *Science* 233:343–346, 1986.

14. Clavel F, Guyader M, Guetard D, et al: Molecular cloning and polymorphism of the human immunodeficiency virus type 2. *Nature* 324:691–695, 1986.

15. Kornfeld H, Riedel N, Viglianti GA, et al: Cloning of HTLV-4 and its relation to simian and human immunodeficiency virus. *Nature* 326:610–613, 1987.

16. Wong-Staal F, Gallo RC: Human T-lymphotropic retroviruses. *Nature* 317:395–403, 1985.

17. Rabson AB, Martin MA: Molecular organization of the AIDS retrovirus. *Cell* 40:477–480, 1985.

18. Arya SK, Guo C, Josephs SF, et al: *Trans*-activator gene of human T-lymphotropic virus type III (HTLV-III). *Science* 229:69–77, 1985.

19. Fisher AG, Feinberg MB, Josephs SF, et al: The *trans*-activator gene of HTLV-III is essential for virus replication. *Nature* 320:367–371, 1986.

20. Rosen CA, Haseltine WA: Selective regulation of HIV gene expression by the *art* gene product. In Franza BR, Cullen BR, Wong-Staal F: *The Control of Human Retrovirus Gene Expression.* Cold Spring Harbor, Cold Spring Harbor Press, 1988, pp 23–27.

21. Guy B, Kieny MP, Riviere Y, et al: HIV F/3′ *orf* encodes a phosphorylated GTP-binding protein resembling an oncogene product. *Nature* 330:266–269, 1987.

22. Ahmad N, Venkatesan S: *Nef* protein of HIV-1 is a transcriptional repressor of HIV-1 LTR. *Science* 241:1481–1485, 1988.

23. Fisher AG, Ensoli B, Ivanoff L, et al: The *sor* gene of HIV-1 is required for efficient virus transmission *in vitro. Science* 237:888–893, 1987.

24. Dalgleish AG, Beverley PCL, Clapham PR, et al: The CD4 (T4) antigen is an essential component of the receptor for the AIDS retrovirus. *Nature* 312:763–767, 1984.

25. Klatzmann D, Champagne E, Chamaret S, et al: T-lymphocyte T4 molecule behaves as the receptor for human retrovirus LAV. *Nature* 312:767–768, 1984.

26. McDougal JS, Mawle A, Cort SP, et al: Cellular tropism of the human retrovirus HTLV III/LAV. I. Role of T cell activation and expression of the T4 antigen. *J Immunol* 135:3151–3162, 1985.

27. Doyle C, Strominger JL: Interaction between CD4 and class II MHC molecules mediates cell adhesion. *Nature* 330:256–259, 1987.

28. Talle MA, Rao PE, Westberg E, et al: Patterns of antigenic expression on human monocytes as defined by monoclonal antibodies. *Cell Immunol* 78:83–99, 1983.

29. Maddon PJ, Dalgleish AG, McDougal JS, et al: The T4 gene encodes the AIDS virus receptor and is expressed in the immune system and the brain. *Cell* 47:333–348, 1986.

30. Lasky LA, Nakamura G, Smith DH, et al: Delineation of a region of the human immunodeficiency virus type 1 gp120 glycoprotein critical for interaction with the CD4 receptor. *Cell* 50:975–985, 1987.

31. Sattentau QJ, Dalgleish AG, Weiss RA, et al: Epitopes of the CD4 antigen and HIV infection. *Science* 234:1120–1123, 1986.

32. Hussey RE, Richardson NE, Kowalski M, et al: A soluble CD4 protein selectively inhibits HIV replication and syncytium formation. *Nature* 331:78–81, 1988.

33. Deen KE, McDougal S, Inacker R, et al: A soluble form of CD4 (T4) protein inhibits AIDS virus infection. *Nature* 331:82–84, 1988.

34. Levy JA, Cheng-Meyer C, Dina D, et al: AIDS retrovirus (ARV-2) clone replicates in transfected human and animal fibroblasts. *Science* 232:998–1001, 1986.

35. Adachi A, Koenig S, Gendelman HE, et al: Productive, persistent infection of human colorectal cell lines with human immunodeficiency virus. *J Virol* 61:209–213, 1987.

36. Nelson JA, Wiley CA, Reynolds-Kohler C, et al: Human immunodeficiency virus detected in bowel epithelium from patients with gastrointestinal symptoms. *Lancet* 1:259–262, 1988.

37. Cheng-Meyer C, Rutka JT, Rosenblum ML, et al: The human immunodeficiency virus (HIV) can productively infect cultured human glial cells. *Proc Natl Acad Sci USA* 84:3526, 1987.

38. Kowalski M, Potz J, Basiripour L, et al: Functional regions of the envelope glycoprotein of human immunodeficiency virus type 1. *Science* 237:1351–1355, 1987.

39. Gallaher WR: Detection of a fusion peptide sequence in the transmembrane protein of human immunodeficiency virus. *Cell* 50:327–328, 1987.

40. Stein BS, Gowda SD, Lifson JD, et al: pH-independent HIV entry into CD4-positive T cells via virus envelope fusion to the plasma membrane. *Cell* 49:659–668, 1987.

41. Pauza CD, Price TM: Human immunodeficiency virus infection of T cells and monocytes proceeds via receptor-mediated endocytosis. *J Cell Biol* 107:959–968, 1988.

42. Bedinger P, Moriarty A, von Borstel RC, et al: Internalization of the human immunodeficiency virus does not require the cytoplasmic domain of CD4. *Nature* 334:162–165, 1988.

43. Porterfield JS. Antibody enhanced viral growth in macrophages. *Immunol Lett* 11:213–217, 1985.

44. Takeda A, Tuazon CU, Ennis FA: Antibody enhanced infection by HIV-1 via Fc receptor-mediated entry. *Science* 242:580–583, 1988.

45. Saag MS, Hahn BH, Gibbons J, et al: Extensive variation of human immunodeficiency virus type-1 *in vivo. Nature* 334:440–444, 1988.

46. Fisher AG, Ensoli B, Looney D, et al: Biologically diverse molecular variants within a single HIV-1 isolate. Nature 334:444–447, 1988.

47. Robinson WE Jr, Montefiori DC, Mitchell WM: Antibody-dependent enhancement of human immunodeficiency virus type-1 infection. *Lancet* 1:790–794, 1988.

48. Shaw GM, Hahn BH, Arya SK, et al: Molecular characterization of human T-cell leukemia (lymphotropic) virus type III in the acquired immune deficiency syndrome. *Science* 226:1165–1171, 1984.

49. Lewis DE, Yoffe B, Bosworth CG, et al: Human immunodeficiency virus-induced pathology favored by cellular transmission and activation. *FASEB J* 2:251–255, 1988.

50. Zagury D, Bernard J, Leonard R, et al: Long-term cultures of HTLV-III infected T cells: a model of cytopathology of T-cell depletion in AIDS. *Science* 231:850–853, 1986.

51. Mosca JD, Bednarik DP, Raj NBK, et al: Herpes simplex virus type-1 can reactivate transcription of latent human immunodeficiency virus. *Nature* 325:67–70, 1987.

52. Nabel GJ, Rice SA, Knipe DM, et al: Alternative mechanisms for activation of human immunodeficiency virus enhancer in T cells. *Science* 239:1299–1302, 1988.

53. Folks TM, Justement J, Kinter A, et al: Cytokine-induced expression of HIV-1 in a chronically infected promonocyte cell line. *Science* 238:800–802, 1987.

54. Quinn TC, Piot P, McCormick JB, et al: Serologic and immunologic studies in patients with AIDS in North America and Africa. *JAMA* 257:2617–2621, 1987.

55. Harper E, Marselle LM, Gallo RC, et al: Detection of lymphocytes expressing human T-lymphotropic virus type III in lymph nodes and peripheral blood from infected individuals by *in situ* hybridization. *Proc Natl Acad Sci USA* 83:772–776, 1986.

56. Lifson JD, Reyes GR, McGrath MS, et al: AIDS retrovirus induced cytopathology: giant cell formation and involvement of CD4 antigen. *Science* 232:1123–1127, 1986.

57. Sodroski J, Goh WC, Rosen C, et al: Role of the HTLV-III/LAV envelope in syncytium formation and cytopathicity. *Nature* 322:470–474, 1986.

58. Lifson JD, Feinberg MB, Reyes GR, et al: Induction of CD4-dependent cell fusion by the HTLV-III/LAV envelope glycoprotein. *Nature* 323:725–728, 1986.

59. Yoffe B, Lewis DE, Petrie BL, et al: Fusion as a mediator of cytolysis in mixtures of uninfected CD4+ lymphocytes and cells infected by human immunodeficiency virus. *Proc Natl Acad Sci USA* 84:1429–1433, 1987.

60. Gruters RA, Neefjes JJ, Tersmette M, et al: Interference with HIV-induced syncytium formation and viral infectivity by inhibitors of trimming glucosidase. *Nature* 330:74–77, 1987.

61. Somasundaran M, Robinson HL: A major mechanism of human immunodeficiency virus-induced cell killing does not involve cell fusion. *J Virol* 61:3114–3119, 1987.

62. Stevenson M, Meier C, Mann AM, et al: Envelope glycoprotein of HIV induces interference and cytolysis resistance in CD4+ cells: mechanism for persistence in AIDS. *Cell* 53:483–496, 1988.

63. Hoxie JA, Alpers JD, Rackowski JL, et al: Alterations in T4 (CD4) protein and mRNA synthesis in cells infected with HIV. *Science* 234:1123–1127, 1986.

64. Siliciano RF, Lawton T, Knall C, et al: Analysis of host-virus interactions in AIDS with anti-gp120 T cell clones: effect of HIV sequence variation and a mechanism for CD4+ cell depletion. *Cell* 54:561–575, 1988.

65. Germain RN: Antigen processing and CD4+ T cell depletion in AIDS. *Cell* 54:441–444, 1988.

66. Wahren B, Morfeldt-Mansson L, Biberfeld G, et al: Impaired specific cellular response to HTLV-III before other immune defects in patients with HTLV-III infection. *N Engl J Med* 315:393–394, 1986.

67. Lyerly HK, Matthews TJ, Langlois AJ, et al: Human T cell lymphotropic virus III B glycoprotein (gp120) bound to CD4 determinants on normal lymphocytes and expressed by infected cells serves as a target for immune attack. *Proc Natl Acad Sci USA* 84:4601–4605, 1987.

68. Stricker RB, McHugh TM, Moody DJ, et al: An AIDS-related cytotoxic autoantibody reacts with a specific antigen on stimulated CD4+ T cells. *Nature* 327:710–713, 1987.

69. Seligmann M, Pinching AJ, Rosen FS, et al: Immunology of human immunodeficiency virus infection and the acquired immunodeficiency syndrome. *Ann Intern Med* 107:234–242, 1987.

70. Lane CH, Masur H, Gelmann EP, et al: Correlation between immunologic function and clinical subpopulations of patients with the acquired immune deficiency syndrome. *Am J Med* 78:417–422, 1985.

71. Zolla-Pazner S, Des Jarlais DC, Friedman SR, et al: Nonrandom development of immunologic abnormalities after infection with human immunodeficiency virus: implications for immunologic classification of the disease. *Proc Natl Acad Sci USA* 84:5404–5408, 1987.

72. Brettler DB, Forsberg AD, Brewster F, et al: Delayed cutaneous hypersensitivity reactions in hemophiliac subjects treated with factor concentrate. *Am J Med* 81:607–611, 1986.

73. Murray HW, Rubin BY, Masur H, et al: Impaired production of lymphokines and immune (gamma) interferon in the acquired immunodeficiency syndrome. *N Engl J Med* 310:883–889, 1984.

74. Lane HC, Depper JM, Greene WC, et al: Qualitative analysis of immune function in

patients with the acquired immunodeficiency syndrome. Evidence for a selective defect in soluble antigen recognition. *N Engl J Med* 313:79–84, 1985.

75. Linette GP, Hartzman RJ, Ledbetter JA, et al: HIV-1-infected T cells show a selective signaling defect after perturbation of CD3/antigen receptor. *Science* 241:573–576, 1988.

76. Lane HC, Masur H, Edgar LC, et al: Abnormalities of B-cell activation and immuno-regulation in patients with the acquired immunodeficiency syndrome. *N Engl J Med* 309:453–458, 1983.

77. Schnittman SM, Lane HC, Higgins SE, et al: Direct polyclonal activation of human B lymphocytes by the acquired immune deficiency syndrome virus. *Science* 233:1084–1086, 1986.

78. Gurney ME, Apatoff BR, Spear GT, et al: Neuroleukin: a lymphokine product of lectin-stimulated T cells. *Science* 234:574–581, 1986.

79. Lee MR, Ho DD, Gurney ME: Functional interaction and partial homology between human immunodeficiency virus and neuroleukin. *Science* 237:1047–1051, 1987.

80. Chaput M, Claes V, Portetelle D, et al: The neurotrophic factor neuroleukin is 90% homologous with phosphohexose isomerase. *Nature* 332:454–455, 1988.

81. Faik P, Walker JIH, Redmill AAM, et al: Mouse glucose-6-phosphate isomerase and neuroleukin have identical 3′ sequences. *Nature* 332:455–457, 1988.

82. Ho DD, Rota TR, Hirsch MS: Infection of monocyte/macrophages by human T-lymphotropic virus type III. *J Clin Invest* 77:1712–1715, 1986.

83. Gartner S, Markovits P, Markovitz DM, et al: The role of mononuclear phagocytes in HTLV-III/LAV infection. *Science* 233:215–219, 1986.

84. Nicholson JKA, Gross GD, Calloway CS, et al: *In vitro* infection of human monocytes with human T-lymphotropic virus type III/lymphadenopathy-associated virus (HTLV III/LAV). *J Immunol* 137:323–329, 1986.

85. Koenig S, Gendelman HE, Orenstein JM, et al: Detection of AIDS virus in macrophages in brain tissue from AIDS patients with encephalopathy. *Science* 233:1089–1093, 1986.

86. Ho DD, Pomerantz RJ, Kaplan JC: Pathogenesis of infection with human immunodeficiency virus. *N Engl J Med* 317:278–286, 1987.

87. Folks TM, Kessler SW, Orenstein JM, et al: Infection and replication of HIV-1 in purified progenitor cells of normal human bone marrow. *Science* 242:919–922, 1988.

88. Smith PD, Ohura K, Masur H, et al: Monocyte function in the acquired immune deficiency syndrome. Defective chemotaxis. *J Clin Invest* 74:2121–2128, 1984.

89. Bender BS, Davidson B, Kline R, et al: Role of the mononuclear phagocyte system in the immunopathogenesis of human immunodeficiency virus infection and the acquired immunodeficiency syndrome. *Rev Infect Dis* 10:1142–1154, 1988.

90. Salahuddin SZ, Rose RM, Groopman JE, et al: Human T lymphotropic virus type III infection of human alveolar macrophages. *Blood* 68:281, 1986.

91. Muller F, Rollag H, Froland SS: Defect macrophage functions in patients with HIV infection. Fourth International Conference on AIDS. Swedish Ministry of Health and Social Affairs, Stockholm, Sweden, Abstract #2065, 1988.

92. Dinarello CA: Interleukin-1 and the pathogenesis of the acute-phase response. *N Engl J Med* 311:1413–1418, 1984.

93. Beutler B, Cerami A: Cachectin and tumour necrosis factor as two sides of the same biological coin. *Nature* 320:584–588, 1986.

94. Lahdevirta J, Maury CPJ, Teppo AM, et al: Elevated levels of circulating cachectin/tumor necrosis factor in patients with acquired immunodeficiency syndrome. *Am J Med* 85:289–291, 1988.

95. Rabeneck L, Boyko WJ, Mclean DM et al: Unusual esophageal ulcers containing enveloped virus-like particles in homosexual men. *Gastroenterology* 90:1882, 1986.

96. Laughon BE, Druckman DA, Vernon A, et al: Prevalence of enteric pathogens in homosexual men with and without acquired immunodeficiency syndrome. *Gastroenterology* 94:984–993, 1988.

97. Quinn TC: Early symptoms and signs of AIDS and the AIDS related complex. In Ebberen P, Briggar RJ, Melbye MM: *AIDS: A Basic Guide for Clinicians.* Copenhagen, Munchgaard, 1984, pp 64–83.

98. Colebunders R, Francis H, Mann JM, et al: Persistent diarrhea, strongly associated with HIV infection in Kinshasa, Zaire. *Am J Gastroenterol* 82:859–864, 1987.

99. Serwadda D, Mugerwa RD, Sewankambo NK, et al: Slim disease: a new disease in Uganda and its association with HTLV-III infection. *Lancet* ii:849–852, 1985.

100. Rene E, Jarry A, Brousse N, et al: Demonstration of HIV infection of the gastrointestinal tract in AIDS patients: relation with symptoms and other digestive infections. Fourth International Conference on AIDS. Swedish Ministry of Health and Social Affairs, Stockholm, Sweden. Abstract #7118, 1988.

101. Overbaugh J, Donahue PR, Quackenbush SL, et al: Molecular cloning of a feline leukemia virus that induces fatal immunodeficiency disease in cats. *Science* 239:906–910, 1988.

102. Hoover EA, Quackenbush SL, Overbaugh JM, et al: Molecularly cloned replication defective immunodeficiency inducing retroviruses are cytopathic for intestinal epithelium as well as T lymphocytes. Fourth International Conference on AIDS. Swedish Ministry of Health and Social Affairs, Stockholm, Sweden. Abstract #2539, 1988.

103. Rodgers VD, Fassett R, Kagnoff MF: Abnormalities in intestinal mucosal T cells in homosexual populations including those with the lymphadenopathy syndrome and acquired immunodeficiency syndrome. *Gastroenterology* 90:552, 1986.

104. McArthur J: Neurologic manifestations of AIDS. *Medicine* 66:407–437, 1987.

105. Craddock C, Bull R, Pasvol G, et al: Cardiorespiratory arrest and autonomic neuropathy in AIDS. *Lancet* ii:16–18, 1987.

106. Lake-Bakaar G, Quadros E, Beidas S, et al: Gastric secretory failure in patients with the acquired immunodeficiency syndrome (AIDS). *Ann Intern Med* 109:502–504, 1988.

107. Kotler DP, Gaetz HP, Lange M, et al: Enteropathy associated with the acquired immunodeficiency syndrome. *Ann Intern Med* 101:421–428, 1984.

108. Gillin JS, Shike M, Alcock N, et al: Malabsorption and mucosal abnormalities of the small intestine in the acquired immunodeficiency syndrome. *Ann Intern Med* 102:619–622, 1985.

109. Janoff EN, Smith PD, Blaser MJ: Acute antibody responses to *Giardia lamblia* are depressed in patients with AIDS. *J Infect Dis* 157:798–804, 1988.

110. Perlman DMN, Ampel NM, Schifman RB, et al: Persistent *Campylobacter jejuni* infection in patients infected with human immunodeficiency virus (HIV). *Ann Intern Med* 108:540–546, 1988.

111. Perrillo RP, Regenstein FG, Roodman ST: Chronic hepatitis B in asymptomatic homosexual men with antibody to the human immunodeficiency virus. *Ann Intern Med* 105:382–383, 1986.

112. Quinn TC, Corey L, Chafee RG, et al: The etiology of anorectal infections in homosexual men. *Am J Med* 71:395–406, 1981.

113. Quinn TC, Stamm WE, Goodell SE, et al: The polymicrobial origin of intestinal infections in homosexual men. *N Engl J Med* 309:576–582, 1983.

114. Gottlieb MS, Groopman JE, Weinstein WM, et al: The acquired immunodeficiency syndrome. *Ann Intern Med* 99:208–220, 1983.

115. Cone LA, Woodard DR, Potts BE, et al: An update on the acquired immunodeficiency syndrome (AIDS). Associated disorders of the alimentary tract. *Dis Colon Rectum* 29:60–64, 1986.

116. Fauci AS, Macher AM, Longo DL, et al: Acquired immunodeficiency syndrome: epidemiologic, clinical, immunologic, and therapeutic considerations. *Ann Intern Med* 100:92–106, 1984.

117. Soave R, Danner RL, Honig CL, et al: Cryptosporidiosis in homosexual men. *Ann Intern Med* 100:504–511, 1984.

118. Modigliani R, Bories C, LeCharpentier Y, et al: Diarrhea and malabsorption in acquired immune deficiency syndrome: a study of four cases with special emphasis on opportunistic protozoan infections. *Gut* 26:179–187, 1985.

119. Current WL, Reese NC, Ernst JV, et al: Human cryptosporidiosis in immunocompetent and immunodeficient persons: studies of an outbreak and experimental transmission. *N Engl J Med* 308:1252–1257, 1983.

120. Shein R, Gelb A: *Isospora belli* in a patient with acquired immunodeficiency syndrome. *J Clin Gastroenterol* 6:525–528, 1984.

121. Clumeck N, Sonnet J, Taelman H, et al: Acquired immune deficiency syndrome in African patients. *N Engl J Med* 310:492–497, 1984.

122. Pape JW, Liautaud B, Thomas F, et al: The acquired immunodeficiency syndrome in Haiti. *Ann Intern Med* 103:674–678, 1985.

123. Malebranche R, Arnoux E, Grerin JM, et al: Acquired immunodeficiency syndrome with severe gastrointestinal manifestations in Haiti. *Lancet* ii:873–878, 1985.

124. Biggar RJ, Bouvet E, Ebbesen P, et al: Clinical features of AIDS in Europe. *Eur J Cancer Clin Oncol* 20:165–167, 1984.

125. Piot P, Quinn TC, Taelman H, et al: Acquired immunodeficiency syndrome in a heterosexual population in Zaire. *Lancet* ii:65–69, 1984.

126. Van de Perre P, Rouvroy D, Lepage P, et al: Acquired immunodeficiency syndrome in Rwanda. *Lancet* ii:62–65, 1984.

127. Klein RS, Harris CA, Small CB, et al: Oral candidiasis in high-risk patients as the initial manifestation of the acquired immunodeficiency syndrome (AIDS). *N Engl J Med* 311:354–357, 1984.

128. Tavitian A, Raufman JP, Rosenthal LE: Oral candidiasis as a marker for esophageal candidiasis in the acquired immunodeficiency syndrome. *Ann Intern Med* 104:54–55, 1986.

129. Welch K, Finkbeiner W, Alpers CE: Autopsy findings in the acquired immunodeficiency syndrome. *JAMA* 252:1152–1159, 1984.

130. Rotterdam H, Sommers SC: Alimentary tract biopsy lesions in the acquired immune deficiency syndrome. *Pathology* 17:181–192, 1985.

131. Lang DJ, Kummer JF, Hartley DP: Cytomegalovirus in semen: persistence and demonstration in extracellular fluids. *N Engl J Med* 291:121–123, 1974.

132. Knapp AB, Horst DA, Eliopoulos G, et al: Widespread cytomegalovirus gastroenterocolitis in a patient with AIDS. *Gastroenterology* 85:1399–1402, 1983.

133. Gertler SL, Pressman J, Price P, et al: Gastrointestinal cytomegalovirus infection in a homosexual man with severe acquired immunodeficiency syndrome. *Gastroenterology* 85:1403–1406, 1983.

134. Meiselman MS, Cello JP, Margaretten W: Cytomegalovirus colitis: report of the clinical, endoscopic, and pathologic findings in two patients with the acquired immune deficiency syndrome. *Gastroenterology* 88:171–175, 1985.

135. Levinson W, Bennetts RW: Cytomegalovirus colitis in acquired immunodeficiency syndrome—a chronic disease with varying manifestations. *Am J Gastroenterol* 80:445–447, 1985.

136. Frank D, Raicht FF: Intestinal perforation associated with cytomegalovirus infection in patients with acquired immune deficiency syndrome. *Am J Gastroenterology* 70:201–205, 1984.

137. Kram HB, Hino ST, Cohen RE, et al: Spontaneous colonic perforation secondary to cytomegalovirus in a patient with acquired immune deficiency syndrome. *Crit Care Med* 12:469–471, 1984.

138. Kavin H, Jonas RB, Chowdhury L, et al: Acalculous cholecystitis and cytomegalovirus infection in the acquired immunodeficiency syndrome. *Ann Intern Med* 104:53–54, 1986.

139. Margulis SJ, Honig CL, Soave R, et al: Biliary tract obstruction in the acquired immunodeficiency syndrome. *Ann Intern Med* 105:207–210, 1986.

140. Emanuel D, Peppard J, Stover D, et al: Rapid immunodiagnosis of cytomegalovirus pneumonia by bronchoalveolar lavage using human and murine monoclonal antibodies. *Ann Intern Med* 104:476–481, 1986.

141. Chachoua A, Dieterich D, Krasinski K, et al: 9-(1,3-dihydroxy-2-propoxymethyl) guanine (Ganciclovir) in the treatment of cytomegalovirus gastrointestinal disease with the acquired immunodeficiency syndrome. *Ann Intern Med* 107:133–137, 1987.

142. Goodell SE, Quinn TC, Mkrtichian E, et al: Herpes simplex virus proctitis in homosexual men: clinical, sigmoidoscopic and histopathologic features. *N Engl J Med* 308:868–871, 1983.

143. Quinnan GV, Masur H, Rook AH: Herpesvirus infections in the acquired immune deficiency syndrome. *JAMA* 252:72–77, 1984.

144. Mata L, Balunos H, Pizarro D, et al: Cryptosporidiosis in children in some highland Costa Rican rural and urban areas. *Am J Trop Med Hyg* 33:24–29, 1984.

145. Hojlyng N, Molbak K, Jepsen S, et al: Cryptosporidiosis in Siberian children. *Lancet* i:738, 1984.

146. Schultz MG: Emerging zoonoses. *N Engl J Med* 301:1285–1286, 1983.

147. Blumberg RS, Kelsey P, Perrone T, et al: Cytomegalovirus and cryptosporidium associated acalculous gangrenous cholecystitis. *Am J Med* 76:1118–1123, 1984.

148. Pitlik SD, Fainstein V, Rios A, et al: Cryptosporidial cholecystitis. *N Engl J Med* 308:967, 1983.

149. Forgacs P, Tarshis A, Ma P, et al: Intestinal and bronchial cryptosporidiosis in an immunodeficient homosexual man. *Ann Intern Med* 99:793–794, 1983.

150. Ma P, Villaneuva TG, Kaufman D, et al: Respiratory cryptosporidiosis in the acquired immune deficiency syndrome. *JAMA* 252:1298–1301, 1984.

151. Bird RG, Smith MD: Cryptosporidiosis in man: parasite life cycle and fine structural pathology. *Am J Pathol* 132:217–233, 1980.

152. Lefkowitch JH, Krumholz S, Feng-Chen KL, et al: Cryptosporidiosis of the human small intestine: a light and electron microscopic study. *Hum Pathol* 14:746–752, 1984.

153. Centers for Disease Control. Update: treatment of cryptosporidiosis in normal and immunodeficient humans with confirmed infections. *J Clin Microbiol* 18:165–169, 1984.

154. Portnoy D, Whiteside ME, Buckley E, et al: Treatment of intestinal cryptosporidiosis with spiramycin. *Ann Intern Med* 101:202–204, 1984.

155. Cook DJ, Kelton JG, Stanisz AM, et al: Somatostatin treatment for cryptosporidial diarrhea in a patient with the acquired immunodeficiency syndrome (AIDS). *Ann Intern Med* 108:708–709, 1988.

156. Fuessl H, Heinlein H, Goebel FD: The treatment of persistent diarrhea in AIDS with the somatostatin analog SMS-201-995. Fourth International Conference on AIDS. Swedish Ministry of Health and Social Affairs, Stockholm, Sweden. Abstract #7125, 1988.

157. Forthal DN, Guest SS: *Isospora belli* enteritis in three homosexual men. *Am J Trop Med Hyg* 33:1060–1064, 1984.

158. Henderson HE, Gillespie GW, Kaplan P: The human isospora. *Am J Hyg* 78:302–314, 1963.

159. DeHovitz JA, Pape JW, Boncy M, et al: Clinical manifestations and therapy of *Isospora belli* infection in patients with acquired immunodeficiency syndrome. *N Engl J Med* 315:87–90, 1986.

160. Soave R: Cryptosporidiosis and isosporiasis in patients with AIDS. *Infect Dis Clin N Am* 2:485–493, 1988.

161. Dobbins WO, Weinstein WM: Electron microscopy of the intestine and rectum in acquired immunodeficiency syndrome. *Gastroenterology* 88:738–749, 1985.

162. Desportes I, LeCharpentier Y, Galian A, et al: Occurrence of a new microsporidian. *Enterocytozoon bieneusi* n.g., n.sp., in the enterocytes of a human patients with AIDS. *J Protozool* 32:250–254, 1985.

163. Ledford DK, Overman MD, Gonzalvo A, et al: Microsporidiosis myositis in a patient with acquired immunodeficiency syndrome. *Ann Intern Med* 102:628–630, 1985.

164. Terada S, Reddy KR, Jeffers LJ, et al: Microsporidan hepatitis in the acquired immunodeficiency syndrome. *Ann Intern Med* 107:61–62, 1987.

165. Hawkins CC, Gold JWM, Whimbey E, et al: *Mycobacterium avium* complex infections in patients with the acquired immunodeficiency syndrome. *Ann Intern Med* 105:184–188, 1986.

166. Jacobson MA. Mycobacterial diseases. Tuberculosis and *Mycobacterium avium* complex. *Infect Dis Clin North Am* 2:465–474, 1988.

167. Stron RL, Gruminger RP: AIDS with *Mycobacterium avium-intracellulare* lesions resembling those of Whipple's disease. *N Engl J Med* 309:1323, 1983.

168. Gillin JS, Urmacher C, West R, et al: Disseminated *Mycobacterium avium-intracellulare* infection in acquired infection in acquired immunodeficiency syndrome mimicking Whipple's disease. *Gastroenterology* 85:1187–1191, 1983.

169. Bermudez LE, Stevens P, Kalowski P, et al: Treatment of *Mycobacterium avium-complex* (MAC) infection in mice with recombinant human interleukin-2 (IL-2) and tumor necrosis factor (TNF). 27th Interscience Conference on Antimicrobial Agents and Chemotherapy, American Society for Microbiology, New York, 1987. Abstract #47.

170. Bermudez LE, Young LS: Augmented intracellular killing of *Mycobacterium avium* complex (MAC) by antibiotics and tumor necrosis factor (TNF). 27th Interscience Conference on Antimicrobial Agents and Chemotherapy, American Society for Microbiology, New York, 1987. Abstract #54.

171. Pitchenik AE, Cole C, Russel BW, et al: Tuberculosis, atypical mycobacterium, and the acquired immunodeficiency syndrome among Haitian and non-Haitian patients in South Florida. *Ann Intern Med* 101:641–645, 1985.

172. Sunderam G, McDonald RJ, Maniatis T, et al: Tuberculosis as a manifestation of the acquired immunodeficiency syndrome (AIDS). *JAMA* 256:362–366, 1986.

173. Centers for Disease Control. Diagnosis and management of mycobacterial infections and disease in persons with human T-lymphotropic virus type III/lymphadenopathy-associated virus infection. *MMWR* 35:448–453, 1986.

174. Graybill JR: Histoplasmosis and AIDS. *J Infect Dis* 158:623–626, 1988.

175. Johnson PC, Khardori N, Najjar AF, et al: Progressive disseminated histoplasmosis in patients with acquired immunodeficiency syndrome. *Am J Med* 85:152–158, 1988.

176. Cappell MS, Mandell W, Grimes MM, et al: Gastrointestinal histoplasmosis. *Dig Dis Sci* 33:353–360, 1988.

177. Gerskin HC, Fanning MM, Read SE, et al: AIDS in a patient with hemophilia receiving mainly cryoprecipitate. *Can Med Assoc J* 131:45–47, 1984.

178. Haggerty CM, Britton MC, Dorman JM, et al: Gastrointestinal histoplasmosis in the acquired immune deficiency syndrome. *West J Med* 143:244–246, 1985.

179. Smith PD, Macher AM, Bookman MA, et al: *Salmonella typhimurium* enteritis and bacteremia in the acquired immunodeficiency syndrome. *Ann Intern Med* 102:207–209, 1985.

180. Nudelman RB, Mathur-Wagh V, Yancovitz SR, et al: *Salmonella* bacteremia associated with the acquired immunodeficiency syndrome (AIDS). *Arch Intern Med* 145:1968–1971, 1985.

181. Glasser JB, Morton-Kute L, Berger SR, et al: A recurrent *Salmonella typhimurium* bacteremia associated with the acquired immunodeficiency syndrome. *Ann Intern Med* 102:189–193, 1985.

182. Jacobs JL, Gold JWM, Murray HW, et al: *Salmonella* infections in patients with the acquired immunodeficiency syndrome. *Ann Intern Med* 102:186–188, 1985.

183. Friedman S, Wright T, Altman D: Kaposi's sarcoma and the gastrointestinal tract: the San Francisco experience. *Gastroenterology* 84:1160, 1983.

184. Lozada F, Silverman S, Migliioratti CA, et al: Oral manifestations of tumors and opportunistic infection in AIDS: findings in 53 homosexual men with Kaposi's sarcoma. *Oral Surg* 56:491–494, 1983.

185. Mitsuyasu RT. Kaposi's sarcoma in the acquired immunodeficiency syndrome. *Infect Dis Clin N Am* 2:511–523, 1988.

186. Knowles DM, Chamulak GA, Subar M, et al: Lymphoid neoplasia associated with the acquired immunodeficiency syndrome (AIDS). *Ann Intern Med* 108:744–753, 1988.

187. Ioachim HL, Cooper MC, Hellman GC: Lymphomas in men at high risk for acquired immune deficiency syndrome (AIDS): a study of 21 cases. *Cancer* 56:2831–2842, 1985.

188. Greenspan JS, Greenspan D, Lennette ET, et al: Replication of Epstein-Barr virus within the epithelial cells of oral "hairy" leukoplakia, an AIDS-associated lesion. *N Engl J Med* 313:1564, 1985.

189. Eversole LR, Jacobsen P, Stone CE, et al: Oral condyloma planus (hairy leukoplakia) among homosexual men: a clinicopathologic study of thirty-six cases. *Oral Surg* 61:249, 1986.

190. Greenspan D, Greenspan JS, Conant M, et al: Oral "hairy" leukoplakia in male homosexuals: evidence of association with both papillomavirus and a herpes group virus. *Lancet* ii:831–834, 1984.

191. Friedman-Kien AE: Viral origin of hairy leukoplakia. *Lancet* 2:694, 1986.

192. Daling JR, Weiss NS, Klopfenstein LL, et al: Correlates of homosexual behavior and the incidence of anal cancer. *JAMA* 247:1988–1990, 1982.

193. Daling JR, Weiss NS, Hislop G, et al: Sexual practices, sexually transmitted diseases, and the incidence of anal cancer. *N Engl J Med* 317:973–977, 1987.

CHAPTER 19

Parasitic Infections

PHILLIP D. SMITH

INTRODUCTION

Parasitic infections are a major cause of intestinal disease in persons throughout the world. Though common in developing nations, they also are an important health problem in developed countries. In contrast to viral and bacterial intestinal infections, which cause primarily diarrhea (see Chapters 20, 21), parasitic pathogens cause a wide spectrum of potentially debilitating symptoms as well as malabsorption. The severity and duration of these manifestations are determined by complex interactions between parasite factors such as virulence and antigenic variation, host immune and nonimmune defense mechanisms, and environmental factors such as intensity of exposure.[1]

Facilitated by rapid advances in the basic sciences, culture technology, and molecular biology, the intimate relationship between the host and enteric parasites has become the subject of intense investigation. Among the enteric parasites receiving the most attention are *Giardia lamblia, Cryptosporidium,* and *Entamoeba histolytica.* These protozoan parasites are the most frequently identified intestinal parasites in the United States. New information regarding their immunobiology addresses important aspects of how the gastrointestinal tract interacts with parasites. For example, the ability of the mucosal parasites *G. lamblia* and *Cryptosporidium* to even elicit an immune response has been appreciated only recently. New evidence also indicates that *G. lamblia* may undergo antigenic variation and that this variation may relate to virulence. Recently, virulence factors were identified in various pathogenic strains of *E. histolytica.* This new information provides the basis for evolving concepts of the immunopathology of *G. lamblia, Cryptosporidium,* and *E. histolytica* and is the subject of this chapter.

GIARDIA LAMBLIA

Giardia lamblia gained wide attention as a potential pathogen of humans in the late 1960s following its identification as the cause of an outbreak of diarrheal illness in Colorado.[2] By 1976, it was the most frequently identified intestinal parasite in the United States,[3] and an unusually high occurrence of water-borne epidemics of giardiasis implicated contaminated drinking water in its transmission.[4] Person-to-person transmission, notably among family members of infants in day-care centers,[5] homosexuals,[6] and residents of mental institutions,[7] indicated that *Giardia* also could be passed by the fecal-oral route. Fecal-oral transmission likely plays an important role in the high prevalence rates in less developed regions of the world.[8,9]

Giardia lamblia is a unicellular protozoan that exists in two stages, the dormant cyst, which, by virtue of its ability to survive in the environment, transmits infection, and the flagellated trophozoite, which causes disease. Normal physiologic conditions within the proximal small intestine including acidity, oxidation-reduction potential, temperature, and carbon dioxide content appear to facilitate excystation after the cyst passes from the stomach into the small intestine where colonization occurs. That the proximal small intestine is a particularly suitable environment for colonization is supported by evidence that bile and biliary lipids promote trophozoite growth in vitro,[10,11] possibly through enhanced membrane lipid (lecithin) uptake.[12] In addition, luminal proteases in the proximal small intestine activate a lectin in *G. lamblia* that is most specific for mannose-6-phosphate,[13] suggesting a novel host-parasite interaction that could facilitate the adherence of trophozoites to the glycosylated microvillous surface of intestinal mucosa. Encystation, the process by which trophozoites become cysts, is poorly understood. However, the ability of high concentrations of bile to induce cyst formation in vitro[14,15] suggests a possible role for bile in this process. During periods of rapid transit of intestinal contents, trophozoites may be excreted, but, unlike cysts, they do not survive in the external environment.

The majority of persons infected with *G. lamblia* are asymptomatic. In developed countries, these individuals include residents of endemic areas,[2,16] homosexual men,[17] and infants in day-care centers.[18] In developing countries, where recurrent exposure is common, persons infected with the parasite also are usually asymptomatic.[19,20] In contrast, persons exposed to *G. lamblia* for the first time or intermittently are more susceptible to symptomatic infection. Such persons include travelers or visitors to endemic regions[21] and persons exposed during water-borne outbreaks.[16,22]

The variability in the clinical manifestation of infection in different populations and among persons exposed to the same isolate may be explained, in part, by the biology of the host-parasite relationship. Nonimmunologic factors may contribute to this variability. As mentioned above, bile and luminal enzymes, which may vary in content among different persons, facilitate trophozoite growth and attachment in vitro. Bile salts also activate lipase, an enzyme that promotes lipolysis of milk lipids, resulting in the release of free fatty acids which have potent giardicidal activity.[23,24] Recent evidence also indicates that *G. lamblia* trophozoites are susceptible to complement lysis.[25] However, the absence of complement on mucosal surfaces suggests that this cytotoxic mechanism may be more important in limiting tissue invasion. Although an earlier study reported the presence of free bile acids in the intestinal lumens of patients with giardiasis and suggested this was the mechanism of *Giardia*-induced steatorrhea,[26] we have shown that the parasite does not deconjugate bile acids.[27] We also have shown that four isolates obtained from persons from several different regions of the world do not secrete a known enterotoxin.[28] However, one of these isolates stimulated the release of prostaglandin E_2 (PGE_2) by macrophages,[29] and other investigators have found increased levels of PGE_2 in the intestinal lumen of mice infected with *Giardia muris*,[30] potentially important findings since prostaglandins may contribute to the pathophysiology of secretory diarrhea. *Giardia lamblia* also may induce mucosal changes ranging from epithelial alterations detectable only at the ultrastructural level[31,32] to intense inflammatory cell infiltration with complete villous atrophy.[33] These changes may affect enterocyte absorptive and secretory function. Indeed, the severity of histologic changes and parasite load correlate with the degree of diarrhea and/or malabsorption in some patients.[34] However, the presence of minimal or absent mucosal changes in many patients with giardiasis implicates additional mechanisms in host susceptibility to symptomatic infection.

The different clinical responses to infection with *G. lamblia* could also be due, in part, to differences in pathogenicity of the parasite. A recent study in which five of ten subjects inoculated with one isolate of *G. lamblia* and none of five inoculated with another isolate developed symptomatic giardiasis underscores the potential role of strain differences in the clinical manifestation of giardiasis.[35] That these differences reflect variation in the parasite's antigenic components is currently under investigation. In the initial characterization of the antigenic components of *G. lamblia*, we identified qualitative and quantitative differences in the protein antigens among strains of *Giardia* from Afghanistan, Oregon, Ecuador, and Puerto Rico.[36] We also have identified a high molecular weight, membrane-derived component, likely a carbohydrate-free proteolipid "excretory-secretory" product, as a potentially important antigen in some isolates.[37] Other surface glycoprotein and cytoskeletal (tubulin) polypeptide antigens are common among *Giardia* isolates.[38,39] However, the dominant antigens recognized by antibodies in human serum appear to be the 31 kD and 30–33 kD surface components, likely corresponding to surface proteins.[40] Analysis of DNA banding patterns following endonuclease restriction indicates the presence of differences in nucleotide sequences among other isolates.[41] The differences in these DNA profiles correlate, to some extent, with the variation in trophozoite surface antigens.[42] Recently, a cysteine-rich 170 kD surface antigen in cloned WB strain trophozoites was shown to undergo changes spontaneously and following selection with monoclonal antibody.[43] This important observation suggests the possibility that antigenic variation occurs in vivo. If new antigens correlate with pathogenicity, they could contribute to the variable clinical response observed among persons exposed to the same isolate. In addition, antigenic variation could provide a mechanism by which trophozoites evade host defense mechanisms in chronically infected persons with an active immune response.[28]

The host immune response likely contributes to the variation in the clinical response to *G. lamblia*. Mucosal changes in the proximal small intestine, the segment colonized by *Giardia*, indicate that in some persons the parasite elicits an inflammatory cell response. These changes, albeit of varying degree, include accumulation of polymorphonuclear leukocytes in the lamina propria, development of shortened villi, loss of the brush border, damage to epithelial cells, and an increase in epithelial cell mitosis and turnover.[44,45] Total villous atrophy, epithelial cell flattening, and dense mononuclear cell infiltration may occur infrequently.[33] The accumulation of inflammatory cells in the mucosa of the small intestine of infected persons suggests participation by these cells in the host immune response to *Giardia.*

The epidemiologic observations that persons repeatedly exposed to *G. lamblia* are more frequently asymptomatic or uninfected than persons episodically exposed suggests that recurrent exposure elicits an immune response that confers at least partial protection. Studies in an animal model of giardiasis have implicated T lymphocytes in this response. Following inoculation of *G. muris* into athymic mice, which are deficient in both circulating T lymphocytes and Peyer's patch T-helper cells, the mice develop chronic giardiasis,[46,47] whereas immunocompetent mice clear the parasite and may even exhibit resistance to reinfection.[48] In chronically infected athymic mice, thymus implantation or reconstitution with syngeneic lymphoid cells from thymus-intact mice causes a progressive reduction in the number of *Giardia,* and this reduction is accelerated further when the reconstituted lymphocytes are from thymus-intact mice previously infected with *Giardia.*[47] In normal mice, infection with *G. muris* is associated with an increase in Peyer's patch lymphocytes, and depletion of T-helper cells leads to chronic infection.[49,50] In uninfected mice, Peyer's patch T cells have been shown to regulate the switch from IgM- to IgA-bearing B cells.[51] Since *G. muris* can induce both a shift in the percentage of Peyer's patch B cells bearing IgA[52] and secretion of antitrophozoite antibodies into the intestinal lumen,[53,54] it is intriguing to speculate that T-helper cells contribute to the clearance of infection by facilitating secretion of parasite-specific antibody.

Since lymphocyte responses require the presentation of antigens by accessory cells, it is reasonable to assume that the host response to *Giardia* involves interaction between the parasite and macrophages. Indeed, macrophages from the mouse, rabbit, and human are capable of phagocytosing *Giardia* trophozoites.[29,55,56] *Giardia* invasion of the mucosa, reported in at least three studies,[32,57,58] and the presence of macrophages in the lamina propria would allow contact between the parasite and antigen-presenting cells. Besides antigen presentation, effector cell function by monocytes-macrophages contributes to host defense mechanisms against many pathogens. In this regard, four reports indicate that human monocytes can kill *G. lamblia,*[59-62] possibly by the production of reactive oxygen intermediates.[61] Although one report has not confirmed these findings,[63] the ability of resident monocytes or monocytes trafficking through the lamina propria to kill *Giardia* could provide a potentially important mechanism for protection against invading trophozoites.

The clinical observations of an increased prevalence of *G. lamblia* in persons with immunoglobulin deficiencies[64-67] underscores the potential importance of antibody in the host's response to this parasite. The presence of circulating antibodies to *Giardia* was first suggested in 1976.[68] Subsequently, we identified the presence of antitrophozoite IgG antibodies, which appeared to be directed to the trophozoite surface, in a high proportion of symptomatic patients.[69,70] Antitrophozoite antibodies of all three major isotypes now have been detected in infected patients. Recently, we showed that patients with AIDS and reduced levels of antitrophozoite antibodies frequently have symptomatic giardiasis, whereas AIDS patients with parasite-specific antibody often have symptoms unrelated to *G.*

lamblia,[71] again suggesting that antibody to *Giardia* may participate in protection. In this regard, in vitro studies have shown that immune serum, purified IgG from immune serum, and IgG antitrophozoite antibodies augment macrophage and neutrophil adherence and/or phagocytosis of *Giardia*.[54,72] Although patients with selective IgA deficiency do not have a higher incidence of giardiasis, IgA antibodies could participate in protection. The presence of secretory IgA antiparasite antibodies in breast milk,[73] particularly when the lactating mother is infected with *Giardia*,[74] may contribute to the apparently lower rate of infection in breast-fed, in contrast to formula-fed, infants in highly endemic regions.[19] We have found that circulating IgA is the most common isotope in persons with acute symptomatic giardiasis.[71,75] Although IgA can participate in antibody-dependent cellular cytotoxic mechanisms, the role that IgA plays in protection is complicated by the fact that serum IgA does not contribute to intestinal IgA.

In summary, the above studies suggest a highly integrated and usually effective system of host defense against *G. lamblia*. Following excystation in the proximal small intestine, trophozoites encounter bile and certain proteases that promote trophozoite growth and attachment. In the event of colonization, nonspecific defense mechanisms such as macrophage effector activity prevent tissue penetration. If the parasite persists, parasite-specific antibodies are elicited, which, acting in concert with cells and possibly complement, provide a second line of protection. However, trophozoites undergoing antigenic variation may evade these mechanisms, survive, and induce disease.

CRYPTOSPORIDIUM

Recent studies of the epidemiology, pathology, and immunology of cryptosporidiosis have expanded traditional concepts of this protozoan parasite. *Cryptosporidium* is a small (2–6 μm) unicellular coccidian that infects the intestinal tract of a variety of animals, birds, reptiles, and fish.[76] The first identification of *Cryptosporidium* in humans was in two persons with farm animal exposure.[77,78] Cryptosporidiosis subsequently gained wide attention as a zoonotic infection transmitted to humans by domesticated farm animals.[79,80] Indeed, a high incidence of symptomatic and, less frequently, asymptomatic cryptosporidiosis occurs among otherwise healthy persons who handle animals, particularly calves. Exposure to fecal material from these reservoir hosts is presumed to be the route of transmission.

Cryptosporidium subsequently was recognized as an important enteric infection in immunocompromised persons, particularly persons with AIDS.[81-83] In the United States, 3–15% of AIDS patients with diarrhea have cryptosporidiosis,[83-85] whereas in Haiti and Africa 50% of symptomatic AIDS patients have the infection.[85] In patients with AIDS, cryptosporidiosis is usually characterized by protracted, often voluminous, watery diarrhea that may be accompanied by abdominal pain, anorexia, weight loss, and occasionally vomiting. Malabsorption may accompany these symptoms. Although spontaneous resolution and the absence of intestinal symptoms may occassionally occur in persons with AIDS,[86,87] the unusually high frequency and marked virulence of *Cryptosporidium* infections in these patients led to the notion that the parasite was an opportunistic pathogen. The marked severity of cryptosporidiosis in AIDS patients is in contrast to that of giardiasis and amebiasis, which are no more severe than in immunocompetent persons.

Recent clinical and epidemiologic studies confirm that in addition to infecting animal handlers and immunocompromised persons, *Cryptosporidium* is an important enteric pathogen in immunocompetent persons throughout the world.[88-91] The parasite is identified frequently in residents of developing countries (3–13%) and in persons in developed countries (0.6–7%).[91] Children are more commonly infected than adults.[92] In contrast to the more virulent form of infection that many AIDS patients experience, cryptosporidiosis in immunocompetent persons is characterized by a self-limited diarrheal illness usually lasting 1–2 weeks.[80,93,94] Symptoms include watery diarrhea in the majority of cases and less often cramping, abdominal pain, low-grade fever, malaise, and weight loss. Infection may be accompanied by *G. lamblia* or other intestinal pathogens.[95] Cryptosporidiosis in the immunocompetent host resolves spontaneously. Water is likely the most common vehicle of transmission worldwide. One large water-borne outbreak of cryptosporidiosis has been documented,[96] and water contamination has been reported in certain regions of the United States.[97] Contaminated drinking water also has been implicated in the cryptosporidiosis acquired by travelers.[98] Person-to-person transmission has been documented among children in day-care centers,[99] family members,[100] and hospital and laboratory personnel[101,102] and likely contributes to the high prevalence rate among homosexual men with AIDS. Thus cryptosporidiosis can be acquired by zoonotic transmission as well as contaminated water and person-to-person contact.

Previously thought to be an extracellular intestinal parasite, electron microscopy has now confirmed the *Cryptosporidia* attach to the mucosa in extracytoplasmic vacuoles just below the epithelial membrane of enterocytes.[103] Thus they are not extracellular organisms, but they also are not fully intracellular. The parasite has been identified in the epithelium of the esophagus, stomach, and entire intestinal tract. In immunocompromised persons, *Cryptosporidium* can occasionally disseminate to the biliary tree, pancreas, and respiratory tract. Resembling the histologic changes associated with infection by *Giardia*, *Cryptosporidium* in immunodeficient persons can induce mild-to-moderate mononuclear cell accumulation and less frequently acute inflammatory cell infiltration, lengthened crypts, and villous atrophy.[103] Incomplete information is available on the histopathology of cryptosporidiosis in immunocompetent persons.

The voluminous loss of fluid associated with the diarrhea of cryptosporidiosis suggests a secretory mechanism.[81] Characterization of this mechanism has eluded investigators. Similarly, the mechanism of the malabsorption of fat and carbohydrates that frequently accompanies infection remains unknown. Although villous atrophy offers one explanation, the presence of malabsorption in patients without a significant loss of surface area suggests the presence of more complex mechanisms. In contrast to *G. lamblia* and *E. histolytica*, which can be cultured in vitro, the lack of a suitable method for culturing *Cryptosporidium* has limited investigation in this area.

The epidemiology of cryptosporidiosis provides important clues into the nature of the defense mechanisms that protect the host against *Cryptosporidium*. The chronicity and increased severity of infection in persons with deficiencies in cellular responses (malignancy, steroid therapy, chemotherapy), humoral responses (hypogammablobulinemia), and both cellular and humoral immunity (AIDS, severe combined immunodeficiency) suggests that humoral and cellular immune mechanisms are involved in host defense. Although limited by the lack of both an animal model and the availability of a source of pure antigen, the contribution of humoral immunity to host defense is currently under investigation. Recent studies indicate that both immunocompetent and certain immunosuppressed persons develop IgG and IgM antibody responses to the parasite, suggesting that antibody does not provide protection.[104,105] However, the increased incidence of severe cryptosporidiosis in persons with hypogammaglobulinemia suggests that antibody at least contributes to protection. The role of cellular responses to *Cryptosporidium* has not been examined. Nevertheless, the studies noted above implicate both cellular and humoral responses in host protection against *Cryptosporidium*.

ENTAMOEBA HISTOLYTICA

Many aspects of the epidemiology of *E. histolytica* are strikingly similar to those of *G. lamblia. Entamoeba histolytica* is estimated to infect 10% of the world's population[106] and 4% of the persons residing in the United States.[107] Infection is more common among certain groups of exposed persons such as residents of developing countries,[108] male homosexuals,[109] residents of mental institutions,[110] and persons from lower socioeconomic settings.[111] The likely reservoir of the parasite is infected humans and not animals. In contrast to giardiasis, the rate of infection with *E. histolytica* increases with age.[112] This suggests that repeated exposure may not provide protection.

Similar to those infected with *G. lamblia,* the majority of persons infected with *E. histolytica* are asymptomatic. When symptoms occur, the gastrointestinal tract is the usual site of disease. Residing in the colon, organisms may induce symptoms ranging from mild diarrhea to severe dysentery characterized by fever, abdominal pain, vomiting, and bloody diarrhea. Children in endemic regions,[113] persons receiving corticosteroid therapy,[114] pregnant and postpartum women,[115] and possibly malnourished persons[116] are more susceptible to invasive intestinal amebiasis. Intestinal amebiasis infrequently may progress to acute toxic megacolon, perforation, and peritonitis. The most common extraintestinal manifestation of infection is liver abscess. This condition is characterized clinically by right upper quadrant abdominal pain; signs of an acute inflammatory process including fever, chills, and leukocytosis; frequent extension across the diaphragm to the lung; and normal transaminase but increased alkaline phosphatase levels. Less frequently, perianal or genital skin involvement and infection at distant sites such as the brain may occur. Local extension of intestinal or hepatic foci may result in cutaneous fistulas. Among South African patients admitted to a university hospital with invasive amebiasis, 60% had intestinal disease, whereas 40% had liver abscess.[117,118] In sharp contrast to the relatively benign clinical course of infection with *G. lamblia* and *Cryptosporidium* in immunocompetent persons, invasive amebiasis in persons in developing countries is associated with mortality rates of 2–13% in modern hospitals and up to 72% in less well-equipped facilities.[119]

Population studies suggest that recurrent exposure to some enteric parasites such as *G. lamblia* protects the host from symptomatic infection. However, the age-specific incidence rates for amebiasis indicate that childhood exposure is not protective. Both recurrent intestinal and hepatic amebiasis occur, although infrequently.[120,121] However, one epidemiologic study has suggested that the incidence of recurrent amebic liver abscess is lower than the expected rate,[122] raising the possibility that invasive hepatic disease may be partially protective against recurrent amebic liver abscess.

The extremely low frequency of invasive amebiasis among some commonly infected populations such as male homosexuals, in contrast to the high incidence of invasive disease among residents of developing countries, indicates that parasite virulence may vary among isolates from different geographic locations. Indeed, the different electrophoretic patterns of four enzymes (zymodemes) of *E. histolytica* isolated from persons with asymptomatic cyst passage versus persons with invasive disease suggests the presence of pathogenic and nonpathogenic strains.[123] As of 1985, 22 distinct zymodemes, 9 of which were from tissue invasive organisms, had been identified in isolates from Mexico, India, and South Africa. Pathogenic organisms were more commonly isolated from men, consistent with the clinical observations of a higher incidence of invasive disease among men. Infrequently, asymptomatic carriers may harbor a pathogenic zymodeme. These persons are 100% seropositive, similar to the seropositivity rate among patients with invasive pathogenic strains. In contrast, only 21% of carriers with a nonpathogenic isolate are seropositive. That pathogenic isolates are more capable of eliciting an antibody response, even in the absence of symptoms, is consistent with tissue penetration by these isolates and consequently the greater likelihood of contact with immune response cells.

The presence of intestinal bacteria may contribute to the virulence of some isolates.[124] This was first suggested by studies in germ-free guinea pigs, which showed that *E. histolytica* did not cause intestinal disease unless bacteria were present.[125] In experimental amebiasis in cats, the incubation period can be shortened and mortality increased by the addition of bacteria. Ameba that loose their virulence through in vitro cultivation may regain it following the addition of certain species of enteric bacteria. The ability of certain bacteria to facilitate amebic adherence, lower the colonic oxidation-reduction potential to a level optimal for amebic growth, or act as a reducing source for amebic metabolic activity may contribute to colonization. Unfortunately, the absence of a reproducible animal model of amebiasis has limited the interpretation of these otherwise intriguing studies.

The ability of *E. histolytica* to adhere to the mucosal surface may play a particularly important role in colonization and possibly mucosal invasion. Two adhesion molecules, or lectins, one inhibited by GalNAc or galactose residues[126] and the other inhibited by GlcNAc polymers,[127] have been identified in in vitro studies as contributing to adherence of ameba to certain target cells. The ability of HM1-IMSS strain amebas to adhere to Chinese hamster ovary cells or neutrophils is more easily inhibited by GalNAc monomers than three less virulent strains (H-303-NIH, H-200-NIH, Larado), indicating a correlation between the presence of GlcNAc-inhibitable adhesins and in vitro virulence among different strains.

Following adherence, ameba can induce cell and tissue destruction. Ameba-induced cytolysis, whether in the intestinal mucosa or liver, is likely multifactorial. The contribution of proteolytic enzymes to cytolysis would require direct contact between the parasite and host cells, because the activity of these enzymes is inhibited by serum. Since many of the enzymes are produced by pathogenic as well as nonpathogenic strains, their role in tissue destruction in vivo is unclear.[128] In addition to enzymes, ameba have been suspected of producing an enterotoxin capable of stimulating secretion by mucosal epithelial cells. In this regard, a non-cytolethal enterotoxin with activity in the rabbit ileal loop has been described,[129] but whether ameba produce an enterotoxin that contributes to human disease is unknown. Recently, one potentially important mechanism of cytolytic action was shown to involve direct cell contact.[130,131] Following contact, a pH-, calcium-, phospholipase A-dependent event may occur causing the release of a pore-forming protein that has lethal consequences for the target cell.[132,133] The role that these cytolytic mechanisms play in the tissue destruction of intestinal and hepatic amebiasis is currently under investigation.

The initial interaction between the host and *E. histolytica* occurs at the level of the intestinal mucosa. In the majority of cases, the parasite does not invade the mucosa but lives as a commensal, reflecting reduced parasite virulence and/or effective host defense. Humoral and cellular immune responses may contribute to this defense. Regarding the humoral responses, the vast majority of patients with invasive intestinal or hepatic disease have circulating IgG antibodies to *E. histolytica*. Although up to 66% of these patients may become seronegative within 6 months, parasite-specific antibodies have been detected 20 years after infection.[134] The presence of IgM antiparasite antibodies indicates active disease.[135] However, the severity of infection does not correlate with the level of antibody response, and invasive amebiasis has been documented in the presence of high titers of antiparasite antibodies. Moreover, the ability of trophozoites to evade the potentially lethal effects of parasite antibodies may be due to membrane redistribution (capping) and spontaneous release of the evaginated caps that contain the surface-bound anti-trophozoite antibody.[136] Thus, although antiparasite antibodies alone do not appear to be protective, they may act with cells or complement to limit infection. A potential role for complement in the host response to *E. histolytica* is suggested by evidence that trophozoites can be lysed by activating both the classical and alternative complement pathways with either immune or nonimmune serum.[137,138] A decrease in C3 and normal C1 levels has been noted in some patients with amebic liver abscess,[139] and amebic virulence as determined by isoenzyme pattern has been shown to correlate with complement resistance.[140] However, the significance of these observations is tempered by the absence of detectable levels of complement on the intestinal mucosa.

Polymorphonuclear neutrophils are frequently identified in the inflammatory reaction that accompanies mucosal ulceration in invasive intestinal amebiasis. In addressing the interaction between human neutrophils and *E. histolytica*, investigators have shown that virulent ameba are capable of lysing neutrophils, whereas less virulent ameba are killed by the neutrophils.[141] This ability to destroy inflammatory cells may contribute to the mucosal invasion by virulent ameba. In addition to killing neutrophils, virulent ameba are capable of killing human monocytes and T lymphocytes.[142] However, following activation with lymphokines, macrophages exhibit contact-dependent, partly oxidative cytotoxic activity for *E. histolytica* trophozoites. Similar to their role in limiting hepatic and metastatic amebiasis in the hamster,[143] activated human macrophages may contribute to limiting tissue invasion by ameba. In addition, lymphocytes obtained from patients after cure for amebic liver abscess can be stimulated with soluble amebic proteins to proliferate and secrete lymphokines that enhance macrophage ameobicidal activity.[144] Moreover, this same soluble amebic protein preparation can stimulate killing by cytotoxic lymphocytes from patients who have recovered from amebic liver abscess. These important observations underscore the potential role that mononuclear cells may play in host defense against this invasive protozoan parasite.

Thus, during the past several years, our concepts of how the host responds to enteric parasites have evolved considerably. As illustrated by one or more of the protozoan organisms described here, parasite factors along with certain physiologic conditions within intestinal lumen facilitate parasite adherence and penetration. Balanced against these factors are nonimmune and immune host defense mechanisms, which serve to limit colonization and promote parasite clearance.

REFERENCES

1. Janoff EN, Smith PD: Perspectives on gastrointestinal infections in AIDS. *Gastroenterol Clin N Am* 17:451–463, 1988.
2. Moore GT, Cross WM, McGuire D, et al: Epidemic giardiasis at a ski resort. *N Engl J Med* 281:402–407, 1969.
3. Centers for Disease Control. Intestinal surveillance—United States 1976. *MMWR* 27:167, 1978.
4. Centers for Disease Control. Waterborne giardiasis—California, Colorado, Oregon, Pennsylvania. *MMWR* 29:121–123, 1980.
5. Polis MA, Tuazon CU, Alling DW, et al: Transmission of *Giardia lamblia* from a day care center to the community. *Am J Public Health* 76:1142–1144, 1986.
6. Schemerin MJ, Jones TC, Klein H: Giardiasis: association with homosexuality. *Ann Intern Med* 88:801–804, 1978.
7. Yoeli M, Most H, Hammond J, et al: Parasitic infections in a closed community: results of a 10-year survey in Willowbrook State School. *Trans R Soc Trop Hyg* 66:764–776, 1972.
8. Hossain MM, Ljungstrom I, Glass RI, et al: Amoebiasis and giardiasis in Bangladesh: parasitological and serological studies. *Trans R Soc Trop Med Hyg* 77:552–554, 1983.
9. Goldsmid JM: Intestinal parasitic infections of man in Tasmania. *Trans R Soc Trop Med Hyg* 75:110–112, 1981.
10. Farthing MJG, Varon SR, Keusch GT: Mammalian bile promotes growth of *Giardia lamblia* in axenic culture. *Trans R Soc Trop Med Hyg* 77:467–469, 1983.
11. Gillin FD, Gault MJ, Hofmann AF, et al: Biliary lipids support serum-free growth of *Giardia lamblia*. *Infect Immun* 53:641–645, 1986.
12. Farthing MJG, Keusch GT, Carey MC: Effects of bile and bile salts on growth and membrane lipid uptake by *Giardia lamblia*. Possible implications for pathogenesis of intestinal disease. *J Clin Invest* 76:1727–1732, 1985.
13. Lev B, Ward H, Keusch GT, et al: Lectin activation in *Giardia lamblia* by host protease. A novel host-parasite interaction. *Science* 232:71–73, 1986.
14. Gillin FD, Reiner DS, Gault MJ, et al: Encystation and expression of cyst antigens by *Giardia lambia* in vitro. *Science* 235:1040–1043, 1987.
15. Schupp DG, Januschka MM, Sherlock LAF, et al: Production of viable giardia cysts *in vitro:* determination by fluorogenic dye staining, excystation, and animal infectivity in the mouse and Mongolian gerbil. *Gastroenterology* 95:1–10, 1988.
16. Istre GR, Dunlop TS, Gaspard B, et al: Waterborne giardiasis at a mountain resort: evidence for acquired immunity. *Am J Public Health* 74:602–604, 1984.

17. Phillips SC, Mildvan D, Williams DC, et al: Sexual transmission of enteric protozoa and helminths in a venereal-disease clinic population. *N Engl J Med* 305:603–606, 1981.

18. Pickering LK, Woodward WE, DuPont HL: Occurrence of *Giardia lamblia* in children in day-care centers. *J Pediatr* 104:522–526, 1948.

19. Islam A, Stoll BJ, Ljungstrom I, et al: *Giardia lamblia* infections in a cohort of Bangladeshi mothers and infants followed for one year. *J Pediatr* 102:996–1000, 1983.

20. Gilman RH, Miranda E, Marquis GS, et al: Rapid reinfection by *Giardia lamblia* after treatment in a hyperendemic third world community. *Lancet* 1:343–345, 1988.

21. Steffen R, Rickenbach M, Wilhelm V, et al: Health problems after travel to developing countries. *J Infect Dis* 156:84–91, 1987.

22. Lopez CE, Dykes AC, Juranek DD, et al: Waterborne giardiasis: a community-wide outbreak of disease and high rate of asymptomatic infection. *Am J Epidemiol* 112:495–497, 1980.

23. Gillin FD, Reiner DS: Human milk kills parasitic intestinal protozoa. *Science* 221:1290–1291, 1983.

24. Hernell O, Ward H, Blackberg L, et al: Killing of *Giardia lamblia* by human milk lipase: an effect mediated by lipolysis of milk lipids. *J Infect Dis* 153:715–720, 1986.

25. Deguchi M, Gillin FD, Gigli I: Mechanism of killing of *Giardia lamblia* trophozoites by complement. *J Clin Invest* 79:1296–1302, 1987.

26. Tandon BN, Tandon RK, Satpathy BK, et al: Mechanisms of malabsorption in giardiasis: a study of bacterial flora and bile salt deconjugation in upper jejunum. *Gut* 18:176–181, 1977.

27. Smith PD, Horsburgh CR, Brown WR: In vitro studies on bile acid deconjugation and lipolysis inhibition by *Giardia lamblia*. *Dig Dis Sci* 26:700–704, 1981.

28. Smith PD, Gillin FD, Spria WW, et al: Chronic giardiasis: studies on drug sensitivity, toxin production and host immune response. *Gastroenterology* 59:790–800, 1982.

29. Smith PD: Pathophysiology and immunology of giardiasis. *Annu Rev Med* 36:295–307, 1985.

30. Ganguly NK, Garg SK, Vasudev V, et al: Prostaglandins E and F levels in mice infected with *Giardia lamblia*. *Indian J Med Res* 79:755–759, 1984.

31. Takano J, Yardley JH: Jejunal lesions in patients with giardiasis and malabsorption. An electron microscopy study. *Bull Johns Hopkins Hosp* 116:413–469, 1964.

32. Morecke R, Parker JP: Ultrastructural studies of the human *Giardia lamblia* and subjacent mucosa in a subject with steatorrhea. *Gastroenterology* 52:151–164, 1967.

33. Levinson JD, Nastro LJ: Giardiasis with total villous atrophy. *Gastroenterology* 74:271–275, 1978.

34. Duncombe VM, Bolin TD, Davis AE, et al: Histopathology in giardiasis: a correlation with diarrhea. *Aust NZ J Med* 8:392–396, 1978.

35. Nash TE, Herrignton DA, Losonsky GA, et al: Experimental infections with *Giardia lamblia*. *J Infect Dis* 156:974–984, 1987.

36. Smith PD, Gillin FD, Kaushal NA, et al: Antigenic analysis of *Giardia lamblia* from Afghanistan, Puerto Rico, Ecuador and Oregon. *Infect Immun* 36:71–719, 1982.

37. Nash TE, Gillin FD, Smith PD: Excretory-secretory products of *Giardia lamblia*. *J Immunol* 131:2004–2010, 1983.

38. Einfeld DA, Stibbes HH: Identification and characterization of a major surface antigen of *Giardia lamblia*. *Infect Immun* 46:377–383, 1984.

39. Tarian BE, Barnes RC, Stephens RS, et al: Tubulin and high molecular weight polypeptides as *Giardia lamblia* antigens. *Infect Immun* 46:152–158, 1984.

40. Taylor GD, Wenman WM: Human immune response to *Giardia lamblia*. *J Infect Dis* 155:137–140, 1987.

41. Nash TE, McCutchan T, Keister D, et al: Restriction-endonuclease analysis of DNA from 15 *Giardia* isolates obtained from humans and animals. *J Infect Dis* 172:64–73, 1985.

42. Nash TE, Keister DB: Differences in excretory-secretory products and surface antigens among 19 isolates of *Giardia*. *J Infect Dis* 172:1166–1171, 1985.

43. Adam RD, Aggurwal A, Lal AA, et al: Antigenic variation of a cysteine-rich protein in *Giardia lamblia*. *J Exp Med* 167:109–118, 1988.

44. Wright SG, Tomkins AM: Quantitative histology in giardiasis. *J Clin Pathol* 31:712–716, 1978.

45. Gillon J, Thamery AL, Ferguson A: Features of small intestinal pathology (epithelial cell kinetics, intraepithelial lymphocytes, disaccharidasis) in primary *Giardia muris* infection. *Gut* 23:498–506, 1982.

46. Stevens DA, Frank DP, Mahmoud, AAF: Thymus dependency of host resistance to *Giardia muris* infection: studies in nude mice. *J Immunol* 120:680–682, 1978.

47. Roberts-Thompson IC, Mitchell GF: Giardiasis in mice. I. Prolonged infection in certain mouse strains and hypothymic (nude) mice. *Gastroenterology* 75:42–46, 1978.

48. Roberts-Thompson IC, Stevens DP, Mahmoud AAF, et al: Acquired resistance to infection in an animal model of giardiasis. *J Immunol* 117:2036–2037, 1976.

49. Carlson JR, Heyworth MF, Owen RL: Response of Peyer's patch lymphocyte subsets to *Giardia muris* infection in BALB/c mice. II. T-cell subsets. *Cell Immunol* 97:44–50, 1986.

50. Heyworth MF, Carlson JR, Ermak TH: Clearance of *Giardia muris* infection requires helper/inducer T lymphocytes. *J Exp Med* 165:1743–1748, 1987.

51. Kawanishi H, Saltzman Le, Strober W: Mechanisms regulating IgA class-specific immunoglobulin production in murine gut-associated lymphoid tissue. I. T cells derived from Peyer's patches that switch sIgM B cells in vitro. *J Exp Med* 157:433–450, 1983.

52. Carlson JR, Heyworth MF, Owen RL: Response of Peyer's patch lymphocyte subsets to *Giardia muris* infection in BALB/c mice. II. B-cell subsets: enteric antigen exposure is associated with immunoglobulin isotype switching by Peyer's patch B cells. *Cell Immunol* 97:51–58, 1986.

53. Snider DP, Gordon J, McDermott MR, et al: Chronic *Giardia muris* infection in anti-IgM treated mice. I. Analysis of immunoglobulin and parasite-specific antibody in normal and immunoglobulin-deficient animals. *J Immunol* 134:4153–4162, 1985.

54. Snider DP, Underdown GJ: Quantitative and temporal analysis of murine antibody response in serum and gut secretions to infection with *Giardia muris*. *Infect Immun* 52:271–278, 1986.

55. Owens RL, Allen CL, Stevens DP: Phagocytosis of *Giardia muris* by macrophages in Peyer's patch epithelium. *Infect Immun* 33:591–601, 1981.

56. Radulescu S, Meyer EA: Opsonization in vitro of *Giardia lamblia* trophozoites. *Infect Immun* 32:852–856, 1981.

57. Brandborg LL, Tankersley CB, Gottieb S, et al: Histological demonstration of mucosal invasion by *Giardia lamblia* in man. *Gastroenterology* 52:143–150, 1967.

58. Saha TK, Gosh TK: Invasion of small intestinal mucosa by *Giardia lamblia*. *Gastroenterology* 73:402–405, 1977.

59. Smith PD, Elson CO, Keister DB, et al: Human host response to *Giardia lamblia*. I. Spontaneous killing by mononuclear leukocytes in vitro. *J Immunol* 128:1371–1376, 1982.

60. Smith PD, Keister DB, Elson CO: Human host response to *Giardia lamblia:* II. Antibody-dependent killing in vitro. *Cell Immun* 82:308–315, 1983.

61. Hill DR, Pearson RD: Ingestion of *Giardia lamblia* trophozoites by human mononuclear phagocytes. *Infect Immun* 55:3155–3161, 1987.

62. Wahl SM, McCartney-Francis N, Hunt DA, et al: Monocyte interleukin 2 receptor gene expression and interleukin 2 augmentation of microbicidal activity. *J Immunol* 139:1342–1347, 1987.

63. Aggarwal A, Nash TE: Lack of cellular cytotoxicity by human mononuclear cells to *Giardia. Am J Trop Med Hyg* 36:325–332, 1987.

64. Brown WR, Butterfield D, Savage D, et al: Clinical, microbiological, and immunological studies in patients with immunoglobulin deficiencies and gastrointestinal disorders. *Gut* 13:589–595, 1972.

65. Ajdukiewicz AB, Youngs GR, Bouchier IAD: Nodular lymphoid hyperplasia with hypogammaglobulinemia. *Gut* 13:589–595, 1972.

66. Ament ME, Ochs HD, Davis DD: Structure and function of the gastrointestinal tract in primary immunodeficiency syndrome: a study of 39 patients. *Medicine* 52:227–248, 1973.

67. Hermans PE, Diaz-Buxo JA, Stobo JD: Idiopathic late-onset immunoglobulin deficiency. Clinical observations in 50 patients. *Am J Med* 61:221–237, 1976.

68. Ridley MJ, Ridley DS: Serum antibodies and jejunal histology in giardiasis associated with malabsorption. *J Clin Pathol* 29:30–34, 1976.

69. Visvesvara GS, Smith PD, Healy GR, et al: An immunofluorescence test to detect serum antibodies to *Giardia lamblia. Ann Intern Med* 93:802–805, 1980.

70. Smith PD, Gillin FD, Brown WR, et al: IgG antibody to *Giardia lamblia* detected by enzyme-linked immunosorbent assay. *Gastroenterology* 80:1476–1480, 1981.

71. Janoff EN, Smith PD, Blaser MJ: Acute antibody responses to *Giardia lamblia* are depressed in patients with the acquired immunodeficiency syndrome. *J Infect Dis* 157:798–804, 1988.

72. Kaplan BS, Uni S, Aikawa M, et al: Effector mechanisms of host resistance in murine giardiasis: specific IgG and IgA cell modulated toxicity. *J Immunol* 32:1975–1981, 1985.

73. Miotti PG, Gilman RH, Pickering LK, et al: Prevalence of serum and milk antibodies to *Giardia lamblia* in different populations of lactating women. *J Infect Dis* 152:1025–1031, 1985.

74. Nayak N, Ganguly NK, Walia BNS, et al: Specific secretory IgA in the milk of *Giardia lamblia*-infected and uninfected women. *J Infect Dis* 155:724–727, 1987.

75. Birkhead G, Janoff EN, Vogt RL, et al: Elevated IgA antibodies to *Giardia lamblia* during a waterborne outbreak of enteric illness. *J Clin Microbiol.* In press.

76. Current WL: *Cryptosporidium* spp. In Genta RM, Walzer PD: *Parasite Diseases in the Immunocompromised Host.* New York, Marcel Dekker Inc., 1988, pp 281–341.

77. Meisel JL, Perera DR, Meligro C, et al: Overwhelming watery diarrhea associated with a cryptosporidium in an immunosuppressed patient. *Gastroenterology* 70:1156–1160, 1976.

78. Nime Fa, Burek JD, Page DL, et al: Acute enterocolitis in a human being infected with the protozoan *Cryptosporidium. Gastroenterology* 70:592–598, 1976.

79. Reese NC, Current WL, Ernst JV, et al: Cryptosporidiosis of man and calf: a case report and results of experimental infections in mice and rats. *Am J Trop Med Hyg* 31:226–229, 1982.

80. Current WL, Reese NC, Ernst JV, et al: Human cryptosporidiosis in immunocompetent and immunodeficient persons: studies of an outbreak and experimental transmission. *N Engl J Med* 308:1252–1257, 1983.

81. Pitlik SD, Fainstein V, Garza D, et al: Human cryptosporidiosis: spectrum of disease: report of six cases and review of the literature. *Arch Intern Med* 143:2269–2275, 1983.

82. Soave R, Danner RL, Honig CL: Cryptosporidiosis in homosexual men. *Ann Intern Med* 100:504–511, 1984.

83. Smith PD, Lane HC, Gill VJ, et al: Intestinal infections in patients with the acquired immunodeficiency syndrome: etiology and response to therapy. *Ann Intern Med* 108:328–333, 1988.

84. Laughon BE, Druckman DA, Vernon A, et al: Prevalence of enteric pathogens in homosexual men with and without the acquired immunodeficiency syndrome. *Gastroenterology* 94:984–993, 1988.

85. DeHovitz JA, Pape JW, Boncy M, et al: Clinical manifestations and therapy of *Isospora belli* infection in patients with the acquired immunodeficiency syndrome. *N Engl J Med* 315:87–90, 1986.

86. Zar F, Geiseler PJ, Brown VA. Asymptomatic carriage of *Cryptosporidium* in the stool of a patient with acquired immunodeficiency syndrome. *J Infect Dis* 151:195, 1985.

87. Berkowitz CD, Seidel S: Spontaneous resolution of cryptosporidiosis in a child with acquired immunodeficiency syndrome. *Am J Dis Child* 139:967, 1985.

88. Bogaerts J, Lepage P, Rouvroy D, et al: *Cryptosporidium* spp., a frequent cause of diarrhea in Central Africa. *J Clin Microbiol* 20:874–876, 1984.

89. Holley HP, Jr., Dover C: *Cryptosporidium:* a common cause of parasitic diarrhea in otherwise healthy individuals. *J Infect Dis* 153:365–368, 1986.

90. Mata L, Bolanos H, Pizarro D, et al: Cryptosporidiosis in children from some highland Costa Rican rural and urban areas. *Am J Trop Med Hyg* 33:24–29, 1984.

91. Janoff EN, Reller LB: Cryptosporidium species, a protean protozoan. *J Clin Microbiol* 23:967–975, 1987.

92. Janoff EN: *Cryptosporidium. Immunocompromised Host* 5:2–11, 1988.

93. Tzipori S, Smith M, Birch C, et al: Cryptosporidiosis in hospital patients with gastroenteritis. *Am J Trop Med Hyg* 32:931–934, 1983.

94. Jokipii L, Phojola S, Jokipii AMM: *Cryptosporidium:* a frequent finding in patients with gastrointestinal symptoms. *Lancet* 1:358–361, 1983.

95. Jokipii L, Pohjola S, Jokipii AMM: Cryptosporidiosis associated with traveling and giardiasis. *Gastroenterology* 89:838–842, 1985.

96. D'Antonio RG, Winn RE, Taylor JP, et al: A waterborne outbreak of cryptosporidiosis in normal hosts. *Ann Intern Med* 103:886–888, 1985.

97. Ongerth JE, Stibbs HH: Identification of *Cryptosporidium* oocysts in river water. *Appl Environ Microbiol* 53:672–676, 1987.

98. Soave R, Ma P: Cryptosporidiosis traveler's diarrhea in 2 families. *Arch Intern Med* 145:70–72, 1985.

99. Alpert G, Bell LM, Kirkpatrick CE: Cryptosporidiosis in a day care center. *N Engl J Med* 311:860–861, 1984.

100. Collier AC, Miller RA, Meyers JD: Cryptosporidiosis after marrow transplantation: person-to-person transmission and treatment with spiramycin. *Ann Intern Med* 101:205–206, 1984.

101. Koch KL, Phillips DJ, Aber RC, et al: Cryptosporidiosis in hospital personnel. Evidence for person-to-person transmission. *Ann Intern Med* 102:593–596, 1985.

102. Blagburn BL, Current WL: Accidental infection of a researcher with human *Cryptosporidium. J Infect Dis* 148:772–773, 1983.

103. Casemore DP, Sands RL, Curry A. *Cryptosporidium* species, a new human pathogen. *J Clin Pathol* 38:1321–1336, 1985.

104. Campbell PN, Current WL: Demonstration of serum antibodies to *Cryptosporidium* spp. in normal and immunodeficient humans with confirmed infections. *J Clin Microbiol* 18:165–169, 1983.

105. Ungar BLP, Soave R, Fayer R, et al: Enzyme immunoassay detection of immunoglobulin M and G antibodies to *Cryptosporidium* in immunocompetent and immunocompromised persons. *J Infect Dis* 153:570–578, 1986.

106. Report of a WHO expert committee. Amebiasis. *WHO Tech Rep Ser* 421:1–52, 1969.

107. Juniper K, Jr.: Amebiasis in the United States. *Bull NY Acad Med* 47:448–461, 1971.

108. Walsh JA: Problems in recognition and diagnosis of amebiasis: estimation of the global magnitude of morbidity and mortality. *Rev Infect Dis* 8:228–238, 1986.

109. Schmerin MI, Gelston A, Jones TC: Amebiasis: an increasing problem among homosexuals in New York City. *JAMA* 238:1386–1387, 1977.

110. Sexton DJ, Krogstad DJ, Spencer HC, et al: Amebiasis in a mental institution: serologic and epidemiologic studies. *Am J Epidemiol* 100:414–423, 1974.

111. Spencer HC, Hermos JA, Healy GR, et al: Endemic amebiasis in an Arkansas community. *Am J Epidemiol* 104:93–99, 1976.

112. Knight R: Surveys of amoebiasis: interpretation of data and their implications. *Ann Trop Med Parasitol* 69:35, 1975.

113. Oyerinde JPO, Ogunbi O, Alonge AA: Age and sex distribution of infections with *Entamoeba histolytica* and *Giardia intestinalis* in the Lagos population. *Int J Epidemiol* 6:231–234, 1977.

114. El-Hennawy M, Abd-Rabbo H: Hazards of cortisone therapy in hepatic amoebiasis. *J Trop Med Hyg* 81:71–73, 1978.

115. Abioye AA: Fatal amoebic colitis in pregnancy and puerperium: a new clinico-pathological entity. *J Trop Med Hyg* 76:97–120, 1973.

116. Singh BN, Srivastava RVN, Dutta GP: Virulence of strains of *Entamoeba histolytica* to rats and the effect of cholestrol, rat cecal and hamster liver on the violence of non-invasive strains. *Indian J Exp Biol* 9:21–27, 1971.

117. Adams EB, MacLeod IN: Invasive amebiasis. Amebic dysentery and its complications. *Medicine* 56:315–323, 1977.

118. Adams EB, Macheod IN: Invasive amebiasis. II. Amebic liver abscess and its complications. *Medicine* 56:324–334, 1977.

119. Martinez-Palomo A, Martinez-Baez M: Selective primary health care: strategies for control of disease in the developing world. X. Amebiasis. *Rev Infect Dis* 5:1093–1102, 1983.

120. Beaver PC, Jung RC, Sherman HJ, et al: Experimental *Entamoeba histolytica* infections in man. *Am J Trop Med Hyg* 5:1000–1009, 1956.

121. Gregory PB: A refractory case of hepatic amoebiasis. *Gastroenterology* 70:585–587, 1976.

122. DeLeon A: Prognostico tardio en el absceso hepatica amibiano. *Arch Invest Med* (Mex) 1:S205–206, 1970.

123. Sargeant PG, Williams JE: Electrophoretic patterns of *Entamoeba histolytica* and *Entamoeba coli*. *Trans R Soc Trop Med Hyg* 72:164–166, 1978.

124. Mirelman D: Ameba-bacterium relationship in amebiasis. *Microbiol Rev* 51:272–284, 1987.

125. Phillips BP, Wolfe PA, Rees CW, et al: Studies on the ameba-bacteria relationship in amebiasis: comparative results of the intracecal inoculation of germfree monocontained, and conventional guinea pigs with *Entamoeba histolytica*. *Am J Trop Med Hyg* 4:678–692, 1955.

126. Ravdin JI, Murphy CF, Solata RA, et al: N-acetyl-D-galactosamine-inhibitable adherence lectin of *Entamoeba histolytica*. I. Partial purification and relation to amoebic virulence *in vitro*. *J Infect Dis* 151:804–815, 1985.

127. Kobiter D, Mirelman D: Adhesion of *Entamoeba histolytica* trophozoites to monolayers of human cells. *J Infect Dis* 144:539–546, 1981.

128. Jarumilinta R, Maegraith BG: Enzymes of *Entamoeba histolytica*. *Bull WHO* 41:269–273, 1969.

129. Lushbaugh WB, Kairalla AB, Cantey JR, et al: Isolation of a cytotoxin-enterotoxin from *Entamoeba histolytica*. *J Infect Dis* 139:9–17, 1979.

130. Ravdin JI, Guerrant RL: Role of adherence in cytopathogenic mechanisms of *Entamoeba histolytica:* study with mammalism tissue culture cells and human erythrocytes. *J Clin Invest* 68:1305–1313, 1981.

131. Ravdin JI, Croft BY, Guerrant RL: Cytopathogenic mechanisms of *Entamoeba histolytica*. *J Exp Med* 152:377–390, 1980.

132. Young JD, Young TM, Lu LP, et al: Characterization of a membrane pore-forming protein from *Entamoeba histolytica*. *J Exp Med* 156:1677–1690, 1982.

133. Lynch EC, Rosenberg IM, Gitler C: An ion-channel forming protein produced by *Entamoeba histolytica*. *EMBO J* 1:801–804, 1982.

134. Patterson M, Healy GR, Shabot JM: Serologic testing for amebiasis *Gastroenterology* 78:136–141, 1980.

135. Jackson TFH, Anderson CB, Simjee AE: Serological differentiation between past and present infection in hepatic amebiasis. *Trans R Soc Trop Med Hyg* 78:342–345, 1984.

136. Calderon J, Munoz ML, Acosta HM: Surface redistribution and release of antibody-induced caps in *Entamoeba*. *J Exp Med* 151:184–193, 1980.

137. Ortiz-Ortiz L, Capin R, Sepulveda B, et al: Activation of the alternative pathway of complement by *Entamoeba histolytica*. *Clin Exp Immunol* 34:10–18, 1978.

138. Calderon J, Schreiber RD: Activation of the alternative and classical complement pathways by *Entamoeba histolytica*. *Infect Immun* 50:560–565, 1985.

139. Capin MR, Jiménez M, Zamacona G, et al: Determinación de complemento y via alterna del complemento en pacientes con absceso hepatico amibiano. *Arch Invest Med* (Mex) 9:S297–302, 1978.

140. Reed SL, Sargeaunt PG, Brande AI: Resistance to lysis by human serum of pathogenic *Entamoeba histolytica*. *Trans R Soc Trop Med Hyg* 77:248–253, 1983.

141. Geurrant RL, Brush J, Ravdin JI, et al: Interaction between *Entamoeba histolytica* and human polymorphonuclear neutrophils. *J Infect Dis* 143:83–93, 1981.

142. Solata RA, Pearson RD, Ravdin RI: Interaction of human leukocytes and *Entamoeba histolytica:* killing of virulent amebae by the activated macrophage. *J Clin Invest* 76:491–499, 1985.

143. Ghadirian E, Meerovitch E, Kongshaven PAL: Role of macrophages in host defense against hepatic amoebiasis in hamsters. *Infect Immun* 42:1017–1019, 1983.

144. Salata RA, Martinez-Paloma A, Murray HN, et al: Patients treated for amebic liver abscess develop cell-mediated immune responses effective in vitro against *Entamoeba histolytica*. *J Immunol* 136:2633–2639, 1986.

CHAPTER 20

Viral Gastrointestinal Infections

CHRISTOPHER CUFF

DONALD H. RUBIN

INTRODUCTION

In the last 5 to 10 years, advances have been made in characterizing viruses that cause diseases in the gastrointestinal (GI) tract. Progress has resulted both from improvements in in vitro isolation and cultivation of virus and from application of molecular biologic techniques for studying GI pathogens. It is now recognized that symptomatic human infection is caused by several distinct groups of viruses. These viral agents include typical (group A) and atypical (groups B–G) rotaviruses, calicivirus, parvovirus, gastrointestinal adenoviruses, and astroviruses. In addition, other agents have been identified as important mammalian GI pathogens, such as breda virus and coronavirus, but the role of these viruses as human pathogens is not yet certain. Thus a systematic classification of diarrhea-causing viruses is beginning to emerge.

With a better classification system of GI viral pathogens, our understanding of the basic mechanisms of pathogenesis of these viral agents has improved concomitantly, including the immune mechanisms involved in protection and resolution of these infections. Basic and applied research of pathogenesis provides a conceptual framework that will lead to effective vaccines (e.g., against rotavirus infection), eradication, or control of GI viral disease. However, problems impede the study: the lack of good animal models of infection for several of the viruses and the continued difficulty of adapting many of these viruses to grow in vitro. These difficulties often limit investigators to the use of exhaustive, technically demanding electron microscopy study.

We thank R. Schafer and E. Eisenberg for critical comments. This work was supported by grants from the Public Health Service (AI 23970) and Veterans Administration. D.H.R. is supported by a career development award from the Veterans Administration.

The aim of this chapter is to review advances in our understanding of mechanisms of viral GI pathogenesis, with a focus on recently described viruses, the nature of immunity, and the pathology associated with infection. In the first part of the chapter, several viruses of known clinical significance will be discussed. In the second part of the chapter, some of our findings and the work of others on the nature of murine reovirus infection of the GI tract will be reviewed. Reovirus is a well-characterized enteric virus that is useful in the study of the cellular and molecular aspects of viral GI pathogenesis and host response. Studies will be reviewed that provide basic insight into viral GI infection and host-immune responses after GI infection.

VIRUSES

Rotavirus

Rotavirus was first detected in 1973 in Australia.[1] Rotavirus infection is the most common cause of severe diarrhea in infants and young children worldwide. The rotavirus contains a double-stranded (ds) RNA genome and is classified as a member of the *Reoviridae* family. Rotaviruses that caused gastroenteritis had previously been found to contain a family-specific serotype (group A) until recently, when atypical rotaviruses, which lack the group A antigens, have been described (Fig. 20–1) (see below).

The exact pathophysiologic mechanisms of rotavirus-induced diarrhea are not completely understood. Histologic examination of rotavirus-infected small bowel

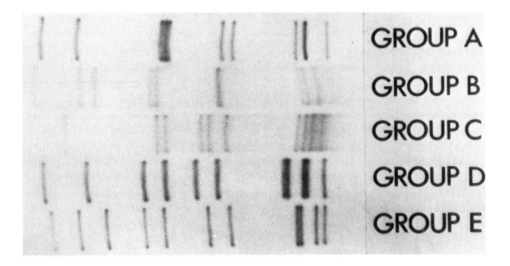

Figure 20–1 dsRNA genome profiles of the type members of rotavirus groups A–E. (From McRae MA: Nucleic acid base analyses of non-group A rotaviruses. In Bishop R: *Novel Diarrhea Viruses.* Ciba Foundation Symposium. Chichester, 1987.)

demonstrates lesions consisting of exfoliation of mature enterocytes with concomitant stunted villi (Fig. 20–2). These stunted villi are thought to result in a loss of absorptive function in the small bowel.[2] Physiologically, a decreased absorption of salt and water, along with carbohydrate malabsorption, occurs.[3] However, in most instances in which dehydration is not severe, oral hydration with World Health Organization (WHO)-recommended solutions containing glucose and sodium chloride is successful in preventing fatal illness.[4] In individuals with severe dehydration, intravenous rehydration is required to preserve fluid balance.

Immunity to rotavirus infection has been studied both in humans and animals. Some common features as well as some conflicting results have been noted. Studies have focused largely on humoral immune responses to virus. The presence of preinoculation serum antibody to rotavirus has been correlated with resistance to diarrheal disease or shedding of rotavirus, suggesting that circulating antibody plays a role in protection against illness.[5,6] Less clear was the relationship of pre-existing local neutralizing activity in intestinal fluid to resistance to infection.

Bishop et al.[7] attempted to assess the effect of neonatal rotavirus infection on subsequent reinfection. These investigators found that infants who were infected

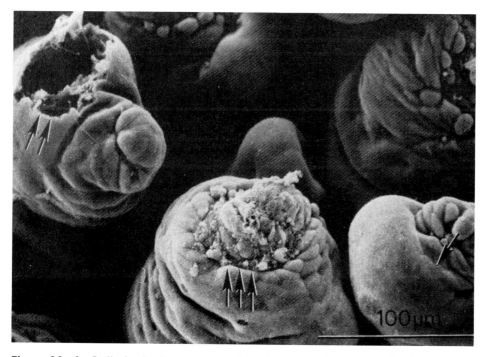

Figure 20–2 Pathologic changes associated with novel rotavirus infection. A scanning electron micrograph of villi from the small intestine of a piglet infected 24 hours previously with a group B rotavirus demonstrates infected and normal villi. The single arrow points to an intact syncytium present on one villus. The double arrow points to a ruptured syncytium on a second villus, and the triple arrow indicates an area of exposed lamina propria on a third villus. Magnification × 350. (From Hall, with permission.)

in the first 14 days of life had less severe subsequent infection. Previous neonatal infection did not confer immunity, since infections still occurred at similar frequencies in children who had never been infected, and in those that had had a previous infection. However, the severity of the disease was reduced in the children previously infected, suggesting that neonatal infection induced partial immunity to reinfection. It is now felt that a rotavirus group A strain, with a unique electrophoretic mobility pattern of the dsRNA segments on polyacrylamide gel electrophoresis (PAGE) (electropherotype),[8] may be relatively specific for the neonatal group. Therefore, partial protection may be explained on the basis of cross reacting epitopes shared by these unique rotavirus strains.

A similar finding was reported in recent clinical trials of a potential vaccine strain derived from an attenuated bovine rotavirus, designated RIT 4237 by Vesikari et al.[9] Although the vaccine did not protect against infection, a significant reduction in clinically detectable rotavirus-associated illness and severe rotavirus-induced diarrhea was observed. Although cross-serotype protection was found, protection against some serotypes seemed to be better than against others.

The role of passive immunity in human rotavirus infection is not clear. It is known that both breast-fed and bottle-fed children develop rotavirus infection and diarrhea. Totterdell et al.[10,11] found that the presence of rotavirus-specific antibody ingested in breast milk was not associated with protection. Other reports[12] have suggested a role for passive immune mechanisms in immunity to rotavirus infection.

Studies in animal infections have provided information about the roles of passive immunity and the immune responses to specific rotavirus gene products. Numerous animal models of rotavirus infection exist. For example, investigators[13,14] have studied rotavirus infection in calves and lambs; however, these animals receive little or no antibody transplacentally, so possible passive-immune mechanisms may not be similar in humans. A mouse model of rotavirus infection has also been described;[15] however, mice are susceptible to rotavirus disease for only a short time after birth, and nonmurine rotaviruses must be used in mouse models because of the difficulty in adapting murine rotaviruses to tissue culture. Nonetheless, studies have demonstrated that in experimental infections of suckling mice with a simian rotavirus, protection was afforded by anti-rotavirus IgA and IgG found in milk from immune mothers.[16] In addition, the role of the product of gene segment 4 in infection has been described,[17] and a protective effect of systemic treatment with monoclonal anti-rotavirus antibody on the disease has been demonstrated.[18]

The development of a rabbit model of rotavirus infection, as described by Conner et al.,[19] is an exciting new advance. This model has numerous advantages and similarities to human infection including an older age of susceptibility to infection, transplacental transfer of antibody, relatively modest cost, and a cultivatible rabbit rotavirus as the pathogen.

For group A rotavirus, most studies support a role for specific antibody in protection against disease. The antibody may lessen the severity of subsequent infections by other rotavirus serotypes. Little is known about cellular immunity, which may play a role in protection. More work needs to be done to elucidate the mechanisms of immunity to increase the chances of developing an effective vaccine against rotavirus.

Novel Rotaviruses

The non-group A rotaviruses have been described as pararotavirus, novel rotavirus, atypical, or antigenically distinct. These viruses exhibit a morphology similar to the rotavirus but lack the group A antigen that is common to previously identified rotaviruses. Currently, serogroups A–F have been identified, and a seventh group (G) has also been tentatively described. Of these serogroups, groups B and C have been found to be responsible for outbreaks of human illness.

Novel rotaviruses contain 11 segments of dsRNA. This feature is common to group A, but the dsRNA electropherotypes differ from group to group (Fig. 20–1). It is hoped that this feature will allow the development of diagnostic characteristics to identify the various groups.

Novel rotaviruses infect a wide spectrum of animals, including rats, calves, and chickens. In humans, a serious form of rotavirus-induced diarrhea caused by group B rotavirus has been described in the People's Republic of China (PRC).[20] In contrast to group A infections, this form of enteritis is very severe in adults, and thus the virus responsible for infection has been referred to as adult diarrhea rotavirus (ADRV). It is estimated that one million people became ill during the 1982–1983 epidemic in the PRC,[20] and the virus continues to cause sporadic outbreaks in that country. It has been suggested that ADRV resulted from a mutation in a group B virus, causing it to become infectious to humans.[21]

The lesions caused by novel rotaviruses are similar to those observed in group A rotavirus infections, with one important difference (Fig. 20–3). In group B infec-

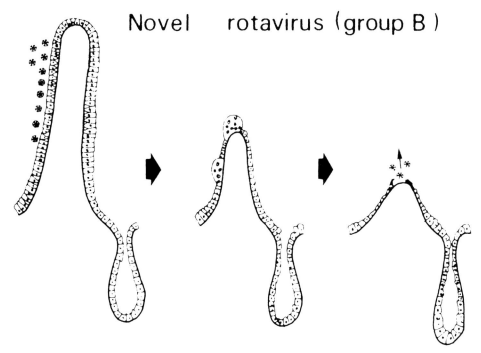

Figure 20–3 Schematic representation of group B rotavirus infection. Syncytia develop in infected enterocytes. (From Hall, with permission.)

tion, syncytia of enterocytes develop on the surfaces of villi of the small intestine.[2] It is not known whether the syncytia formation is pathognomonic for all atypical rotavirus infections, but it does appear to be characteristic of group B infection.

Immunity to novel rotaviruses was studied by Hung et al.:[22] 9.5 – 20% of healthy people from nonendemic areas were found to have significant antibody titers to ADRV. In subjects from an area where a previous ADRV epidemic had occurred, 41% of healthy subjects (who had never had enteritis) and 53% of individuals who had become ill had positive antibody titers to ADRV. In addition to human studies, it has also been reported that no cross-protection is observed between two group B viruses after experimental animal infection.[23] The roles of local humoral and cellular immunity to atypical rotaviruses have not yet been determined.

Norwalk-Like viruses

A small round virus (SRV) producing significant GI disease was first identified by immune electron microscopy (IEM) in fecal specimens obtained during a 1968 outbreak of gastroenteritis in Norwalk, Ohio.[24] Subsequent analysis of similar outbreaks of epidemic diarrheal disease has indicated that similar SRV particles are present in the feces of symptomatic adults and older children.[25] Many of these outbreaks may also be due to viruses that are morphologically and serologically similar to the Norwalk virus; thus the agents responsible for these outbreaks are referred to as "Norwalk-like" viruses. This group of viruses has been difficult to study because it cannot be propagated in vitro and because currently no animal model of infection exists for human isolates. However, recent molecular biologic and serologic data suggest that SRV that have been considered Norwalk-like are members of two different viral groups, the caliciviruses and the parvoviruses.[26]

Caliciviruses contain single-stranded (ss) RNA as their genome. This group of viruses has a broad range of virion sizes, but the average is 31 – 35 nm (Fig. 20 – 4). The caliciviruses are known to cause diarrhea in other mammalian species, including cats. Outbreaks of calicivirus infection in humans, in addition to the initial Norwalk virus outbreak, have been reported by several investigators.[25,26]

Parvoviruses, which contain a DNA genome, have been implicated in enteritis and several other human diseases, including red cell aplastic crises of sickle cell anemia, hydrops fetalis, and erythema infectiosum. The caliciviruses and parvoviruses that induce diarrhea invoke similar symptoms.

A characteristic lesion caused by Norwalk-like viruses has been reported in the small intestine and stomach of infected humans.[27-29] Biopsies of small intestines, 2 days after oral administration of Norwalk-like virus, reveal shortened villi and an infiltration of the lamina propria by lymphocytes. By 6 days postinfection, crypts become hypertrophied, and vacuolated cytoplasm in epithelial cells is observed. Interestingly, tissues were antigen-negative by immunohistochemical techniques during these studies, so the exact location of virus replication in humans is unknown. Since no animal model of human infection exists, little is known about the dissemination of the virus through the GI tract or systemic circulation. However, based upon animal studies, it is quite likely that the Norwalk-like human parvoviruses induce pathologic changes due to infection of immature crypt cells and may have a cycle of infection similar to reovirus type 1 (see below).

A peculiar paradox concerning immunity to Norwalk-like viruses is emerging. First, it should be reiterated that Norwalk-like viruses rarely cause symptomatic

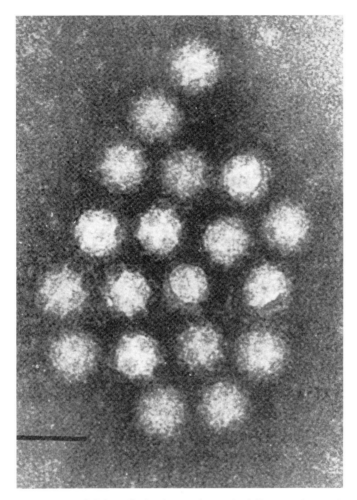

Figure 20 – 4 Human calicivirus displaying a characteristic cup-shaped surface morphology. Bar = 50 nm. (From Cubitt W, et al: Antigenic relationships between human calciviruses and Norwalk virus. *J Infect Dis* 156:806–814, 1987, with permission.)

illness in infants or young children, but generally may cause disease in children and adults. In an often cited study by Parrino et al.,[30] human volunteers infected with Norwalk-like virus were found to be immune without detectable antibody to the Norwalk-like virus. In this study 6 of 12 volunteers became ill when experimentally infected. Significant increases in antibody were found in these six patients. In contrast, the six volunteers who remained well had little or no increase in serum antibody titers. Twenty seven to forty two months later, the 12 volunteers were reinoculated. The same six volunteers who became ill following the first infection became sick following the second inoculation. Four to eight weeks later, four of the six volunteers were inoculated for a third time. Following this inoculation, only one of four became clinically ill. Thus, those people who did not develop antibody titers did not become ill, and those who did develop antibody titers did become ill. The reason for this unusual pattern of susceptibility is not yet known. Several explanations have been proposed, including genetic predisposition to infection, and a requirement for repeated exposure to the infectious agent to develop illness.[25] Although the latter hypothesis is consistent with the observation that the disease develops in adults, it does not explain why the volunteers were resistant to a third challenge shortly after infection. Several more recent reports have verified the observation that a rise in antibody titers to Norwalk-like virus is associated with the development of gastroenteritis in naturally occurring infection.[31-33] In contrast, there are reports that have shown an association between pre-existing antibody levels and protection from illness.[34,35] The major difference between these studies appears to be that those reporting protection associated with higher antibody titers are from patient populations in underdeveloped countries. Thus there may be a difference in immunity when children are exposed to a panoply of infectious agents, or are subject to a larger number of exposures to other viruses such as calici- or parvoviruses. As is the case with rotavirus, the role of cellular immunity in resistance to Norwalk-like viruses has not been adequately addressed, primarily because of the inability to cultivate the viruses. Because the efficacy of specific immune responses to Norwalk-like viruses in the control of the disease is questionable, the prospect for developing a vaccine is bleak, especially in developed countries. If specific immunity can protect populations in underdeveloped countries, where the prevalence is greater than in developed countries, the chance of developing an effective vaccine may be better.

Astrovirus

Astrovirus is an SRV that contains a positive ssRNA genome and is acid-stable and resistant to inactivation by alcohol. These viruses are approximately 27–30 nm in size and were named astrovirus by Madeley and Cosgrove in 1975 because of their characteristic star-like morphology on electron microscopy.[36] Both human and animal astroviruses have been described.

Astrovirus has been responsible for a number of outbreaks of gastroenteritis, mainly in children. Astrovirus does not appear to cause widespread illness in adults. In an experimental infection described by Kurtz et. al.,[37] astrovirus was found to cause illness in only 3 of 17 volunteers given fecal filtrates containing astrovirus. In those infected with astrovirus, systemic symptoms such as anorexia, headache, and fever can occur. In contrast to Norwalk-like viruses, which have a short incubation time, the symptoms associated with astrovirus typically occur several days after ingestion of virally contaminated foods. In at least one outbreak, symptoms consistent with dual infection of Norwalk-like virus and astrovirus occurred, suggesting that interference between various groups does not occur. This may indicate that different cells in the GI tract (e.g., epithelial villus cells or M cells) become infected.

Two different pathologic lesions may result from astrovirus infection of animals. In lambs, astrovirus appears to infect mature enterocytes followed by exfoliation of enterocytes and crypt hypertrophy.[38] In contrast, calves experimentally infected with astrovirus display no infection of enterocytes by virus. Infection is restricted to M cells, the specialized cells in the dome epithelium of Peyer's patches.[2,39] The site of infection in calves is similar to that seen in mice infected with reovirus type 1 (see below).

In contrast to Norwalk-virus infection, volunteers who are antibody-positive do not develop diarrhea after experimental infection; thus the development of astro-virus-specific antibody seems to correlate with protection from symptoms.

Enteric Adenovirus

The adenovirus group is nonenveloped and contains a DNA genome. Adenoviruses are classified into 6 subgenera and 41 serotypes. Of these, groups A–E (39 sero-types) may be cultivated in cultures of human embryo kidney or heteroploid cell lines. Serotypes 40 and 41, which constitute group F, are able to grow in Chang conjunctiva cells[40] or the 293 cell line.[41] The two serotypes in group F, AD40 and AD41, have been shown to cause severe infantile diarrhea.[42,43]

Using electron microscopy, Flewett[44] identified large numbers of adenovirus particles that failed to grow in tissue culture in stools from patients with gastritis. Since then, numerous studies[45–47] have detailed the epidemiology and clinical features of infantile diarrhea caused by adenovirus. Adenovirus consistently causes moderate illness with long-lasting diarrhea (> 10 days). In addition, no significant seasonal variation has been reported. Although cases of adult infection have been reported, most cases involve infants and young children. Precise mechanisms of immunity have not been elucidated. However, serotype-specific neutralizing antibodies do develop after postinfection, and it is thought that these antibodies may play a role in preventing serious reinfection.[48]

Pathologic examination of intestine from experimental[49] and natural infection[50] shows evidence of stunted villi in jejunum and ileum. Infection of mature entero-cytes occurs and intranuclear inclusions develop in infected enterocytes which then degenerate and lyse (Fig. 20–5). The lamina propria of the intestinal villus becomes infiltrated with mononuclear cells, and the crypts hypertrophy. The detection of intranuclear inclusions in villus enterocytes appears to be characteristic of adenovirus infection.[2]

Human adenovirus has also been implicated in the pathogenesis of celiac disease.[51] A comparison has been made between a wheat protein, A-gliadin, which is known to activate celiac disease in susceptible individuals, and the 54-kD E1b protein of human adenovirus type 12 (Ad12, group A). A region of homology exists between the 12 AA sequence in E1b and A-gliadin. In addition, antibody raised against the E1b protein cross reacts with A-gliadin. Thus adenovirus infection may play an important role in the pathogenesis of celiac disease.

Hepatitis A

Several enteric viruses are known to enter the host through the gut and spread to other organ systems. Included in this group are the enteroviruses: coxsackievirus, ECHO, poliovirus, and hepatitis A virus. These viruses typically cause mild if any GI disease, and their most profound pathogenic manifestations are evidenced at specific organ sites, such as the anterior horn cells of the spinal cord for poliovirus and the hepatocytes for hepatitis A virus. Because the scope of this chapter emphasizes diseases of the GI tract and liver, a brief discussion of hepatitis A virus is warranted.

Hepatitis A virus is a 27–32-nm icosahedral particle that contains a positive ssRNA genome. Six polypeptides have been identified in highly purified hepatitis A

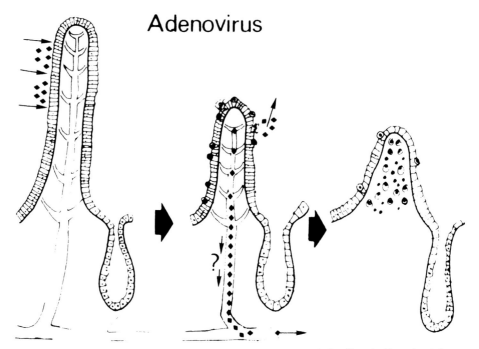

Adenovirus

Figure 20–5 Schematic representation of adenovirus infection in the pig. Intranuclear inclusions develop in infected enterocytes. Infected enterocytes degenerate and rupture, resulting in stunted villi, hypertrophied crypts, and an infiltration of the lamina propria by inflammatory cells. (From Hall BA: Comparative pathology of infections by novel diarrhea viruses. In Bishop R: *Novel Diarrhea Viruses.* Ciba Foundation Symposium. Chichester, 1987.)

particles, four of which are structural proteins. The basic structural proteins of the virus closely resemble those found within the *Picornaviridae* family.

Infection with hepatitis A is characterized by fever, vomiting, nausea, and abdominal pain. Jaundice and hepatosplenomegaly follow the generalized symptoms. Infections caused by hepatitis A virus are similar to infections due to Norwalk-like viruses and ADRV in that they are usually more severe in adolescents and adults. Hepatitis A infection occurs at any time of the year, but most commonly in temperate zones in winter and autumn. Hepatitis A infections are usually transmitted by the oral-fecal route. Both food-borne and water-borne sources have been implicated in infections. In addition, it has been documented that infected primates have transmitted the disease to humans.[52]

Antibody to hepatitis A virus develops less than 5 weeks after exposure to the virus and reaches peak levels 8–12 weeks postexposure.[53,54] Following infection, immunity is long-lasting and may persist for life.[55] In addition to a systemic immune response (IgM and IgG), IgA coproantibodies are detected during the early phases of infection in stools of patients with severe hepatitis A infection and may provide local immunity.[56] Furthermore, IgA antibodies to hepatitis A are only found for the first 3–4 months following infection and may therefore provide, along with serum IgM titers, a serologic marker for acute infection.

Little is known about the pathogenesis of hepatitis A except that infection impairs liver functions. Hepatitis A virus is released from infected hepatocytes and is spread to the feces through bile. While many enteroviruses are presumed to replicate in the intestinal epithelium, the exact mode of intestinal pathogenesis is still unknown. For hepatitis A virus, enterocytes are not observed to contain virus after oral inoculation of experimentally infected marmosets.[57] Therefore virus passage to new hosts may occur predominantly or exclusively via passage in the bile (see reovirus type 1 below).

Feinstone[58] has reported that marmosets infected with hepatitis A virus develop histopathologic and biochemical evidence of disease within 1 week of infection. Approximately 3 weeks after infection, a second phase of disease develops, which results in necrosis of hepatocytes and prominent inflammation. It was suggested that an immunopathic component of hepatitis A-induced pathology may be responsible for the second phase of the disease.

REOVIRUS AS A MODEL FOR STUDYING VIRAL PATHOGENESIS

Reoviruses have been implicated in some cases of mild respiratory and gastrointestinal tract infections in young children.[59] In addition, a role for reovirus in neonatal biliary atresia has been suggested.[60-61] Although the importance of reovirus in human disease is unclear, reovirus remains an important model system for studying viral pathogenesis in a murine model.

Reovirus causes a number of diseases in mice, particularly in neonatal mice. These characteristics have made it ideal for studying both cellular and molecular aspects of viral pathogenesis. Of particular interest are the diseases caused by reovirus serotypes 1 and 3. Reovirus serotype 1 can cause disease of the GI tract as well as a central nervous system (CNS) infection of ependymal cells that results in hydrocephalus. In addition, serotype 1 has been implicated in murine diabetes mellitus and other autoimmune diseases.[62] Reovirus serotype 3 can cause active chronic hepatitis,[63] a highly lethal encephalitis with destruction of neuronal cells,[64,65] biliary atresia, and a fatal GI disease.[66]

Structure and Function

Reoviruses contain ten segments of dsRNA that are divided into three groups, designated L (large), M (medium), and S (small). The gene products encoded by these RNA segments are designated by the Greek symbols for each letter — λ, μ, and σ. The mammalian reoviruses fall into three serotypes, 1, 2, and 3, based on hemagglutination inhibition and neutralization tests.[67] The σ1-polypeptide, the viral hemagglutinin, is a minor polypeptide component and is present in approximately 48 copies per virion.[68] Recent data suggests that the viral hemagglutinin extends upon a flexible stalk when exposed to the small intestine environment. In this state, the hemagglutinin is capable of binding to cellular receptors to promote viral entry into the host cell.[69]

Infection of the GI Tract by Reovirus Serotypes 1 and 3

Recent work on reovirus infection of the GI tract has used the stability of reovirus serotype 1 in the intestinal milieu.[70] Reovirus type 1 specifically binds to the M cells overlying Peyer's patches in the small intestine and utilizes these cells to enter the host.[71,72] A hypothetical route of infection has been developed, as illustrated in Figure 20-6.

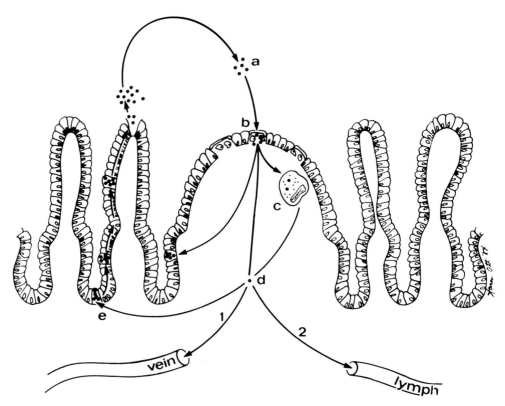

Figure 20–6 Hypothetical model of reovirus infection of the gut. Reovirus in the lumen (a) is transported into the host via M cells (b) to the macrophage-rich sube-pithelial region overlying a Peyer's patch. From the lymphoid follicle, the virus is either endocytosed (c) and carried intracellularly or flows freely to the basal crypt epithelial cells. Dissemination of virus occurs (d) by vein (1) or by lymphatic efferents (2) to the blood stream, where it is circulated to systemic or intestinal sites supportive of viral replication, thereby resulting in infection of crypt cells distant to the Peyer's patch. In the intestine, the infected basal crypt cell (e) migrates toward the villus type during maturation into an absorptive enterocyte; lysis or exfoliation releases free virus into the intestinal lumen. (From Rubin DH, et al: Reovirus serotype 1 intestinal infectinal: a novel replicative cycle with ileal disease, *J Virol* 53:391–398, 1985, with permission.)

Figure 20–7 Reovirus binding to isolated intestinal epithelial cells. Reovirus types 1/L or 2/J were incubated with intestinal epithelial cells, and the cells were examined for virus binding by indirect immunofluorescence. Isolated villus (A1, A2) or crypt cells (B1, B2) incubated with reovirus type 1/L and villus cells incubated with reovirus 2/J (C1, C2) demonstrate immunofluorescence on the basolateral membranes. Brush border (B) is visible with light microscopy, and virus-specific binding is evident by immunofluorescence (V). Controls consisting of virus-adsorbed cells followed by an-ticoxsackievirus serum (E1, E2), or rabbit antireovirus serum alone are also shown. Magnification ×510 (From Rubin DH, et al: Reovirus serotype 1 binds to the basolat-eral membrane of intestinal epithelial cells. *Microb Pathogen* 3:215–217, 1987.)

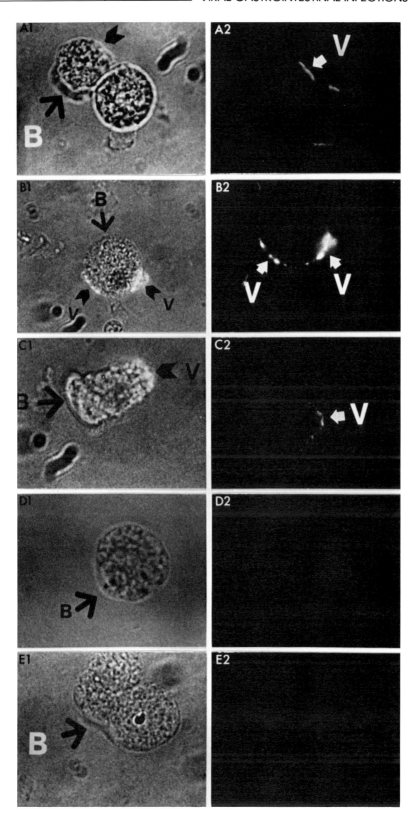

Recent data supports the hypothesis that reovirus infects susceptible crypt epithelium by binding to receptors localized to the basolateral portion of the cell[73-75] (Fig. 20–7). Therefore the virus must first enter the host before it can infect the epithelial cells in the crypts of Lieberkuhn of the ileum.[73] In this manner, reovirus infection is a model for diarrhea-causing astrovirus and parvovirus (see above) as well as the enteric viruses that cause systemic disease. Based upon this model of virus entry prior to epithelial cell infection, a further hypothesis would predict that humoral IgG may be as protective of the epithelial cells as IgA. Experiments are now in progress to test this hypothesis.

With reovirus type 1, large doses of virus ($10^8 - 10^9$ PFU [plaque forming unit]) induce an inflammatory cell response in the lamina propria, hyperplasia of crypts, and a loss of nuclear polarity restricted to the ileum. Inoculation with 10^{10} PFU results in perforation of the ileum with fibrosis of the lamina propria. The presence of large numbers of antigen-positive cells surrounding the lesions suggest that the virus plays a direct role in the induction of this lesion.[73] However, since the binding of virus to cellular receptors does not appear to be restricted to a particular region of the intestine, the mechanism of antigen localization to a particular region of intestinal mucosa is still unknown. Reovirus serotype 3 induces GI pathologic lesions that are present in the lamina propria of the small intestine and proximal colon. The epithelial cells do not appear to be a target of infection with this virus, although diarrhea can be induced by high intravenous inocula (10^{10} PFU). Further studies are in progress to understand the relationship of GI pathology to reovirus type 3 infection.

Genetic Studies: Identification of Virulence Factors

The genetics of the reovirus has been studied in detail and characterized using recombinants generated by coinfection of cells with reoviruses of different serotypes. These reassortments have made it possible to identify viral gene segments that are responsible for reovirus pathogenesis.[76] Using these recombination techniques, it was found that the S1 gene product (σ-1 polypeptide) determines virus tropism. Reovirus σ-1 polypeptide determines the homing pattern of virus to organs that contain viral-specific receptors. For reovirus type 1, this includes ependymal cells of the central nervous system (CNS),[77] pituitary gland,[62] lung,[78] and intestine.[74,75] Reovirus type 3 binds to receptors localized to neuronal cells and

Figure 20–8 Reovirus type 1 but not reovirus type 3 binds to isolated intestinal cells via the virus hemagglutinin. Reovirus types 1/L, 3/D, reassortant 3.HA-1, or reassortant 1.HA-3 were incubated with cells followed by treatment with rabbit antireovirus antiserum and FITC-labeled goat anti-rabbit antibody. Isolated villus cells were incubated with reovirus type 1/L (A1, A2), or were incubated with reovirus reassortant 3.HA-1 (B1, B2) and demonstrate immunofluorescence on the basolateral membranes. No immunofluorescence is observed with reovirus type 3 (C1, C2) or reovirus reassortant 1.HA-3 incubated with isolated intestinal cells (D1, D2). Brush border (B) is visible with light microscopy. Magnification ×600. (From Weiner HL, et al: Molecular basis of reovirus virulence: role of the S1 gene. *Proc Natl Acad Sci USA* 74:5744–5748, 1977, with permission.)

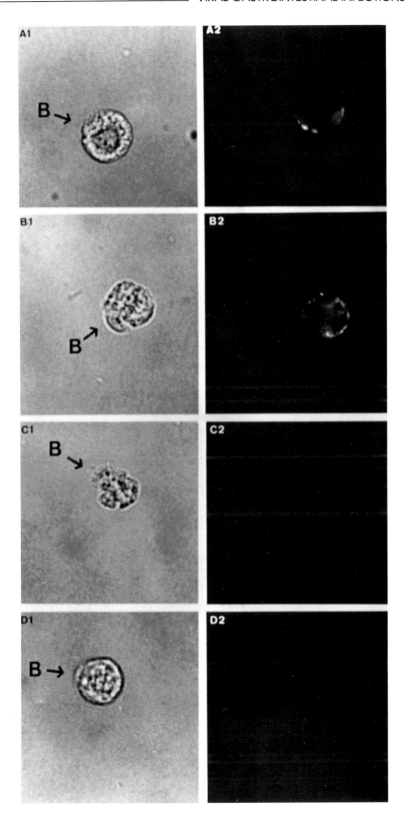

Table 20–1 PARENTAL ORIGIN OF GENOME SEGMENTS[a]

Serotype or reassortant	Outer capsid[b]				Core[b]				NS[b]		Cell[c]	
	S1	L2	M2	S4	L1	L3	M1	S2	M3	S3	I	L
1	1	1	1	1	1	1	1	1	1	1	+	+
3.HA-1	1	3	3	3	3	3	3	3	3	3	+	+
3	3	3	3	3	3	3	3	3	3	3	−	+
1.HA-3	3	1	1	1	1	1	1	1	1	1	−	+

[a] Isolated villus epithelial cells or L-cells were absorbed with 10^6 particles/cell of reovirus type 1,3, or reassortants 3.HA-1 or 1.HA-3, and binding was visualized using fluorescent techniques. Fluorescent staining of cells was restricted by the presence of the reovirus type 1 hemagglutinin to villus cells, but not to L-cells.

[b] Physical location of viral polypeptides encoded by each genome segment. NS, nonstructural proteins are encoded by these genome segments.

[c] Cell types used for binding. I, dispersed intestinal villus cells; L, L-929 cells.

[From Ref. 75 with permission.]

to lymphocytes. Both serotypes are bound to M cells in the intestine, whereas only reovirus type 3 adsorbs to the surface of adsorptive epithelial cells. However, the binding of reovirus type 3 to the intestinal cell surface is lost if cells are dispersed in EDTA-containing media, suggesting that the binding may be due to a removable substance such as mucin (Fig. 20–8, Table 20–1). In neonatal mice, the binding of reovirus type 3 to mucin may result in entry of the virus and subsequent infection of enterocytes, whereas in adult mice there is no evidence that mice inoculated with reovirus type 3 develop productively infected enterocytes. In addition, studies describe the M2 gene product, a proteolytic-sensitive polypeptide, as important both in GI pathogenesis and neurovirulence.[70,79]

Finally, during the course of systemic infection of reovirus, occasional hepatocytes that contain viral antigen as well as an accumulation of viral particles within Kupffer cells are seen.[80] Virus is passaged into the intestinal lumen during the systemic phase of infection via the bile. Therefore reovirus type 1 shares a mode of egress from the host similar to that of the hepatitis A virus. Studies have determined that uptake by Kupffer cells is essential for biliary transmission of virus. In addition, the expression of the major histocompatibility complex (MHC) antigen I-A is further required.[81] Exactly how Kupffer cells participate in virus transport is unknown. However, experiments have focused on two possible mechanisms: 1) a direct association between MHC I-A antigen-bearing cells and virus; or 2) factors released by these cells [e.g., interleukin-1 (IL-1)], which may affect the metabolism of the hepatocytes (Fig. 20–9).

Immunity

Although serotype-specific neutralizing antibodies have been shown to be specific for the σ1-polypeptide and are type-specific,[82] Hayes et al.[83] reported that monoclonal antibodies against reovirus type 3 could neutralize the infectivity of reovirus type 1, strain Lang (type 1/L), and type 2, strain Jones, as well as type 3 Dearing (type 3/D). It was also found that monoclonal antibodies against λ2 (L2 gene product) can inhibit hemagglutination as well as neutralize infectivity across serotypes. These results suggest that cross-protection to disease can be induced, a notion that is now supported by experimental results (see below).

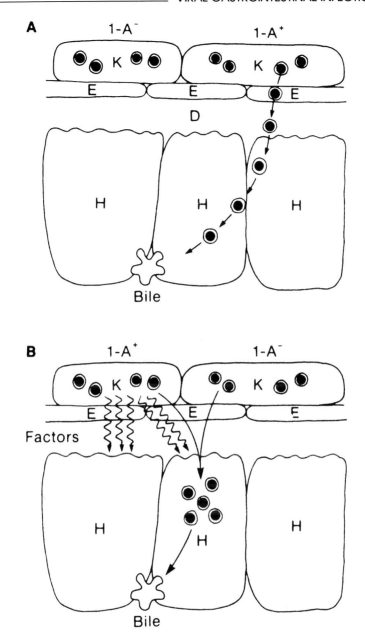

Figure 20 – 9 Possible roles of I-A bearing cells in the secretion of reovirus type 1/L. **A:** The I-A antigen-bearing Kupffer cell (K) directly interacts with reovirus and serves as a conduit for passage of the virus into the space of Disse (D) for presentation of the virus to hepatocytes (H) and passage to the bile. The endothelial cells (E) do not concentrate virus or participate in the passage of the virus. **B:** Soluble factors from I-A antigen-bearing cells induced by reovirus uptake affect the transport of reovirus through a second cell (i.e., a hepatocyte). (From Rubin DH, et al: Transport of infections reovirus into bile: class II major histocompatibility antigen-bearing cells determine reovirus transport. *J. Virol* 61:3222–3226, 1987, with permission.)

In addition to humoral immune responses, cellular immune responses are also induced following reovirus infection. Virus-specific cytotoxic T-lymphocyte (CTL) activity can be detected after infection with reovirus. These CTLs kill reovirus-infected cells in an antigen-specific, major histocompatibility complex MHC-restricted manner. A controversy about the specificity of these CTLs has recently developed. The first report[84] suggested that the σ-polypeptide was the major viral component recognized by CTLs. Thus CTLs were thought to be essentially serotype-specific. A more recent paper[85] has demonstrated CTL activity that is not serotype-specific, but is reovirus-specific and MHC-restricted, suggesting that the σ1-polypeptide is not the dominant antigen in a CTL response. Therefore CTLs generated during infection with one serotype of reovirus may participate in the immune response to a second serotype.

Although vigorous humoral and cellular virus-specific immune responses can be detected following infection, the role of specific immunity to reovirus was questioned in a paper by Letvin et al.[86] In this report, the role of T-cell mediated immunity to type 1 virus in C3H/HeJ mice was investigated. It was found that mice irradiated with ultraviolet light or athymic "nude" mice were no more susceptible to infection (as measured by virus titer in specific organs) than normal controls following intragastric administration of virus. These results suggested to the investigators that nonspecific immunity mediated by natural killer (NK)-cells or activated macrophages may be more important than specific immunity to reovirus in adult mice. It should be pointed out that tissue titers were evaluated 7–14 days after infection, and all of the titers were positive. Recent data from our laboratory utilizing a severe combined immunodeficient (SCID) mouse model suggest that functional T and B cells are necessary for protection (Kost, unpublished results). The SCID mice, which have functional macrophages and NK cells, but lack functional B and T cells, develop a localized inflammatory response surrounding antigen-positive hepatocytes. Functional T and B cells protect SCID mice from this disease. Therefore specific B- and T-lymphocyte subsets may play a role in resolution of infection. Furthermore, the restriction in replication of reovirus in adult mice is only in part due to immune mechanisms, while cellular target restrictions in replication probably account for the major barrier to infection in adult mice.

We have undertaken studies to determine the roles of reovirus-specific immune responses in a neonatal mouse model of infection. In these experiments, a highly virulent strain of reovirus type 3 (designated DH9 or type 3/mouse) is used to infect neonatal mice perorally. Reovirus type 3/mouse can induce a fatal encephalitis characterized by a meningoencephalitis. In contrast to reovirus type 3/D, type 3/mouse causes the encephalitis following peroral inoculation of 2–3-day-old mice.[79] Maternal immunization protects pups from lethal reovirus infection. Female mice were hyperimmunized with viable type 1/L or type 3/D by the subcutaneous or oral routes. The females were mated with noninfected, normal males, and the resulting offspring were infected 2 days after birth with 3×10^6 PFU of reovirus type 3/mouse intragastrically. The infected pups were observed for the development of neurologic disease and death. In addition, some pups were sacrificed 4 days after infection, and virus titers were determined from small intestine, liver, and brain. The results are summarized in Table 20–2.

We inferred from the results that passive immunity was responsible for the protection from death. In addition, immunity was partially serotype-nonspecific

Table 20–2 PASSIVELY ACQUIRED IMMUNITY TO REOVIRUS INFECTION

Treatment[b]	Day 4 Virus Titers[a]			
	Gut	Liver	Brain	Death
Normal	+	+	+	+
T1 SubQ	+	+	−	−
T1 PO	+	+	−	−
T3 SubQ	+	−	−	−
T3 PO	−	−	−	−

[a] Virus titers were determined by sacrificing three pups 4 days after infection and assaying tissues by plaque assay. +, positive virus titer; −, no detectable virus.

[b] Female mice were immunized with two treatments 1 week apart of 1×10^7 PFU of either type 1 (T1-serotype 1/Lang) or type 3 (T3-serotype 3/Dearing) reovirus by the oral (PO) or subcutaneous (SubQ) routes. Two weeks after the second treatment, the females were mated with normal males. The offspring were infected with 3×10^6 PFU type 3 (mouse strain) reovirus 2 days after birth.

because the pups from type 1 immune mothers did not die, although dissemination of virus to the liver was observed at day 4, and some mice developed histologic evidence of encephalitis. The type 3 immune mothers conferred immunity to the pups that limited virus replication to the gut (type 3 subcutaneous) or inhibited replication completely (type 3 peroral). These results indicate that cross-serotype immunity develops in hyperimmunized adults and that oral immunization of the mothers with the same serotype as the virus used to infect the pups is more effective than subcutaneous immunization. It is not yet known if neonatal immunity is related to unique features of neonatal gut permeability or is related to passively transferred antibody.

The results indicate that serotype-specific immunity to reovirus infection in neonatal infection is not necessary to protect from lethal disease. However, the consequences of a nonlethal encephalitis may be a deficit in neurologic function. This system clearly has relevance to other systems (e.g., rotavirus), in which protection from disease, but not necessarily infection, is provided by heterotypic (nonserotype identical) immunization. Further studies are in progress to define the exact role of cellular and humoral immunity in protection against infection.

CONCLUSIONS

Numerous disease-causing viruses of the GI tract have been described. The diseases that they induce range from subclinical to fatal GI or systemic organ infection. Recent advances in molecular biology and virus culture techniques, as well as improvements in animal models of these infections, have increased our understanding of the pathologic processes associated with these viruses.

While our overall understanding of these viruses has improved to the extent that many more viruses can be identified as pathogens, we are still a long way from achieving a thorough understanding of the pathogenesis of viral infection, the mechanisms that mediate immunity.

REFERENCES

1. Bishop RF, Davidson GP, Holmes IH, et al: Virus particles in epithelial cells of duodenal mucosa from children with acute non-bacterial gastroenteritis. *Lancet* ii:1281–1283, 1973.
2. Hall BA: Comparative pathology of infections by novel diarrhea viruses. In Bishop R: *Novel Diarrhea Viruses*. Ciba Foundation Symposium. Chichester 128:192–217, 1987.
3. Sack DA, Rhoads M, Molla A, et al: Carbohydrate malabsorption in infants with rotavirus diarrhea. *Am J Clin Nutr* 36:1112–1118, 1982.
4. Marin L, Saner G, Sokucu S, et al: Oral rehydration therapy in neonates and young infants with infectious diarrhea. *Acta Pediatr Scand* 76:431–437, 1987.
5. Kapikian AZ, Wyatt RG, Levine MM, et al: Oral administration of human rotavirus to volunteers: induction of illness and correlates of resistance. *J Infect Dis* 147:95–106, 1983.
6. Wyatt RG, Kapikian AZ, Greenberg HB, et al: Prospects for development of a vaccine against rotaviral diarrhea. In Holmes T, Holmgren J, Merson MH, et al: *Proceedings of Third Nobel Conference. Acute Enteric Infections in Children. New Prospects for Treatment and Prevention*. New York, Elsevier North-Holland, 1981, p 502.
7. Bishop RF, Barnes GL, Cipriani E, et al: Clinical immunity after neonatal rotavirus infection. A prospective longitudinal study in children. *N Engl J Med* 309:72–76, 1983.
8. Gorziglia M, Green K, Nishikawa K, et al: Sequence of the fourth gene of human rotaviruses recovered from asymptomatic or symptomatic infections. *J Virol* 62:2978–2984, 1988.
9. Vesikari T, Isolauri E, Ruuska T et al: Clinical trials of rotavirus vaccines. In Bishop R: *Novel Diarrhea Viruses*. Ciba Foundation Symposium. Chichester 128:218–231, 1987.
10. Totterdell BM, Chrystie IL, Banatvala JE: Cordblood and breast milk antibodies in neonatal rotavirus infection. *Br Med J* 280:828–830, 1980.
11. Totterdell BM, Nicholson KG, Macleod J, et al: Neonatal rotavirus infection: role of lacteal neutralizing alpha-anti-trypsin and non-immunoglobulin activity in protection. *J Med Virol* 10:37–44, 1982.
12. McLean BS, Holmes IH: Effects of antibodies, trypsin, and trypsin inhibitors on susceptibility of neonates to rotavirus infection. *J Clin Microbiol* 13:22–29, 1981.
13. Wyatt RG, Yolken RH, Vrrutia JJ, et al: Rotaviral immunity in gnotobiotic calves: heterologous resistance to human virus induced by bovine virus. *Science* 203:548–550, 1979.
14. Snodgrass DR, Wells PW: Rotavirus infection in lambs: studies on passive protection. *Arch Virol* 52:201–205, 1976.
15. Offit PA, Clark HF, Kornstein MJ, et al: A murine model for oral infection with a primate rotavirus (simian S11). *J Virol* 51:233–236, 1984.
16. Offit PA, Clark HF: Protection against rotavirus-induced gastroenteritis in a murine model by passively acquired gastrointestinal but not circulating antibodies. *J Virol* 54:58–64, 1985.
17. Offit PA, Blavat G, Greenberg HB, et al: Molecular basis of rotavirus virulence: role of gene segment 4. *J Virol* 57:46–49, 1986.
18. Offit PA, Shaw RD, Greenberg HB: Passive protection against rotavirus-induced diarrhea by monclonal antibodies to VP3 and VP7. *J Virol* 58:700–703, 1986.
19. Conner MG, Estes MK, Graham DY: Rabbit model of rotavirus infection. *J Virol* 62:1625–1633, 1988.
20. Hung T, Chen GM, Wang CA, et al: Rotavirus-like agent in adult non-bacterial diarrhea in China. *Lancet* ii:1078–1079, 1983.

21. Chen GM, Hung T, Bridger JC, et al: Chinese adult rotavirus is a group b rotavirus. *Lancet* ii:1123–1124, 1985.
22. Hung T, Chen G, Wang C, et al: Seroepidemiology and molecular epidemiology of the Chinese rotavirus. In Bishop R: *Novel Diarrhea Viruses*. Ciba Foundation Symposium. Chichester 128:49–62, 1987.
23. Saif LJ, Theil KW: Antigenically distinct rotaviruses of human and animal origin. In Tzipori S: *Infectious Diarrhoea in the Young: Strategies for Control in Humans and Animals*. Amsterdam, Excerpta Medica, 1985, p 208.
24. Kapikian AZ, Wyatt RG, Dolin R, et al: Visualization by immune electron microscopy of a 27nm particle associated with acute infectious non-bacterial gastroenteritis. *J Virol* 10:1075–1081, 1972.
25. Cukor G, Blacklow NR: Human viral gastroenteritis. *Microbiol Rev* 48:157–179, 1984.
26. Cubitt W, Blacklow N, Herrman JE, et al: Antigenic relationships between human caliciviruses and Norwalk virus. *J Infect Dis* 156:806–814, 1987.
27. Schreiber DS, Blacklow NR, Trier JS: The mucosal lesion of the proximal small intestine in acute infectious nonbacterial gastroenteritis. *N Engl J Med* 288:1318–1323, 1973.
28. Widerlite L, Trier JS, Blacklow NR, et al: Structure of the gastric mucosa in acute infectious non-bacterial gastroenteritis. *Gastroenterology* 68:425–430, 1975.
29. Agres SG, Dolin R, Wyatt RG, et al: Acute infectious non-bacterial gastroenteritis: intestinal histopathology: histologic and enzymatic alterations during illness produced by the Norwalk agent in man. *Ann Intern Med* 79:18–25, 1973.
30. Parrino TA, Schreiber DS, Trier JS, et al: Clinical immunity in acute gastroenteritis caused by Norwalk agent. *N Engl J Med* 297:86–89, 1977.
31. Jenkins S, Horman JT, Israel E, et al: An outbreak of Norwalk-related gastroenteritis at a boy's camp. *Am J Dis Child* 139:187–189, 1985.
32. Griffin MR, Surowiec JJ, McCloskey DI, et al: Foodborne Norwalk virus. *Am J Epidemiol* 115:178–184, 1982.
33. Koopman JS, Eckert EA, Greenberg AB, et al: Norwalk virus enteric illness acquired by swimming exposure. *Am J Epidemiol* 115:173–177, 1982.
34. Black RE, Greenberg HB, Kapikian AZ, et al: Acquisition of serum antibody to Norwalk virus and rotavirus and relation to diarrhea in a longitudinal study of young children in rural Bangladesh. *J Infect Dis* 145:483–489, 1982.
35. Ryder RW, Singh N, Reever WC, et al: Evidence of immunity induced by naturally acquired rotavirus and Norwalk virus infection on two remote Panamanian islands. *J Infect Dis* 151:99–105, 1985.
36. Madely CR, Cosgrove BP: 28nm particles in faeces in infantile gastroenteritis. *Lancet* ii:451–452, 1975.
37. Kurtz JB, Lee TW, Craig JW, et al: Astrovirus infection in volunteers. *J Med Virol* 3:221–230, 1979.
38. Gray EW, Angus KW, Snodgrass DR: Ultrastructure of the small intestine in astrovirus-infected lambs. *J Gen Virol* 49:71–82, 1980.
39. Woode GN, Pohleng JF, Gourlay NEK, et al: Astrovirus and Breda virus infections of dome cell epithelium of bovine ileum. *J Clin Microbiol* 19:623–630, 1984.
40. Kidd AH, Madely CR: *In vitro* growth of some fastidious adenoviruses from stool specimens. *J Clin Pathol* 34:213–216, 1981.
41. Takiff HE, Strauss SE, Garon LF: Propagation and *in vitro* studies of previous non-cultivable enteral adenovirus in 293 cells. *Lancet* ii:832–834, 1981.
42. Johansson ME, Uhnoo I, Kidd AH, et al: Direct identification of enteric adenoviruses, a

candidate new serotype associated with infantile gastroenteritis. *J Clin Microbiol* 12:95–100, 1980.

43. Uhnoo I, Wadell G, Svensson L, et al: Two serotypes of enteric adenovirus causing infantile diarrhoea. *Dev Biol Stand* 53:311–318, 1983.

44. Flewett TH, Bryden AS, Davies H: Epidemic viral enteritis in a long-stay children's ward. *Lancet* i:4–5, 1975.

45. Brandt CD, Kim HW, Rodriguez WJ, et al: Adenoviruses and pediatric gastroenteritis. *J Infect Dis* 151:437–443, 1985.

46. Uhnoo I, Olding-Stenkvist E, Kreuger A: Clinical features of acute gastroenteritis associated with rotavirus, enteric adenoviruses, and bacteria. *Arch Dis Child* 61:732–738, 1986.

47. Middleton PJ, Szymanski MT, Petric M: Viruses associated with acute gastroenteritis in young children. *Am J Dis Child* 131:733–737, 1977.

48. Uhnoo I, Wadell G, Svensson L, et al: Importance of enteric adenovirus 40 and 41 in acute gastroenteritis in infants and young children. *J Clin Microbiol* 20:365–372, 1984.

49. Ducatelle R, Coussement W, Hoorems J: Sequential pathological study of experimental porcine adenovirus enteritis. *Vet Pathol* 19:179–189, 1982.

50. Coussement W, Ducatelle R, Charlie G, et al: Adenovirus enteritis in pigs. *Am J Vet Res* 42:1905–1911, 1981.

51. Kagnoff MF, Austin RK, Hubert JJ, et al: Possible role for a human adenovirus in the pathogenesis of celiac disease. *J Exp Med* 160:1544–1557, 1984.

52. Coulepis AG, Anderson BN, Gust ID: Hepatitis A. *Adv Vir Res* 32:129–169, 1987.

53. Locarnini SA, Ferris AA, Lehmann NI, et al: The antibody response following hepatitis A infection. *Intervirology* 8:309–318, 1977.

54. Krugman S: Effect of human immune serum globulin on infectivity of hepatitis A virus. *J Infect Dis* 134:70–74, 1976.

55. Krugman S, Friedman H, Lattimer C: Viral hepatitis type A: identification by specific complement fixation and immune adherence tests. *N Engl J Med* 292:1141–1143, 1975.

56. Locarnini SA, Coulepis AG, Kador J, et al: Coproantibodies in hepatitis A: detection by enzyme-linked immunosorbent assay and immune electron microscopy. *J Clin Microbiol* 11:710–716, 1980.

57. Mathison LR, Moller AM, Purcell RH: Hepatitis A virus in the liver and intestine of marmosets after oral inoculation. *Infect Immun* 28:45–48, 1980.

58. Feinstone SM: Hepatitis A. *Prog Liver Dis* 8:299–310, 1986.

59. Stanley NF: Diagnosis of reovirus infections—comparative aspects. In Kurstak E, Kurstak K: *Comparative Diagnosis of Viral Disease.* New York, Academic Press, 1977, p 385.

60. Stanley NF, Joske RA: Animal model of human disease: chronic biliary obstruction caused by reovirus type 3. *Am J Pathol* 80:185–187, 1975.

61. Bangaru BE, Morecki R, Glaser JH, et al: Comparative studies of biliary atresia in the human newborn and reovirus-induced cholangitis in weanling mice. *Lab Invest* 43:456–462, 1980.

62. Onedra T, Toniolo A, Ray UR, et al: Virus induced diabetes mellitus XX. polyendocrinopathy and autoimmunity. *J Exp Med* 153:1457–1473, 1981.

63. Stanley NF, Joske RA: Animal model of human disease: chronic murine hepatitis induced by reovirus type 3. *Am J Pathol* 80:181–184, 1975.

64. Raine CS, Fields BN: Reovirus type III encephalitis—a virologic and ultrastructural study. *J Neuropathol Exp Neurol* 32:19–33, 1973.

65. Margolis G, Kilham L, Gonatas NK: Reovirus type III encephalitis: observations of

virus-cell interactions in neural tissue I. Light microscopy studies. *Lab Invest* 24:91–100, 1971.

66. Morecki R, Glaser JH, CMo S, et al: Biliary atresia and reovirus type 3 infection. *N Engl J Med* 307:481–484, 1982.

67. Rosen L: Serologic groupings of reoviruses by hemagglutination-inhibition. *Am J Hyg* 71:243–249, 1960.

68. Weiner HL, Ramig RF, Mustoe TA, et al: Identification of the gene coding for the hemagglutinin of reovirus. *Virology* 86:581–584, 1978.

69. Furlong DB, Neibert ML, Fields B: Sigma 1 protein of mammalian reovirus extends from surfaces of viral particles. *J Virol* 62:246–256, 1988.

70. Rubin DH, Fields BN: Molecular basis of reovirus virulence: role of the M2 gene. *J Exp Med* 152:853–868, 1980.

71. Wolf JL, Kauffman RS, Finberg R, et al: Determinants of reovirus interaction with the intestinal cells and absorptive cells of murine intestine. *Gastroenterology* 85:291–300, 1983.

72. Wolf JL, Rubin DH, Finberg R, et al: Intestinal M cells: a pathway for entry of reovirus into the host. *Science* 212:471–472, 1981.

73. Rubin DH, Kornstein MJ, Anderson AO: Reovirus serotype 1 intestinal infection: a novel replicative cycle with ileal disease. *J Virol* 53:391–398, 1985.

74. Rubin DH: Reovirus serotype 1 binds to the basolateral membrane of intestinal epithelial cells. *Microb Pathogen* 3:215–217, 1987.

75. Weiner DB, Giradrd K, Williams WV, et al: Reovirus type 1 and type 3 differ in their binding to isolated intestinal epithelial cells. *Microb Pathogen* 5:29–40, 1988.

76. Sharpe AH, Fields B: Pathogenesis of viral infections. *N Engl J Med* 312:486–497, 1985.

77. Weiner HL, Drayna D, Averill DR Jr, et al: Molecular basis of reovirus virulence: role of the S1 gene. *Proc Natl Acad Sci USA* 74:5744–5748, 1977.

78. Verdin EM, Lynn SP, Fields B, et al: Uptake of reovirus serotype 1 by the lungs from the bloodstream is mediated by the viral hemagglutinin. *J Virol* 62:545–551, 1988.

79. Hrdy DB, Rubin DH, Fields BN: Molecular basis of reovirus neurovirulence: role of the M2 gene in avirulence. *Proc. Natl Acad Sci USA* 79:1298–1302, 1982.

80. Rubin DH, Eaton MA, Costello T: Reovirus type 1 is secreted into the bile. *J Virol* 60:726–728, 1986.

81. Rubin DH, Costello T, Witzleben CL, et al: Transport of infectious reovirus into bile: class II major histocompatibility antigen-bearing cells determine reovirus transport. *J Virol* 61:3222–3226, 1987.

82. Weiner HL, Fields BN: Neutralization of reovirus: the gene responsible for neutralization antigen. *J Exp Med* 146:1305–1310, 1977.

83. Hayes EC, Lee Pwk, Miller SE, et al: The interaction of a series of hybridoma IgGs with reovirus particles. *Virology* 108:147–155, 1981.

84. Finberg R, Weiner HL, Fields BN, et al: Generation of cytolytic T-lymphocytes after reovirus infection: role of S1 gene. *Proc Natl Acad Sci USA* 76:442–446, 1979.

85. London SD, Rubin DH, Cebra JJ: Gut mucosal immunization with reovirus serotype 1/L stimulate virus specific cytotoxic T-cell precursors as well as IgA memory cells in Peyer's patches. *J Exp Med* 165:830–847, 1987.

86. Letvin N, Kauffman RS, Finberg R: T-lymphocyte immunity to reovirus: cellular requirements for generation and role in clearance of primary infection. *J Immunol* 127:2334–2338, 1981.

CHAPTER 21

Bacterial Infections

W. LANCE GEORGE

INTRODUCTION

Acute infectious diarrheal diseases are among the most prevalent of all illnesses and are particularly common in developing countries. In general, effective means for preventing these diseases do not exist; although effective treatment exists for most of the bacterial enteritides, the cost of treatment and the incidence of morbidity and mortality of these illnesses are unacceptable. It is quite evident that development of effective vaccines for prevention of infection by certain enteric pathogens would represent a major advance in medicine.

Investigation of the immunologic interactions between the human gut and potentially enteropathogenic bacteria is extremely difficult for several reasons, including the relative inaccessibility of the human gastrointestinal tract to direct study, the presence of an enormous (and therefore, confounding) resident or normal bacterial flora in the colon, and the variety of pathogenic mechanisms by which different types of potentially harmful bacteria may attack the gastrointestinal tract of both the normal and the impaired host.

In considering the bowel and bacterial infections, one must recognize several relatively different types of disease processes[1] (Table 21–1); the nature of these illnesses usually depends more on the properties of the bacterium than on the host or host defenses. Some bacterial enteropathogens cause dysfunction of the mucosal cell but do not damage the cell, *e.g.*, the enterotoxigenic (heat-labile-toxin-producing) organisms, *Escherichia coli* and *Vibrio cholerae*. Other enteropathogens may cause injury to, and dysfunction of, the mucosal cell. Most of these "invasive" organisms do not invade the host beyond the bowel wall, *e.g.*, *Campylobacter jejuni*, enteroinvasive *E. coli*, and *Shigella*, sp. A few invasive enteropathogens, such as *Salmonella* sp. (particularly *Salmonella typhi*), *Vibrio vulnificus*, and *Yersinia enterocolitica* are relatively likely to produce disseminated or metastatic infection.

Table 21–1 POSSIBLE MECHANISMS OF DISEASE PRODUCTION BY ENTEROPATHOGENIC BACTERIA[a]

Mechanism	Action
Toxins	
Heat-labile enterotoxins	Cause increased fluid secretion and/or decreased fluid absorption by small bowel without causing cell injury; causal factor in diarrhea due to 01 *V. cholerae* and certain *E. coli;* also found in many other enteropathogens, but role in disease unclear
Heat-stable enterotoxins	Produce disease similar to that caused by heat-labile toxins but act by different mechanisms and are not immunologically related to heat-labile toxins; causal factor in diarrhea due to certain *E. coli* strains and present in other enteropathogens
Cytotoxins	Many different types, but role in disease not always clear (examples include *C. difficile* cytotonic toxin, *Shigella* Verotoxins, *Salmonella* cytotoxin, *Aeromonas* cytolytic toxin, etc.)
Invasive properties	Invasive *E. coli* and *Shigella* possess similar plasmids that code for ill-defined invasive properties; invasiveness of *Y. enterocolitica* is mediated by a 41-MD plasmid, and certain *Salmonella* strains possess a plasmid that permits replication within the reticuloendothelial system
Mucosal cell attachment	Attachment necessary for disease production by some enteropathogens, but attachment per se does not cause disease (e.g. heat-labile, toxin-producing *E. coli*) Enteroadherence per se by some strains of "enteropathogenic" *E. coli* possibly appears to alter mucosal function, thereby causing diarrhea; three different types of enteroadherence have been described

[a] (Modified from Gorbach SL (ed): Infectious diarrhea. *Infect Dis Clin N Am* 2:557–676, 1988)

Certain bacteria can also cause disease of the gut by producing a toxin that is then ingested by the host; this type of disease is often referred to as bacterial food poisoning because the toxin is produced in food contaminated by the bacterium. Because many enteropathogenic bacteria can be, and frequently are, transmitted by contaminated foods, it is more appropriate (and less confusing) to refer to disease caused by toxin ingestion as an intoxication; most of these, such as *Staphylococcus aureus* or *Bacillus cereus* (food poisoning) are self-limited diarrheal diseases. An important exception, however, is botulism; the diarrhea that may occur in botulism can initially confuse the clinician by overshadowing the potentially lethal systemic effects of the toxin.

It is important to appreciate that the bowel may also be the source of disseminated illness in the patient who is immunocompromised as a consequence of corticosteroid or cytotoxic chemotherapy. In this type of individual, the gastrointestinal tract serves as the portal of entry for bacteremia caused by organisms that are not enteropathogenic; the most common example of this is gram-negative bacillary bacteremia due to organisms such as *Pseudomonas aeruginosa*, *Enterobacter* sp., *Klebsiella pneumoniae,* and other members of the family Enterobacteriaceae.

NONIMMUNOLOGIC HOST DEFENSES

There are several nonimmunologic host factors that are important in providing protection against bacterial pathogens[2] (Table 21–2). Personal hygiene is obviously a major defense against bacterial enteric infections because virtually all such infections arise following ingestion of the pathogen. The state of nutrition is a major determinant of the integrity of both the immunologic and the nonimmunologic host defenses; our understanding of how nutrition affects these defenses is, unfortunately, fragmentary.

A low gastric pH is extremely important for prevention of infection with *V. cholerae* and probably for many other organisms, because exposure to an acidic environment is often lethal. The rise in gastric pH associated with antacid or H_2 antagonists, hypo- or achlorhydria, or even the ingestion of food may allow the enteric pathogen to escape exposure to the deleterious effects of stomach acid. The harmful effects of pancreaticobiliary secretions upon potential enteric pathogens has not been well studied but may represent another host defense. Two physical barriers to potential pathogens that are of major importance to the host are gastrointestinal mucus, which can bind or entrap bacteria (thereby preventing them from gaining access to the mucosa), and the integrity of the mucosa itself (which prevents bacteria from gaining access to deeper tissues and thereby prevents possible dissemination of infection). Intestinal motility (and possibly even hypermotility resulting from infection) serve to expel pathogens from the gut, thereby reducing their numbers and the concentrations of their "toxic" products; this expulsive effect helps to protect the host when a potential pathogen is ingested or to limit the severity of disease when infection cannot be prevented.

Another host factor that is an important determinant of susceptibility to infection is the presence or absence of mucosal receptors. Host species-specific mucosal receptors for antigens of the attachment organelles [e.g., K88, K99, and colonization factors (CFI and CFII)] of enterotoxigenic *E. coli* are thought to be essential for disease production; for example, K88 antigen-producing strains of *E. coli* that cause lethal diarrhea in suckling piglets are incapable of causing diarrhea in humans because human gut mucosal cells do not express a receptor for the K88 antigen. Similarly, (human) enteropathogenic strains of *E. coli* that have lost their ability to produce CFI or CFII are no longer able to cause significant diarrhea in humans because they cannot attach to the gut mucosa and "deliver" toxin directly to the site of action. Certain bacterial toxins are also known to bind to mucosal

Table 21–2 NONIMMUNOLOGIC ENTERIC HOST DEFENSES

Hygiene
State of nutrition
Gastric acidity
Gastrointestinal mucus
Physical integrity of the mucosa
Bowel motility
Presence/absence of intestinal receptors
Colonization resistance (colonic microflora)
Age

"receptors" (e.g., cholera toxin to Gm_1 ganglioside); such toxin-binding sites have not been found to be toxin- or species-specific, however. A complete understanding of the mechanisms by which bacteria and their toxins bind to host mucosal cells is essential for vaccine development; manipulation of the immune system so as to prevent these "binding" events is the key to development of an effective vaccine for any of the bacterial enteric pathogens.

The contents of the distal colon normally contain a total of at least 100 billion bacterial cells per gram of material, which may represent 300–400 different bacterial species or variants;[3] viruses, yeasts, and protozoa do not appear to be an important component of the normal human enteric flora. The flora of the mid- and proximal colon is somewhat less complex, but still resembles that of the distal colon.[4] The remainder of the bowel lacks a normal flora but probably often contains low counts of bacteria that are present transiently. The normal colonic flora is extremely stable and resistant to colonization by nonresident bacteria.

Based on clinical and laboratory observations, it appears that the normal flora represents a major deterrent to intestinal infection by certain bacteria. For example, diarrhea due to *Clostridium difficile* rarely, if ever, occurs in the absence of antimicrobial therapy; antibiotics are thought to alter the protective properties of the colonic flora in the adult, thereby permitting *C. difficile* (if present) to proliferate, produce toxins, and cause diarrhea. The frequent presence of this organism and its toxins in the gut of asymptomatic neonates, however, is contradictory and presently not explained.[5]

Hentges[6] in a summary of his work and that of others, noted that components of the normal colonic flora inhibited intestinal colonization by *Salmonella*, *Shigella*, and *V. cholerae* in laboratory animals; one must appreciate, however, that the disease produced by each one is different in terms of pathogenesis and site of attack in the gastrointestinal tract. These and other data, however, support the thesis that the "colonization resistance" provided by the normal flora of the colon is an important host defense against colonic infection by certain enteric pathogens.

Age is an important factor in susceptibility to infection by certain types of pathogens, such as enteropathogenic *E. coli*. The susceptibility of the infant or young child to enteric infection is complex and probably represents age-related differences in gut mucus, cell surface factors (such as receptors), resident microbial flora, environmental exposure to potential pathogens, and incomplete development of gut-related immunity.

Clearly, a number of nonimmunologic factors are important in the prevention or amelioration of bacterial enteric infections. The vital role of gut-related immunity in helping the host to deal with such infections is quite evident, however, when one considers the impaired ability, or complete inability of the immunodeficient patient to defend against a variety of enteric pathogens that cause self-limited disease in the immunocompetent individual. The most extreme example of this is the patient infected with the human immunodeficiency virus (HIV).

IMMUNOLOGIC RESPONSE OF THE HOST TO THE NORMAL BOWEL FLORA

As indicated above, the human colon always contains prodigious numbers of bacteria that are considered to be normal flora. A potentially important aspect of the host's defense against enteric infection is the extent to which the immune system recognizes indigenous gram-negative bacteria, particularly *E. coli,* as non-self; this is an important issue, in that many enteric pathogens (e.g., *Salmonella, Shigella,* and *E. coli*) are members of the family Enterobacteriaceae and have a number of similar biochemical components, such as surface lipopolysaccharide. In a recent review, Berg[7] noted that several investigators have found IgG, IgA, and IgM reacting with *E. coli* in the sera of healthy volunteers; moreover, several investigators have reported the presence of secretory IgA, which reacted with *E. coli* and other enteric bacteria in human colostrum and intestinal secretions. In addition, he noted that one group of investigators had found that various species of Enterobacteriaceae in the feces of normal human subjects were coated with "intestinal" IgA.

The difficulty in interpreting these data in regard to intestinal infection is that one cannot determine to which epitopes these antibodies were directed. In other words, it is unclear whether or not the normal bacterial flora confers a certain basic level of "intrinsic" immunity upon the host; there is indirect evidence to suggest that this is not an important factor in resistance to enteric infection. For example, it is generally believed that an individual is immune to the strains of heat-labile, toxin-producing *E. coli* that are prevalent in his or her area of residence, presumably as a consequence of prior exposure to, or infection by such strains; a person traveling to a different geographic area does not possess effective immunity to the environmental strains of pathogenic *E. coli* prevalent in that area and is, therefore, known to be at significant risk for developing diarrhea ("travelers' diarrhea").

IMMUNOPATHOLOGY OF BACTERIAL ENTERIC INFECTIONS

The number of known or suspected enteric bacterial pathogens is quite extensive (Table 21-3). A great deal is known regarding the immunopathology of infection by some, but not all, of these bacterial species. The aspects of immunity that are

Table 21-3 POTENTIAL BACTERIAL ENTERIC PATHOGENS

Bacterium	Comment
Vibrio cholerae	
Noncholera *Vibrio*	Many species
Escherichia coli	Seven possible mechanisms for causing diarrhea
Shigella	Four species
Salmonella	Approximately 1,500 serotypes
Yersinia enterocolitica	
Campylobacter	At least seven species
Aeromonas	10-12 DNA homology groups, each of which may represent a separate species
Plesiomonas shigelloides	
Bacillus cereus[a]	
Clostridium botulinum[a]	
Clostridium difficile	
Clostridium perfringens[a]	
Staphylococcus aureus[a]	

[a] An agent of food poisoning or intoxication.

important for enteric pathogens can be appreciated by assessing the published literature for certain selected organisms. The development of effective vaccines for each of the important enteric pathogens requires an understanding of the pathogenesis of the disease produced by the organism in question.

Vibrio cholerae

Attempts to determine the exact nature of naturally acquired immunity to cholera (that is, immunity resulting from naturally acquired infection, as opposed to infection produced by challenge of a volunteer with the pathogen) date back at least 50 years;[8] many studies involved investigation of the organisms in various animal models.[8] The ligated rabbit ileal loop assay was developed in the 1950s and demonstrated the usefulness of animal models for the study of bacterial enteric disease. Despite years of research, however, the currently licensed parenteral cholera vaccine does not prevent asymptomatic infection (i.e., colonization of the gut); it reduces diarrhea in approximately 50% of vaccinees and provides immunity for a relatively brief duration (3–6 months).[1] Thus the currently available parenteral vaccine(s) is impractical for the prevention or control of cholera epidemics.

Part of the difficulty in developing an effective vaccine for cholera, however, was the heavy reliance placed upon studies in various animal models; a thorough study published by Holmgren et al. in 1975[9] led to the conclusion that "toxoid vaccination, particularly by the s.c. [subcutaneous] route may be useful for improved immunoprophylaxis against cholera." Holmgren's group subsequently reported[10] that there was a close correlation between the magnitude of intestinal synthesis of specific antitoxic IgA following immunization by various routes and protection against intestinal challenge with cholera toxin; neither serum nor intestinal IgG or IgM were found to be protective. It is important to appreciate that the cholera toxin molecule consists of five circularly arranged B subunits, an A_2 subunit, and an A_1 subunit; the B subunit serves to bind the toxin molecule to mucosal Gm_1 ganglioside, the A_1 subunit is responsible for activating adenylate cyclase (which is the diarrhea-inducing step), and the A_2 subunit is thought merely to bind A_1 to the B subunits. Thus antitoxic immunity acquired as a consequence of natural disease conceivably could be directed against any or all of these toxin components.

Recurrent symptomatic infections by *V. cholerae* appear to be uncommon, a finding suggesting that natural infection is highly protective, in contrast to the relatively poor protection conferred by standard vaccines. The concept that prior infection is highly protective is supported by a large surveillance study done in East Pakistan (an area in which cholera is highly prevalent) from 1963 to 1970; only 14 cases of reinfection by *V. cholerae* were documented during this period.[11] In an excellent study published in 1981, Levine et al.[12] showed that four volunteers were immune to rechallenge with either homologous or heterologous serotypes of *V. cholerae* 33–36 months after initial infection; none developed diarrhea, and only one was found to excrete the organism after rechallenge. Interestingly, secretory IgA was not detectable in jejunal fluid from the "cholera veterans" prior to rechallenge, nor was it detectable in the control subjects prior to initial challenge. Two of the four "cholera veterans" and one of the control subjects did, however, have appreciable rises in secretory IgA by day 8 postchallenge; interestingly, the control subject who had a rise in secretory IgA was the only one of the five controls who did not develop diarrhea. All of the controls and two of the four "veterans" also had appreciable rises in serum titers of vibriocidal antibody. These data suggest that natural immunity to cholera is complex and may be due to a synergistic protective effect of both antibacterial and antitoxic activities.

The most reasonable explanation for the mechanism of acquired anticholera immunity involves adherence of *V. cholerae* or cholera antigens to intestinal "M cells"; the organism (and its important antigens, such as lipopolysaccharide, adhesin, and flagellar and toxin antigens) is transported to subepithelial lymphocytes that enter the circulation, are "processed" at a distant site, and then return to the lamina propria (and other mucosal tissues) to produce IgG and secretory IgA.[13-17] The exact mechanisms involved in immunity are difficult to unravel because the important antigen-antibody interactions are undoubtedly occurring at the mucosal surface; measuring antibodies in the gut, particularly within a few microns of the epithelium, is difficult because of potential interactions with intestinal mucus and hydrolysis by luminal proteolytic enzymes.

Presently available data[18] suggest that the best candidate vaccine is a combined B subunit-whole cell vaccine.

Escherichia coli

Consideration of the immunopathology of *E. coli* enteric infections is difficult because of the several different mechanisms of disease production. With the exception of enteroinvasive *E. coli,* however, the disease processes are probably similar to those of cholera, because they occur primarily at the mucosal surface. Of the *E. coli*-induced diarrheas, the disease caused by heat-labile-toxin-producing strains is best understood; this toxin resembles cholera toxin, both in structure and mechanism of action. A recent study[19] in which approximately 50,000 Bangladeshi children and women were given either a combined cholera B subunit-whole cell killed vaccine or the whole cell killed vaccine alone (by mouth) evaluated the development of diarrhea due to *V. cholerae* and to heat-labile-toxin-producing *E. coli*. The rationale for such a study was that the B subunits of cholera and *E. coli* toxin are antigenically similar, and vaccination with a preparation containing the B subunit of one toxin might confer protection against the other. These investigators found marked short-term (3 months) protection against *E. coli* diarrhea, but no protection was noted during the subsequent 9 months. These data suggest that it may be possible to augment the response to a B subunit-containing vaccine to the point that longer-lasting immunity can be achieved. In addition to causing travelers' diarrhea, heat-labile, toxin-producing *E. coli* are a major cause of morbidity and mortality in infants and small children in developing countries.

Toxigenic strains of *E. coli* may produce a heat-stable toxin (STa) either instead of, or in addition to, heat-labile toxin. This toxin acts via activation of guanylate cyclase, produces fluid accumulation in the suckling mouse assay, but not in the rabbit ligated ileal loop assay, and is poorly immunogenic. Relatively little is known about the immunopathology of diarrhea due to this toxin.

Strains of *E. coli* previously known as enteropathogenic *E. coli* have recently been found to possess unusual properties and are more aptly termed enteroadherent *E. coli*. These organisms belong to serogroups that have been linked epidemiologically to diarrhea (particularly in infants) but lack the enteric pathogenic properties of other *E. coli* strains, such as heat-labile or heat-stable toxin production, or the invasiveness of *Shigella*. Studies in adult volunteers have affirmed the ability of these organisms to cause diarrhea. These enteroadherent *E. coli* bind closely to the mucosal cell membrane, and there may be destruction of the underlying microvilli;

evidence of invasion is not seen. The actual mechanism(s) by which these organisms cause diarrhea is not known, but recently published studies have shed light on the enteropathogen-host mucosal cell interaction.[13] One type of enteroadherent *E. coli,* called RDEC-1, causes diarrhea in rabbits. This organism differs from *V. cholerae* in that it is not transported through the M cell to the subepithelial lymphoid tissues; such transport is considered to be essential for subsequent production of secretory IgA in the bowel mucosa. Inman et al.,[20] using recombinant techniques, generated two different strains of RDEC-1 *E. coli;* one strain expressed a *Shigella flexneri* somatic antigen, was readily transported to the underlying lymphoid tissue by the M cell, and was appreciably less virulent than the other strain, which possessed the original RDEC-1 *E. coli* 015 somatic antigen. These findings suggested that the virulence of RDEC-1 *E. coli* is related to the inability of the M cell to transport it to subepithelial lymphoid tissue. In other words, if M-cell transport does not occur, there is a blunted or absent mucosal immune response, and the organism is able to proliferate unchecked on the mucosal surface; this unrestrained proliferation allows large numbers of enteroadherent *E. coli* to attach to absorptive cells and, by a yet unknown mechanism, cause diarrhea.

Recently, *E. coli* 0157:H7 has been found to be a cause of hemorrhagic colitis. This serotype and certain other serotypes of *E. coli* produce a Vero or Shiga-like toxin or toxins. These toxins are capable of inactivating 60S ribosomal subunits in rabbit cells and can cleave ribosomal RNA. In addition, they contain a plasmid that encodes for an antigen that mediates attachment to intestinal epithelial cells in vitro.[1] Medically, there are two important aspects to this organism. First, although it is not invasive, the organism is capable of causing a hemorrhagic colitis by virtue of a cytolytic toxin. Second, and perhaps more important, Vero toxin-producing *E. coli* and Shiga toxin-producing *Shigella* species have been implicated as causal agents of the hemolytic-uremic syndrome. Preliminary studies have suggested that vascular endothelial cells may be a target of the toxin in this disease. Prevention of infection could be achieved possibly by development of a vaccine to attachment antigens.

Enteroinvasive *E. coli* invade the intestinal mucosa and produce a disease clinically indistinguishable from shigellosis. Virulence is plasmid-mediated, and there is appreciable homology between the invasiveness plasmid of enteroinvasive *E. coli* and *Shigella.*

Shigella Species

Classical shigellosis is a biphasic illness in which voluminous watery diarrhea is followed by the development of bloody mucoid stools that frequently contain large numbers of granulocytes; the former phase of disease is thought to involve abnormalities of fluid resorption in the small bowel, whereas the later stage represents invasion of the colonic mucosa. Keusch and Jacewicz[21] reported the production by *Shigella* of a cytolytic toxin that was lethal to HeLa cells; this cytolytic toxin was produced by *S. sonnei, S. flexneri,* and *S. dysenteriae* type 1 and was distinct from the Shiga toxin. Some investigators have speculated that the watery diarrhea seen early in shigellosis might be caused by the cytotoxin; data to support this contention are sparse, however. The essential virulence characteristic of *Shigella* is mucosal cell invasiveness. The invasive properties of virulent strains are associated with several proteins encoded by a 140-MD plasmid.[22] Epidemiologic data suggest that at least partial immunity is conferred by natural infection. Reed and Williams[23] found that fecal antibodies of the IgG, IgA, and IgM classes were increased following naturally acquired shigellosis. Moreover, these antibodies possessed anti-*Shigella* activity. Lowell and colleagues[24] studied serum and peripheral blood lymphocytes, monocytes, and granulocytes from normal subjects and individuals convalescing from shigellosis. They found that the in vitro anti-*Shigella* activity of cellular elements required immune serum but not complement; this process of inhibition of bacteria by Fc receptor-bearing cells in the presence of antibody (but absence of complement) was termed antibody-dependent cell-mediated antibacterial activity and is similar to antibody-dependent cell-mediated cytotoxicity. The mucosal surface and tissues of the gut are relatively rich in immunoglobulin and mononuclear cells but are deficient in complement. Lowell and coworkers theorized that Fc receptor-bearing lymphocytes, monocytes, and granulocytes, in the presence of appropriate antibody, might therefore be an important host defense against enteric pathogens such as *Shigella.*

The study by Inman et al.[20] mentioned above may also provide an indication of another potential virulence factor for *Shigella* and other invasive enteropathogens. The ability of the M cell to bind and transport a virulent enteric pathogen into the submucosa might carry significant risks for the host, because in effecting such transport the protective "barrier" properties of the intact mucosa would be bypassed. The mechanisms by which the defenses of the submucosa might either kill or limit the proliferation of a pathogen have not been defined; thus M cell transport might be one of the first steps in mucosal invasion.[13]

A recent clinical trial suggested that prevention of shigellosis by vaccination might be possible. Black et al.[25] created a bivalent oral vaccine by transferring a 120-MD plasmid of *Shigella sonnei* that encodes for O lipopolysaccharide antigen into an attenuated strain of *Salmonella typhi.* Significant protection for the vaccinees against subsequent challenge with *S. sonnei* was noted, as was the presence of serum and local intestinal immune responses. Part of the rationale for this approach is related to some unique properties of the *S. typhi* used. This *Salmonella* has shown efficacy as an oral vaccine against typhoid fever; more important, however, is the fact that this strain crosses the mucosa of the small intestine and is ingested by macrophages but is not immediately killed. This allows the attenuated *Salmonella* strain to bring antigens into direct contact with lymphoid tissues and may permit it to evoke a stronger immune response than does a carrier strain that does not leave the bowel lumen.

Salmonella Species

Consideration of the pathogenesis and immunopathology of *Salmonella* infection is an extremely difficult task. In the United States from 1975 to 1985, approximately 370,000 isolations of *Salmonella* were reported to the Centers for Disease Control. Approximately 35% of these isolates were *Salmonella typhimurium.* Nine other serotypes each accounted for from 1.5% to 8% of the total; the remaining isolates constituted approximately 29% of the total and probably represented at least 40 different serotypes. Thus we might want to consider approximately 50 different serotypes of *Salmonella* in order to evaluate the role of this genus in human disease in the United States. Our difficulties are compounded by the fact that the diseases these serotypes may produce in humans range from typhoid fever to a self-limited enteritis to asymptomatic carriage. There appears to be a variety of potential virulence factors among the various serotypes; moreover, these organisms are often highly adapted to their primary host species and may infect humans only incidentally.

After ingestion, the organism proliferates in the small bowel lumen and probably penetrates the mucosa in the distal ileum and proximal large bowel; some authorities have suggested that this may occur through the M cell,[1,13] as was suggested above for *Shigella.* The mechanism of diarrhea production is not known; some have suggested that the invading organisms interact with polymorphonuclear cells that then release prostaglandins, thereby causing diarrhea, whereas others have suggested that "*Salmonella* enterotoxins" are elaborated.[1,26]

After the organism has penetrated the mucosa, it may multiply in Peyer's patches and then spread to regional lymph nodes; this is probably the usual extent of infection. However, when the organism is *S. typhi,* or less commonly another species of *Salmonella,* there may be spread to the systemic circulation through the thoracic duct and dissemination of the organism to virtually any tissue.

There are many factors that may contribute to the virulence of *Salmonella.*[1] The lipopolysaccharide O antigen can activate C3, resulting in phagocytosis; the presence of the virulence antigen (Vi) on *S. typhi* apparently prevents the binding of C3, thereby inhibiting phagocytosis. Probably one of the most important virulence factors of *Salmonella* is its ability to survive within the macrophage following ingestion, permitting the organism to persist and even proliferate in the host and to remain in a site that shields it from the other host defenses. Some investigators have suggested that virulence plasmids may allow the organism to persist and multiply within phagocytes,[1] but this has not been substantiated for most species. Hornick et al.[27] have suggested that endotoxin release may be responsible for many of the systemic findings of typhoid fever; such release has not been clearly established despite a number of studies that have attempted to implicate continued circulation of endotoxin as a major aspect of pathogenesis.

As indicated previously, an attenuated strain of *S. typhi* has been successful as an oral vaccine in protecting against development of typhoid fever.[25] Immunization with this strain (*S. typhi* Ty21a) evokes a specific secretory IgA response to both lipopolysaccharaide and flagellar antigens after oral administration;[28] it is thought that these responses are important for development of immunity.

Yersinia enterocolitica

This is a rather unique organism that may produce a variety of diseases, the most common of which are enteritis and mesenteric lymphadenitis.[1] The organism penetrates the intestinal mucosa and proliferates in the lymphoid tissues. Several virulence factors appear to be plasmid-encoded and exhibit a marked temperature dependence for expression. Such factors include invasiveness (in certain animal models), autoagglutinability, resistance to the bactericidal activity of human serum, and synthesis of a unique surface antigen (VW antigen). The VW antigen confers resistance to phagocytosis by polymorphonuclear leukocytes as well as certain other traits. Many strains also produce a heat-stable toxin that resembles the heat-stable enterotoxin of *E. coli,* but its importance in disease production is unknown.

Campylobacter Species

Although there are several species of *Campylobacter* that may infect or colonize the gastrointestinal tract of humans, those that have received the greatest attention recently are *C. jejuni* and *C. pylori (C. pyloridis); C. fetus* is an important organism because of its propensity to cause disseminated infection in the setting of immunodepression. Because the role, if any, of *C. pylori* in human gastroduodenal disease is unclear, it will not be discussed here; there are several excellent review papers that address the potential role in disease of this organism.[29,30]

Campylobacter jejuni is one of the most commonly detected bacterial enteric pathogens and affects both children and adults. It appears, however, that there are marked differences in the host-parasite interaction in various parts of the world. In industrialized countries, ingestion of *C. jejuni* is usually associated with development of both systemic and gastrointestinal symptoms of infection. Clinically, the organism appears to possess invasive properties manifested by the presence of fecal leukocytes and occult blood in the stool; in some patients the illness may be that of an overt colitis or dysentery. Regardless, the illness is invariably self-limited in the immunocompetent host, although relapse with subsequent resolution may occasionally occur. Chronic carriage in industrialized countries is uncommon.[1] In contrast, there is an appreciable incidence of asymptomatic carriage in parts of the Indian subcontinent and Africa and a tendency for the illness to be less severe than it is in industrialized countries.[1,31-33] Blaser et al.[33] assessed *C. jejuni*-specific serum immunoglobulins in children from Bangladesh and the United States and found significantly higher levels in the former group. In Bangladeshi children, specific serum IgA levels rose linearly with age, IgG peaked in the 2–4-year-old age group and then fell, and IgM levels peaked in the 2–4-year-old age group and then leveled off; these findings were somewhat unexpected. Blaser and colleagues speculated that repeated exposure to the organism might explain the elevated serum IgA (one presumes that secretory IgA was also elevated) and that the presence of such antibodies might prevent tissue invasion by the organism; they postulated that this protective effect might result in a decline in specific serum IgG (presuming that serum IgG reflected a response to invasion) with age. Serum levels of IgM specific for *C. jejuni* tended to plateau in children from both countries; they suggested that this finding might reflect a certain amount of cross-reactivity between *C. jejuni* and members of the normal bowel flora. These hypotheses are attractive and could help to explain the age-related decline in asymptomatic carriage, the lesser frequency of fever and bloody diarrhea, and the generally milder form of illness in Bangladeshi children than in children in the United States. The presence of at least partial gut immunity (which can be inferred from the higher specific serum immunoglobulin levels) would also explain the frequent lack of symptoms or mild form of illness observed in older children and adults in Bangladesh, in comparison with the United States. Similar findings were noted in a rural community in Thailand.[34]

Our understanding of the mechanism of disease production by *C. jejuni* is quite poor.[1] Several investigators have detected a heat-labile toxin of *C. jejuni* that behaves like cholera toxin (i.e., causes fluid accumulation in an animal ligated ileal loop model and elongation of Chinese hamster ovary cells in tissue culture) and that can be neutralized in assay systems by cholera antitoxin; the medical implications of these findings are potentially quite significant because of the potential for producing a vaccine that would be active against *C. jejuni, V. cholerae,* and heat-labile, toxin-producing *E. coli*. It must be remembered, however, that *C. jejuni* can also produce an invasive colitis; thus the significance of a cholera-like toxin in regard to disease production and vaccine development is not clear. Other investigators have described a cytotoxin that is active against Vero and HeLa cells.[1] Although *C. jejuni*-induced illness in the immunologically naive individual resembles shigellosis, a mechanism or marker for invasiveness (such as the invasiveness plasmid of *Shigella*) has not been described.

Kiehlbauch et al.[35] have suggested an additional virulence mechanism of *C. jejuni*. These investigators found that human peripheral blood monocytes would rapidly ingest *C. jejuni* in the absence of opsonins but that the organisms were able to survive intracellularly for at least 6 days, whereas the organism survived for only 1–2 days extracellularly. The relevance of this in vitro study to gastrointestinal tract infection is unclear but certainly warrants further attention.

It is possible that in industrialized countries the disease process is due both to a cholera-like enterotoxin (hence the watery diarrhea) and to invasive properties that lead to mucosal destruction; in developing countries, however, there may be sufficient existing immunity to prevent invasion of the mucosa but not to prevent the effects of a cholera-like enterotoxin. This hypothesis, however, is contrary to our present knowledge regarding the immune response to invasiveness properties and enterotoxins.

Although *C. jejuni* enteritis is a self-limited disease in immunocompetent individuals, Dworkin et al.[36] reviewed reports of 12 immunodeficient patients with "chronic diarrhea" due to this organism and noted that the usual underlying process was hypo- or agammaglobulinemia. Although these data are anecdotal, they indicate the potential importance of antibody in eradicating this organism from the gastrointestinal tract.

Campylobacter fetus is usually isolated from blood or other extraintestinal sites (but rarely from feces), whereas *C. jejuni* is rarely recovered from sites outside the gastrointestinal tract. Clinical data suggest that the portal of entry for *C. fetus* is the gut and that a history of antecedent diarrheal illness can often be obtained from patients with *C. fetus* bacteremia. Blaser et al.[37] reported significant differences in the serum susceptibilities of the two species. *C. fetus* was found to be highly resistant to normal human serum, whereas *C. jejuni* demonstrated complement- and antibody-mediated serum sensitivity. This differential serum susceptibility may explain the rarity with which *C. jejuni* is found in blood and the (relative) frequency of *C. fetus* bacteremia.

Other Bacterial Enteric Pathogens

There are a number of other important bacterial enteric pathogens (see Table 21–3), but information regarding the immunopathology of infections in humans by these agents is relatively sparse. A meaningful review of host-parasite interactions for many enteric pathogens therefore, is not possible.

Whipple's Disease

This fascinating disease probably holds the keys to some of the immunologic mysteries of bacterial enteric infections. The four most prominent symptoms are weight loss, diarrhea, arthralgia, and abdominal pain.[38] Histologically, the disease is characterized by peculiar macrophages in virtually all organs. These cells stain intensely with the periodic acid-Schiff reagent and have been shown to contain intracellular bacterial-like organisms that have been termed the Whipple bacillus; the bacillus can be found in a wide variety of other host cells, including intestinal epithelial cells, lymphatic and capillary endothelial cells, smooth muscle cells, polymorphonuclear leukocytes, plasma cells, mast cells, and intraepithelial lymphocytes. Although the organism cannot be cultivated in vitro or in an animal model, the response in most patients to treatment with antibiotics supports the belief that the disease is a bacterial infection. These findings have led to the belief that the Whipple bacillus is an intracellular pathogen and that Whipple's disease is a disseminated bacterial infection that originates in the gastrointestinal tract.

CONCLUSIONS

There is an enormous volume of literature on immunologic aspects of the bacterial enteritides; unfortunately, much of it focuses on systemic immunity rather than gut-associated immunity or else is based on animal studies. Admittedly, the assessment of local (mucosal) immune responses in humans to bacterial pathogens is extremely difficult; however, determining the extent to which animal models of enteric disease can be applied to human illness is even more difficult, if not impossible. Conley and Delacroix, in a recent review,[39] pointed out several differences between the rat and the human in regard to production, distribution, and catabolism of IgA. The fact that there is not even one vaccine for a bacterial enteric infection that confers relatively long-term immunity is quite remarkable and a true indication of our ignorance of such infections. The very recent and significant progress in vaccine development validates the thesis that these diseases must also be studied in humans (not just in laboratory animals) and is a measure of the value of molecular and cellular biology in the study of these diseases.

The available data indicate that M-cell transport and production of secretory IgA are major aspects of defense against enteropathogens that interfere with mucosal cell function; the role of cellular elements in this type of process is less clear. Enteroinvasive pathogens may utilize the M cell as one means for traversing the mucosal cell layer to enter the submucosa; once the submucosa has been entered and there has been proliferation of the pathogen, the full array of humoral and cellular defenses are undoubtedly brought into play. The mechanisms by which intracellular pathogens (such as *S. typhi*) avoid destruction by mononuclear cells is unclear. It is evident that local immunity may prevent subsequent mucosal invasion by many pathogens following either immunization or naturally acquired infection.

REFERENCES

1. Gorbach SL (ed): Infectious diarrhea. *Infect Dis Clin N Am* 2:557–676, 1988.
2. Guerrant RL: Principles and definition of syndromes. In Mandell GL, Douglas RG Jr, Bennett JE: *Principles and Practice of Infectious Diseases,* ed 2. New York, John Wiley & Sons, 1985, p 635.
3. Finegold SM, Sutter VL, Mathisen GL: Normal indigenous intestinal flora. In Hentges

DJ: *Human Intestinal Microflora in Health and Disease.* New York, Academic Press, 1983, p 3.

4. George WL, Finegold SM: Clostridia in the human gastrointestinal flora. In Borriello SP: *Clostridia in Gastrointestinal Disease.* Boca Raton, FL, CRC Press, 1985, p 2.

5. Cooperstock M: *Clostridium difficile* in infants and children. In Rolfe RD, Finegold SM: *Clostridium difficile: Its Role in Intestinal Disease.* San Diego, Academic Press, 1988, p 46.

6. Hentges DJ: Role of the intestinal microflora in host defense against infection. In Hentges DJ: *Human Intestinal Microflora in Health and Disease.* New York, Academic Press, 1983, p 311.

7. Berg RD: Host immune response to antigens of the indigenous intestinal flora. In Hentges DJ: *Human Intestinal Microflora in Health and Disease.* New York, Academic Press, 1983, p 101.

8. Freter R: Coproantibody and bacterial antagonism as protective factors in experimental enteric cholera. *J Exp Med* 104:419–426, 1956.

9. Holmgren J, Svennerholm A-M, Ouchterlony O, et al: Antitoxic immunity in experimental cholera: protection, and serum and local antibody responses in rabbits after enteral and parenteral immunization. *Infect Immun* 12:1331–1440, 1975.

10. Svennerholm A-M, Lange S, Holmgren J: Correlation between intestinal synthesis of specific immunoglobulin A and protection against experimental cholera in mice. *Infect Immun* 21:1–6, 1978.

11. Woodward WE: Cholera reinfection in man. *J Infect Dis* 123:61–66, 1971.

12. Levine MM, Black RE, Clements ML, et al: Duration of infection-derived immunity to cholera. *J Infect Dis* 143:818–820, 1981.

13. Sneller MC, Strober W: M cells and host defense. *J Infect Dis* 154:737–741, 1986.

14. Pierce NF, Gowans JL: Cellular kinetics of the intestinal immune response to cholera toxoid in rats. *J Exp Med* 142:1550–1563, 1975.

15. Owens RL, Pierce NF, Apple RT, et al.: M cell transport of *Vibrio cholerae* from the intestinal lumen into Peyer's patches: a mechanism for antigen sampling and for microbial transepithelial migration. *J Infect Dis* 153:1108–1118, 1986.

16. Elson CO, Ealding W: Generalized systemic and mucosal immunity in mice after mucosal stimulation with cholera toxin. *J Immunol* 132:2736–2741, 1984.

17. Jones GW, Freter R: Adhesive properties of *Vibrio cholerae:* nature of the interaction with isolated rabbit brush border membranes and human erythrocytes. *Infect Immun* 14:240–245, 1976.

18. Svennerholm A-M, Jertborn M, Gothefors L, et al: Mucosal antitoxic and antibacterial immunity after cholera disease and after immunization with a combined B subunit-whole cell vaccine. *J Infect Dis* 149:884–893, 1984.

19. Clemens JD, Sack DA, Harris JR, et al: Cross-protection by B subunit-whole cell cholera vaccine against diarrhea associated with heat-labile toxin-producing enterotoxigenic *Escherichia coli:* results of a large-scale field trial. *J Infect Dis* 158:372–377, 1988.

20. Inman LR, Cantley JR, Formal SB: Colonization, virulence, and mucosal interaction of an enteropathogenic *Escherichia coli* (strain RDEC-1) expressing shigella somatic antigen in the rabbit intestine. *J Infect Dis* 154:742–751, 1986.

21. Keusch GT, Jacewicz M: The pathogenesis of *Shigella* diarrhea. VI. Toxin and antitoxin in *Shigella flexneri* and *Shigella sonnei* infections in humans. *J Infect Dis* 135:552–556, 1977.

22. Hale TL, Oaks EV, Formal SB: Identification and antigenic characterization of virulence-associated, plasmid-coded proteins of *Shigella* species and enteroinvasive *Escherichia coli. Infect Immun* 50:620–629, 1985.

23. Reed WP, Williams RC Jr: Intestinal immunoglobulins in shigellosis. *Gastroenterology* 61:35–45, 1971.

24. Lowell GH, MacDermott RP, Summers PL, et al: Antibody-dependent cell-mediated antibacterial activity: K lymphocytes, monocytes, and granulocytes are effective against *Shigella. J Immunol* 125:2778–2784, 1980.

25. Black RE, Levine MM, Clements ML, et al: Prevention of shigellosis by a *Salmonella typhi-Shigella sonnei* bivalent vaccine. *J Infect Dis* 155:1260–1265, 1987.

26. Stephen J, Wallis TS, Stark WG, et al: Salmonellosis: in retrospect and prospect. In: *Microbial Toxins and Diarrhoeal Disease.* Ciba Foundation Symposium 112, London, 1985, p 175.

27. Hornick RB, Greisman SE, Woodward TE, et al: Typhoid fever: pathogenesis and immunologic control. *New Engl J Med* 283:686–691, 739–746, 1970.

28. Cancellieri, Fara GM: Demonstration of specific IgA in human feces after immunization with live Ty21a *Salmonella typhi* vaccine. *J Infect Dis* 151:482–484, 1985.

29. Blaser MJ: Gastric *Campylobacter*-like organisms, gastritis, and peptic ulcer disease. *Gastroenterology* 93:371–383, 1987.

30. Bartlett JG: *Campylobacter pylori:* fact or fancy? *Gastroenterology* 94:229–238, 1988.

31. Blaser MJ, Glass RI, Huq MI, et al: Isolation of *Campylobacter fetus* subsp. *jejuni* from Bangladeshi children. *J Clin Microbiol* 12:744–747, 1980.

32. Rajan DP, Mathan VI: Prevalence of *Campylobacter fetus* subsp. *jejuni* in healthy populations in southern India. *J Clin Microbiol* 15:749–751, 1982.

33. Blaser MJ, Black RE, Duncan DJ, et al: *Campylobacter jejuni*-specific serum antibodies are elevated in healthy Bangladeshi children. *J Clin Microbiol* 21:164–167, 1985.

34. Blaser MJ, Taylor DN, Echeverria P: Immune response to *Campylobacter jejuni* in a rural community in Thailand. *J Infect Dis* 153:249–254, 1986.

35. Kielbach JA, Albach RA, Baum LL, et al: Phagocytosis of *Campylobacter jejuni* and its intracellular survival in mononuclear phagocytes. *Infect Immun* 48:446–451, 1985.

36. Dworkin B, Wormser GP, Abdoo RA, et al: Persistence of multiply antibiotic-resistant *Campylobacter jejuni* in a patient with the acquired immune deficiency syndrome. *Am J Med* 80:965–970, 1986.

37. Blaser MJ, Smith PF, Kohler PF: Susceptibility of *Campylobacter* isolates to the bactericidal activity of human serum. *J Infect Dis* 151:227–236, 1985.

38. Dobbins WO III: Whipple's disease. In Mandell GL, Douglas RG Jr, Bennett JE: *Principles and Practice of Infectious Diseases,* ed 2. New York, John Wiley & Sons, 1985, p 695.

39. Conley ME, Delacroix DL: Intravascular and mucosal immunoglobulin A: two separate but related systems of immune defense? *Ann Intern Med* 106:892–899, 1987.

CHAPTER 22

Prospects for Oral Vaccines for Enteric Bacterial Infections

Edgar C. Boedeker

INTRODUCTION

The prospects for the development of effective oral vaccines against enteric bacterial pathogens have never been greater. There are several reasons for optimism. First, over the past 10 years, there has been a tremendous expansion in our knowledge of the "molecular pathogenesis" of enteric bacterial infections.[1,2] We now understand many of the specific bacterial (and host) determinants of enteric colonization and virulence at the level of gene regulation, gene expression, and mechanisms of action of gene products. For many recognized bacterial virulence factors, such as colonization factors and toxins, complete protein and gene sequence data are available. Thus we have increased knowledge of the antigenic targets for vaccine development.[3]

Second, our expanded molecular knowledge has also increased our ability to more readily diagnose enteric pathogens.[4] Such specific reagents as monoclonal antibodies and gene probes, which have been designed to detect specific virulence factors, are now being used in combination with improved, or simplified, culture techniques. When appropriate tests are used, etiologic agents can now be ascribed to a majority of cases of diarrhea. With the exception of rotavirus, most of the agents responsible for epidemic diarrhea, infantile diarrhea, and diarrhea of travelers have proved to be limited to a few bacterial pathogens, which can now account for the majority of cases. These include *Shigella*, *Vibrio cholerae*, enterotoxigenic *Escherichia coli*, *Salmonella*, and *Campylobacter jejuni*.

The views expressed herein are those of the author and not necessarily those of the United States Army or the Department of Defense.

Third, vaccine development for bacterial enteric infections seems to be a realistic, if as yet largely unrealized, goal since, for many of these infections, active enteric infection confers protective immunity.[5] This has been shown directly by volunteer studies[3], and suggested in epidemiologic studies in endemic areas. The protective mechanism has not been definitively proved, but it is widely assumed to be mucosally produced and secreted immunoglobulin of the IgA class.[6] In addition, for a number of analogous enteric bacterial pathogens of animals, passively administered intraluminal antibody (as colostrum) has been shown to protect young animals against these analogous enteric infections, suggesting that a mucosal antibody response should be sufficient for protection.[7,8] This principle was recently extended to passive antibody protection of human enteric disease when it was shown that hyperimmune cow's milk immunoglobulin concentrate could protect against challenge of volunteers with virulent enterotoxigenic *E. coli*.[9]

Finally, as illustrated throughout this volume, recognition of the independent nature of the mucosal immune system, and knowledge of its function and regulation, have been expanding in parallel with the expansion of knowledge of bacterial virulence mechanisms. This knowledge strongly suggests that oral (or other mucosal) immunization is the preferred method to stimulate gut mucosal secretory immunity. The challenge is to effectively combine our knowledge of bacterial pathogenesis and mucosal immunity to actively immunize susceptible hosts, and to maintain that immunity, in order to prevent enteric bacterial infection. This will require strategies for antigen selection and delivery that will stimulate local immunity, avoid local suppression, and also avoid the production of disease.

This chapter will review the very limited number of currently available vaccines for enteric bacterial infections; describe the desired characteristics of oral vaccines; discuss recent and current research efforts in enteric vaccine development for individual pathogens; and suggest future approaches to the solution of this important problem.

CURRENTLY AVAILABLE VACCINES

Currently available vaccines for public health use in the United States against enteric bacterial infections are limited to vaccines for *Salmonella typhi,* the agent of typhoid fever, and *V. cholera.* Both of these generally available vaccine preparations are killed whole cell vaccines for parenteral use. Of these two, only the *V. cholerae* vaccine qualifies primarily as a vaccine against an enteric infection, but its use is seldom recommended.

The parenteral heat-phenol killed (L) or acetone killed (K) typhoid vaccines have provided good protection (60% efficacy in field trial studies) against typhoid fever,[10] which is a systemic disease acquired through enteric exposure, via Peyer's patch and/or mucosal invasion. Its protective efficacy is probably related to systemic, cell-mediated immunity against somatic antigens.[11,12] Its ability to protect against typhoid, but not other salmonellae, stems from the homogeneity of the somatic antigens of typhoid strains, and the great diversity of other salmonella serotypes.

The killed whole cell cholera vaccine still available is based on a mixture of the major cholera serotypes and biotypes, but without cholera toxin. This vaccine induces serum vibriocidal, but not antitoxic, activity that correlates with protection in residents of endemic areas. Since parenteral vaccines may also boost mucosal responses, this may be the mechanism whereby the currently available killed whole cell cholera vaccine enhances immunity in endemic areas, where populations have been primed enterically by environmental exposure. Field trials of this vaccine indicated 50% efficacy in reducing clinical illness from cholera for 3–6 months. It is no longer required by the Public Health Service (PHS) for travelers coming to the United States from cholera endemic areas, nor is it recommended by the World Health Organization (WHO) for travelers to endemic areas.[13]

DESIRABLE CHARACTERISTICS OF ORAL VACCINES

As exemplified by the limited utility of the existing parenteral cholera vaccine, parenteral vaccines have not been, and are not likely to be, effective primary inducers of mucosal immunity. This is because of the well-documented requirement to populate the lamina propria with effector cells by homing events initiated in the organized lymphoid tissue of the gut (Peyer's patch). Oral, or other mucosally administered, vaccines are likely to be superior for priming for mucosal immune system.

As presently conceived, oral vaccines may take the form of either living, attenuated, or avirulent strains of microorganisms (bacteria or viruses), or nonliving antigenic material. Live bacterial vaccine strains have been produced by mutagenesis of pathogens and are currently being developed through the more directed approach of genetic engineering to delete virulence determinants, to modify them, or to transfer their expression to other carrier organisms. Nonliving vaccines under development range from killed whole bacterial cells to isolated virulence factors to specific peptide epitopes coupled to carriers and/or adjuvants.

The two alternative methods of antigen delivery into the gut have their own advantages and disadvantages. Living vaccines are much more economical to produce in quantity than purified nonliving material, and they have the distinct advantage of replication to increase the antigenic load. In practice, however, with live vaccines, it has been much more difficult to achieve a reproducible phenotype through production scale-up and formulation, to avoid lot-to-lot variability in production, and to reproducibly reconstitute in the field. Nonliving material is subject to degradation by the digestive process.

In order for an oral vaccine of either type to induce an effective primary mucosal sIgA immune response, it may be helpful if it shares some of the properties of enteric pathogens. Oral vaccines must resist the acid environment of the stomach and the proteolytic activity of pancreatic and brush border enzymes. Many live oral vaccine strains can survive passage through the stomach (to divide and colonize the gut and be shed in the feces) if administered with acid-neutralizing agents or inhibitors of acid secretion. Such antacid protection may not be sufficient for nonreplicating vaccines, which are susceptible to hydrolysis. These may require specific methods of protection such as encapsulation or other antigen delivery systems.

Ideal oral vaccines should be targeted for delivery to the organized lymphoid tissue of the Peyer's patch, as is the case for virulent cholera, *Salmonella, Shigella, E. coli,* and *C. jejuni.* The portal of entry is the specialized antigen-sampling M cell in the lymphoepithelium over the dome of the patch.[14] In this regard, live oral vaccines seem to have a great advantage; the work of Owen[15] has suggested that live organisms are much more effectively taken up by M cells (either specifically or permissively) than killed ones. In addition, live organisms might be engineered to express specific molecules that target them to the M cell. M-cell targeting of nonliving vaccine material may be achievable by presenting it in particles of a certain size, or in association with molecules (such as monoclonal antibodies) that recognize M cell surface components.

Oral vaccines should include or express appropriate "protective" protein or carbohydrate antigens characteristic of virulent strains. Since passively administered luminal antibody can prevent enteric infection,[7-9] the desired effector response to vaccination is a mucosal secretory IgA response directed at critical bacterial antigens. Target antigens of choice may be colonization factor antigens or invasion antigens that are involved in the initial stages of pathogenesis, or other surface molecules, such as outer membrane proteins or lipopolysaccharide (LPS) components, which are universally expressed by pathogenic strains. Bacterial exotoxins are additional logical targets since they are required for virulence of many pathogens. These antigens may be administered expressed by living strains, as intact proteins, or as selected epitopes.

Distinct protein or carbohydrate B-cell epitopes will be required to select appropriate Peyer's patch B-cell precursors for proliferation, differentiation to IgA antibody-producing cells, and migration to the lamina propria. B-cell epitopes are likely not to be linear but to depend on tertiary protein structure; they may now be mimicked, however, by novel means such as anti-idiotypic antibodies.[16] The target antigens should also include appropriate linear, amphipathic T-cell peptide epitopes for presentation to the T-cell receptor in association with class II molecules on antigen-presenting cells[17,18] in order to stimulate antigen-specific Peyer's patch T-cell help for antibody synthesis and secretion. Ideally, the immunizing T and B epitopes would be linked to provide directed T-cell help for specific antibody synthesis and secretion.[19] It is not clear whether T-cell cytotoxic mechanisms play a role in defense against nonsystemic enteric bacterial infections, as they are likely to against virally infected cells, although Tagliabue has suggested a role for IgA-mediated bacterial cytotoxicity.[20,21]

Although there is general agreement that mucosal antibody is the primary effector, it is not clear whether protection conferred by natural enteric infection is provided by maintaining some minimal levels of luminal antibody at the mucosal surface or in the bile (perhaps through repeated subclinical exposure to pathogens or through booster immunizations), or whether protection is achieved by establishing sufficient mucosal memory so that the host is capable of initiating a rapid and strong secondary immune response upon subsequent exposure to the pathogen. Such a secondary response would have to be extremely rapid in order to prevent infection, instead of simply contributing to more rapid clearance of infecting organisms. If a rapidly effective secondary response can occur, it is likely to be achieved by local stimulation and proliferation of primed B- and T-cell populations in the lamina propria at the site of antigen exposure (although it might also be reinforced by recruitment of cells homing from the organized lymphoid tissue). This suggests that vaccines for booster immunizations might be designed differently from those for primary immunization, to target the lamina propria rather than the organized lymphoid tissue. They could be designed for uptake across the absorptive epithelium to the lamina propria, providing epitopes for presentation by lamina propria macrophages, by class II-positive B cells or perhaps by epithelial cells, to stimulate T-cell help to B-cell proliferation and secretion of antibody. As an additional strategy, booster vaccines might include only T-cell epitopes to permit them to avoid immune exclusion by pre-existing antibody within the lumen.

BACTERIA VACCINES, CURRENT DEVELOPMENT AND PROSPECTS

Priorities for vaccine development have been guided by the definition of important pathogens through epidemiologic studies. Current efforts are focused on *Shigella* (five groups, multiple serotypes), which are epidemic in Asia, frequently antibiotic-resistant, and associated with multiple systemic complications; on *V. cholerae*, which is responsible for a continuing pandemic (two serotypes, two biotypes); and on the enterotoxigenic *E. coli* (multiple serotypes, several colonization factor antigens), which are responsible for infantile diarrhea in developing countries and remain the single most important cause of traveler's diarrhea. Other pathogens also demand attention. *Campylobacter jejuni* is emerging as a frequent cause of infant and traveler's diarrhea; *Yersinia enterocolitica* is increasingly recognized in cold climates, and enteropathogenic *E. coli*, which is responsible for childhood diarrhea, is also beginning to receive renewed attention as its pathogenesis is better understood. If effective vaccines could be developed for these agents (as well as for rotavirus), the majority of lethal and disabling diarrheal diseases would be controlled.

Not all of the above agents are equal candidates for vaccine development. The likelihood of successful vaccine development for a given pathogen is increased if there is little antigenic drift in essential antigens, if there is one, or only a few, clones of the pathogen responsible for most cases of disease, or if there are shared essential virulence determinants among the several clonal types. Development is also encouraged if there is evidence that infection with a pathogen confers a degree of protective immunity. Based on such criteria, the Institute of Medicine has predicted that vaccines for international use for *S. typhi, Shigella, V. cholerae,* and enterotoxigenic *E. coli* species will be available within the next ten years.[22] This review will focus on these organisms. In contrast, the multiplicity of non-typhoidal salmonella serotypes, inadequate knowledge of common pathogenic mechanisms, and mildness of illness, makes it unlikely that a vaccine against non-typhoid salmonellae will be forthcoming in the near future. Rapid advances are being made in understanding the virulence determinants of *Campylobacter, Yersinia* and enteropathogenic *E. coli* that may advance the development of vaccines, but these organisms are beyond the scope of this review.

In contrast to the increased understanding of the antigen requirements for regulating the mucosal immune response and achieving T-B cooperation, the development of enteric vaccines has been somewhat empiric. Selection of new antigens for inclusion in vaccines is currently based on knowledge of the role of these antigens in pathogenesis. This role is frequently defined in in vitro systems, such as cell or organ culture, using genetically engineered strains to define virulence determinants. It is increasingly apparent that antigen expression by bacteria is dependent on culture conditions; therefore antigens prominently expressed in vitro may not be expressed in vivo, or may be only transiently expressed. This is particularly true for antigens involved in particular stages of pathogenesis.[1,2] Choice of a particular antigen for vaccine development is supported by the demonstration that this same antigen is recognized by antibody produced during infection. Frequently, only convalescent serum antibody is available from epidemiologic studies, although breast milk IgA and sIgA from intestinal purges have occasionally been utilized.[23] Recently it has been shown possible to detect IgA antibody-producing B cells in the circulation following enteric infection or immunization. These cells presumably represent B cells migrating from the organized lymphoid tissue of the gut en route to the lamina propria.[24] This methodology should be important both to define antigens and to determine vaccine immunogenicity. Methods for defining relevant antigens, using immune serum or secretions, range from bacterial agglutination to Western blots against electrophoretically separated antigens[25,26] to enzyme-linked immunosorbent assays (ELISA) against purified antigens, including peptide epitopes. Vaccines need not be limited to such naturally immunogenic epitopes, since it is theoretically possible to induce antibody, by vaccination, to a protective epitope, which might not be recognized during natural infection.

Once a vaccine product has been developed, demonstrations of safety, immunogenicity, and efficacy against challenge are required. When animal models of human enteric infections are available, they are extremely useful to screen for these required properties of vaccines. Unfortunately, most of the important enteric bacterial infections are limited in their host range to humans (or occasionally to humans and other higher primates). This is true for *Shigella*, for those enterotoxigenic *E. coli* strains that infect humans, and to a large extent for *V. cholera*. Thus animal models of enteric bacterial infection frequently involve extensive manipulation designed to inactivate host clearance mechanisms[27] to permit colonization of nonnatural hosts. These models are useful, but one must be aware that such manipulations may also obscure the role of bacterial adherence or other virulence mechanisms in causing disease, rendering protection either excessively difficult to achieve, or irrelevant to natural infections. Infections of primates have also been a useful stage of vaccine development, but disease processes may differ even in these animals. For example, *Shigella* strains infect monkeys only at doses much higher than those required to infect humans. For these reasons, development of antibacterial enteric vaccines has relied heavily on human volunteer challenge studies, often as the initial test of efficacy. The lack of good animal models has slowed the development process. To date, nonliving oral vaccines have tended to be safe, but poorly immunogenic. This may relate to inadequate protection against proteolysis and poor M-cell uptake. Living oral vaccines based on attenuated pathogenic strains, or on the expression of virulence determinants in nonpathogens, have often failed to achieve the appropriate balance between safety and immunogenicity.

Recent vaccine development has produced two oral vaccines, one living attenuated strain and one nonliving combination vaccine, which provide alternatives to the current parenteral typhoid and cholera vaccines, respectively. The production of a safe, immunogenic, and effective live oral typhoid vaccine (strain Ty21a)[28] has had broad implications for oral vaccine development, since this vaccine strain has been recognized as a carrier for other immunizing antigens.

Typhoid Vaccines Against *S. typhi:* Bacteria That Invade and Produce Systemic Infection

Salmonella typhi is not primarily important as a cause of diarrhea.[12] It is responsible for typhoid fever, which is an enterically acquired systemic illness predominantly affecting school age children. Although two effective parenteral typhoid vaccine formulations (based on heat-killed or formalin-treated whole organisms) have been long available, development of alternate vaccines was stimulated by the high incidence of side effects of parenteral whole cell vaccines, particularly local reactions with painful swelling at the injection site accompanied by fever.[10] An additional parenteral vaccine based on highly purified Vi capsular polysaccharide (which is universally present on blood isolates) has been developed, tested, and found to have few adverse reactions and to be effective with single-dose regimens in providing protection against typhoid fever.[29]

The live attenuated Ty21a strain of *S. typhi* was successfully developed by Germanier and Furer[28] as an oral typhoid vaccine by introducing a mutation in the virulent parent strain. This strain was not designed to be defective in any specific virulence determinants, but only in survival ability. Ty21a has a chemically induced mutation in the enzyme UDP galactose-4-epimerase (galE), which was felt to account for its inability to survive in mammalian tissues. In the absence of galactose the strain is unable to express its LPS O antigen and is susceptible to cell-mediated killing. In the presence of galactose the strain accumulates toxic amounts of galactose-1-phosphate and UDP-galactose, and lyses. These assumptions have apparently proved to be oversimplifications of the actual attenuating lesions, since Hone et al.[30] have shown that a genetically engineered mutation in galE did not eliminate the pathogenic potential of *S. typhi*. Nevertheless, Ty21a appears to achieve its immunizing effect, which is primarily cell-mediated, by being capable of sufficient invasion to achieve antigen exposure, but only limited survival in tissue. It is now an established vaccine that is safe and effective.

Testing of the efficacy of the Ty21a vaccine in different endemic areas has provided insight into the difficulties encountered in standardizing formulation, production, and administration of live oral bacterial vaccines in order to provide significant protection in the field. Thus, in an initial double-blind field trial in Egypt,[31] the vaccine achieved 96% protection when the reconstituted, lyophilized vaccine was administered in three doses following gastric neutralization by bicarbonate. In contrast, when the lyophilized vaccine was administered in Chile in enteric-coated capsules,[32] or in gelatin capsules with bicarbonate (but not reconstituted), it achieved only 67% protection. A direct comparison of encapsulated versus reconstituted preparations is now being undertaken. Increased numbers of doses appear to give increasing protection, but also increase the expense of administration.[10]

Stocker[33] has prepared an attenuated *S. typhi* vaccine strain 541Ty by introducing mutations in the chromosomal genetic loci termed aroA and purA. These mutations render the strain auxotrophic for paramino benzoate and adenine, respectively, which can be supplied in growth media but which are not available as substrates in the human host. The strain should be capable of only limited replication in the human host, but still capable of mimicking the initial stage of natural infection. The combination of two mutations in the strain should markedly decrease the chance of reversion to virulence by back mutation. In contrast to Ty21a, there should be no alterations in the expression of surface antigens. This strain has been demonstrated to be safe in human volunteers,[34] and it induced cell-mediated immunity against *S. typhi,* but little humoral immunity. It is suggested that the requirement for adenine reduced both tissue survival and live-vaccine efficacy, and that strains blocked only in aromatic biosynthesis may be more effective oral vaccines. Such vaccines are now in preparation. These *Salmonella* mutant strains might also be useful as carriers of antigens, and similar mutations might be introduced in other pathogens.

Curtiss et al.[35] have developed avirulent mutants of *S. typhimurium,* a parent strain that induces only diarrheal disease in humans but causes a systemic typhoid-like illness in mice. Their strategy has been to induce deletion mutations in the cya and crp chromosomal genetic loci, which determine production of adenylate cyclase and the cyclic AMP receptor. These strains have been utilized to deliver streptococcal antigens.

The Ty21a strain, and subsequently developed attenuated *Salmonella* strains, have acquired particular importance to the field of enteric vaccine development, since they may serve as potential carriers of heterologous antigens relevant to other enteric infections. Several such "bivalent" candidate vaccines have been produced by techniques of genetic engineering, including vaccines for malaria,[36] dental caries,[35] cholera,[37] enterotoxigenic *E. coli,*[38] and shigellosis.[39]

Shigella and Enteroinvasive *E. coli:* Bacteria That Invade and Proliferate in Epithelial Cells

There are currently no acceptable vaccines for shigellosis or enteroinvasive *E. coli,*[40] although a number of candidates have been produced. Of the 30 *Shigella* serotypes, most cases of shigellosis are caused by *Shigella sonnei* (in industrialized nations), *Shigella flexneri* 2a and 3 (in developing nations), and *Shigella dysenteriae* 1, which is responsible for the current epidemics in southern Asia and Africa. Enteroinvasive *E. coli* are genetically homologous to *Shigella,* share *Shigella* virulence mechanisms, and also have a limited number of different serogroups.

There is evidence for serotype-specific immunity to shigellosis; therefore attenuation of virulent shigellae to provide serotype-specific immunity (to selected prevalent serotypes) offers one long-standing approach to vaccine development. Spontaneous avirulent mutants of *S. flexneri* that are noninvasive have been used to provide serotype-specific protection in monkeys, but high doses were required.[41] In Yugoslavia,[42] noninvasive streptomycin-dependent mutants have been utilized with some success in clinical trials. These strains required high doses and repeated boosting; an additional disadvantage of these strains is their instability, with the possibility of reversion to full virulence. Recently Lindberg et al.[43] have produced aromatic auxotrophic *Shigella* mutants that require aromatic substances for growth. These organisms have invasive properties but poor survival in tissue. It is also hoped that these organisms will provide cross-protection against multiple serotypes by choosing an LPS for surface expression that consists of a component common to many serotypes. These vaccines are now being prepared for clinical trial.

A large body of work[44] has related specific genetic loci in *shigellae* (and their products) to the stages of *Shigella* virulence, thereby offering an additional approach to vaccine development.[39,45] Both plasmid and chromosomal genes, and their products, are involved in *Shigella* virulence. Virulent shigellae invade and multiply in colonic epithelial cells (or tissue culture cells), in a process that can be divided into several stages, including attachment, penetration, uptake in vacuoles, lysis of vacuoles, intracellular multiplication, and invasion of adjacent cells.

Chromosomal genes are involved in the production of full virulence in animal models including the induction of an inflammatory conjunctivitis in the eye of the guinea pig (Sereny test) (the kcp locus, cotransducible with purE) and in the production of fatal disease in starved guinea pigs (a locus near the xyl-rha region encoding an aerobactin system for iron binding). Although organisms lacking any of these regions can still invade cultured cells, it is presumed that these chromosomal determinants are related to the ability of the invading organisms to survive in tissues. Organisms that do not express O antigen (rough strains) are also avirulent. Serogroup-specific O antigen expression is a chromosomally determined property located near the His region in *S. flexneri* and *S. sonnei* but is, in part, a plasmid-regulated property in *Shigella dysenteriae*.

Invasion is determined by genes encoded on large (120 *S. flexneri* or 140 *S. sonnei* MD) virulence plasmids.[46] Studies of the expression of plasmid-encoded *Shigella* proteins in minicell systems have shown that these plasmids encode at least seven *Shigella* outer membrane proteins that appear to be related to attachment and uptake. Other plasmid-encoded regions are responsible for survival in epithelial cells and lysis of endocytic vacuoles.

An additional virulence determinant of *Shigella* strains is the production of shiga toxin, at high levels, by *S. dysenteriae*, and at lower levels by strains of other serogroups. Shiga toxin is a protein exotoxin that interferes with protein synthesis. It is not directly associated with invasiveness, but its production has been associated with extraintestinal manifestations of shigellosis, including hemolytic-uremic syndrome. Shiga toxin production should be eliminated from any candidate vaccine strain.

Because of the genetic similarity between *Shigella* and *E. coli*, it has been possible to produce partially or fully virulent *Shigella* by transfer of *Shigella* chromosomal or plasmid-associated virulence regions into *E. coli*[47,48] or, conversely, by replacing *Shigella* virulence genes with corresponding loci from *E. coli*. The aim of such transfers in vaccine development is to maintain sufficient invasiveness and survival capacity to induce an immune response, but insufficient virulence to cause disease. This has been a difficult balance to achieve.

Several vaccines based on transfer of the above virulence regions between *E. coli* and *Shigella* have been developed. An invasive vaccine was produced by Formal et al.[49] by transferring the xyl-rha region of *E. coli* K12 into *S. flexneri* 2a. This vaccine strain invaded cultured cells, survived poorly in tissue, and protected monkeys against challenge, but also caused diarrhea in human volunteers. A more recent vaccine candidate (EC104) has been produced by transferring the 140 MD *S. flexneri* 2a invasion plasmid, as well chromosomal His and Pro regions, into *E. coli* K-12.[50] This strain produces transient mucosal invasion and expresses the *S. flexneri* 2a serotype. It provided some degree of protection to monkeys without adverse reactions; however, human volunteers receiving this strain experienced some symptoms.[39]

Since protection is associated with somatic antigen immunity, a further approach was to transfer the *S. sonnei* O antigen genes into the Ty21a invasive carrier strain.[39] This was achieved by transfer of the *S. sonnei* plasmid. This hybrid vaccine has protected monkeys against *S. sonnei* challenge, but it has been difficult to produce reproducible lots of the vaccine for human studies;[51] thus field trials have not been undertaken. A similar construct has been produced bearing the *S. flexneri* type and group antigen genes in Ty21a.[52]

Vibrio cholera and Enterotoxigenic *E. coli:* Bacteria That Adhere and Produce Cytotonic Toxins

These organisms share pathogenic mechanisms. They are completely noninvasive, but colonize mucosal surfaces, a process aided by the production of surface adhesins. Although cholera and enterotoxigenic *E. coli* (ETEC) adhesins are unrelated, both types of organism produce analogous heat-labile toxins that induce fluid secretion by epithelial cells without cytotoxic effects. ETEC also produce a family of heat-stabile toxins. Both the adhesive factors and toxins are potential immunogens and candidates for vaccine development.

Vibrio cholerae

Pathogenic cholera vibrios are of only two major serotypes (Ianaba and Ogawa) within two biotypes (classical and El Tor), all of which are contained in the available heat- and formalin-inactivated parental vaccine.[3,13] In addition, they all produce cholera toxin, composed of one A (active, the proenzyme form of ADP-ribosyl-transferase) and five B (GM_1 ganglioside-binding) subunits. Cholera toxin is not present in the parenteral vaccine. Volunteer challenge studies demonstrate that immunity can persist for over 3 years following initial infection.[53] Immunity is both vibriocidal and antitoxic, the antitoxic immunity being directed primarily toward the 103 amino acid B subunit, which contains multiple B cell epitopes.[54] However, vibriocidal immunity, directed to LPS, flagellar, outer membrane protein (OMP), hemagglutinin, and perhaps pilus antigens, is more important than antitoxic immunity, which alone is insufficient to protect against clinical disease.

Nonliving Cholera Vaccines

Over 25 years ago, Freter showed that oral immunization of humans with killed cholera vibrios induced antibody in stools more readily than did parenteral injection.[55] Over the last 5 years, Clemens et al.[56,57] have developed, tested, and proved the efficacy of a nonliving oral combination vaccine consisting of killed whole vibrios (2×10^{11}) administered with 5 mg of the purified B subunit of cholera toxin. Administration of three doses of this oral combination vaccine was not associated with adverse reactions, but induced both serum and intestinal antibody against both toxin and bacteria. This combination vaccine was demonstrably efficacious (64%) in both North American volunteer challenge studies (performed at 4 weeks after vaccination),[58,59] and in field trials in an endemic area (Bangladesh), where it was 85% protective in the population after 6 months[57] and remained 62% effective after 1 year.[56] At 6 months there was apparent advantage to the combination vaccine (with B subunit) as opposed to whole cells alone, but this advantage was no longer apparent at 1 year. The vaccine was less effective in children immunized at less than 5 years of age. The duration of protective immunity beyond 1 year is currently unknown, although Jertborn et al.[60] reported a memory response to revaccination in Swedish volunteers at 5 years following initial immunization.

These vaccine results represent a new standard against which alternative cholera vaccines must now be compared, and their analysis has important implications for future development of vaccines. These studies provide strong support for oral immunization as a means of protecting against cholera, both in endemic areas and in western populations. They also tend to confirm some importance for enterotoxigenic immunity in protection against cholera, since the addition of B subunit increased initial protection over whole cells alone.

Cholera toxin and its subunits are themselves immunogens and antigens, but the holotoxin also has strong immunostimulant and adjuvant properties. Cholera toxin has been shown to promote antibody production to, and prevent the development of oral tolerance to, simultaneously administered antigens.[61,62] Lycke and Strober[63] have recently shown that cholera toxin promotes B-cell differentiation to IgA isotype-producing cells, a property apparently shared by the B subunit alone. It is clearly not practical to administer native cholera toxin (CT) for its immunostimulant properties, since native CT is diarrheogenic in humans. Since the binding (B) subunit alone may share some of the immunostimulatory properties of the whole toxin,[63] it remains a possibility that the effect of added B subunit in the combination vaccine was due to a stimulatory effect on mucosal IgA production. These considerations suggest, however, that natural infection with cholera has a unique immunostimulating property because of the production of cholera toxin. It may be possible to utilize some of this immunizing capacity in vaccines that contain B subunit only but lack active cholera toxin. Cholera toxin components may be useful additions to any mucosal vaccine.

Recently Langevin-Perriat and co-workers[64] have attempted to improve delivery of cholera components by oral administration of LPS-outer membrane protein complexes administered in enteric-coated microgranules. They have induced secretory and serum antibody to cholera surface components. The immunogenicity of this preparation was not directly compared with that of the orally administered killed whole cell vaccine.

To permit better selection of cholera-associated antigens, Richardson et al.[65] have examined the antigen specificity of serum and secretory immune responses of human subjects challenged with classical *V. cholerae* by performing immunoblots against outer membrane antigens expressed on homologous and heterologous organisms grown both in vivo (in isolated ileal loops) and in vitro. Their aim was to determine the basis for heterologous protective immunity. They found reactivity with protein antigens common to homologous and heterologous strains, including antigens uniquely expressed on organisms grown in vivo. Similar results had previously been suggested by Kabir[66] in studies in rabbits.

Cholera toxin itself may also be a target antigen. Studies by Finklestein's group,[54] using a battery of monoclonal antibodies, have shown that potentially protective B-subunit epitopes (which block in vitro production of adenylate cyclase in cell culture) may be, but are not necessarily, related to the GM_1 ganglioside binding site. Although GM_1 binding may not be contained in a single linear epitope, it was reported that the 30–50 fragment of CTB blocks GM_1 binding. Jacob and coworkers[67,68] have utilized a peptide fragment (designated CTP3) consisting of residues 50–64 of the B subunit conjugated either to tetanus toxoid, or to polyalanyl polylysine, to induce neutralizing antibody to cholera toxin, and to prime for antibody production upon subsequent exposure to cholera toxin. These results are of particular interest since this peptide was not naturally immunogenic following exposure to the holotoxin. Administration of this and other peptide antigens remains a particular problem since, in Jacob's studies, immunization required adjuvant, or direct Peyer's patch injection.

Sanchez and Holmgren[69] recently reported the development of a recombinant system for overexpression of cholera toxin B subunit in *V. cholerae* as a basis for vaccine development. In their system, they introduced a plasmid containing cloned genes for B subunit under the influence of a strong promoter (tacP) into nontoxigenic classical and El Tor *V. cholerae*. They suggest that their strain will be immediately useful as a source of killed whole cells containing large amounts of B subunit, but the principle might also be used to produce live vaccine strains. Currently the expense of preparation of purified B subunit is a limiting factor in the use of the combination B subunit/killed whole cell vaccine. Moreover, the plasmid construct is designed to permit the introduction of genes for additional peptide antigens (fusions) adjacent to the B subunit, thereby permitting the production of a series of hybrid proteins for oral vaccine use.

Live Oral Vaccines

The use of chemical mutagenesis for attenuation of virulent cholera strains is best exemplified by "Texas Star," an EL Tor Ogawa strain selected by Honda and Finkelstein[70] for its ability to produce B subunit but not A subunit. This strain proved to be immunogenic in volunteers, providing 61% protection (18/25 versus 4/19), but it proved an unacceptable vaccine candidate because it caused mild diarrhea in 24% of volunteers.[71] The cause of this diarrhea was not defined, although it appeared clinically different from toxin-induced diarrhea. This may have been due to colonization alone, but might have been due to other unrecognized accessory virulence factors. The unmasking of unrecognized virulence factors is a major problem in vaccine development from clinical isolates, since the problem may not be discovered until the stage of human testing. Moreover, since the specific genetic lesions in Texas Star were not defined, concern remained that the vaccine strain could revert to full virulence.

Genetic engineering now offers improved methods of producing defined live oral cholera vaccines that can be constructed so as to make reversion to virulence extremely unlikely; however, the possibility of persisting, unrecognized virulence determinants remains a problem for this approach. As reviewed in detail by Kaper,[72] two basic genetic engineering approaches have been used to date to develop live oral cholera vaccines. These include the introduction of specific, nonreverting deletions in *V. cholera* to produce attenuated strains, and the expression of cholera antigens in heterologous nonpathogenic (carrier) organisms, as described below:

ATTENUATED CHOLERA STRAINS: ENTEROTOXIN-DEFICIENT MUTANTS. Kaper et al. have produced a series of enterotoxin-deficient vaccine strains (JBK70, CVD101, CVD 103, and CVD 103-HgR) by deleting genes encoding subunits of cholera toxin. This was accomplished by cloning the genes encoding cholera toxin, determining their sequence, cutting out essential subunit sequences with restriction enzymes, recloning the altered sequences, mobilizing them into pathogenic *V. cholerae,* and selecting for strains in which native subunit genes were replaced by altered genes. Strains JBK 70 and CVD 101 were both prepared from virulent El Tor Inaba. Strain JBK 70 lacks both A and B subunits, whereas strain CVD 101 lacks only the A subunit, leaving the B subunit structural genes and promoter intact and functional to permit the development of antitoxic immunity. When tested in volunteers, both strains were immunogenic, generating strong vibriocidal antibody titers, whereas CVD 101 also induced the expected antitoxic response. Both strains were equally protective against cholera challenge, again indicating the primary importance of vibriocidal immunity. Unfortunately, both strains also had a high incidence (50%) of mild-to-moderate diarrhea, similar to that seen with the earlier Texas Star.[73] To overcome this unacceptably high incidence of diarrheal side effects, the A subunit deleted (B+) strains CVD 103 (and its mercury-resistant variant CVD 103−HgR) were prepared from classical Inaba strain 569B. This parent was known to differ from the previous parent strain in that it did not produce any detectable shiga-like toxin, a suggested accessory virulence factor. These strains were shown to be immunogenic and protective against challenge in North American volunteers.[74] These vaccines are currently candidates for expanded clinical trials in endemic areas. The introduction of mercury resistance as a marker in CVD-HgR is an acceptable alternative to the antibiotic resistance markers frequently used for genetic manipulations. Antibiotic resistance is not an acceptable property of a live vaccine strain.

ATTENUATED CHOLERA STRAINS: COLONIZATION FACTOR MUTANTS. The determinants of *V. cholerae* colonization remained largely undefined until the discovery by Taylor et al.[75,76] of a gene cluster involved in the assembly of a pilus colonization factor (termed TCP for toxin coregulated pilus) of cholera. This colonization factor is regulated by the toxR gene product, which regulates toxin production, and is a member of the broad family of N-methylphenylalanine pili with N-terminal sequences shared by pseudomonas, neisseriae, moraxella, bacteroides, and vibrios.[2] Strains were constructed, following cloning of the tcp operon, which overproduce the TCP pilus (20% of available protein) as well as only the B subunit of cholera toxin. It remains to be determined whether live, colonizing mutants of this type will be useful as live oral vaccines or whether knowledge of this operon can be used to produce either attenuated colonization-defective or super-colonizing mutants. Studies by Pierce et al.[77] of virulent and mutant *V. cholerae* in rabbits indicated that the prime determinant of immunizing capacity of a strain was its colonizing capacity; however, studies of other organisms have suggested that colonization alone may also be sufficient to cause diarrheal disease. Nevertheless, killed strains of this type should be expected to improve the current killed whole cell vaccine, which contains little CTB or TCP.

Heterologous strains expressing cholera antigens.

ATTENUATED CHOLERA STRAINS: OTHER CONSTRUCTS. Forrest et al.[77] have introduced genes encoding the putative protective O antigens of *V. cholerae* Inaba and of Ogawa into the established *S. typhi* vaccine strain Ty21a. The O antigen genes were introduced on a plasmid that was stabilized by using a thymine-dependent Ty21a recipient, and by including genes for thymine independence on the transforming plasmid. The hybrid vaccine expressed both *S. typhi* and cholera O antigens but when tested in volunteers yielded a higher IgA response to the *Salmonella* determinants than to the cholera LPS; nevertheless these responses were similar to those seen after feeding the killed whole cell cholera vaccine. Efficacy studies of this vaccine construct in human volunteers have recently been undertaken.

Newton et al.[37] have introduced a synthetic oligonucleotide encoding the immunogenic (and in vitro protective) CTP3 epitope[67,68] (residues 50−64) of cholera toxin B subunit into a cloned *Salmonella* flagellin gene. The cloned gene produced functioning flagella containing the CTP3 epitope when transformed into *E. coli* or when transformed into an aromatic auxotrophic (aroA) mutant of *Salmonella dublin*. Moreover, antibody responses to the CTP3 epitope could be elicited in laboratory animals by administering either the live aroA vaccine strain, killed flagellate bacteria, or isolated flagella from the strain. Although there may be constraints on the size or type of epitope that could be introduced in this system, while still retaining flagellar function, the system is potentially adaptable to relevant protective epitopes from other pathogens.

In a variation on this theme, Dasgupta et al.[79] developed "cell surface leaky" phenotype mutants in a commensal *E. coli* strain by transposon mutagenesis and then introduced plasmids encoding complete CT or B subunit only. These "leaky" strains have the property of releasing toxin, or B subunit, into the medium at increased rates. Since cholera toxin B subunit is not normally expressed on the surface, nor normally transported from the periplasm in *E. coli*, these leaky mutants represent an alternative to surface expression of an antigen in a vaccine strain.

Enterotoxigenic Escherichia coli

ETEC are the most common agents causing the self-limited traveler's diarrhea frequently experienced by Europeans or North Americans visiting developing nations. In the developing countries, ETEC are a frequent (several episodes per individual per year) cause of often severe or fatal infantile diarrhea, but episodes decrease in survivors, suggesting a degree of acquired immunity with continuing exposure in endemic areas. This epidemiologic situation suggests that different vaccine strategies may be required to protect the two target populations of ETEC, adult travelers and infants in the third world. Other analogous, but serologically distinct, ETEC strains cause economically important diarrheal disease in newborn pigs, calves, and sheep. These veterinary diseases have been successfully prevented by passively administered intraluminal antibody in milk or colostrum from immunized sows or dams.[7,8] Active mucosal immunization is a goal for prevention of ETEC-associated traveler's diarrhea. Third world infants may be protected by passive antibody, perhaps through a program of maternal immunization and encouragement of breast feeding.

The pathogenesis of ETEC-induced disease is similar to that of cholera. ETEC adhere to normal small intestinal absorptive epithelium. There they secrete toxins that stimulate intestinal secretion. The major virulence determinants of ETEC include surface adhesive molecules or adhesins, which are typically expressed on nonflagellar protein appendages termed pili (or fimbriae)[80] and the heat-labile and/or heat-stable enterotoxins. The adhesins expressed by ETEC isolates of human origin have been termed colonization factor antigens (CFAs). Both CFAs and toxins are being explored as target antigens for vaccine development.[81]

The genes encoding most ETEC adhesins and toxins are located on virulence plasmids, rather than the chromosome, although exceptions to this rule are emerging. In some cases, structural genes are located on the chromosome, and regulatory genes are present on plasmids. The net result is that virulence is plasmid-associated. The virulence plasmids are not randomly transferable to other commensal *E. coli*. As a result, each CFA type is expressed in strains of only a limited number of characteristic serotypes within serogroups; thus the infecting strains represent widely distributed clones.

Even though serogroup-specific secretory immunity may be protective against ETEC,[27,82] the total number of serotypes represented among ETEC is too large to permit group (O)- and type (O:H:K)-specific antigens to be practical targets of vaccine development. These serogroups may be shared by nonpathogenic, commensal *E. coli*. In addition, theoretical concern has been raised that induction of active mucosal immunity to these determinants might be associated with systemic unresponsiveness to the same antigens.

The unique studies of Stoll et al.[23] defined mucosal antibody responses to ETEC antigens in naturally acquired ETEC diarrhea in an endemic area. These investigators obtained representative mucosal antibody using an intestinal lavage technique and studied the reaction of each patient to his own isolate. Eighty percent of heat-labile toxin (LT)+ patients responded to LT, 63% of CFA+ patients responded to the same CFA, and 78% of ETEC patients responded to the serogroup-specific LPS O antigen of their infecting strain with a mucosal IgA response. These results are similar to those previously found in volunteer challenge studies[3] and confirm these antigens as appropriate targets.

Antipilus Immunity

Calves and pigs can be passively protected against ETEC disease if they receive immunoglobulin directed against pilus adhesins (K88, K99, or 987) in the milk or colostrum of immunized dams or sows.[7,8] Similar protection can be achieved by administering monoclonal antibodies against pili. This experience strongly supports a protective role for anti-pilus immunity in ETEC infections. Additional data supporting this concept come from animal models[82] and, in particular, from human volunteer challenge studies conducted by Levine et al.[83] Volunteers orally immunized with live, piliated, nontoxigenic organisms (which were spontaneous mutants) were protected when subsequently challenged with virulent toxigenic ETEC strains, expressing the same pili, but of an unrelated O serotype.

The increasing number of CFAs recognized on ETEC, and their variation with geographic region, increases the difficulty of providing appropriate and efficacious antipilus immunity. If antipilus protection can be achieved for any one type of CFA, it should be possible to immunize with a mixture of CFAs. Alternatively, common determinants in the CFA types may be exploited for cross-reactive vaccine development. Three major CFAs are expressed by human ETEC strains, i.e., CFA/I, CFA/II, and CFA/IV (pcf8775). ETEC strains expressing these adhesins account for the majority of disease-related ETEC; however, a significant minority of strains have other adhesins, or do not express recognized adhesins. The simplest case is CFA/I, which has a typical pilus (fimbrial) structure, i.e., a hair-like macromolecular aggregate of identical repeating protein (pilin) structural subunits. The situation is more complex for CFA/II- and CFA/IV (pcf8775)- positive strains. Each of these typically consists of two different surface protein structures. Each strain typically expresses one of several antigenically distinct types of pili (CS1 or CS2 in CFA/II strains; CS4 or CS5 in CFA/IV strains). These are expressed together with finer "fibrillar" structures that are also composed of repeating protein subunits (termed CS3 in CFA/II strains and CS6 in CFA/IV strains). Although in some *E. coli* pili [e.g., the Pap pili of urinary tract isolates[84] and type I or common pili], the actual adhesive molecule is on a minor subunit, which presents an additional target for vaccine development, such a situation has not yet been described for ETEC CFAs.

The structural gene for the CFA/I pilin subunit has been cloned, and its complete amino acid sequence is known, permitting prediction of immunogenic epitopes.[80] Sequence data are now available for the pilin subunits of CS2, CS4, and the fibrillar subunit of CS3, permitting comparisons of common, or shared epitopes. CFA/I, CS2, and CS4 share extensive common N-terminal sequences, whereas CS3 is quite different, as would be expected from its different morphologic appearance. Recent evidence[85] suggests that immunization with a common epitope of several CFA pili induces antibodies that will recognize the intact pili. The converse may not be the case, however, since antibody recognition is dependent on the three-dimensional structure of the pilus aggregates. Karch[86] has shown that antibodies raised to intact pili do not often recognize dissociated pilin subunits.

Purified pilus vaccines have achieved a degree of protection against challenge with virulent ETEC.[87] Oral administration of purified pili has not satisfactorily primed the mucosal immune system in human volunteers, probably because of intraluminal degradation[83]; however, a combination of low-dose parenteral priming followed by oral boosting achieved some protective effect.[86] In these cases, oral administration of pili was preceded by neutralization of gastric acidity with bicarbonate and/or histamine (h_2) blockers. This may not have provided sufficient protection against intraluminal degradation of the antigens. Direct intraduodenal administration of antigen yielded a better mucosal immune response. Future approaches to oral pilus immunization may require microencapsulation to protect against degradation and/or targeting to the Peyer's patch.

The introduction of pilus expression in live carrier strains is currently a favored approach. Yamamoto[38] et al. have demonstrated the possibility of expressing both CFA/I and enterotoxin in the Ty21a *S. typhi* carrier, but this concept has not yet been utilized to prepare an acceptable vaccine candidate. Current work is focused on the definition of the genetics of ETEC CFAs and the availability of improved carrier strains in view of major problems encountered in fielding Ty21a/*Shigella* constructs as vaccines. The *Salmonella* typhi aromatic mutants being developed may be good candidates for carriers.

Antitoxin Immunity

The *E. coli* heat-labile toxin (LT) is analogous to CT of *V. cholerae*. The toxins share 75% nucleotide and 70–80% amino acid homology. They have A (active) and B (binding) subunits with similar mechanisms of action. The *E. coli* heat-stable (ST) toxins belong to a group with no counterparts in *V. cholerae*. They are a family of poorly immunogenic small peptides (from 2 to 5 kD) that activate guanylate cyclase. Their activity resides in a common C-terminal 18 amino acid segment.[88] Most ETEC strains produce ST. Many also produce LT. LT only strains are least frequent.

The structural similarities between *E. coli* LT and cholera toxin, and antibody neutralization data, raised the possibility of immunization with cholera B subunit to cross-protect against ETEC LT + strains. Holmgren et al.[89] recently reported the converse, i.e., that ETEC diarrhea caused by LT-producing strains primes the mucosal immune system of humans for an anamnestic response to cholera B subunit. This group has also obtained data suggesting that following administration of the cholera whole cell/B subunit vaccine, the incidence of clinically severe ETEC diarrhea was reduced.[90] However, in an animal model of ETEC diarrhea, LT or B subunit mucosal immunization provided less protection than did serotype-specific antibody.[27]

Efforts to induce immunity to ST have used synthetic ST peptides covalently linked to carrier proteins, such as ovalbumin for veterinary use,[91] native LT B subunit,[92] or a 26 amino acid epitope of the LT B subunit for human use[93] to enhance their immunogenicity. The veterinary study, however, suggested that the anti-ST antibody that developed gave protection that was inferior to antipilus immunity. The cross-linked toxoids[92] and the completely synthetic peptide LT/ST construct[93] prepared by Klipstein both induced intestinal IgA and serum IgG responses to both toxins in human volunteers; however, the efficacy of these vaccines in human volunteer challenge studies has not yet been reported.

CONCLUSIONS

The previous sections have described some desireable characteristics of an oral vaccine, reviewed the successful development of the attenuated Ty21a oral typhoid vaccine, and outlined the current work in progress toward the production of oral vaccines for *Shigella, V. cholera,* and enterotoxigenic *E. coli.* The demonstrable efficacy of the oral killed whole cell/B subunit combination cholera vaccine gives encouragement to the concept of oral immunization against enteric infection, but much work remains to be done.

On the basis of the available evidence, some generalizations can be made about the choice of antigens as immunogens, and of the means of antigen delivery, for future vaccine development.

Selection of antigen as immunogen. Virulence determinants are currently commonly selected as vaccine components. The choice of virulence determinants as immunizing antigens represents a two-edged sword, since their inclusion in a vaccine may induce disease, yet these are the very molecules that define disease and whose function should be inhibited to prevent disease. Fortunately for this approach, no single virulence determinant is usually sufficient to render even a live organism virulent; thus this approach will be likely to remain a mainstay of vaccine development. This approach is facilitated by the choice of only portions of the virulence factor for immunization. This is best exemplified by the successful cholera vaccine expressing only the B subunit of cholera toxin (strain CVD 103-HgR).[73] It is expected that future vaccines will be developed by selecting only those structures that are antigenic, immunogenic, and appropriate for B- and T-cell stimulation. Difficulties arise when the inclusion of a virulence antigen in a living strain is intended to permit the limited colonization, or invasion, necessary for immunogenicity. This is a very difficult balance to achieve, as exemplified by the multiple *Shigella* vaccine candidates that have been developed. It remains to be seen whether this concern will limit the usefulness of carrier strains expressing fully functional colonization factor antigens of *E. coli.* There is some evidence that small bowel colonization alone can cause disease, but knowledge of the genetic determinants of CFA expression should soon permit the expression of only the common immunogenic and protective epitopes of these structures.

Attempts to induce serotype-specific immunity provide a reliable approach to protection in most cases of invasive and noninvasive disease. This approach is most applicable to pathogens that have a limited number of serotypes, such as *Shigella* and cholera; it is least applicable to *E. coli.* A variation of this approach is the definition of commonly expressed surface protein antigens that may not be directly related to virulence, such as outer membrane proteins. Selection of appropriate antigens will be aided by definition of those antigens that are expressed in vivo during the early stages of disease.

Selection of means of delivery: live versus nonliving vaccines. The success of the killed whole cell/B subunit vaccine trails has boosted confidence in nonliving vaccines, particularly when they are intended to enhance protection in endemic areas. This approach required that large amounts of material be administered in repeated doses. This became a problem when purified antigen, in this case the B subunit of cholera toxin, was required; however, techniques for expression of genetically engineered material in quantity should provide technical solutions. Improved methods of antigen delivery, protecting the antigen, and targeting the mucosal immune system need to be developed. It remains to be determined whether delivery of carefully selected protein epitopes will provide the protection seen with administration of whole organisms. The inclusion of cholera toxin B subunit, for its cross-reactivity with *E. coli* toxins, or for its own potential immunomodulatory effects, in other vaccines deserves further study. Other orally effective adjuvants and immunomodulators await development.

The successful development of the Ty21a attenuated *S. typhi* has improved the likelihood of rapid development of a number of live oral vaccines. This strain has the potential to serve as the carrier for any of a number of defined bacterial antigens whose genes have been cloned. The fact that this strain has already been extensively tested, and proved safe, gives it a great advantage over strains yet to be developed. However, difficulties in formulation and large-scale preparation as well as uncertainty about its actual attenuating lesions(s) have caused some workers to approach its use as a carrier with caution. These problems have emerged with the *S. sonnei*-Ty21a vaccine candidate. A current favored approach is aromatic mutations of *S. typhi* or of other pathogens, but the ability of such strains to induce a protective immune response has yet to be demonstrated. The selection, and testing, of appropriate carrier strains for vaccine antigens is becoming a major field of activity. The field will be greatly advanced by the development of valid animal models.

REFERENCES

1. Falkow S: Molecular Koch's postulates applied to microbial pathogenicity. *Rev Infect Dis* 10:S274–S276, 1988.
2. Finlay BR, Falkow S: Common themes in microbial pathogenicity. *Microbiol Rev* 53:210–230, 1989.
3. Levine MM, Kaper B, Black RE, et al: New knowledge on pathogenesis of bacterial enteric infections as applied to vaccine development. *Microbiol Rev* 47:510–550, 1983.
4. Boedeker EC, McQueen CF: Laboratory investigation of childhood enteric infections. *Front Gastrointest Res* 16:169–219, 1989.
5. Boedeker EC, McQueen CF: Intestinal immunity to bacterial and parasitic infections. *Immunol Allergy Clin N Am* 8:393–421, 1989.
6. Fubara ES, Freter R: Protection against enteric bacterial infection by secretory IgA antibodies. *J Immunol* 111:395–403, 1973.
7. Acres SD, Isaacson RE, Babiuk K, et al: Immunization of calves against enterotoxigenic colibacillosis by vaccinating dams with purified 99 antigen and whole cell bacterins. *Infect Immun* 2:121–112, 1979.

8. Rutter M, Jones GW, Brown GTH, et al: Antibacterial activity in colostrum and milk associated with protection of piglets against enteric disease caused by K88 positive *Escherichia coli. Infect Immun* 13:667–676, 1976.

9. Tackett CO, Losonsky G, Link H, et al: Protection by milk immunoglobulin concentrate against oral challenge with enterotoxigenic *Escherichia coli. N Engl J Med* 318:1240–1244, 1988.

10. Levin MM, Ferreccio C, Black RE: Progress in vaccines against typhoid fever. *Rev Infect Dis* 11:S552–S567, 1989.

11. Robbins JD, Robbins B: Reexamination of the protective role of the capsular polysaccharide (Vi antigen) of *Salmonella typhi. J Infect Dis* 150:436–449, 1984.

12. Robbins JB, Schneerson R, Aharya II, et al: Protective roles of mucosal and serum immunity against typhoid fever. *Monogr Allergy* 24:315–320, 1988.

13. Anonymous: Leads from the MMWR, Cholera Vaccine. *JAMA* 260:2489–2490, 1988.

14. Sneller MC, Strober W: M cells and host defense. *J Infect Dis* 154:737–741, 1986.

15. Owen RL, Pierce NF, Apple RT, et al: M cell transport of *Vibrio cholerae* from the intestinal lumen into Peyer's patches: a mechanism for antigen sampling and for microbial transepithelial migration. *J Infect Dis* 153:1108–1118, 1986.

16. Ertl HCJ, Bona CA: Criteria to define anti-idiotypic antibodies carrying the internal image of an antigen. *Vaccine* 6:80–84, 1988.

17. Unanue ER, Allen PM: The basis for the immunoregulatory role of macrophages and other accessory cells. *Science* 236:551–557, 1987.

18. Berzofsky JA: Features of T-cell recognition and antigen structure useful in the design of vaccines to elicit T-cell immunity. *Vaccine* 6:89–93, 1988.

19. Celada F, Sercarz EE: Preferential pairing of T-B specificities in the same antigen: the concept of directional help. *Vaccine* 6:94–98, 1988.

20. Tagliabue A, Nencioni L, Carrena A, et al: Cellular immunity against *Salmonella typhi* after live oral vaccine. *Clin Exp Immunol* 62:242–247, 1985.

21. Tagliabue A, Nencioni L, Villa L, et al: Antibody dependent cell-mediated antibacterial activity of intestinal lymphocytes with secretory IgA. *Nature* 306:184–186, 1983.

22. Jordan WS: Impediments to the development of additional vaccines: vaccines against important disease that will not be available in the next decade. *Rev Infect Dis* 11:S603–S612, 1989.

23. Stoll B, Svennerholm AM, Gothefors L, et al: Local and systemic antibody responses to naturally acquired enterotoxigenic *Escherichia coli* diarrhea in an endemic area. *J Infect Dis* 153:527–534, 1986.

24. Lycke N, Lindolm L, Holmgren J: Cholera antibody production in vitro by peripheral blood lymphocytes following oral immunization of humans and mice. *Clin Exp Immunol* 62:39–45, 1985.

25. Winsor DK Jr, Mathewson JJ, DuPont HL: Western blot analysis of intestinal secretory immunoglobulin A response to *Campylobacter jejuni* antigens in patients with naturally acquired *Campylobacter* enteritis. *Gastroenterology* 90:1217–1222, 1986.

26. Dunn BE, Blaser MJ, Snyder EL: Two-dimensional gell electrophoresis and immunoblotting of *Campylobacter* outer membrane proteins. *Infect Immun* 55:1564–1572, 1987.

27. Sack RB, Kline RL, Spira WM: Oral immunization of rabbits with enterotoxigenic *Escherichia coli* protects against intraintestinal challenge. *Infect Immun* 56:387–394, 1988.

28. Germanier R, Furer E: Isolation and characterization of GalE mutant Ty21a of *Salmonella typhi:* a candidate for a live oral typhoid vaccine. *J Infect Dis* 131:553–558, 1975.

29. Acharya IL, Lowe CU, Thapa R, et al: Prevention of typhoid fever in Nepal with the Vi capsular polysaccharide of *Salmonella typhi. N Engl J Med* 317:1101–1104, 1987.

30. Hone DM, Attridge SR, Forrest B, et al: A galE via (Vi antigen negative) mutant of *Salmonella typhi* Ty2 retains virulence in humans. *Infect Immun* 56:1326–1333, 1988.

31. Wahden MH, Serie C, Cerisier Y, et al: A controlled field trial of live *Salmonella typhi* strain Ty21a oral vaccine against typhoid: three year results. *J Infect Dis* 145:292–296, 1982.

32. Levine MM, Ferreccio C, Black RE, et al: Large-scale field trial of Ty21A live oral typhoid vaccine in enteric-coated capsule formulation. *Lancet* I:1049–1052, 1987.

33. Stocker BAD: Auxotrophic *Salmonella typhi* as live vaccine. *Vaccine* 6:141–145, 1988.

34. Levine MM, Herrington D, Murphy JR, et al: Safety, infectivity, immunogenicity and in vivo stability of two attenuated auxotrophic mutant strains of *Salmonella typhi*, 541ty and 543ty, as live oral vaccines in man. *J Clin Invest* 79:888–902, 1987.

35. Curtiss RW, Goldschmidt RM, Fletchall NB, et al: Avirulent *Salmonella typhimurium* delta-cya, delta-crp oral vaccine strains expressing a streptococcal colonization and virulence antigen. *Vaccine* 6:155–160, 1988.

36. Sadoff JC, Ballou WR, Baron LS: Oral *Salmonella typhimurium* vaccine expressing circumsporozoite protein protects against malaria. *Science* 240:336–338, 1988.

37. Newton SMC, Jacob CO, Stocker BAD: Immune response to cholera toxin epitope inserted in *Salmonella* flagellin. *Science* 244:70–72, 1989.

38. Yamamoto T, Tamura Y, Yokota T: Enteroadhesion fimbriae and enterotoxin of *Escherichia coli:* genetic transfer to streptomycin-resistant mutant of the galE oral-route live-vaccine *Salmonella typhi* Ty21a. *Infect Immun* 50:925–928, 1985.

39. Formal SB, Baron LS, Kopecko DJ, et al: Construction of a potential bivalent vaccine strain: introduction of *Shigella sonnei* form I antigen genes into the galE *Salmonella typhi* Ty21a typhoid vaccine strain. *Infect Immun* 34:746–750, 1981.

40. Formal SB, Hale TL: Shigella vaccines. *Rev Infect Dis* 11:S547–S551, 1989.

41. Formal SB, LaBrec EH, Palmer A, et al: Protection of monkeys against experimental shigellosis with attenuated vaccines. *J Bacteriol* 90:63–68, 1965.

42. Mel DM, Gangarosa EJ, Radovanovic ML: Studies on vaccination against bacillary dysentery. 6. Protection of children with oral immunization using streptomycin-dependent Shigella strains. *Bull WHO* 45:457–464, 1974.

43. Lindberg AA, Karnell A. Stocker BAD: Development of an auxotrophic oral live *Shigella flexneri* vaccine. *Vaccine* 6:146–150, 1988.

44. Hale TL, Formal SB: Genetics of virulence in *Shigella*. *Microbiol Pathogen* 1:511–518, 1986.

45. Mills SD, Sekizaki T, Gonzalez-Carrero MI, et al: Analysis and genetic manipulation of *Shigella* virulence determinants for vaccine development. *Vaccine* 6:116–122, 1988.

46. Sansonetti PJ, Kopecko DJ, Formal SB: Involvement of a plasmid in the invasive ability of *Shigella flexneri*. *Infect Immun* 3:852–860, 1982.

47. Formal SB, Gemski P, Baron EH, et al: Genetic transfer of *Shigella flexneri* antigens to *Escherichia coli* K-12. *Infect Immun* 1:279–286, 1970.

48. Sansonetti PJ, Hale TL, Dammin GJ, et al: Alterations in the pathogenicity of *Escherichia coli* K-12 after transfer of plasmid and chromosomal genes from *Shigella flexneri*. *Infect Immun* 39:1392–1402, 1983.

49. Formal SB, Kent TH, May HC, et al: Protection of monkeys against experimental shigellosis with a living, attenuated oral polyvalent dysentery vaccine. *J Bacteriol* 92:17–22, 1969.

50. Formal SB, Hale TL, Kapfer C, et al: Oral vaccination of monkeys with an invasive *Escherichia coli* K-12 hybrid expressing *Shigella flexneri* 2a somatic antigen. *Infect Immun* 46:465–469, 1984.

51. Black RE, Levine MM, Clements ML, et al: Prevention of shigellosis by a *Salmonella typhi-Shigella sonnei* bivalent vaccine. *J Infect Dis* 155:1260–1265, 1987.

52. Baron LS, Kopecko DJ, Formal SB, et al: Introduction of *Shigella flexneri* 2a type and group antigen genes into oral typhoid vaccine strain *Salmonella typhi* Ty21a. *Infect Immun* 55:2797–2801, 1987.

53. Levine MM, Black RE, Clements ML, et al: Duration of infection derived immunity to cholera. *J Infect Dis* 143:818–820, 1981.

54. Finkelstein RA, Burks MF, Zupan A, et al: Epitopes of the cholera family of enterotoxins. *Rev Infect Dis* 9:544–561, 1987.

55. Freter R: Detection of coproantibody and its formation after parenteral and oral immunization of human volunteers. *J Infect Dis* 111:37–48, 1962.

56. Clemens JD, Harris JD, Sack DA, et al: Field trial of oral cholera vaccines in Bangladesh: results of a one year follow up. *J Infect Dis* 158:60–69, 1988

57. Clemens JD, Sack DA, Harris JR, et al: Field trial of oral cholera vaccines in Bangladesh. *Lancet* II: 124–127, 1986.

58. Black RE, Levine MM, Clements ML, et al: Protective efficacy in humans or killed whole-vibrio oral cholera vaccine with and without the B subunit of cholera toxin. *Infect Immun* 55:1116–1120, 1987.

59. Levine MM, Kaper JB, Herrington D, et al: The current status of cholera vaccine development and experience with cholera vaccine trials in volunteers. *SE Asian J Trop Med Public Health* 19:401–415, 1988.

60. Jertborn M, Svennerholm A-M, Holmgren J: Five year immunologic memory in Swedish volunteers after oral cholera vaccination. *J Infect Dis* 157:374–377, 1988.

61. Lycke N, Holmgren J: Strong adjuvant properties of cholera toxin on gut mucosal immune responses to orally presented antigens. *Immunology* 59:301–308, 1986.

62. Elson CO, Ealing W: Cholera toxin feeding did not induce oral tolerance in mice and abrogated oral tolerance to an unrelated protein antigen. *J Immunol* 133:2892–2897, 1984.

63. Lycke N, Strober W: Cholera toxin promotes B cell isotype differentiation. *J Immunol* 11:3781–3787, 1989.

64. Langevin-Perriat A, LaFont S, Vincent C, et al: Intestinal secretory antibody response induced by an oral cholera vaccine in human volunteers. *Vaccine* 6:509–512, 1988.

65. Richardson K, Kaper JB, Levine MM: Human immune response to *Vibro cholerae* 01 whole cells and isolated outer membrane antigens. *Infect Immun* 57:495–501, 1989.

66. Kabir S: Immunological responses of rabbits to various somatic and secreted antigens of *Vibrio cholerae* after intraduodenal inoculation. *J Med Microbiol* 24:29–40, 1987.

67. Jacob CO, Grossfeld S, Sela M, et al: Priming immune response to cholera toxin induced by synthetic peptides. *Eur J Immuno* 16:1057–1062, 1986.

68. Jacob CO, Vaerman JP: Induction of rat secretory IgA antibodies against cholera toxin by a synthetic peptide. *Immunology* 59:129–133, 1986.

69. Sanchez J, Holmgren J: Recombinant system for overexpression of cholera toxin B subunit in *Vibrio cholerae* as a basis for vaccine development. *Proc Natl Acad Sci USA* 86:481–485, 1989.

70. Honda T, Finkelstein RA: Selection and characterization of a *Vibrio cholerae* mutant lacking the A (ADP-ribosylating) portion of the cholera enterotoxin. *Proc Natl Acad Sci USA* 76:2052–2056, 1984.

71. Levine MM, Black RE, Clements ML, et al: Evaluation in humans of attenuated *Vibrio cholerae* El Tor Ogawa strain Texas Star-SR as a live oral vaccine. *Infect Immun* 43:515–522, 1984.

72. Kaper JB: *Vibrio cholerae* vaccines. *Rev Infect Dis* 11:S568–S569, 1989.

73. Levine MM, Kaper JB, Herrington D, et al: Safety, immunogenicity and efficacy of recombinant live oral cholera vaccines, CVD 103 and CVD 103–HgR. *Lancet* II:467–470, 1988.

74. Levine MM, Kaper JB, Herrington D, et al: Volunteer studies of deletion mutants of *Vibrio cholerae* 01 prepared by recombinant techniques. *Infect Immun* 56:161–167, 1988.

75. Taylor RK, Miller VL, Farley DB, et al: Use of pho gene fusions to identify a pilus colonization factor coordinately regulated with cholera toxin. *Proc Natl Acad Sci USA* 84:2833–2837, 1987.

76. Taylor R, Shaw C, Peterson K, et al: Safe, live *Vibrio cholerae* vaccines? *Vaccine* 6:151–154, 1988.

77. Pierce NF, Kaper JB, Mekalanos JJ, et al: Determinants of the immunogenicity of live virulent and mutant *Vibrio cholerae* 01 in rabbit intestine. *Infect Immun* 55:477–481, 1987.

78. Forrest DB, LaBrooy JT, Attridge SR, et al: Immunogenicity of a candidate live oral typhoid/cholera hybrid vaccine in humans. *J Infect Dis* 159:145–146, 1989.

79. Dasgupta U, Guhathakurta I, Das J: Excretion of cholera toxin from *Escherichia coli:* a potential oral vaccine for cholera. *Biochem Biophys Res Commun* 153:967–972, 1988.

80. Klemm P: Fimbrial adhesins of *Escherichia coli*. *Rev Infect Dis* 7:321–340, 1985.

81. Kaper JB, Levine MM: Progress towards a vaccine against enterotoxigenic *Escherichia coli*. *Vaccine:* 197–199, 1988.

82. Ahren CA, Svennerholm A-M: Experimental enterotoxin-induced *Escherichia coli* diarrhea and protection induced by previous infection with bacteria of the same adhesin or enterotoxin type. *Infect Immun* 50:255–261, 1985.

83. Levine M, Morris JG, Losonsky G, et al: Fimbriae (pili) as vaccines. In Lark, DL: *Protein-Carbohydrate Interactions in Biological Systems*. New York, Academic Press, 1986, p. 143.

84. Lind B, Lindberg F, Marklund B-I: Tip proteins of pili associated with pyelonephritis: new candidates for vaccine development. *Vaccine* 6:110–112, 1988.

85. Reid R, Engler R, Ferren P, et al: Primary in vitro antibody response to N-terminal peptide of CFA/I recognizes the pilus protein. *Gastroenterology* 94:A372, 1988.

86. Karch H, Leying H, Buscher K-H, et al: Three dimensional structure of fimbriae determines specificity of the immune response. *Infect Immun* 50:517–522, 1985.

87. Evans DG, Graham DY, Evans DJ Jr: Administration of purified colonization factor antigens (CFA/I, CFA/II) of enterotoxigenic *Escherichia coli* to volunteers. Response to challenge with virulent enterotoxigenic *Escherichia coli*. *Gastroenterology* 87:934–940, 1984.

88. Chan S-K, Giannella RA: Amino acid sequence of heat stable enterotoxin produced by *Escherichia coli* pathogenic for man. *J Biol Chem* 26:7744–7746, 1981.

89. Holmgren J, Svennerholm A-M, Gothefors L, et al: Enterotoxigenic *Escherichia coli* diarrhea in an endemic area prepares the intestine for an anamnestic immunoglobulin A antitoxin response to oral cholera B subunit vaccination. *Infect Immun* 56:230–233, 1988.

90. Clemens JD, Sack DA, Harris JR, et al: Cross protection by B subunit-whole cell cholera vaccine against diarrhea associated with heat-labile toxin-producing enterotoxigenic *Escherichia coli:* results of a large-scale field trial. *J Infect Dis* 158:372–377, 1988.

91. Frantz JC, Bhatnagar PK, Brown AL, et al: Investigation of synthetic *Escherichia coli* heat-stable enterotoxin as an immunogen for swine and cattle. *Infect Immun* 55:1077–1084, 1987.

92. Klipstein FA, Engert RF, Clements JD, et al: Protection against human and porcine enterotoxigenic strains of *Escherichia coli* in rats immunized with a cross-linked toxoid vaccine. *Infect Immun* 40:924–929, 1983.

93. Klipstein FA, Engert RF, Houghten RA: Immunisation of volunteers with a synthetic peptide vaccine for enterotoxigenic *Escherichia coli*. *Lancet* I:471–473, 1986.

CHAPTER 23

Inflammatory Bowel Disease

RICHARD P. MacDERMOTT

WILLIAM F. STENSON

INTRODUCTION

The etiologic agents for ulcerative colitis and Crohn's disease have not been identified. A large number of microbial and dietary agents have been put forth as candidates for etiologic roles in these diseases, but none has been proved to cause disease. Mechanisms for the spontaneous exacerbations and remissions characteristic of these diseases are also undefined. Although the etiologic agents are unknown, recent studies have provided valuable insights into the mechanisms for amplification of the inflammatory response that results in the histologic and clinical changes characteristic of the inflammatory bowel diseases.

In ulcerative colitis, there are mucosal ulcers and infiltration of the mucosa and submucosa with neutrophils, macrophages, and lymphocytes. In Crohn's disease, the inflammatory infiltrate frequently contains granulomas and extends through all layers of the bowel wall, rather than being confined to the mucosa and submucosa as in ulcerative colitis. Both diseases have been viewed as "chronic" inflammatory diseases because of their prolonged clinical courses and because their inflammatory infiltrates contain lymphocytes and macrophages, a histologic picture that is characteristic of chronic inflammation. However, both diseases also have a less well recognized, but equally prominent "acute" component marked by a constant flux of neutrophils out of the circulation, into inflamed mucosa, through the epithelium, and then into the intestinal lumen.

Inflammatory responses in the intestine can be induced by disorders of immunoregulation (e.g., systemic lupus erythematosus); infectious colitis (e.g., shigellosis); impaired circulation (e.g., ischemic colitis); or toxic compounds (e.g., acetic

This work was supported in part by USPHS grants DK-33165, DK-21474, DK-33487, and by grants from the National Foundation for Ileitis and Colitis acid colitis). There are striking similarities in clinical and morphologic manifestations among the diseases marked by intestinal inflammation. The likely explanation for these similarities is that the clinical and histologic manifestations of each of these diseases arise, not from directed, target cell injury, but rather from "innocent bystander" effects due to the soluble mediators of inflammation that are generated as part of the inflammatory process. The functional and histologic changes seen in inflammatory bowel disease (IBD) are thus due to soluble mediators of inflammation. Neutrophil and macrophage infiltration, for example, suggests the presence of soluble chemotactic agents that cause neutrophils and monocytes in the circulation to migrate into the mucosa. Mucosal edemal and hyperemia reflect the presence of soluble mediators that induce enhanced vascular permeability and vasodilation.

As advances have been made in understanding the immune system and as investigative techniques have become increasingly sophisticated, IBD investigators have been able to carry out studies that have provided new information on the immunopathogenesis of ulcerative colitis and Crohn's disease.[1-4] Moreover, this new information is beginning to translate into promising therapeutic leads.

GENETIC MARKERS

The frequent finding of IBD in more than one family member and association with defined ethnic groups has led to a search for a genetic marker. Studies of IBD in family members have shown incidences ranging from 10 to 35%,[5] a rate many times higher than would be predicted by the prevalence of IBD in the general population. However, examination of the standard HLA-A, -B, -C, and -DR antigens[6-8] has not shown a clear or uniform correlation with the occurrence of IBD. Even within families, patients with IBD do not necessarily have the same HLA type. On the other hand, HLA-B27 is more frequent in the subset of patients with IBD who have ankylosing spondylitis. Furthermore, extensive analysis and summation of many different studies[9] revealed an increased association in Caucasians of Crohn's disease with HLA-2, and ulcerative colitis with HLA-B27 and HLA-Bw35. In contrast, there was an increased association of ulcerative colitis with HLA-B5 in Japanese.[9] In addition, IBD is quantitatively associated with several genetic disorders, such as Turner's syndrome.

A genetic alteration could be responsible for an inability to mount an adequate immune response to a particular agent, or could lead to the inability to shut down an appropriate intestinal immune response to common inciting agents. Genetic influences could also affect the transition from immune activation to inflammation — a step in the pathogenesis of inflammatory bowel disease that has not been well characterized. Polygenic influences, variability of penetrance, and incomplete recognition of mild or subclinical disease states could all tend to obscure correlation of tissue typing results with patterns of inheritance in IBD.

ALTERATIONS OF PERIPHERAL BLOOD LYMPHOCYTE FUNCTION

Because of accessibility, peripheral blood lymphocytes have usually been the starting point for studies of immune alterations in IBD. However, immunologic abnormalities exhibited by peripheral blood mononuclear cells (MNC) from patients with IBD have often proved to be nonspecific and secondary in nature and not to represent primary abnormalities related to disease pathogenesis. The duration and severity of IBD, adequacy of nutrition, and therapeutic medications all have a major influence on tests of cell-mediated immune function.[1,3]

Early studies[10,11] disagreed as to the quantitative peripheral blood lymphocyte subpopulation changes seen in Crohn's disease. The conflicting results from many studies were clarified when Auer and coworkers[12,13] divided their patients with Crohn's disease into two groups: 1) patients in whom the disease was newly diagnosed and who had never been treated with steroids; and 2) patients in whom the disease was of long duration and who had been treated with sulfasalazine and/or steroids. It was the second group, the patients who had had long-term disease and who had been treated, in whom significant total lymphocytopenia and a decrease in T cells occurred.[12] In contrast, minimal changes were seen in untreated patients with recent onset Crohn's disease, because secondary influences on the immune system were minimized. Auer and coworkers[13] have also presented evidence that the secondary influences causing the total and T-cell lymphocytopenia were related to the chronicity and activity of the Crohn's disease, rather than the effect of therapy. Thus total lymphocyte numbers as well as T-cell numbers are decreased in a subset of patients with Crohn's disease who have had active disease of long duration; this is a secondary rather than a primary event, since it is not observed in patients with recent onset disease who have not been treated. Finally, in studies using monoclonal antibodies, Selby and Jewell[14] and Yuan et al.[15] found no significant differences between IBD patients and controls with regard to the proportions of circulating T lymphocytes or their subsets.

Recently Raedler and coworkers[16] reported that in active Crohn's disease an elevated percentage (24.3%) of peripheral blood T lymphocytes are T9$^+$. In contrast, patients with inactive Crohn's disease exhibited only 9.9% T9$^+$ peripheral blood T cells.[16] They have also observed a significantly increased number of Fc alpha receptor-positive cells within the subset of T9$^+$ cells.[17] Elevated percentages of Fc alpha-bearing T cells were uniquely found in Crohn's disease and were not found in patients with systemic lupus erythematosus, rheumatoid arthritis, sarcoidosis, or infectious gastroenteritis.[17] These studies provide intriguing evidence for the activation of discrete peripheral blood mononuclear cell subpopulations as part of the alterations in the immune response of inflammatory bowel disease patients.

SERUM ANTIBODIES AND CLASS II ANTIGENS

Broberger, Perlmann, and coworkers[18-21] demonstrated anticolon antibodies that were: 1) directed against epithelial cells; 2) cross-reactive with *Escherichia coli* 014; and 3) present in sera from 56% of patients with ulcerative colitis (UC) and 67% of patients with Crohn's disease. It was hypothesized that anticolon antibodies were produced by sensitization with *E. coli* 014 and functioned as an initiating or perpetuating factor in IBD.[18-21] Subsequent studies, however, provided evidence against a role for anticolon antibodies in IBD. Broberger and Perlmann[22] observed that sera from patients with ulcerative colitis, in the presence of complement, did not kill fetal colonic cells. Rabin and Rogers[23] immunized rabbits with intestinal tissue, resulting in circulating anticolon antibodies, but did not observe any pathologic tissue damage in the intestine. Deodhar et al.[24] provided evidence for the lack of disease specificity of anticolon antibodies by observing that 28 of 54 patients with autoimmune diseases had anticolon antibodies, but that none of these patients had evidence of IBD. The lack of disease specificity of anticolon antibodies was conclusively demonstrated by Carlsson and coworkers,[25] who examined 1,310 sera samples and found that, although 60% of ulcerative colitis patients and 61% of Crohn's disease patients had serum titers of anticolon antibodies greater than 1:16, so too did 69% of patients with urinary tract infections, 53% of patients with multiple polyposis, 62% of patients with cirrhosis, 50% of patients with salmonellosis, 47% of patients with gastroenteritis, and 47% of patients with irritable bowel syndrome. Finally, Heddle and Shearman[26] measured serum antibody titers against enterobacterial common antigen, *E. coli* 014, and five other *E. coli* serotypes, and found that patients with ulcerative colitis had the same levels of antibodies as did control subjects. Thus the lack of disease specificity and the lack of pathogenic capability argue strongly against a primary role for anticolon antibodies in IBD and suggest that they arise secondary to the disease process.

Korsmeyer and coworkers[27,28] found that lymphocytotoxic antibodies occur in approximately 40% of IBD patients, 40% of household contacts of patients with IBD, 50% of spouses of patients with IBD, and 34% of relatives of patients with IBD. Furthermore, lymphocytotoxic antibodies were found both in patients with IBD and family members.[28] Strickland and coworkers[29] characterized IBD lymphocytotoxic antibodies as being predominantly cold-reactive, with 60% of the antibodies being directed against both T and B cells, while 20% were directed against T cells alone and 20% against B cells alone.

We found cold-reactive antilymphocyte antibodies in 40% of patients with ulcerative colitis and 41% of patients with Crohn's disease, as opposed to only 10% of controls.[1,3] Antilymphocyte antibodies against B cells were present at 37°C, as well as 20°C and 4°C, indicating the presence of IgG, warm-reactive, as well as IgM cold-reactive antilymphocyte antibodies.[1,3] The sera were extensively absorbed with platelets, after which lymphocytotoxic antibodies were found to react exclusively with B cells and macrophages.[1,3] The lymphocytotoxic antibodies were not directed against any particular HLA antigens, but a number did react to DR antigens.[1,3] Interestingly, the DR specificities were broad, with most of the lymphocytotoxic antibodies reacting against two, or sometimes three, DR specificities, perhaps representing supertypic determinants.[1,3] Reactivity was commonly seen against combinations of DRW types (i.e., 3, 5, plus 6, or 4 plus 7). Because IBD lymphocytotoxic antibodies were directed against a wide variety of DRW antigen types,[1,3] sensitization to DR antigens may be involved in their development.

Class II (HLA-DP, -DQ, -DR) molecules have two chains (alpha and beta), each with a single constant domain and a single variable region. CD4 (helper, inducer) T cells recognize soluble antigens in conjunction with class II molecules present on macrophages and B cells. Class II antigens on intestinal epithelial cells may play an important role in antigen processing within the intestinal immune compartment. Scott and coworkers[30] demonstrated that class II molecules are present on normal human small intestinal but not normal human colonic epithelial cells, and also observed that class II antigen expression on small intestinal epithelial cells is retained in patients with Crohn's disease.[31] They speculated that HLA-DR molecules on human intestinal epithelial cells may be involved in antigen-induced triggering of intraepithelial lymphocytes.[31] Subsequently, Selby and coworkers demonstrated that marked enhancement of colon epithelial cell HLA-DR staining occurred in active ulcerative colitis and Crohn's colitis.[32]

Hirata and coworkers[33] used anti-human HLA-DR antibodies and observed staining of a number of different cell types in normal intestine, including lamina propria mononuclear cells, dendritic cells, and fibroblasts, as well as both vascular and lymphatic endothelial cells. The most marked change noted in inflammatory bowel disease was the intense staining by anti-HLA-DR antibodies of epithelial cells from diseased tissue, indicating the induction of HLA-DR antigens on epithelial cells.[33] Activation of cells of a variety of types will lead to the induction of HLA-DR antigens on their surfaces. Helper T cells are capable of recognizing foreign antigens in the presence of HLA-DR molecules.[34] Polymorphism of the major histocompatibility complex provides the potential for presenting antigen in different contexts and may allow the expansion of autoreactive T cells.[34,35] Sensitization to antigens in conjunction with self-HLA-DR molecules by T cells could result in T cells activated to recognize the same antigen presented by self-HLA-DR components at future times.[35] The state of activation of lymphocytes and the relationship of lymphocyte activation to class II antigen expression by intestinal epithelial cells is therefore currently an area of intense study.

Pallone and coworkers have demonstrated that early activation markers are increased in the peripheral blood and intestinal lamina propria of active Crohn's disease patients.[36] Only in patients who have had resections of intestine involved with Crohn's disease, without disease recurrence, is the number of early activation antigen-bearing cells within normal range.[36] Thus Crohn's disease patients have an increased number of preactivated rather than fully activated lymphocytes in the peripheral blood and intestine, suggesting a state of chronic immune activation.[36] Fais and coworkers have demonstrated that in diseased intestine of patients with elevated early activation markers, there is increased expression of MHC class II antigens (HLA-DR molecules) on the surface of intestinal epithelial cells.[37]

McDonald and Jewell have observed that although HLA-DR antigens are not present on normal control epithelial cells, colonic epithelial cells stained positively for HLA-DR antigens not only in patients with ulcerative colitis and Crohn's disease, but also in patients with infectious colitis.[38] Therefore the induction of HLA-DR antigens on intestinal epithelial cells is a nonspecific response to inflammation.[38] The nonspecific presentation of autoantigens by HLA-DR-bearing epithelial cells induced during inflammation could lead to subsequent chronic activation of specifically sensitized effector B and T lymphocytes.[39] Indeed, it has been shown that cytotoxic T lymphocytes, sensitized by defined antigens in combination with cell surface HLA-DR antigens, results in an expansion of cells bearing T-cell receptor idiotypes with cross-reactive potential for normal tissue components.[40]

In recent studies, Mayer and Shlien[41] have demonstrated that human intestinal epithelial cells, obtained from resected specimens, are capable of processing and presenting antigens in vitro. They observed that freshly isolated human intestinal epithelial cells are capable of functioning as accessory cells in the immune response.[41] Class II antigen-bearing human epithelial cells can act as stimulators of the mixed leukocyte reaction and are able to present a soluble antigen (tetanus toxoid) to tetanus-primed T cells.[41] In healthy persons, the major group of T cells responding to epithelial cell antigen presentation is a subpopulation of T cytotoxic suppressor cells.[41] In contrast, in IBD patients, Mayer and Eisenhardt have observed that T-helper cells were the major responding T-cell subclass to IBD intestinal epithelial cells.[42] Furthermore, IBD intestinal epithelial cells failed to stimulate antigen-nonspecific suppressor cells.[42] The subsequent lack of T-suppressor cell induction could in turn lead to increased expression of class II antigens in diseased bowel.[42] Intestinal epithelial cell DR determinants that are amplified during the inflammatory process[30-33,36-39] could result in both anticolon[18-26] and antilymphocyte[27-29] antibodies. It is, therefore, possible that antilymphocyte antibodies arise as part of a "networking" phenomenon that also involves anticolonic antibodies. Formation of anticolonic antibodies directed against DR antigens on epithelial cells could lead to antibodies capable of reacting with DR antigens on B cells and monocytes and thereby may modulate immune function. Sensitized T cells capable of recognizing DR antigens and autoantigens on intestinal epithelial cells may be induced and then play a subsequent immunoregulatory or effector role in IBD.

CELL-MEDIATED CYTOTOXICITY

Perlmann and Broberger[43] observed that exposure of fetal human colon cells to peripheral blood MNC from children with ulcerative colitis, but not control subjects, led to target cell death. Shorter and coworkers[44] demonstrated that peripheral blood mononuclear cells from patients with Crohn's disease, as well as ulcerative colitis, were capable of killing adult allogeneic human colon epithelial target cells. Shorter observed that the cytotoxic effector cells were T cells; that the cytotoxicity diminished 10 days after intestinal resection; and that a 4-day incubation with either E. coli 0119:B14, lipopolysaccharide (LPS), or the IgM fraction of sera from patients with IBD could induce normal peripheral blood MNC to become cytotoxic for colon cells. Stobo and coworkers[45] showed that the cytotoxic capabilities of UC peripheral blood MNC were present in the non-T, non-B, Fc receptor-bearing class of lymphocytes (K cells). It was proposed[45] that antigen-antibody complexes containing anticolon antibodies could arm Fc receptor-bearing K cells in patients with IBD and lead to killing via antibody-dependent cytotoxicity (ADCC) mechanisms. However, controlled and blinded cytotoxicity experiments using peripheral blood MNC from patients with autoimmune disorders, chronic liver diseases, infectious diarrheal illnesses, and other intestinal diseases were not performed. If, indeed, anticolon antibodies are prearming cells, patients without IBD, who have anticolon antibodies, could have prearmed cytotoxic K cells or, alternatively, could exhibit altered natural killer (NK) activity against colonic epithelial cell targets.

A number of experimental observations have led investigators to question cell-mediated cytotoxicity as the primary cause of IBD. First, in contrast to peripheral blood MNC, we and others have observed that both normal and IBD intestinal MNC are poor mediators of cytotoxicity against cell line targets in both ADCC and spontaneous cell-mediated cytotoxicity (SCMC) assays.[46,47] Second, Auer and coworkers[48,49] have demonstrated that peripheral blood MNC from patients with Crohn's disease have decreased cytotoxic capabilities against noncolonic cell line targets, in both SCMC and ADCC systems and that patients with infectious diarrheal illnesses exhibit similar cytotoxicity defects. We not only observed decreased cytotoxicity by peripheral blood MNC from IBD patients but also found that peripheral blood cell-mediated cytotoxicity was only partially restored after induction by lectins or interferon.[50,51] Finally, Gibson et al.[52] have clearly demonstrated that spontaneously cytotoxic as well as LAK cells are unlikely to play a role in the generation of colonic epithelial cell injury by direct cytotoxicity in IBD. It therefore appears that there is generalized defective K cell and NK cell function in patients with active Crohn's disease.

It is intriguing that in comparison with control peripheral blood MNC, intestinal MNC from both control and IBD specimens are poor mediators of both SCMC and ADCC with cell lines as targets.[46,47,50,51] Although lectins and interferon can induce cell-mediated cytotoxicity by intestinal MNC, IBD intestinal MNC are hyporesponsive to activation by lectins or interferon.[50] Lymphocytes in a solid organ compartment, such as the intestine, thus appear to differ from peripheral blood lymphocytes and have their own unique biologic and functional capabilities.[51] Inactive cytotoxic effector cells may serve an important role as a pool of cells that can be called upon to participate in host mucosal defense mechanisms without nonspecifically causing damage to the surrounding tissue. Intestinal MNC thus must be activated to become efficient effector cells.[47,50,51] Examination of intestinal cytotoxic cell precursor subpopulations is thus of great interest because of the opportunity to understand effector capabilities that are markedly different from peripheral blood MNC.

Fiocchi and coworkers[53] and Hogan and coworkers[54] have observed that interleukin 2 (IL-2) will induce control, as well as IBD intestinal MNC to lyse cell line targets. In their studies, intestinal lamina propria mononuclear cells were unable to mediate spontaneous cell-mediated cytotoxicity and were devoid of NK cells, but after incubation in culture with IL-2 for 3–4 days, lymphokine-activated killer cells were observed.[53,54] Shanahan and coworkers[55] have demonstrated the presence of distinct subpopulations of cytotoxic effector cells in human intestine and have shown that natural killer and lymphokine-activated killer cells are both present in human gut mucosa. In recent studies, Shanahan et al.[56] have observed that antibodies to the CD3 complex of the human T-cell receptor complex trigger T-cell cytotoxicity in normal (noninflamed) mucosal MNC populations. They have postulated that anti-CD3-triggered lysis may be a marker of in vivo primed mucosal T cells of undetermined antigen specificity.[56] Future studies delineating the cytokines, cytotoxic cell types, and cytotoxic effector molecules involved in normal mucosal immune defense mechanisms and the alterations associated with IBD will provide valuable insights into the mechanisms of protection as well as injury that are present in the intestinal immune system.

ALTERATIONS IN IMMUNOGLOBULIN SYNTHESIS AND SECRETION

Long-standing IBD is characterized by a mixed cellular infiltrate composed predominantly of B cells and T cells. The B cells are arrayed in follicles or in areas subjacent to ulcerations, while the T cells are found around granulomas, in perifollicular zones, and in deep areas of lesions. IgG-containing cells are increased more than other plasma cell types and are present in deeper tissue layers. Other inflammatory cells present in lesions of IBD include neutrophils, eosinophils, mast cells, and macrophages. The latter are a large component of the granulomas in Crohn's disease. The cellular infiltrate in IBD does not explain the origin of the lesion and may be similar to that found in any long-standing intestinal infection.

The intestine contains numerous immunogenic substances, to which the mucosal immune system must respond and mount a protective response. The normal ongoing intestinal immune response must be effective and yet controlled. In IBD, on the other hand, the mucosal immune system may evidence altered immune responses because of defective or altered immunoregulation. Stevens and coworkers demonstrated diminished tetanus-specific immunoglobulin G production in vitro by peripheral blood mononuclear cells from patients with Crohn's disease, 7 days after immunization with tetanus toxoid,[57] and proposed that in IBD the inability to generate effectively a normal humoral response to potential pathogens could lead to persistent infection and chronic inflammation.

Elson et al. found that pokeweed mitogen (PWM)-stimulated peripheral blood MNC from Crohn's disease patients revealed "covert" suppressor T cells capable of marked IgM suppression.[58] They subsequently described two patients in whom the development of common variable hypogammaglobulinemia followed the development of Crohn's disease.[59] James and coworkers[60] characterized the covert suppressor T cells in Crohn's disease patients as having a unique (LEU-2a[+], HNK-1[+]) cell surface phenotype. They found that T cells from both peripheral blood and lamina propria of Crohn's disease patients were similar to normal peripheral blood T cells in their ability to provide help for IgM synthesis.[61] When suppressor cell function was assessed, neither peripheral blood nor lamina propria T cells from patients with Crohn's disease or control patients caused inhibition of IgA synthesis. Elson and coworkers[62] also found that lamina propria of control and Crohn's disease intestines contain T cells that are able to exhibit excellent helper function, but do not exhibit suppressor cell capabilities. Additional evidence for a central role of CD4 T cells and an intact immune response in the pathogenesis of Crohn's disease has recently been provided by the report by James[63] of a patient with an 18-year history of Crohn's disease who developed a complete remission after human immunodeficiency virus infection and development of progressive immunodeficiency.

However, studies by Selby and coworkers[64] of the T-cell subsets present in IBD lesions demonstrated that T4/T8 ratios are similar to those in control intestinal tissue, leading them to conclude that an imbalance of mucosal immunoregulatory T cells as defined by monoclonal antibodies does not occur in IBD. Furthermore, in examination of active IBD patient peripheral blood MNC, Selby and Jewell[14] and Yuan et al.[15] found no differences between IBD patients and controls with regard to circulating T lymphocytes or their subsets.

It is now evident that in IBD there are major changes in spontaneous immunoglobulin secretion by intestinal and peripheral blood mononuclear cells, particularly with regard to IgA and IgG subclasses.[65,66] Our studies have demonstrated that the peripheral blood mononuclear cells of patients with new onset, untreated IBD display a strikingly high level of spontaneous synthesis and secretion of IgA as well as IgG and IgM.[67,68] This pattern of markedly elevated spontaneous immunoglobulin secretion coupled with PWM-induced suppression is not unique to IBD peripheral blood MNC; we have also observed it with peripheral blood MNC of patients with systemic lupus erythematosus and Henoch-Schonlein purpura, as well as with normal human rib bone marrow MNC.[68-70] Intestinal MNC from control specimens also spontaneously secrete large amounts of IgA, which is suppressed by

PWM.[67,71] In IBD patients, intestinal MNC exhibit decreased spontaneous IgA secretion,[67,71] but have increased IgG secretion compared with control intestinal MNC.[72,73] Intestinal MNC have unique capabilities and differ in their functional characteristics when compared with peripheral blood MNC.[47,50,51,67,68,71,72] Furthermore, changes in peripheral blood MNC function are not specific for IBD and often reflect secondary events. We have, therefore, focused our attention on spontaneous antibody secretion by intestinal MNC.

Control intestinal MNC secrete 61% of their IgA as IgA_1, whereas intestinal MNC from IBD specimens exhibit an increase of 71–74% of their IgA as IgA_1.[71] These changes are consistent with the migration of monomeric IgA- and IgA_1-secreting cells from peripheral blood into the diseased intestine and could represent a normal mucosal response to intestinal antigens or pathogens. Alternatively, with overall decreased IgA production[67,71] and an increased percentage of monomeric IgA and IgA_1 being produced, a local dimeric IgA and IgA_2 deficiency may occur in IBD,[73] which could lead to impairment of mucosal immune defense mechanisms.

When compared with control intestinal MNC, a marked increase in spontaneous secretion of IgG is observed from IBD MNC.[72] The greatest increase in spontaneous IgG secretion is seen with ulcerative colitis intestinal MNC, due to the secretion of large amounts of IgG_1 with a concomitant increase in IgG_3 secretion. Crohn's disease intestinal MNC exhibit increased IgG secretion primarily due to IgG_2.[72] We have recently observed similar alterations in IgG subclass concentrations in the sera of active, untreated, IBD patients.[74]

That IBD intestinal MNC should exhibit increased total IgG and IgG subclass secretion in vitro is consistent with previous observations[75-79] of increased numbers and altered ratios of intestinal lymphocytes and plasma cells in IBD. The total lymphocyte number has been observed to be four times greater than normal in intestinal specimens from patients with both ulcerative colitis and Crohn's disease,[75-79] with the major increase occurring in IgG-containing cells. Compared with control specimens, numbers of IgG-containing cells were 30 times greater, while numbers of IgA-containing cells were two times greater and those of IgM-containing cells five times greater than normal. Van Spreeuwel et al.[80] have found that in comparison with IBD biopsies, significantly fewer IgG-containing cells were found in biopsies of patients with acute infectious colitis.[80] The status of IgG-containing cells in the mucosa[80] may thus provide an important marker in the delineation of differences between IBD and acute infectious colitis. The increased secretion of total IgG and IgG subclasses from IBD intestinal MNC, therefore, is most likely related to the increased percentage of IgG-containing cells present in vivo in inflamed mucosa. Indeed, Kett et al.[81] have observed increased IgG_1-containing cells in ulcerative colitis patients and increased IgG_2-containing cells in Crohn's disease patients.[81] Furthermore, Kett and coworkers[82] have observed decreased J-chain expression in both IgA_1- and IgA_2-producing cells in colonic mucosa from patients with ulcerative colitis and Crohn's disease. Finally, Badr-El-Din et al.[83] have also recently provided evidence for defective IgA production in ulcerative colitis.

Traditionally, IgA has been viewed as the major protective mucosal immunoglobulin of the intestine. Now it appears that, for inflammatory bowel disease at least, IgG and its subclasses also need to be carefully examined. Because elevated levels of serum IgG_1 have been associated with a number of potentially autoimmune disorders,[84-89] it could be speculated that IgG_1 contributes locally to tissue autoimmune events in patients with ulcerative colitis. Different antigens and mitogens induce antibody responses restricted to particular IgG subclasses in both murine and human systems.[85,90-93] IgG_1 and IgG_3 antibodies account for the predominant IgG response to proteins and T cell-dependent antigens.[85,88,89] Both IgG_1 and IgG_3 are better complement pathway activators and opsonins than IgG_2 and IgG_4.[85,88,89] Delineation of the stimuli and antigens that induce the increased secretion of IgG subclasses in IBD may provide insight into possible etiologic and immunopathogenic aspects.[73] In this regard, it is important to note the recent evidence provided by Kaulfersch et al.[94] that both the B-cell and T-cell populations in IBD lamina propria MNC populations are polyclonal in nature. IgG_2 provides the predominant IgG response to carbohydrates and many bacterial antigens. IgG_2 and IgG_4 deficiencies[85-89] have been detected in patients with recurrent bacterial infections (e.g., otitis media, pneumococcal respiratory tract infections, pericarditis, meningococcal infections) and in some inherited immunodeficiency disorders (such as ataxia telangiectasia and Wiskott-Aldrich syndrome). The increased production of IgG_2 in Crohn's disease may represent an appropriate immune response that might partially contain, but not eradicate, a chronic infectious process.[73]

Therefore, it is now apparent that: 1) major alterations occur with regard to spontaneous antibody secretion in IBD; 2) PWM-induced suppression is a nonspecific and irrelevant phenomenon; 3) the peripheral blood compartment reflects mainly secondary phenomena in IBD; 4) intestinal MNC comprise a unique immunologic compartment with distinct immunobiologic capabilities; and 5) it is within the intestine involved with disease that major alterations in antibody secretion are occurring, particularly with regard to the IgA and IgG subclasses.[67-74]

GRANULOCYTE AND MACROPHAGE FUNCTION

Inflammatory bowel disease has long been viewed as a disorder of chronic inflammation — a view that is reinforced by the large numbers of lymphocytes and histiocytes in the diseased mucosa and submucosa. Both ulcerative colitis and Crohn's disease also have histologic characteristics of acute inflammation: there is intense infiltration of the mucosa and submucosa with neutrophils. Large numbers of neutrophils leave the blood stream and enter the inflamed mucosa and submucosa of the bowel. Some neutrophils migrate across the epithelium into the lumen and are passed in the stool, whereas others are destroyed in the inflamed tissue before they have a chance to migrate into the lumen. This constant flux of neutrophils implies the presence of chemotactic agents in the inflamed mucosa. As markers of acute inflammation, the abundant neutrophils indicate that there is a large acute component to inflammatory bowel disease that coexists with a chronic disease state.

Investigators have examined polymorphonuclear leukocyte (PMN) function, including migration, chemotaxis, adherence, and phagocytosis, in IBD. Rhodes et al.[95] demonstrated decreased random migration and decreased chemotaxis of normal peripheral blood leukocytes exposed in vitro to drugs frequently used in the treatment of IBD (prednisone, sulfasalazine, and 5-aminosalicylic acid). By the skin window chamber technique, random migration of PMNs was found to be suppressed in Crohn's disease in vivo.[96] Inhibitors directed against both chemotactic factors and leukocytes in sera from patients with Crohn's disease and ulcerative colitis were described by Rhodes et al.[97] On the other hand, chemotaxis induced by zymosan-activated serum or casein has been found to be normal in patients with IBD, and phagocytosis by PMNs from patients with IBD has been shown to be no different from control subjects.[96-98]

Saverymuttu et al. have carried out important studies on the in vivo assessment of granulocyte migration to diseased bowel.[99,100] Patients' peripheral blood granulocytes were isolated in vitro and radiolabeled by incubation with [111]Indium tropolonate. The radiolabeled granulocytes were injected intravenously with the patient positioned beneath a gamma camera. In 20 of 22 Crohn's disease patients, the radiolabeled granulocytes accumulated rapidly in the inflamed bowel.[99] A similar study done in ulcerative colitis showed no delayed migration in any of the 15 patients tested.[100] In addition to establishing the absence of a defect of migration in IBD, these studies emphasize the importance of granulocytes in the mediation of inflammation in IBD.[99,100] Refinements in labeling techniques have been reported by Scholmerich et al., who have demonstrated the usefulness of technetium 99m-hexamethyl propylene amine oxine as a leukocyte label in the scanning of Crohn's disease patients.[101] Although few studies have been performed on macrophage function in IBD, the demonstration by Pullman et al.[102] that technetium 99m-stannous colloid labeling of both mononuclear phagocytes (macrophages) and leukocytes can be used to provide an objective assessment of disease activity in IBD also gives evidence for macrophage chemotaxis and transmigration into inflamed intestine of both ulcerative colitis and Crohn's disease patients. Thus the in vivo evaluation of granulocyte and macrophage function in IBD patients will lead in the future to important basic and clinical studies.

PRODUCTS OF THE COMPLEMENT PATHWAY

Complement activation is one of the major effector mechanisms of the immune system. Investigators have proposed pathogenic roles in IBD for complement system molecules, but the nature and extent of their involvement in IBD is still undefined. Some of the disease's clinical and histologic changes are consistent with the biologic activities of C3b and C5a. Opsonization by complement leading to particle coating with C3b is an important step in phagocytosis, enabling the necessary contact between phagocyte (neutrophil or macrophage) and particle through specific cellular receptors. Phagocytosis of bacteria and cellular debris occurs at an accelerated rate in intestinal inflammation, irrespective of the cause. Abnormalities in phagocytosis could influence the intensity of the inflammatory response. C5a, like LTB_4, is a potent chemotactic agent for neutrophils and increases vascular permeability.[103] The large numbers of neutrophils in IBD mucosa suggest the presence of a chemotactic agent in IBD, and the presence of mucosal edema suggests the presence of a soluble mediator that enhances vascular permeability. Thus some of the functional and histologic changes seen in IBD are consistent with the biologic activities of C3b and C5a.

Several studies have found normal levels of C3 and C4 in the circulation in IBD. Incubation of serum with zymosan or nylon fibers activates the alternative pathway with production of C3b and C5a. The state of activation of the alternative pathway in IBD has variously been described as decreased, normal, and increased.

In support of decreased activation of the alternative pathway is a study in which depression of properidin and properidin convertase, along with diminished consumption of C3–C9 after reaction with cobra venom were seen in sera from patients with Crohn's disease and ulcerative colitis.[104] In other experiments that also demonstrated decreased activation of the alternative pathway in IBD, sera from healthy persons and patients with Crohn's disease was incubated with zymosan or nylon fibers,[105] and the amount of C5a-related chemoattractant activity was assayed. C5a activity was diminished in Crohn's sera compared with healthy individuals, there was decreased consumption of the major complement component C3, and the generation of C5a was reduced in Crohn's disease patients treated with steroids.[105]

In a similar study with different results,[106] the alternative pathway was activated by incubation of serum with zymosan, and the opsonization of zymosan with C3b was quantitated. Binding of C3b to zymosan was greater in the Crohn's sera than in healthy individuals, whereas consumption of C3, the precursor of C3b, was similar in the two groups.[106] Thus this study[106] suggests that the activation of the alternative pathway in Crohn's disease is normal, but the degradation of C3b is impaired.

Finally, there are studies indicating an increased level of activation of the complement pathways in IBD.[107–109] Radioiodinated C3 was injected intravenously into healthy persons and patients with IBD, and both the synthesis and catabolism of C3 were enhanced in patients with Crohn's disease and ulcerative colitis, suggesting an enhanced state of activation.[107,108] The levels of a C3 split product, C3c, were assayed in plasma from healthy persons and untreated outpatients with Crohn's disease and ulcerative colitis.[109] The levels of C3c in the Crohn's patients were tenfold greater than those in the healthy persons or ulcerative colitis patients. C3c levels did not correlate with disease activity in Crohn's disease. Elevated levels of C3c in Crohn's disease suggest hypercatabolism of C3 and activation of the complement cascade.

PROSTAGLANDINS AND LEUKOTRIENES

Some of the functional and macroscopic changes seen in IBD, including mucosal hyperemia and edema, are typical of changes seen in any inflammatory state, no matter what organ system is involved. These changes are the products of soluble mediators released in the process of inflammation. They cause tissue edema by increasing vascular (postcapillary venule) permeability to albumin and other macromolecules; hyperemia results from mediators that induce vasodilation. Other functional changes (including diminished salt and water absorption) that are characteristic of intestinal inflammation are probably also the result of soluble mediators, but their pathogenesis is less clear. Progress has been made in characterization of the soluble mediators of inflammation and their role in the amplification of the immune response in IBD. Although study of mediators of inflammation is not likely to provide any insight into the events that initiate the disease, there are two reasons for defining their pathogenic role in IBD. First, the soluble mediators appear to be largely responsible for the clinical and histologic changes seen in the disease. Second, the drugs that have proven to be beneficial for ulcerative colitis and Crohn's disease appear to exert their therapeutic effect by blocking the synthesis of those mediators. As will be expanded upon below, corticosteroids and sulfasalazine block the synthesis of prostaglandins and leukotrienes in vivo and in vitro.[110,111] Furthermore, until the etiologic agents of IBD are identified, it is likely that advances in medical therapy for IBD will be in the area of regulation of the synthesis of soluble mediators of inflammation.

Arachidonic acid is metabolized through the cyclooxygenase pathway to prostacyclin, thromboxanes, and prostaglandins. Prostaglandins are produced by almost all mammalian cells, including intestinal epithelium and cells associated with inflammatory events (i.e., mast cells, macrophages, and platelets).[112,113] Prostaglandins, particularly those of the E series, have biologic properties that are proinflammatory (i.e., enhanced vascular permeability, vasodilation, and production of pain).[112,113] Prostaglandins also have specific functional effects on the intestine. They induce mucosal secretion of water and electrolytes in the small intestine.[114] The effects of prostaglandins on secretory function in the colon are less well defined; pharmacologic doses may impair salt and water transport in the colon, but physiologic doses have little effect.[115]

There is no question that IBD is associated with increased levels of prostaglandin production. Elevated levels of prostaglandins (primarily PGE_2) are found in the stool, venous blood, and rectal mucosa in IBD.[116-118] Elevated levels of prostaglandin metabolites are found in the urine.[118] When incubated in vitro, pieces of rectal mucosa from patients with ulcerative colitis synthesize increased amounts of PGE_2 and thromboxane B_2.[116] An in vivo estimate of prostaglandin synthesis by rectal mucosa is achieved by use of bags of dialysis tubing, which are filled with buffer and placed in the patient's rectum. After a period of hours, the bag is removed and the concentration of prostaglandins in the bag measured by bioassay or radioimmunoassay.[119] Studies using this technique reveal elevated levels of PGE_2 in the rectal dialysates of patients with ulcerative colitis. Prostaglandin levels in IBD, whether in mucosa, serum, or rectal dialysate, correlate with disease activity, and successful medical management results in a reduction in prostaglandin levels. In inactive UC, prostaglandin levels are not significantly different from normal controls.[120]

The source of the prostaglandins in colonic mucosa in IBD is not well defined; both epithelial cells and mononuclear inflammatory cells produce prostaglandins. Definition of relative rates of synthesis by epithelial and mononuclear cells requires physical separation of the cell types with all the attendant artifacts of the separation system. Despite these difficulties, it appears that intestinal mononuclear cells are responsible for as much, or more, prostaglandin synthesis than are intestinal epithelial cells.[121] This finding is consistent with studies of inflammation in other organ systems in which inflammatory cells were found to be the major source of prostaglandin synthesis.[112,113]

IBD is clearly associated with elevated prostaglandin levels and enhanced prostaglandin synthesis. Furthermore, prostaglandins have proinflammatory biological properties that could account for some of the histologic and functional changes seen in IBD. Alternatively, enhanced prostaglandin synthesis in IBD may be a nonspecific product of intestinal inflammation that has little to do with the pathogenesis of the disease. Some insight into this question comes from studies of the effects of drug therapy on prostaglandin levels in IBD. Sulfasalazine and its cleavage product, 5-aminosalicylate, inhibit cyclooxygenase in vitro.[116] Moreover, when patients are treated with sulfasalazine, prostaglandin synthesis in the rectal mucosa diminishes. Corticosteroids induce the synthesis of a protein, lipomodulin, which inhibits phospholipase A_2.[110] The rate-limiting step in the synthesis of prostaglandins and other arachidonic acid metabolites is the release of arachidonate from phospholipids by phospholipase A_2. Inhibition of phospholipase A_2 synthesis by lipomodulin results in diminished synthesis of prostaglandins. Measurement of PGE_2 levels in rectal dialysates from patients with UC reveals that even a brief course of therapy with oral prednisolone results in a marked decrease in PGE_2 production.[119] Thus data from both in vitro and in vivo studies with sulfasalazine and corticosteroids are consistent with the suggestion that prostaglandins are major mediators of inflammation in IBD and, moreover, that the therapeutic actions of sulfasalazine and corticosteroids are achieved by inhibition of prostaglandin synthesis.

However, there is substantial evidence against a significant role for prostaglandins as mediators of inflammation in IBD. This evidence comes from a few small clinical studies of nonsteroidal antiinflammatory drugs (e.g., NSAIDs), particularly indomethacin, in IBD.[118,122,123] Indomethacin and other NSAIDs are potent inhibitors of cyclooxygenase. Use of these drugs in rheumatoid arthritis and other inflammatory diseases results in both decreased prostaglandin synthesis and diminished clinical activity. It is this clinical improvement in response to treatment with NSAIDs that helped establish a role for prostaglandins as important mediators of inflammation in rheumatoid arthritis. In contrast to their usefulness in rheumatoid arthritis, NSAIDs have no role in the medical management of IBD. Small trials of indomethacin administered orally[119] and rectally[122,123] revealed no improvement in ulcerative colitis. There is even some suggestion that indomethacin may cause clinical deterioration in ulcerative colitis, despite causing a decrease in prostaglandin production.[118,123] Another NSAID, flurbiprofen, has also been shown to cause clinical deterioration in ulcerative colitis.[124,125] The failure of NSAIDs to induce clinical improvement in IBD, despite their inhibition of prostaglandin production, suggests that prostaglandins do not play important roles as mediators of inflammation in IBD. Moreover, these studies suggest that corticosteroids and sulfasalazine exert their therapeutic effects in IBD by a mechanism other than inhibition of prostaglandin synthesis.

Attention has now turned to lipoxygenase products in IBD. The cyclooxygenase pathway is present in effectively all mammalian cells, but the 5-lipoxygenase pathway exists primarily in cells of bone marrow origin involved in the inflammatory process (i.e., mast cells, neutrophils, monocytes, and macrophages).[126] The major products of the 5-lipoxygenase pathway are 5-hydroxy-6,8,11,14-eicosatetraenoic acid (5-HETE) and leukotrienes B_4, C_4, D_4, and E_4 (LTB_4, LTC_4, LTD_4, and LTE_4). Neutrophils metabolize arachidonate to 5-HETE and LTB_4.[120] The sulfidoleukotrienes (LTC_4, LTD_4, and LTE_4), along with 5-HETE and LTB_4, are products of mast cells and macrophages.[126] LTB_4 and, to a lesser extent, 5-HETE are potent chemotactic agents for neutrophils. LTB_4, in the presence of neutrophils, also induces enhanced vascular permeability. The sulfidoleukotrienes induce smooth muscle contraction in the lung, blood vessels, and the gastrointestinal tract.[113,126]

The lipoxygenase pathway was described much more recently than the cyclooxygenase pathway.[127] As a result, there are fewer studies on the role of lipoxygenase products in IBD than on the role of prostaglandins. The studies on the role of the lipoxygenase pathway in IBD have focused on LTB_4. Incubation of IBD mucosa with radiolabeled arachidonic acid results in the synthesis of large quantities of LTB_4 and 5-HETE and smaller quantities of PGE_2 and thromboxane B_2.[128] IBD mucosa produces larger quantities of lipoxygenase and cyclooxygenase products than normal mucosa. Patterns of arachidonate metabolism are similar for ulcerative colitis and Crohn's disease. Lipid extracts of IBD mucosa contain large amounts of LTB_4: 250 ng/g of IBD mucosa as compared with less than 5 ng/g of normal mucosa.[125] A concentration of 250 ng/g of mucosa is the equivalent of a solution of 5×10^{-7}M, a concentration well within the range of biologic activity of LTB_4.

The results of this in vitro study were confirmed by an in vivo study using rectal dialysis. Lauritsen and coworkers measured the levels of PGE_2 and LTB_4 in rectal dialysates from healthy persons and patients with ulcerative colitis. Levels of both PGE_2 and LTB_4 were markedly higher in rectal dialysates from the UC patients.[119] Moreover, treatment of UC patients with a short course of prednisolone resulted in a decline in PGE_2 and LTB_4 almost to normal levels.

The presence of large numbers of neutrophils in IBD mucosa suggests that there is a chemotactic factor (or factors) present in IBD mucosa that induces neutrophils to migrate out of the circulation and into the tissue. LTB_4 is a potent chemoattractant for human neutrophils[129]; there are, however, other chemotactic compounds that are likely to be present in IBD mucosa. Among these compounds are C5a, a product of the complement pathway[130] and formylmethionylleucylphenylalanine (FMLP), a product of *E. coli*.[131] In an attempt to sort out the contributions of various chemotactic factors to neutrophil infiltration in IBD, a study was done using homogenized IBD mucosa as the chemotactic stimulus for ^{51}Cr-labeled neutrophils in a Boyden chamber.[132] IBD mucosa had far more chemotactic activity than normal mucosa. Moreover, lipid extracts of the IBD mucosa had 65–90% of the chemotactic activity of the whole mucosa, indicating that among the compounds contributing to the neutrophil chemotactic activity in IBD mucosa are one or more lipids. The lipid extract from IBD mucosa was fractionated by reverse-phase high-performance liquid chromatography (HPLC) and the fractions assayed for chemotactic activity. The only fraction with significant chemotactic activity was the fraction coeluting with LTB_4. Moreover, the chemotactic activity in the lipid extract of IBD mucosa was totally ablated with antiserum raised against LTB_4. These data indicate that LTB_4 is the major neutrophil chemotactic agent in IBD mucosa. If the findings using the in vitro assay for neutrophil chemotaxis in the Boyden chamber can be extrapolated to the in vivo situation, one could argue that LTB_4 is the mediator that is primarily responsible for neutrophils leaving the circulation and entering the intestinal tissue in IBD. The generation of LTB_4 is certainly not the initiating event in IBD, nor is it specific for IBD. However, inhibition of the process of neutrophil migration into the mucosa and submucosa in IBD would diminish the intensity of the inflammatory response and, in turn, the degree of clinical disease activity. In this case, drugs that inhibit LTB_4 synthesis, or block LTB_4 binding to neutrophil receptors, might be expected to diminish the inflammatory response and disease activity in IBD.

Although the role of LTB_4 in IBD has been the most extensively studied, there are preliminary reports of a possible role for the sulfidoleukotrienes (LTC_4, LTD_4, LTE_4). Colonic mucosa obtained at surgery was chopped and incubated in the presence and absence of the calcium ionophore A23187. The sulfidoleukotrienes released into the media were assayed by radioimmunoassay. Crohn's colitis mucosa produced three times as much sulfidoleukotrienes as normal mucosa in both the stimulated and unstimulated conditions.[133] The predominant sulfidoleukotriene found was LTE_4, suggesting that released LTC_4 is rapidly degraded by peptidases. Sulfidoleukotrienes cause smooth muscle contraction, vasoconstriction, plasma exudation, and mucus release. Each of these biologic effects could be relevant to IBD: for example, effects on smooth muscle may be associated with increased intestinal motility.

IMMUNOPHARMACOLOGY

The medications used to treat ulcerative colitis and Crohn's disease most likely exert their effects through the immune system. Corticosteroids have been the mainstay of therapy, markedly improving symptoms in the acute phases of the disease, but their long-term use can cause significant complications. Sulfasalazine is beneficial for mild Crohn's colitis and is useful for inducing and maintaining remissions in ulcerative colitis. For the most part, the effects of these drugs on arachidonate metabolism have been studied in vitro, and many of these findings may not carry over into in vivo situations. As mentioned above, both sulfasalazine and 5-aminosalicylic acid (5-ASA) inhibit cyclooxygenase and, thus, prostaglandin synthesis. The ID_{50} for cyclooxygenase is about 1 mM for both compounds. In addition, sulfasalazine, but not 5-ASA, inhibits thromboxane synthetase in both platelets[134] and colon. Sulfasalazine has also been shown to inhibit 5-lipoxygenase and LTB_4 synthesis in human peripheral blood neutrophils and in inflamed colon.[135] The ID_{50} of sulfasalazine for neutrophil 5-lipoxygenase is about 1 mM. 5-ASA also has an effect on the 5-lipoxygenase pathway, but the nature of that effect has not yet been elucidated.[135]

Defining the mechanism of action of sulfasalazine is a particular problem. The stool concentrations of sulfasalazine and its cleavage product, 5-ASA, are extraordinarily high, i.e., 2×10^{-3} M and 9×10^{-3} M, respectively. However, the serum concentration of sulfasalazine is 5×10^{-5} M and that of 5-ASA is 7×10^{-6} M.[111] Thus the colonic epithelial cells are exposed to a high drug concentration on the luminal surface and a much lower concentration on the basolateral surface. The concentrations of these drugs in the inflamed mucosa in IBD is not known. This is an important issue in that the inhibitory effects of sulfasalazine and 5-ASA on arachidonate metabolism described in vitro occur at concentrations around 1 mM, which is well within the range of concentrations in the colonic lumen but far higher than the concentrations in the circulation. Whether or not these concentrations are achieved in the inflamed mucosa is not known. Another difficulty in defining the mechanisms of action of sulfasalazine in IBD is the large number of in vitro effects of sulfasalazine that might be related to its therapeutic efficacy. The effects of sulfasalazine and 5-ASA on arachidonate metabolism are enumerated above; however, sulfasalazine and 5-ASA also have in vitro effects unrelated to arachidonate metabolism, including inhibition of chemotactic peptide binding to neutrophils,[136] inhibition of neutrophil chemotaxis, inhibition of platelet activating factor synthesis,[137] inhibition of antibody secretion,[138] and inhibition of oxygen radical generation as well as functioning as an oxygen radical scavenger.[139] Any or all of these biologic properties may contribute to the therapeutic efficacy of sulfasalazine.

Corticosteroids, like sulfasalazine, have a number of biologic properties that may be related to their therapeutic effects in IBD. These include effects on lymphocyte differentiation, lymphokine synthesis, and interferon production. Corticosteroids, like sulfasalazine, also have effects on arachidonic acid metabolism that may relate to their therapeutic effects in IBD. As noted earlier, corticosteroids promote the synthesis of a protein, lipomodulin,[110] which inhibits phospholipase A_2 and thus blocks the release of arachidonic acid from phospholipids. The inhibition of arachidonic acid release would block the synthesis of both cyclooxygenase and lipoxygenase products. As mentioned above, Lauritsen and coworkers found markedly elevated levels of LTB_4 and PGE_2 in rectal dialysates of UC patients.[119] When these patients were given a short course of oral prednisolone, the levels of both mediators fell almost to normal. One could interpret this as the result of the induction of lipomodulin synthesis by corticosteroids. Alternatively, one could argue that corticosteroids diminished the inflammatory response by some other mechanism, and the decline in LTB_4 and PGE_2 is a nonspecific manifestation of diminished inflammation.

CONCLUSIONS

Extensive investigation for more than two decades has failed to uncover the cause of either ulcerative colitis or Crohn's disease. Moreover, no coherent underlying mechanism has emerged to elucidate the role of the immunologic abnormalities identified to date. There is sufficient convincing evidence, however, to conclude that immunologic processes are involved in the pathogenesis of these diseases.

The initiating factors and activation events in IBD are currently receiving increased attention (Fig. 23–1). The search continues for an infectious agent against which an inflammatory response is elicited. The list of candidates for that role includes viruses, bacteria, and mycobacteria. One potential candidate as an etiologic agent in Crohn's disease is a variant of *Mycobacterium paratuberculosis*.[140-144] However, there is insufficient evidence to definitively implicate mycobacteria at this time.[145] An infectious theory would suggest that the host mounts an appropriate immune response against a pathogenic organism but is unable to eradicate the organism. Most of the candidate organisms have fastidious culture requirements, and it is suggested that the inability to consistently isolate them is related to the difficulties of in vitro culture. A second possibility is that the initiating agent is a common agent, either dietary or bacterial, against which the patient mounts an inappropriately vigorous and prolonged inflammatory response. The epithelial cell could play an important role in this process by the presentation of cell surface autoantigens or antigens in the intestinal tract, with subsequent triggering of macrophages and release of IL-1 (Fig. 21–1).

Both ulcerative colitis and Crohn's disease are largely confined to the gastrointestinal tract. There appear to be no systemic immune abnormalities, which suggests that immune recognition and memory processes are intact and are directed specifically against the intestine (Fig. 23–2). Cell-mediated components of the intestinal immune system could be directing a cytotoxic response against a normal component cell within the intestine, most likely the epithelial cell, which may have antigenic cross-reactivity with microbial antigens. Alternatively, the epithelial cell may express new antigens (such as DR antigens), perhaps in response to infection or inflammation, and the immune response could be directed against one or more of these cell surface antigens.

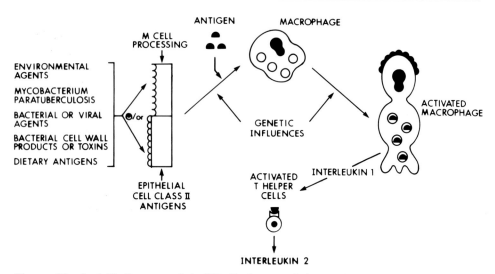

Figure 23 – 1 Initiating events in IBD. Environmental agents, mycobacteria, infectious agents, bacterial cell wall products or toxins, or dietary antigens may be processed by M cells followed by antigen presentation in conjunction with class II antigens on intestinal epithelial cells resulting in an intestinal immune response in patients with inflammatory bowel disease. In a genetically predisposed host, macrophages may then activate the immune response through the production of cytokines such as interleukin-1. Subsequent activation of helper T cells and interleukin-2 production may then initiate cell-mediated events in IBD. Although the precise infectious agents or lumenal antigens that play a role in IBD remain unclear, the initiation of a mucosal immune response may be an appropriate host defense mechanism against a pathogenic agent that is unable to eradicate the organism. Alternatively, the IBD patient may be mounting an inappropriately vigorous and prolonged inflammatory response against common bacterial or dietary antigens.

Constant stimulation of the secretory IgA system results in the priming and activation of B cells for accelerated production of IgA_1 and monomeric IgA (Fig. 23 – 2). In IBD patients, a break in the mucosal barrier and/or failure of IgA_2 and dimeric IgA to control pathogens result in increased synthesis and secretion of IgG — with a preferential increase of IgG_1 and IgG_3 in ulcerative colitis and an increase of IgG_2 in Crohn's disease (Fig. 23 – 2). IgG antibodies, by autoimmune cross-reactivity and/or complement activation (Fig. 23 – 3), may contribute in a primary or secondary fashion to the pathogenesis of the disease. Alternatively, it is possible that altered secretion patterns of IgA and IgG (and their subclasses) reflect a normal mucosal immune response to infectious agents or stimulatory molecules, which augment or perpetuate the intestinal inflammatory process. Identification of the antigens against which antibodies of IgG and IgA subclasses are directed in IBD may provide important information regarding the altered immunobiology that underlies ulcerative colitis and Crohn's disease.

The inability to identify specific antigens or agents triggering the immune response in IBD may reflect the limitations of the methods used to look for the antigens or may reflect the transience of the agents. The antigen or agent may be present only briefly, but a sensitized, immune response persists. It is also possible

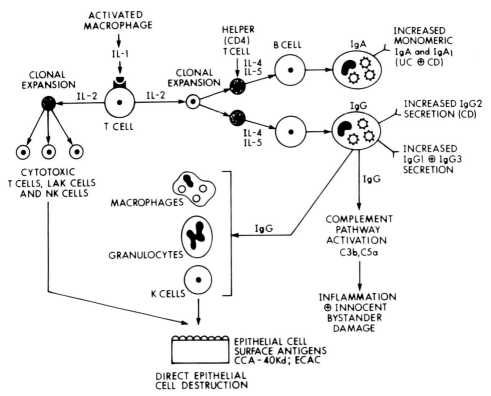

Figure 23–2 Cell-mediated events in IBD. After antigen processing and presentation of antigens to T lymphocytes in combination with IL-1 (Fig. 23–1), a population of sensitized and activated T cells capable of IL-2 secretion can stimulate expansion of specific helper T cells (CD4). Increased helper T cell-B cell function may lead to increased antibody secretion due to the release of additional cytokines, such as IL-4 and IL-5. Preferential expansion of monomeric IgA and IgA subclass 1 secreting cells occurs in both ulcerative colitis and Crohn's disease tissues. In contrast, marked expansion of different subclass expressing IgG plasma cells occurs with IgG subclass 1 markedly increased in ulcerative colitis and IgG subclass 2 increased in Crohn's disease. The IgG subclass antibodies as opposed to IgA antibodies are capable of complement activation and induction of cytotoxicity as well as mediation of opsonic activity. Antigen-specific destruction of epithelial cells by cytotoxic mechanisms, activation of macrophages, or antibody plus complement due to autoantigens on epithelial cells may then occur. Cell-mediated memory events may be an important component of the recurrent organ-specific damage that characterizes ulcerative colitis and Crohn's disease.

that there is no specific antigen but that IBD is an inappropriate activation of the immune system in the intestine to a variety of common intestinal stimuli. More likely is the possibility that there is a specific antigen involved in the initiation of the immune response, but the antigen-specific clonal expansion is overwhelmed by the nonspecific cytokine and inflammatory mediator-driven amplification of the immune response so that the specific component cannot be identified. Thus IBD may be the result of an inability to mount an appropriate immune response to a

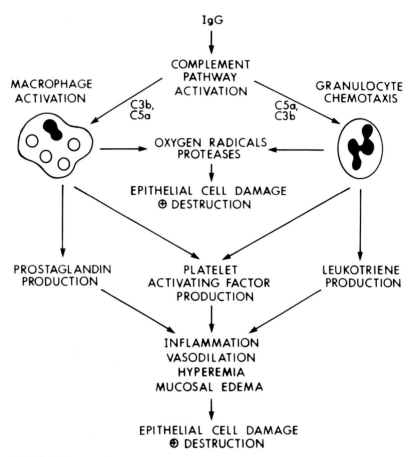

Figure 23 – 3 Inflammatory events in IBD. Effector mechanisms in IBD involve not only specific memory cell-mediated events (Fig. 23–2), but also nonspecific inflammatory events in which the intestine is damaged by virtue of being an innocent bystander to the ongoing inflammatory events. Subsequent to secretion of IgG in increased amounts in ulcerative colitis and Crohn's disease (Fig. 23–2) complement activation may occur with release of chemotactic molecules such as C3b and C5a with a resultant influx of neutrophils and macrophages. The influx of neutrophils in turn leads to enhanced production of leukotrienes with further chemotaxis and enhanced neutrophil influx. Neutrophil and macrophage activation with release of proteases and other enzymes capable of mediating intestinal damage as well as the production and release of oxygen radicals in turn results in increased epithelial cell injury. Activation of macrophages will lead to a variety of inflammatory mediators being produced including prostaglandins and platelet activating factor. The inflammatory mediators then lead to vasodilation, enhanced vascular permeability, hyperemia, and mucosal edema. Mediators of the inflammatory response lead to the majority of the observed pathologic and clinical alterations observed in inflammatory bowel disease. The inflammatory process could also be part of a normal protective response against pathogenic organisms, injurious agents, or triggering antigens.

specific antigen, such that the immune system is activated but fails to destroy the offending antigen and, as a result, we see the histologic and clinical manifestations of a prolonged but ineffective immune response. Alternatively, the defect in IBD may be a problem in turning off the immune response. In that case, what we see is an effective immune response that has destroyed the triggering antigen, but that has not been shut down at the appropriate time. Available data do not allow the choice of one of these explanations over the other.

Critical steps in the pathogenesis of IBD involve the transition from immune activation to inflammation and nonspecific destructive processes. Inflammatory responses in the intestine can be induced by disorders of immunoregulation (e.g., systemic lupus erythematosus); infectious colitis (e.g., shigellosis); impaired circulation (e.g., ischemic colitis); or toxic compounds (e.g., acetic acid colitis). There are striking similarities in clinical and morphologic manifestations among the diseases marked by intestinal inflammation. The likely explanation for these similarities is that the clinical and histologic manifestations of each of these diseases arise, not from the etiologic agents, but from the soluble mediators of inflammation that are generated in the inflammatory process. Much recent progress in IBD research has come in the area of the characterization of mediators of inflammation in IBD and their role in the amplification of the immune response (Fig. 23–3). Although studies in this area are not likely to give insight into the specific initiating event in IBD, they are likely to give a better understanding of how the inflammatory response is promulgated and preserved. The mechanism accounting for much of the observed intestinal damage in IBD is the generation of soluble mediators. Hyperemia, edema, and neutrophil infiltration are all products of soluble mediators.

Crohn's disease and ulcerative colitis are diseases marked by chronic immune activation of the intestinal tract. Insight into the pathogenesis of those diseases is most likely to come from a better understanding of normal immune regulation in the gastrointestinal tract — with particular attention to the ability of the intestinal immune system to suppress the generation of an inflammatory response to the multiple antigens normally present in the intestinal lumen. Progress in therapy is likely to come from a better understanding of the role of soluble mediators of inflammation in IBD.

REFERENCES

1. MacDermott RP: Cell mediated immunity in gastrointestinal disease. *Hum Pathol* 17:219–233, 1986.
2. MacDermott RP, Stenson WF: The immunology of idiopathic inflammatory bowel disease. *Hosp Pract,* November 15:97–116, 1986.
3. MacDermott RP, Stenson WF: Alterations of the immune system in ulcerative colitis and Crohn's disease. *Adv Immunol* 42:285–328, 1988.
4. Elson CO: The immunology of inflammatory bowel disease. In JB Kirsner, RG Shorter: *Inflammatory Bowel Disease,* ed 3, Philadelphia, Lea and Febiger, 1988.
5. Farmer RG, Michener WM, Sivak DS: Studies of family history in inflammatory bowel disease. In Pena AS, Weterman IT, Booth CC, Strober W: *Developments in Gastroenterology,* vol. 1: *Recent Advances in Crohn's Disease.* The Hague, Martinus Nijhoff, 1981, p 213.
6. Burnham WR, Gelsthorpe K, Langman MJS: HLA-D related antigens in inflamma-

tory bowel disease. In Pena AS, Weterman IT, Booth CC, Strober W: *Developments in Gastroenterology*, vol. 1: *Recent Advances in Crohn's Disease*. The Hague, Martinus Nijhoff, 1981, p 192.

7. Asakura H, Tsuchiya M, Aiso S, et al: Association of the human lymphocyte-DR2 antigen with Japanese ulcerative colitis. *Gastroenterology* 82:413, 1982.

8. Smolen JS, Gangl A, Polterauer P, et al: HLA antigens in inflammatory bowel disease. *Gastroenterology* 82:34–38, 1982.

9. Biemond I, Burnham WR, D'Amaro J, et al: HLA-A and HLA-B antigens in inflammatory bowel disease. *Gut* 27:934–91, 1986.

10. Strickland RG, Korsmeyer S, Soltis RD, et al: Peripheral blood T and B cells in chronic inflammatory bowel disease. *Gastroenterology* 67:569–577, 1974.

11. Thayer WR, Charland C, Field CE. The subpopulations of circulating white blood cells in inflammatory bowel disease. *Gastroenterology* 71:379–384, 1976.

12. Auer IO, Wechsler W, Ziemer E, et al: Immune status in Crohn's disease. I. Leukocyte and lymphocyte subpopulations in peripheral blood. *Scand J Gastroenterol* 13:561–571, 1978.

13. Auer IO, Gotz S, Ziemer E, et al: Immune status in Crohn's disease. 3. Peripheral blood B lymphocytes, enumerated by means of F(ab)2-antibody fragments, null and T lymphocytes. *Gut* 20:261–268, 1979.

14. Selby WS, Jewell DP: T lymphocyte subsets in inflammatory bowel disease: peripheral blood. *Gut* 24:99–105, 1983.

15. Yuan SZ, Hanauer SB, Kluskens LF, et al: Circulating lymphocyte subpopulations in Crohn's disease. *Gastroenterology* 85:1313–1318, 1983.

16. Raedler A, Fraenkel S, Klose G, et al: Involvement of the immune system in the pathogenesis of Crohn's disease. Expression of the T9 antigen on peripheral immunocytes correlates with the severity of the disease. *Gastroenterology* 88:978–983, 1985.

17. Raedler A, Fraenkel S, Klose G, et al: Elevated numbers of peripheral T cells in inflammatory bowel diseases displaying T9 antigen and Fc alpha receptors. *Clin Exp Immunol* 60:518–524, 1985.

18. Broberger O, Perlmann P: Autoantibodies in human ulcerative colitis. *J Exp Med* 110:657–673, 1959.

19. Broberger O, Perlmann P: Demonstration of an epithelial antigen in colon by means of fluorescent antibodies from children with ulcerative colitis. *J Exp Med* 115:13–26, 1962.

20. Lagercrantz R, Hammarstrom S, Perlmann P, et al: Immunological studies in ulcerative colitis. III. Incidence of antibodies to colon-antigen in ulcerative colitis and other gastro-intestinal diseases. *Clin Exp Immunol* 1:263–276, 1966.

21. Lagercrantz R, Hammarstrom S, Perlmann P, et al: Immunological studies in ulcerative colitis. IV. Origin of autoantibodies. *J Exp Med* 128:1339–1352, 1968.

22. Broberger O, Perlmann P: In-vitro studies of ulcerative colitis. I. Reactions of patients serum with human fetal colonic cells in tissue culture. *J Exp Med* 117:705–715, 1963.

23. Rabin BS, Rogers SJ: Nonpathogenicity of anti-intestinal antibody in the rabbit. *Am J Pathol* 83:269–277, 1976.

24. Deodhar SD, Michener WM, Farmer RG: Study of the immunological aspects of chronic ulcerative colitis and transmural colitis. *Am J Clin Pathol* 51:591–597, 1969.

25. Carlsson HE, Lagercrantz R, Perlmann P: Immunological studies in ulcerative colitis. VIII. Antibodies to colon antigen in patients with ulcerative colitis, Crohn's disease, and other diseases. *Scand J Gastroenterol* 12:707–714, 1977.

26. Heddle RJ, Shearman DJC: Serum antibodies to *Escherichia coli* in subjects with ulcerative colitis. *Clin Exp Immunol* 38:22–30, 1979.

27. Korsmeyer SJ, Williams Jr RC, Wilson ID, et al: Lymphocytotoxic antibody in inflammatory bowel disease. A family study. *N Engl J Med* 293:1117–1120, 1975.

28. Korsmeyer SJ, Williams Jr RC, Wilson ID, et al: Lymphocytotoxic and RNA antibodies in inflammatory bowel disease: a comparative study in patients and their families. *Ann NY Acad Sci* 278:574–585, 1976.

29. Strickland RG, Friedler EM, Henderson CA, et al: Serum lymphocytotoxins in inflammatory bowel disease. Studies of frequency and specificity for lymphocyte subpopulations. *Clin Exp Immunol* 21:384–393, 1975.

30. Scott H, Solheim BG, Brandtzaeg P, et al: HLA-DR-like antigens in the epithelium of the human small intestine. *Scand J Immunol* 12:77–82, 1980.

31. Scott H, Brandtzaeg P, Solheim BG, et al: Relationship between HLA-DR-like antigens and secretory component (SC) in jejunal epithelium of patients with celiac disease or dermatitis epideformis. *Clin Exp Immunol* 44:233–238, 1981.

32. Selby WS, Janossy G, Mason DY, et al: Expression of HLA-DR antigens by colonic epithelium in inflammatory bowel disease. *Clin Exp Immunol* 53:614–618, 1983.

33. Hirata I, Berrebi G, Austin LL, et al: Immunohistological characterization of intraepithelial and lamina propria lymphocytes in control ileum colon and in inflammatory bowel disease. *Dig Dis Sci* 31:593–603, 1986.

34. Flavell RA, Allen H, Burkly LC, et al: Molecular biology of the H-2 histocompatibility complex. *Science* 233:437–443, 1986.

35. Goverman J, Hunkapiller T, Hood L: A speculative view of the multicomponent nature of T cell antigen recognition. *Cell* 45:475–484, 1986.

36. Pallone F, Fais S, Squarcia O, et al: Activation of peripheral blood and intestinal lamina propria lymphocytes in Crohn's disease. In vivo state of activation and in vitro response to stimulation as defined by the expression of early activation antigens. *Gut* 28:745–753, 1987.

37. Fais S, Pallone F, Squarcia O, et al: HLA-DR antigens on colonic epithelial cells in inflammatory bowel disease: I. Relation to the state of activation of lamina propria lymphocytes and to the epithelial expression of other surface markers. *Clin Exp Immunol* 68:605–612, 1987.

38. McDonald GB, Jewell DP: Class II antigen (HLA-DR) expression by intestinal epithelial cells in inflammatory diseases of colon. *J Clin Pathol* 40:312–317, 1987.

39. Bland P: MHC class II expression by the gut epithelium. *Immunol Today* 9:174–176, 1988.

40. Strominger JL: Biology of the human histocompatibility leukocyte antigen (HLA) system and a hypothesis regarding the generation of autoimmune diseases. *J Clin Invest* 77:1411–1415, 1986.

41. Mayer L, Shlien R: Evidence for function of Ia molecules on gut epithelial cells in man. *J Exp Med* 166:1471–1483, 1987.

42. Mayer L, Eisenhardt L: Defect in immunoregulatory intestinal epithelial cells in inflammatory bowel disease, current status and future approach. In RP MacDermott: *Excerpta Medica*, International Congress Series, 775:9–16, 1988.

43. Perlmann P, Broberger O: In-vitro studies of ulcerative colitis. II. Cytotoxic action of white blood cells from patients on human fetal colon cells. *J Exp Med* 117:717–733, 1963.

44. Shorter RG, Spencer RJ, Huizenga KA, et al: Inhibition of in-vitro cytotoxicity of lymphocytes from patients with ulcerative colitis and granulomatous colitis for allogenic colon epithelial cells using horse anti-human thymus serum. *Gastroenterology* 54:227–231, 1968.

45. Stobo JD, Tomasi TB, Huizenga KA, et al: In-vitro studies of inflammatory bowel

disease. Surface receptors of the mononuclear cell required to lyse allogeneic colonic epithelial cells. *Gastroenterology* 70:171–176, 1976.

46. Bookman MA, Bull DM: Characteristics of isolated intestinal mucosal lymphoid cells in inflammatory bowel disease. *Gastroenterology* 77:503–510, 1979.

47. MacDermott RP, Franklin GO, Jenkins KM, et al: Human intestinal mononuclear cells. I. Investigation of antibody-dependent, lectin-induced, and spontaneous cell-mediated cytotoxic capabilities. *Gastroenterology* 78:47–56, 1980.

48. Auer IO, Ziemer E, Sommer H: Immune status in Crohn's disease. Decreased in-vitro natural killer cell activity in peripheral blood. *Clin Exp Immunol* 42:41–49, 1980.

49. Auer IO, Ziemer E: Immune status in Crohn's disease. IV. In-vitro antibody dependent cell mediated cytotoxicity in peripheral blood. *Klin Wochensch* 58:779–787, 1980.

50. MacDermott RP, Bragdon MJ, Kodner IJ, et al: Deficient cell mediated cytotoxicity and hyporesponsiveness to interferon and mitogenic lectin activation by inflammatory bowel disease peripheral blood and intestinal mononuclear cells. *Gastroenterology* 90:6–11, 1986.

51. MacDermott RP: Human intestinal mononuclear cells (MNC) isolated from normal and inflammatory bowel disease (IBD) specimens are a functionally unique lymphoid population. In Pena AS, Weterman IT, Booth CC, Strober W: *Recent Advances in Crohn's Disease*. The Hague, Martinus Nijhoff, 1981, pp 439–444.

52. Gibson PR, Van De Pol E, Pullman W, et al: Lysis of colonic epithelial cells by allogeneic mononuclear and lymphokine activated killer cells derived from peripheral blood and intestinal mucosa: evidence against a pathogenic role in inflammatory bowel disease. *Gut* 29:1076–1084, 1988.

53. Fiocchi C, Tubbs RR, Youngman K: Human intestinal mucosal mononuclear cells exhibit lymphokine-activated killer cell activity. *Gastroenterology* 88:625–637, 1985.

54. Hogan PG, Hapel AJ, Doe WF: Lymphokine-activated and natural killer cell activity in human intestinal mucosa. *J Immunol* 135:1731–1738, 1985.

55. Shanahan F, Brogan M, Targan S: Human mucosal cytotoxic effector cells. *Gastroenterology* 42:1951–1957, 1987.

56. Shanahan F, Deem R, Nayersina R, et al: Human mucosal T cell cytotoxicity. *Gastroenterology* 94:960–967, 1988.

57. Stevens R, Oliver M, Brogan M, et al: Defective generation of tetanus-specific antibody-producing B cells after in vivo immunization of Crohn's disease and ulcerative colitis. *Gastroenterology* 88:1860–1866, 1985.

58. Elson CO, Graeff AS, James SP, et al: Covert suppressor T cells in Crohn's disease. *Gastroenterology* 80:1513–1521, 1981.

59. Elson CO, James SP, Graeff AS, et al: Hypogammaglobulinemia due to abnormal suppressor T-cell activity in Crohn's disease. *Gastroenterology* 86:569–576, 1984.

60. James SP, Neckers LM, Graeff AS, et al: Suppression of immunoglobulin synthesis by lymphocyte subpopulations in patients with Crohn's disease. *Gastroenterology* 86:1510–1518, 1984.

61. James SP, Giocchi C, Graeff AS, et al: Immunoregulatory function of lamina propria T cells in Crohn's disease. *Gastroenterology* 88:1143–1150, 1985.

62. Elson CO, Machelski E, Weiserbs DB: T cell-B cell regulation in the intestinal lamina propria in Crohn's disease. *Gastroenterology* 89:321–327, 1985.

63. James SP: Remission of Crohn's disease after human immunodeficiency virus infection. *Gastroenterology* 95:1667–1669, 1988.

64. Selby WS, Janossy G, Bofill M, et al: Intestinal lymphocyte subpopulations in inflammatory bowel disease: an analysis by immunohistological and cell isolation techniques. *Gut* 25:32–40, 1984.

65. MacDermott RP: Altered secretion patterns of IgA and IgG subclasses by IBD intestinal mononuclear cells. In H Goebell, BM Peskar, H Malchow: *Inflammatory Bowel Diseases — Basic Research and Clinical Implications,* MTP Press Limited, Falcon House, Lancaster, England, pp 105–111, 1988.

66. MacDermott RP, Stenson WF: The role of the immune system in inflammatory bowel disease in gut and intestinal immunology. *Immunol Allergy Clin North Am* 8:521–542, 1988.

67. MacDermott RP, Nash GS, Bertovich MJ, et al: Alterations of IgM, IgG, and IgA synthesis and secretion by peripheral blood and intestinal mononuclear cells from patients with ulcerative colitis and Crohn's disease. *Gastroenterology* 81:844–852, 1981.

68. MacDermott RP, Beale MG, Alley CD, et al: Synthesis and secretion of IgA, IgM, and IgG by peripheral blood mononuclear cells in human disease states, by isolated human intestinal mononuclear cells, and by human bone marrow mononuclear cells from ribs. In McGhee JR, Mestecky J: *The Secretory Immune System.* New York, *NY Acad Sci* 409:498, 1983.

69. Beale MG, Nash GS, Bertovich MJ, et al: Similar disturbances in B cell activity and regulatory T cell function in Henoch-Schonlein purpura and systemic lupus erythematosus. *J Immunol* 128:486–491, 1982.

70. Alley CD, Nash GS, MacDermott RP: Marked in-vitro spontaneous secretion of IgA by human rib bone marrow mononuclear cells. *J Immunol* 128:2804–2808, 1982.

71. MacDermott RP, Delacroix DL, Nash GS, et al: Evidence for the migration of B-cells secreting monomeric IgA and IgA subclass 1 (IgA1) from peripheral compartments into the intestine in inflammatory bowel disease. *Gastroenterology* 91:379–385, 1986.

72. Scott MG, Nahm MH, Macke K, et al: Spontaneous secretion of IgG subclasses by intestinal mononuclear cells: differences between ulcerative colitis, Crohn's disease, and controls. *Clin Exp Immunol* 66:209–215, 1986.

73. MacDermott RP, Nahm MH: Expression of human immunoglobulin G subclasses in inflammatory bowel disease. *Gastroenterology* 93:1127, 1987.

74. MacDermott RP, Nash GS, Auer IO, et al: Alterations in serum IgG subclasses in patients with ulcerative colitis and Crohn's disease. *Gastroenterology* 94:A275, 1988.

75. Brandtzaeg P, Baklien K, Fausa O, et al: Immunohistochemical characterization of local immunoglobulin formation in ulcerative colitis. *Gastroenterology* 66:1123–1136, 1974.

76. Baklien K, Brandtzaeg P: Comparative mapping of the local distribution of immunoglobulin-containing cells in ulcerative colitis and Crohn's disease of the colon. *Clin Exp Immunol* 22:197–209, 1975.

77. Rosekrans PCM, Meijer CJLM, Van der Wal AM, et al: Immunoglobulin containing cells in inflammatory bowel disease of the colon: a morphometric and immunohistochemical study. *Gut* 21:941–947, 1980.

78. Scott BB, Goodall A, Stephenson P, et al: Rectal mucosal plasma cells in inflammatory bowel disease. *Gut* 24:519–524, 1983.

79. Keren DF, Appelman HD, Dobbins WO, et al: Correlation of histopathologic evidence of disease activity with the presence of immunoglobulin-containing cells in the colon of patients with inflammatory bowel disease. *Hum Pathol* 15:757–763, 1984.

80. Van Spreeuwel JP, Lindeman J, Meijer CJLM: A quantitative study of immunoglobulin containing cells in the differential diagnosis of acute colitis. *J Clin Pathol* 38:774–777, 1985.

81. Kett K, Rognum TO, Brandtzaeg P: Mucosal subclass distribution of IgG-producing cells is different in ulcerative colitis and Crohn's disease of the colon. *Gastroenterology* 93:919, 1987.

82. Kett K, Brandtzaeg P, Fausa O: J-chain expression is more prominent in immunoglobulin A2 than in immunoglobulin A1 colonic immunocytes and is decreased in both subclasses associated with inflammatory bowel disease. *Gastroenterology* 94:1419–1425, 1988.

83. Badr-El-Din S, Trejdosiewicz LK, Heatley RV, et al: Local immunity in ulcerative colitis: evidence for defective secretory IgA production. *Gut* 29:1070–1075, 1988.

84. Yount WJ, Dorner MM, Kunkel HG, et al: Studies on human antibodies. VI. Selective variation in subgroup composition and genetic markers. *J Exp Med* 127:633, 1968.

85. Skakib F, Stanworth DR: Human IgG subclasses in health and disease. A review. Part II. *Ricerca Clin Lab* 10:561, 1980.

86. Yount WJ: IgG2 deficiency and ataxia-telangiectasia. *N Engl J Med* 306:541–543, 1982.

87. Waldmann TA, Broder S, Goldman CK, et al: Disorders of B cells and helper T cells in the pathogenesis of the immunoglobulin deficiency of patients with ataxia telangiectasia. *J Clin Invest* 71:282–295, 1983.

88. Heiner DC: Significance of immunoglobulin G (IgG) subclasses. *Am J Med* 76:1, 1984.

89. Oxelius VA: Immunoglobulin G (IgG) subclasses and human disease. *Am J Med* 76:7–18, 1984.

90. Gronowicz E, Couthino A: Heterogeneity of B cells: direct evidence of selective triggering of distinct subpopulations by polyclonal activators. *Scand J Immunol* 5:55, 1976.

91. Slack JH, Der-Balian G, Nahm MH, et al: Subclass restriction of murine antibodies. II. The IgG plaque forming cell response to thymus independent type 1 and type 2 antigens in normal mice and mice expressing and X-linked immunodeficiency. *J Exp Med* 151:853, 1980.

92. McKearn JP, Paslay JW, Slack JH, et al: B cell subsets and differential responses to mitogens. *Immunol Rev* 64:10, 1982.

93. Scott MG, Nahm MH: Mitogen-induced IgG subclass expression. *J Immunol* 135:2454–2460, 1984.

94. Kaulfersh W, Fiocchi C, Waldmann TH: Polyclonal nature of the intestinal mucosal lymphocyte populations in inflammatory bowel disease. *Gastroenterology* 95:364–370, 1988.

95. Rhodes JM, Bartholomew TC, Jewell DP: Inhibition of leukocyte motility by drugs used in ulcerative colitis. *Gut* 22:642–647, 1981.

96. Wandall JH, Binder V: Leukocyte function in ulcerative colitis. *Gut* 23:758–765, 1982.

97. Rhodes JM, Potter BJ, Brown DJC, et al: Serum inhibitors of leukocyte chemotaxis in Crohn's disease and ulcerative colitis. *Gastroenterology* 82:1327–1334, 1982.

98. Morain CO, Segal AA, Walker D, et al: Abnormalities of neutrophil function do not cause the migration defect in Crohn's disease. *Gut* 22:817–822, 1981.

99. Saverymuttu SH, Peters AM, Lavender JP, et al: In vivo assessment of granulocyte migration to diseased bowel in Crohn's disease. *Gut* 26:378–383, 1985.

100. Saverymuttu SH, Chadwick VS, Hodgson HJ: Granulocyte migration in ulcerative colitis. *Eur J Clin Invest* 15:60–68, 1985.

101. Scholmerich J, Schmidt E, Schumichen C, et al: Scintigraphic assessment of bowel involvement and disease activity in Crohn's disease using technetium 99m hexamethyl propylene amine oxine as leukocyte label. *Gastroenterology* 95:1287–1293, 1988.

102. Pullman WE, Sullivan PJ, Barratt PJ, et al: Assessment of inflammatory bowel disease activity by technetium 99m phagocyte scanning. *Gastroenterology* 95:989–996, 1988.

103. Wilkinson PC: *Chemotaxis and Inflammation,* ed 2. Edinburgh, Churchill Livingstone, 1982, p 93.

104. Lake AM, Stitzel AE, Urmson JR, et al: Complement alterations in inflammatory bowel disease. *Gastroenterology* 76:1374–1379, 1979.

105. D'Amelio R, Rosi P, Le Moli S, et al: In vitro studies on cellular and humoral chemotaxis in Crohn's disease using the under agarose gel technique. *Gut* 22:566–570, 1981.

106. Elmgreen J, Berkowicz A, Sorensen H: Defective release of C5a related chemo-attractant activity from complement in Crohn's disease. *Gut* 24:525–531, 1983.

107. Simonsen T, Elmgreen J: Defective modulation of complement in Crohn's disease. *Scand J Gastroenterol* 20:883–886, 1985.

108. Hodgson HJF, Potter BJ, Jewell DP: C3 metabolism in ulcerative colitis and Crohn's disease. *Clin Exp Immunol* 28:490–495, 1977.

109. Elmgreen J, Berkowicz A, Sorensen H: Hypercatabolism of complement in Crohn's disease — assessment of circulating C3c. *Acta Med Scand* 214:403–407, 1983.

110. Flower RJ, Blackwell CJ: Anti-inflammatory steroids induce biosynthesis of a phospholipase A2 inhibitor which prevents prostaglandin generation. *Nature* 278:456–459, 1979.

111. Stenson WF: Pharmacology of sulfasalazine. *Viewpoints Dig Dis* 16:13–16, 1984.

112. Bach MK: Mediators of anaphylaxis and inflammation. *Ann Rev Microbiol* 36:371–413, 1982.

113. Parker CW: Mediators: release and function. In Paul WE: *Fundamental Immunology.* New York, Raven Press, 1984, pp 697–750.

114. Bukhave K, Rask Madsen J: Saturation kinetics applied to in vitro effects of low prostaglandin E2 and F2alpha concentrations on ion transport across human jejunal mucosa. *Gastroenterology* 78:32–42, 1980.

115. Milton-Thompson GJ, Cummings JH, Newman A, et al: Colonic and small intestinal response to intravenous prostaglandin F2alpha and E2 in man. *Gut* 16:42–46, 1975.

116. Sharon P, Ligumsky M, Rachmilewitz D, et al: Role of prostaglandins in ulcerative colitis. Enhanced production during active disease and inhibition by sulfasalazine. *Gastroenterology* 75:638–640, 1978.

117. Gould SR: Assay of prostaglandin-like substances in faeces and their measurement in ulcerative colitis. *Prostaglandins* 11:489–497, 1981.

118. Gould SR, Brash AR, Conolly ME, et al: Studies of prostaglandins and sulphasalazine in ulcerative colitis. *Prostaglandins Leukotrienes Med* 6:165–182, 1981.

119. Lauritsen K, Laursen LS, Bukhave K, et al: Effects of systemic prednisolone on arachidonic acid metabolites determined by equilibrium in vivo dialysis of rectum in severe relapsing ulcerative colitis (Abstr). *Gastroenterology* 88:1466, 1985.

120. Rampton DS, Sladen GE, Youlten LY: Rectal mucosal prostaglandin E2 release and its relation to disease activity, electrical potential difference and treatment in ulcerative colitis. *Gut* 21:591–596, 1980.

121. Zifroni A, Treves AJ, Sachar DB, et al: Prostanoid synthesis by cultured intestinal epithelial and mononuclear cells in inflammatory bowel disease. *Gut* 24:659–664, 1983.

122. Gilat T, Ratan J, Rosen P, et al: Prostaglandins and ulcerative colitis. *Gastroenterology* 77:1083, 1979.

123. Campieri M, Lanfranchi GA, Bazzochi G, et al: Prostaglandins, indomethacin, and ulcerative colitis. *Gastroenterology* 78:193, 1980.

124. Levy N, Gaspar E: Rectal bleeding and indomethacin suppositories. *Lancet* 1:577, 1975.

125. Rampton DS, Sladen GE: The relationship between rectal mucosal prostaglandin production and water and electrolyte transport in ulcerative colitis. *Digestion Intern* 30:13–22, 1984.

126. Stenson WF, Parker CW: Leukotrienes. *Adv Intern Med* 30:175–199, 1984.

127. Borgeat P, Samuelsson B: Transformation of arachidonic acid by rabbit polymorpho-nuclear leukocytes. *J Biol Chem* 254:2643–2646, 1979.

128. Sharon P, Stenson WF: Enhanced synthesis of leukotriene B4 by colonic mucosa in inflammatory bowel disease. *Gastroenterology* 86:453–460, 1984.

129. Ford-Hutchinson AW, Bray MA, Doig MV, et al: Leukotriene B, a potent chemotactic and aggregating substance released from polymorphonuclear leukocytes. *Nature* 266:264–265, 1984.

130. Wilkinson PC: *Chemotaxis and Inflammation*, ed 2. Edinburgh, Churchill Livingstone, 1982, p 93.

131. Schiffman E, Corcoran BA, Wahl SA: N-formylmethionyl peptides as chemoattract-ants for leukocytes. *Proc Natl Acad Sci* USA 72:1059–1062, 1975.

132. Stenson WF: Role of lipoxygenase products in inflammatory bowel disease. In Rach-milewitz D: *Inflammatory Bowel Diseases*. The Hague, Martinus Nijhoff, in press.

133. Peskar BM, Dreyling KW, Hoppe U, et al: Formation of sulfidopeptide-leukotrienes (SP-LT) in normal human colonic tissue, colonic carcinoma, and Crohn's disease (Abstr). *Gastroenterology* 88:1537, 1985.

134. Stenson WF, Lobos EA: Inhibition of platelet thromboxane sythetase by sulfasalazine. *Biochem Pharmacol* 33:2205–2209, 1983.

135. Stenson WF, Lobos E: Sulfasalazine inhibits the synthesis of chemotactic lipids by neutrophils. *J Clin Invest* 69:494–497, 1982.

136. Stenson WF, Mehta J, Spilberg I: Sulfasalazine inhibits the binding of formyl-methio-nylleucylphenylalanine (FMLP) to its receptor on human neutrophils. *Biochem Phar-macol* 33:407–412, 1984.

137. Eliakim R, Karmeli F, Razin E, et al: Role of platelet-activating factor in ulcerative colitis. Enhanced production during active disease and inhibition by sulfasalazine and prednisone. *Gastroenterology* 95:1167–1172, 1988.

138. MacDermott RP, Schloemann SR, Bertovich MJ, et al: Inhibition of antibody secre-tion by 5-aminosalicylic acid. *Gastroenterology* 94:A275, 1988.

139. Miyachi Y, Yoshioka A, Imamura S, et al: Effect of sulfasalazine and its metabolites on the generation of reactive oxygen species. *Gut* 28:190–195, 1987.

140. Chiodini RJ, Van Kruiningen HJ, Thayer WR, et al: Possible role of mycobacteria in inflammatory bowel disease. I. An unclassified mycobacterium species isolated from patients with Crohn's disease. *Dig Dis Sci* 29:1073–1079, 1984.

141. Thayer WR, Coutu JA, Chiodini RJ, et al: Possible role of mycobacteria in inflamma-tory bowel disease. II. Mycobacterial antibodies in Crohn's disease. *Dig Dis Sci* 29:1080–1085, 1984.

142. Chiodini RJ, Van Kruiningen HJ, Thayer WR, et al: In vitro antimicrobial susceptibil-ity of a mycobacterium species isolated from patients with Crohn's disease. *Antimicrob Agents Chemother* 26:930–932, 1984.

143. Chiodini RJ, Van Kruiningen HJ, Merkal RS, et al: Characteristics of an unclassified mycobacterium species isolated from patients with Crohn's disease. *J Clin Microbiol* 20:966–971, 1984.

144. Van Kruiningen HJ, Chiodini RJ, Thayer WR, et al: Experimental disease in infant goats induced by a mycobacterium isolated from a patient with Crohn's disease. *Dig Dis Sci* 31:1351–1360, 1986.

145. Hampson SJ, McFadden JJ, Hermon-Taylor J: Mycobacteria and Crohn's disease. *Gut* 29:1017–1019, 1988.

CHAPTER 24

Celiac Disease

MARTIN F. KAGNOFF

INTRODUCTION

Celiac disease (gluten-sensitive enteropathy, celiac sprue, or nontropical sprue) is characterized by damage to the small intestinal mucosa and malabsorption. Symptoms commonly appear during the first 3 years of life, after the introduction of cereals into the diet, with a second peak occurring during the third decade.[1] Clinical manifestations predominantly reflect the consequences of malabsorption. Although celiac disease was noted in earlier centuries,[2,3] a striking decrease in celiac disease was observed in Holland during the wheat-deprived years of World War II, followed by an increase in incidence after that period. This suggested an association between celiac disease and the ingestion of wheat-containing products.[4,5]

The pathogenesis of celiac disease appears to involve interactions between environmental, genetic, and immunologic factors. It is well recognized that disease can be activated by defined proteins present in several dietary grains (wheat, rye, barley, and oats). The major genetic association of celiac disease has been with genes and gene products of the class II region of the major histocompatibility locus (HLA-D region genes) on chromosome 6. Many studies are currently focusing on the role of the immune system in this disease.

PATHOLOGY

Celiac disease mainly affects the small intestine. The small intestinal lesion is characterized by mucosal villous atrophy and crypt hyperplasia, with a decrease in the villous-to-crypt ratio. This is accompanied by an increased plasma cell and lymphocyte infiltration of the lamina propria, abnormalities in the surface epithe-

487

lial cells (which, instead of being columnar, become flattened or cuboidal), and the apparent infiltration of the epithelium with intraepithelial lymphocytes (IEL) (Fig. 24–1). Pathology usually is most marked in the duodenum and jejunum, but the extent of the lesion varies between individuals. Depending on the severity of disease, the entire small intestine can be involved. In mild disease, the lesion can be subtle. Similar histologic changes can be seen in other diseases, including tropical sprue, soy and milk protein allergy, diffuse intestinal lymphoma, giardiasis, Zollinger-Ellison syndrome, and viral gastroenteritis.[6]

Following oral gluten challenge, increased infiltration of the mucosa with IEL can be seen within hours, even in the absence of other overt histologic changes. Recent studies also have reported increased numbers of mucosal mast cells.[7] By electron microscopy, fewer microvillous intramembrane particles and abnormal tight junctions between epithelial cells are seen. Such findings parallel alterations in intestinal permeability and disaccharidase deficiency in celiac disease.

EPIDEMIOLOGY

Celiac disease is common in Ireland and northern Europe, but is not restricted to that region.[6] The reported prevalence of celiac disease in specific geographic areas increased after 1960, paralleling the widespread use of the small intestinal mucosal biopsy for diagnosis. Accurate epidemiologic data on celiac disease is difficult to obtain because asymptomatic disease makes ascertainment of true prevalence rates problematic. Nonetheless, the high incidence of celiac disease in western Ireland appears to have decreased significantly (~60%) over the past 20 years. Although not necessarily causally related, this decrease has occurred at a time when there has been an increase in breast feeding and an increase in the age at which first gluten feeding takes place among that population. Concurrently, there have been changes in the formulation of cows' milk formulas.

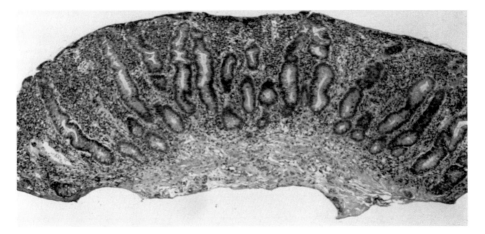

Figure 24–1 Pathology of the small intestinal mucosa in celiac disease. Note the flat mucosal surface, absent villi, and hyperplastic crypts, accompanied by increased cellularity of the lamina propria. There is a loss of normal columnar surface epithelial cells, which are replaced by cuboidal and squamoid cells.

PATHOGENESIS

The major models of disease pathogenesis view celiac disease as an immunologic disease in which environmental, genetic, and immunologic factors contribute to the disease process. However, historically, several competing hypotheses have been put forth to explain the etiology and pathogenesis of this disease. The possibility that celiac disease is due to abnormal small intestinal peptidase activity does not appear likely;[8] the small intestinal mucosa is known to contain multiple peptide hydrolases with overlapping substrate specificities, and biochemical abnormalities usually return to normal when patients are treated with a gluten-free diet. Based on the observation that gliadin treated with a carbohydrase enzyme did not activate disease in several patients, carbohydrate side chains on the gliadins were postulated to be important in disease pathogenesis.[9] This notion does not appear likely, however, as several major α-gliadin components known to activate celiac disease lack carbohydrate side chains.[10] In addition, there is little evidence to support the hypothesis that purified gluten has lectin-like properties or that lectin-like properties of gluten are important in disease pathogenesis.[11,12] The hypothesis that a primary defect in intestinal mucosal permeability is responsible for celiac disease[13] also seems unlikely in that abnormal mucosal permeability may normalize on a gluten-free diet.[14]

Environmental Factors

Grain Proteins

Celiac disease is activated when a susceptible host ingests food products that contain wheat, rye, barley, or oats. It is the gliadin fraction of wheat gluten and similar alcohol-soluble proteins in the other grains (termed *prolamins*) that are associated with the development of the intestinal damage.

Cereal grains belong to the grass family (Gramineae). The grains other than wheat that activate celiac disease (e.g., rye and barley) bear a close taxonomic relationship to wheat (Fig. 24–2). Oats, which in large quantities are thought to

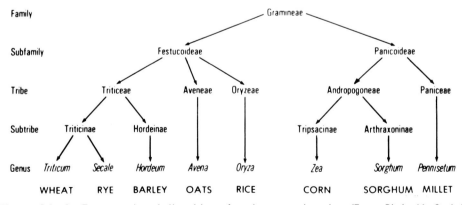

Figure 24–2 Taxonomic relationships of major cereal grains. (From Bietz JA: Serial prolamin evolution and homology revealed by sequence analysis. *Biochem Genet* 20:1039–1053, 1982; with permission.)

activate disease, are further removed from wheat, rye, and barley. Grains that do not activate disease (e.g., rice and corn) are still further separated from wheat in terms of their derivation from the primitive grasses.[15-17]

Common bread wheats developed relatively recently in evolution (in the last 10,000 years) and have a hexaploid genome (genome content AABBCC). Durum wheat, commonly used in the production of pasta, is tetraploid (genome content AABB), whereas rye and barley are diploid.[15] Gene clusters that code for the gliadins are present on chromosomes of homologous groups 1 and 6.[18] Because gliadins are encoded on more than one chromosome,[19-21] the breeding of wheat varieties devoid of disease-activating properties has not been practical.[22]

Gluten is a major component of the wheat endosperm and serves as a source of nitrogen for the germinating wheat embryo.[15,16] Its elastic properties are important in the production of bread. Gliadins and glutenins (mostly the low molecular weight glutenins) are the major protein components of gluten, but only the gliadins have been clearly demonstrated to activate celiac disease. Minor constituents that contaminate gluten extracts (e.g., wheat albumins, globulins, membrane proteins, lipids, and carbohydrates) do not appear to be important in disease activation. In rye, barley, and oats, the alcohol-soluble proteins associated with the activation of disease are termed secalins, hordeins, and avenins, respectively.

Gliadins are single polypeptide chains that range in molecular weight from 30,000 to 75,000. They have a low charge[16] and a high glutamine and proline content (32–56 glutamine and 15–30 proline residues per 100 amino acid residues). Gliadin from a single variety of wheat can be shown to contain 40 or more different but closely related components.[16] By gel electrophoresis, gliadins can be categorized into four major electrophoretic fractions: α-gliadins, β-gliadins, γ-gliadins, and ω-gliadins.[16,23] Each fraction, in turn, contains several subcomponents (β_1-, β_2-, β_3-gliadins; γ_1-, γ_2-, γ_3-gliadins; ω_1-, ω_2-, ω_3-, and ω_4-gliadins).[24] Gliadins of the α, β, and γ_1 fractions share a similar amino acid composition and NH_2-terminal sequence (i.e., α-type sequence).[15,16,25,26] γ_2-, γ_3-, and ω-Gliadins differ markedly from the α-type sequence in their amino acid composition and NH_2-terminal sequence (i.e., γ-type sequence).[27-30]

When α-gliadins from suitable wheat varieties are ultracentrifuged, a precipitate of aggregatable α-gliadins, termed A-gliadin, is formed.[26,31] This major α-gliadin fraction is known to activate disease.[15,32,33] Recently, the complete primary amino acid sequence of A-gliadin was determined from amino acid sequencing,[34] and other α-gliadin sequences have been deduced from sequencing of cDNA clones.[27,34,35] Such information will be important for studies to define which amino acid sequences in gliadin are responsible for disease activation.

The question of which wheat gliadin fractions are capable of activating disease is controversial. Early reports suggested that only α-gliadins activate celiac disease.[36] Later studies suggested that β- and perhaps γ-, but not ω-gliadins might also activate disease.[37] Because ω-gliadins have the highest content of glutamine and proline, the high content of those amino acids alone is not thought to be the determining factor in disease activation. However, recent studies suggested that all gluten fractions might activate disease.[38-40] Complete hydrolysis of gliadin destroys its disease-activating properties.

Controversy over which gliadin fractions activate celiac disease may stem in part from heterogeneity among patients in sensitivity to different gliadin fractions; differences in the timing among studies when small intestinal biopsies are obtained after in vivo gliadin challenge; the use of different clinical and diagnostic end points to assess mucosal damage after in vivo gliadin challenge; using impure gliadin preparations for in vivo or in vitro challenge studies; or an erroneous assumption that abnormalities in in vitro assays equate to disease activation.

Relevance of Adenovirus 12

Studies of monozygotic twins have indicated a lack of complete concordance for celiac disease. We suggested, therefore, that environmental factors other than dietary grains may also be important in the pathogenesis of this disease.[41] To explore that possibility, known protein sequences were examined for amino acid sequence similarity with A-gliadin, the α-gliadin component discussed above, which is known to activate disease. The 31,000-dalton A-gliadin molecule was shown to have a region of amino acid sequence similarity with the 54-kD E1b protein of human adenovirus serotype 12 (Ad12).[41] This region of similarity spans 12 amino acids and includes 8 amino acid residue identities and an identical penta-peptide (Fig. 24–3). A-gliadin has 32 glutamines and 15 prolines per 100 amino acid residues.[34] However, the region of sequence similarity with the E1b protein in-volves domain V of A-gliadin, a domain that lacks repeating sequences with a high glutamine and proline content.[34] In addition, the region includes only a single glutamine and proline residue in the Ad12 E1b protein. This amino acid similarity between these proteins is probably due to chance, as A-gliadin and the Ad12 E1b protein are unrelated functionally and are not likely to share a common ancestry.

The region of sequence similarity between A-gliadin and the Ad12 E1b protein is hydrophilic in both proteins, suggesting that those sequences may be located on the exterior of the respective proteins.[41] Further studies have indicated that antisera raised to the 54-kD Ad12 E1b protein specifically cross reacts with A-gliadin and a heptapeptide of A-gliadin (FRSPQQN) spanning residues 211–217. Although the E1b protein from Ad5 is highly homologous with the Ad12 E1b protein,[42,43] it does not share a region of sequence similarity with A-gliadin, and antisera to Ad5 E1b do not cross react with A-gliadin or the synthetic heptapeptide. Taken together, these studies indicate that antibody raised to the native 54-kD Ad12 E1b protein can specifically cross react with A-gliadin in the region of shared sequence.

Ad12 is a double-stranded DNA virus that usually is isolated from the human intestinal tract and that has been detected in stool samples as early as the first 1–2

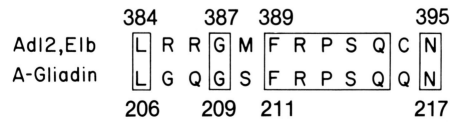

Figure 24–3 Amino acid sequence of the adenovirus 12 E1b protein (Ad12, E1b) and A-gliadin, beginning at amino acid residues 384 and 206, respectively. The re-gion of homology includes 8 of 12 residue identities, including an identical penta-peptide. The single-letter code for amino acids is used. (From Kagnoff MF, et al: Possible role for a human adenovirus in the pathogenesis of celiac disease. *J Exp Med* 160:1544, 1984, with permission.)

years of life.[44,45] Ad12 has not been implicated previously as a cause of human disease but has been studied extensively because of its ability to transform mammalian cell lines.[44] Thus, cells transformed by Ad12 induce tumors in rodents at a high frequency within a relatively short time period.[46] The transforming activity of Ad12 has been assigned to the left-hand 11% of the viral genome (i.e., early region I), which contains two transcriptional units, E1a and E1b in a 3.9-kb DNA segment.[47,48] Those units are the first to be expressed during lytic infection of human cells by Ad12. Note that the 54-kD protein is not a structural protein of Ad12. However, the 54-kD protein does represent the predominant virus-encoded protein expressed in the cytoplasm of mammalian cell lines that have been transformed by Ad12.[44]

Evidence for Prior Exposure to Adenovirus 12
Patients with celiac disease were tested for evidence of prior infection with adenovirus 12 using Ad12 neutralizing antibody as an indicator of past exposure to Ad12. Ad12 neutralizing antibody was chosen since it is directed to determinants on the structural hexon (ϵ) protein of Ad12,[49] a protein that is not related to the Ad12 E1b protein or A-gliadin. As shown in Figure 24–4, 89% (16/18) of a group of untreated celiac disease patients from London had neutralizing antibody to Ad12.[50,51] In contrast, such antibody was present in only 17% (6/35) of disease controls from the same institution (Fig. 24–4). Antibody to Ad12 in the celiac disease subjects did not appear to reflect a general increase in antibody titers to multiple viruses in those individuals. Thus there was not a significant difference in the prevalence of neutralizing antibody to echovirus 11 among individuals with celiac disease, compared with disease controls (Fig. 24–4). In addition, there was no significant difference in the presence of neutralizing antibody to Ad18, an adenovirus closely related to Ad12, between subjects with untreated celiac disease and controls.[50,51] Although antibody to Ad18 was present in a greater number of untreated adult celiac disease subjects compared with controls, the data did not achieve statistical significance.[50] The prevalence of Ad18 neutralizing antibody in control populations previously reported[52] approximated that noted among several control groups we have studied and has ranged from 5 to 20%.

Among patients with treated celiac disease in San Diego County, approximately one-third have had positive Ad12 neutralizing antibody titers. Similar results have also been obtained among treated celiac disease children in London. The prevalence of antibody to Ad12 in our control adults and children, including those with intestinal disorders other than celiac disease, has approximated the 0–15% prevalence noted before by others for Ad12 neutralizing antibody among different control populations.[51,52] The prevalence of neutralizing antibody to Ad12 is greater in untreated than in treated celiac disease patients and may reflect more recent infection with Ad12, although studies have not directly addressed this issue. Note, however, that the above results do not exclude the possibility that celiac disease patients may be more likely than controls to acquire Ad12 infection.

The region of sequence similarity between A-gliadin and the Ad12 E1b protein has been shown to act as an antigenic determinant in assays of antibody recognition[50] and assays of cell-mediated immunity.[53,54] Parenthetically, we note that patients with dermatitis herpetiformis (DH), a skin disease, also have a significantly increased prevalence of Ad12 neutralizing antibody (M. Kagnoff and I. Gigli, personal communication). This latter finding is of interest, since most DH

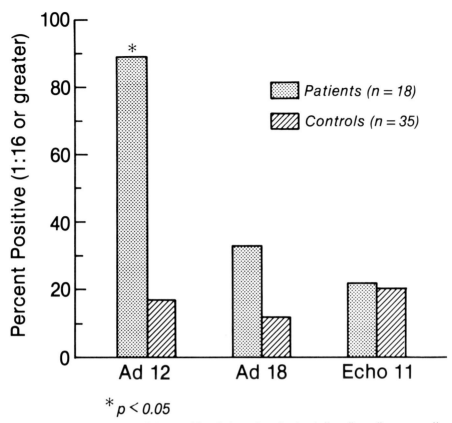

Figure 24–4 Virus-neutralizing antibody in untreated adult celiac disease patients and controls. n, number of subjects in each group; positive subjects defined as titers of 1:16 or greater. *, value significantly different from control group. Kagnoff MF: Celiac disease: a model of an immunologically mediated intestinal disease. *Immunol Clin N Am* 8:505–520, 1988.

patients have a celiac disease-like intestinal lesion that responds to gluten withdrawal from the diet. Like celiac disease, there is a marked association of DH with an HLA haplotype marked by the -DR3 and -DQw2 serologic specificities.[55,56]

Ad12 may play a role in the pathogenesis of celiac disease because of chance immunologic cross-reactivity between shared epitopes on an Ad12 encoded protein and components of the α-gliadin fraction of wheat gluten. If shared epitopes between these proteins have a role in disease pathogenesis by virtue of such molecular mimicry, this most likely occurs at the level of T-cell recognition. As discussed later, a striking feature of celiac disease is its association with a specific HLA haplotype. Presumably peptide fragments of gliadin or the viral protein associate with specific HLA class II molecules on antigen-presenting cells and form a bimolecular complex that is recognized by the receptor for antigen on CD4 T cells. Such CD4 T cells could help in the induction of antibody responses to the antigenic determinants in the region of shared sequence, as well as to determinants on other parts of the α-gliadin molecule. The latter antibodies may cross react with epitopes on γ- and ω-gliadins and barley or rye prolamins, as is commonly seen in patients with celiac disease.[57] The mechanisms by which antigliadin antibodies may play a role in the pathogenesis of celiac disease are discussed later in the section on humoral immunity. Alternatively, it is possible that the peptide sequence shared by the E1b protein and A-gliadin could act as part of a target structure that is recognized on cells of the intestinal mucosa by cytotoxic lymphocytes.

Genetic Factors

Families and Twins

There is an increased prevalence of celiac disease among asymptomatic first-degree relatives of celiac disease patients compared with the general population. This prevalence has ranged as high as 10–20% in some studies[58] but has been substantially lower in other reports.[59] Thus, when all 100 first-degree relatives of 32 Swedish patients were examined,[59] only 2 individuals had convincing celiac disease; others have reported celiac disease in less than 5% of family members.

At least 24 pairs of identical twins with celiac disease have been reported,[60] of which 18 (75%) were concordant for disease. Not all had monozygosity unequivocally proven, and some twin pairs have not undergone sufficient long-term follow-up to be certain that disease will not develop at a later age. Nonetheless, there appears to be a number of instances of discordance for celiac disease among monozygotic twins. Assuming that monozygotic twins ingest similar dietary grains, such discordance suggests that additional environmental factors are important in disease expression (see prior section). Alternatively, because of the gene rearrangements that take place in the immunoglobulin and T-cell receptor loci to generate diversity of immunoglobulin and T-cell receptor molecules, monozygotic twins may not be identical in terms of their repertoire of antibodies and T-cell receptors for antigen.

HLA and Non-HLA Markers

Celiac disease has a striking association with an extended HLA haplotype. This haplotype is characterized telomerically by the class I HLA-B-8 antigen and, more centromerically, the class III SCO1 complotype and the class II HLA-DR52a, -DR3, and DQw2 antigens.[6,61] The strongest association of celiac disease is with proteins encoded in the HLA class II D region. The association of celiac disease with class I and III region genes is thought to be secondary to linkage disequilibrium between genes for specific allelic markers in those regions and in the HLA class II D region (Fig. 24–5).

The HLA-D region is organized into several distinct subregions, including the -DR, -DQ, and -DP subregions. The α and β genes in these subregions code for the respective -DR, -DQ, and -DP molecules that are expressed constitutively on cells of the immune system (e.g., B cells, activated T cells, macrophages, dendritic reticular cells) or can be induced to be expressed on several other cell types, including intestinal epithelial cells. HLA-DR, -DQ, and -DP molecules are highly polymorphic (i.e., exist between individuals in multiple allelic forms).

A striking finding is that the HLA-D region molecules, HLA-DR52a, -DR3, and -DQw2 are present on the cells of 80–90% of Northern European Caucasians with celiac disease, compared with 20–25% of the normal Caucasian population. Nonetheless, the latter population also ingests gliadin without developing celiac disease.

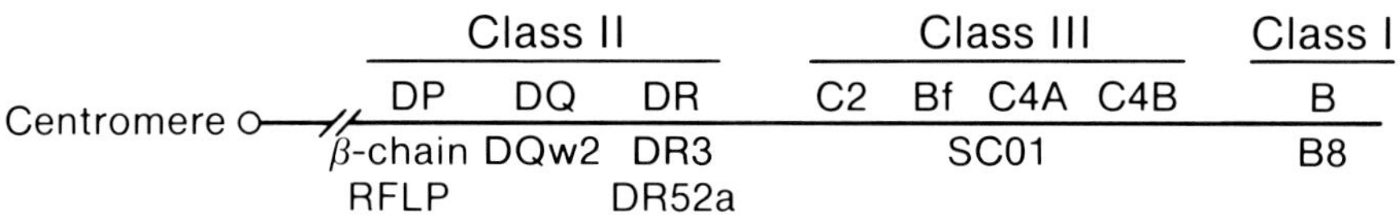

	Class II			Class III				Class I
	DP	DQ	DR	C2	Bf	C4A	C4B	B
Centromere o——//	β-chain	DQw2	DR3		SC01			B8
	RFLP		DR52a					

Figure 24–5 Celiac disease HLA haplotype on chromosome 6.

To investigate whether or not there are subtle differences between the HLA class II D region genes in celiac disease and healthy individuals having the same serologic markers, we use the approach of restriction fragment length polymorphism (RFLP) analysis. Using the restriction endonuclease Rsa I and HLA class II region cDNA probes, we found a polymorphic 4.0-kb genomic DNA fragment that occurred in over 90% of HLA-DR3/DQw2 celiac disease patients but in less than 30% of -DR3/DQw2 controls. This 4.0-kb fragment thus provided a means to distinguish the class II HLA haplotype of celiac disease patients from that of serologically matched controls.[62,63] In further studies, we isolated an HLA-D region gene containing the 4.0-kb Rsa I fragment from a bacteriophage genomic library constructed from the DNA of a celiac disease patient.[63] Based on restriction mapping and differential hybridization with different class II D region cDNA and oligonucleotide probes, this gene was identified as one encoding an HLA-DP β-chain. This celiac disease-associated HLA-DP β-chain gene was flanked by HLA-DP α-chain genes and therefore was probably in its normal chromosomal location.

The joint segregation of an HLA-DP β-chain gene with those encoding the -DR52a, -DR3, and -DQw2 serologic specificities in celiac disease indicates that the class II HLA haplotype associated with this disease is extended throughout the entire HLA-D region (Fig. 24–5). Furthermore, celiac disease susceptibility genes may reside on this haplotype as far centromeric as the HLA-DP subregion.[63] Normally there is a high recombination frequency between the -DQ and -DP subregions. Thus our findings could indicate that the HLA-D region haplotype associated with celiac disease has an unusual degree of linkage disequilibrium that extends centromerically from the HLA-DR subregion to the HLA-DP subregion. Alternatively, the cosegregation of this constellation of D-region alleles in celiac disease may result, not from a decreased recombination frequency between the regions encoding these alleles, but from selection by the disease for this haplotype. If this is the case, the susceptibility to celiac disease associated with the HLA locus may be multigenic with, for example, obligatory roles for HLA-DP, and -DQ and/or -DR genes. In more recent studies, we have shown that the high frequency of the DP β-chain RFLP in celiac disease reflects the striking increase of a specific constellation of DP alleles in this disease.[64]

Polymorphism of the expressed class II D region molecules is determined, to a large extent, by the high degree of polymorphism in the amino-terminal extracellular domain of those molecules. Such polymorphism explains the varying ability of specific peptides to bind to different class II molecules. The receptor for antigen on CD4 T cells recognizes a bimolecular complex consisting of a peptide antigen in conjunction with an HLA class II molecule. The HLA-DR, -DQ, and -DP α and β genes that encode the expressed polymorphic domains of the celiac disease associated HLA class II D region molecules have now been cloned and sequenced in our laboratory. Such studies appear to provide insights, at a structural level, as to the possible basis for the association of celiac disease with a specific constellation of class II D region genes on an extended haplotype.[64,65]

In several populations[60] celiac disease has been associated with a heterozygous phenotype that includes the -DR3/DQw2 haplotype described above on one chromosome and the HLA-DR7 serologic marker, or a haplotype having HLA-B44, HLA-DR7, and the FC31 complotype[61] on the other chromosome. It is not yet known if the genes on the chromosome having -DR7 contribute to celiac disease susceptibility by *trans*-complementation of a β-chain gene from the -DR7 haplotype with an α-chain gene on the other chromosome, or by another mechanism.

Among sibling pairs affected with celiac disease, all share one or both HLA haplotypes.[66] However, only 28 or 40% of siblings who share one or two HLA haplotype(s) with a propositus, respectively, develop celiac disease. Differences in the concordance rates for celiac disease between monozygotic twins ($\sim 75\%$) and presumed HLA-identical siblings ($\sim 40\%$) suggest that genes outside the HLA locus also confer susceptibility to celiac disease. The observation that celiac disease occurs more frequently in family members who share the HLA susceptibility haplotype than in nonfamily members who appear to have the same haplotype further supports that notion. Studies reporting HLA identity depended in the past largely on serologic testing for markers at one or more HLA loci and did not document HLA identity across the entire HLA class II D region. It is now recognized that some siblings assumed to be HLA-identical by serologic testing may not be identical when detailed studies examining HLA genes are used.

It has been proposed that genes coding for immunoglobulin heavy chain allotype markers on human IgG heavy chain mark for a second genetic region that may be important in the pathogenesis of celiac disease.[67–69] Such allotype markers, termed Gm markers, reflect inherited differences between individuals in the amino acid composition of the chromosome 14-encoded IgG heavy chain constant regions. The G2m(n) allotype marker, a marker on IgG2, has been associated with the persistence of antigliadin antibody in celiac disease patients maintained on gluten-free diets,[69] and other studies have suggested that a particular Gm phenotype, Gm(f;n;b) may be a predisposing factor to celiac disease among some individuals.[68,70]

Humoral and Cell-Mediated Immunity

Humoral Immunity

Important insights into the regulation of antibody responses to wheat gliadins have been derived from studies in mice demonstrating that the antibody response to A-gliadin is governed by genes that map to the murine major histocompatibility complex (termed H-2) and the immunoglobulin heavy chain region. Further studies in mice have indicated that limited regions of the A-gliadin molecule are important in the activation of T-helper cell responses.[24,67,71]

Serum antibodies to whole gliadin and its major electrophoretic fractions can be detected in most celiac disease patients with active disease[72] and in many with inactive disease.[57] Furthermore, IgG antigliadin antibody, at low levels, can persist for long periods (up to 20 years) in clinically asymptomatic patients maintained on a "gluten-free diet".[69] Such antibody may be directed against any one, or as many as all four (α, β, γ and ω) of the major electrophoretic fractions of gliadin.[57] The small intestinal lamina propria in celiac disease contains an increased number of plasma cells. This correlates with the increase in immunoglobulin production noted in the mucosa of these patients.

Antigliadin antibody could play a role in disease pathogenesis by one of several mechanisms. For example, antigliadin antibody complexed with gliadin to form immune complexes could activate tissue-damaging effector mechanisms, including the complement cascade. Alternatively, antigliadin antibody could cause intestinal injury via a cell-mediated cytotoxic reaction in which antigliadin antibody recognizes gliadin peptides bound to mucosal structures and directs a killer (K)-cell-mediated, antibody-dependent, cell-mediated cytotoxic reaction. In support of the above possibilities, cells producing IgG antibody capable of mediating such reactions are markedly increased in the lamina propria during active disease,[73] and organ culture studies have demonstrated increased local production of antigliadin antibody in celiac small intestinal mucosa after gliadin challenge.[74] Nonetheless, current evidence neither documents nor refutes a major role for antigliadin antibody in the pathogenesis of this disease.

Many celiac disease patients have serum antibodies against other food proteins, including milk, egg, and soya proteins. Such antibodies to dietary proteins may simply reflect increased permeability of the intestinal mucosa in this disease. Thus IgG antigliadin antibodies can also be found in approximately 15% of Crohn's disease patients, in whom the small intestinal mucosa is disrupted.[69] However, enhanced absorption may not be a complete explanation, since antigliadin antibodies can also be found in small numbers of apparently normal individuals, and in healthy (i.e., biopsy-negative) relatives of celiac disease patients. The possible role in disease of other antibodies, including antireticulin antibodies, antiendomysial antibodies, and circulating immune complexes containing a mannose-rich, 90-kD glycoprotein, is unknown at present.[75-77]

Cell-Mediated Immunity

Cell-mediated immune mechanisms may play a role in the pathogenesis of celiac disease, although, like antibody responses, their precise importance in this disease requires greater definition. Leukocyte migration assays using gluten components,[78] α-gliadin, or a 12-amino acid peptide of A-gliadin similar to the AD12/E1b protein[41] have documented lymphocyte sensitization to gliadin proteins, as well as other food proteins, in celiac disease patients.[53,54,79] Other studies have demonstrated that soluble factors active in leukocyte migration inhibition assays are produced when intestinal biopsy specimens from celiacs with active disease are cultured with α-gliadin or gluten fractions.[80] Polyclonal stimulation of peripheral blood lymphocytes with the mitogen phytohemagglutinin has been reported as normal or altered in celiac disease.

Intraepithelial lymphocytes in celiac disease patients, as in normal individuals, predominantly have the CD8 (OKT8, T8, Leu2) surface antigen usually associated with class I restricted T cells (i.e., T cells that mediate suppressor or cytotoxic functions), and small intestinal biopsy specimens from celiac disease patients that are cultured with gluten are reported to develop an increase in CD8-bearing intraepithelial lymphocytes.[81] Such lymphocytes produce lymphokines and could be directly responsible for epithelial damage, although this has not been formally demonstrated. The T-cell infiltrate is increased in the lamina propria in celiac disease, although the ratio of CD4 (class II restricted, helper/inducer phenotype) to CD8 (class I restricted, suppressor/cytotoxic phenotype) T cells in the intestinal mucosa and circulation has not differed between celiac disease patients and controls.[82] Some evidence suggests impaired suppressor-cell function in celiac disease, whereas other studies suggest that the fraction of CD4 T cells (i.e., putative helper/inducer cells) in the lamina propria that are activated is increased in this disease.[83]

During active celiac disease, there is an increase in the expression and an alteration in the distribution of HLA class II-DR molecules on small intestinal epithelial cells.[84] Whether this is secondary to increased lymphokine production (e.g., γ-interferon) by mucosal T cells and whether intestinal epithelial cells have an important role in this disease by presenting antigen (for example, gliadin) to mucosal lymphocytes are not known. Finally, the similarity between small intestinal mucosal villous atrophy and crypt hyperplasia in mice undergoing a graft-versus-host reaction[85] or infection with the parasite *Trichinella spiralis*[86] and celiac disease is worth noting. Such findings suggest that immune mechanisms in those diseases can lead to a pattern of intestinal tissue injury similar to that observed in celiac disease, although such murine experimental lesions lack the epithelial cell abnormalities characteristic of human celiac disease.

In summary, the pathogenesis of celiac disease appears to involve the immune system. Interactions between the gene products of the HLA class II D region on chromosome 6 and the gliadin proteins, possibly because of their homology with an intestinal viral protein, are probably important. A logical extension of these findings would hypothesize that T cells, particularly CD4 T cells, must play a key role in the pathogenesis of celiac disease by virtue of their recognition of peptides in conjunction with HLA class II D region molecules.

The precise mechanisms by which the HLA class II genes and their products in the periphery or the thymus contribute to celiac disease is not known. Our studies suggest that the HLA association of this disease has a structural basis reflecting the presence of certain amino acid residues in the hypervariable first domain of several class II D region molecules on the celiac disease-associated HLA class II haplotype. Whether or not a regulatory abnormality in the expression of HLA class II D region genes and/or abnormal *cis* or *trans*-complementation of HLA class II α- and β-chains (creating new and novel class II structures on the cell surface) also contribute to disease pathogenesis is not known. Furthermore, the precise peptide sequence in gliadin that interacts with the relevant HLA class II D region molecule(s) is not known. Finally, the role of CD4 T cells in the pathogenesis of celiac disease, either directly or indirectly via their ability to regulate other T-cell subsets and antibody-producing B cells, remains to be defined. Furthermore, additional genes and environmental factors that may be important for disease susceptibility and the full expression of the disease phenotype await discovery.

CLINICAL FEATURES

Clinical manifestations of celiac disease are protean and vary markedly with the age of the patient, the duration and extent of disease, and the presence of extraintestinal pathology. A disease spectrum that ranges from minor nutritional deficiencies to more striking weight loss, steatorrhea, and malnutrition can be seen. Although celiac disease remits clinically during the teenage years, whether or not the disease disappears is not certain. Persistent hematologic and morphologic abnormalities in some patients suggest that perhaps symptoms, rather than the disease, remit.[6,51]

Associated Diseases

Insulin-dependent diabetes mellitus[87] (the majority of cases are heterozygous for HLA-DR3 and HLA-DR4 haplotypes) and abnormalities in thyroid function can be seen in association with celiac disease. In addition, the majority of patients with DH have a celiac disease-like enteropathy.[56] In DH, the small intestinal lesion is often patchy, rather than diffuse, and gluten ingestion may be required to provoke the histologic abnormalities. DH patients with granular-type IgA deposits in the skin usually have an HLA-DR3 haplotype. Thus HLA class II genes appear to mark for a common link between susceptibility to celiac disease and DH. Although there are many reports of associations between celiac disease and diseases in other organ systems, further studies are required to show that such associations are more than simply coincidental.

Diagnosis

Small intestinal mucosal biopsy is the cornerstone for diagnosis. The finding of a loss of duodenal folds, at endoscopy, may suggest the presence of villous atrophy.[88] A series of biopsies, the first performed at the onset of illness to demonstrate characteristic mucosal abnormalities, a second biopsy performed while the patient is on a gluten-free diet to demonstrate improvement, and a third biopsy performed after deliberate gluten challenge, avoids misdiagnosis (European Society for Pediatric Gastroenterology diagnostic criteria). Whether or not three biopsies and supervised gluten rechallenge are necessary or advisable in all patients is a matter of debate. In children, such a detailed evaluation seems valid, since the corollary of diagnosis is commitment to a life-long gluten-free diet. In adults, one biopsy at the time of initial diagnosis and a second following a gluten-free diet is warranted. The potential benefit for diagnosis of gluten rechallenge and rebiopsy does not seem sufficiently high to warrant the additional risk. However, controlled gluten challenge seems justifiable in adults who are thought to have celiac disease and have been placed on a gluten-free diet, if they have not had a prior biopsy.

Noninvasive screening tests for celiac disease currently lack adequate validation to warrant widespread clinical application. Measurement of serum antibody to purified wheat gliadin fractions can be useful in following the course of dietary therapy in celiac disease. However, measures of antigliadin antibody lack sufficient specificity to substitute for the gold standard of intestinal biopsy in the diagnoses of celiac disease. Nonetheless, a decrease in antibody titers in conjunction with a clinical response to a gluten-free diet can obviate the need for additional biopsies. Studies of antireticulin antibodies reveal a high degree of specificity for celiac disease but low sensitivity. Studies of IgA antiendomysial antibodies[75] have not yet been validated on a sufficiently wide-scale basis for general clinical use.

Celiac mucosa is impermeable to small polar molecules (monosaccharides) but not to intermediate-sized polar molecules (disaccharides). Thus determination of disaccharide compared with monosaccharide absorption (for example, cellobiose versus mannitol, or lactulose versus mannitol)[89] has been proposed as a more specific test for celiac disease than the absorption of monosaccharides like D-xy-lose.[90] The chromium EDTA absorption test has been used to show that abnormal permeability of the small intestinal mucosa can persist in patients with celiac disease, despite clinical and apparent histologic remission.[91,92] However, the specificity of abnormal mucosal permeability for celiac disease is not known, and wide variability in test results has been reported.

Complications

Celiac disease may be associated with complications other than nutritional deficiency. Neoplastic disease is seen in as many as 10% of older patients. In one study of 259 malignancies in 235 patients with histologically confirmed celiac disease,[93] approximately one-half of the tumors were lymphomas (mainly malignant histiocytosis), most commonly in the small intestine. The malignant cells, which resemble histiocytes by morphology, may have T-cell markers on their surface,[94] although clear proof of their lineage requires further study. Of the nonlymphomatous tumors, approximately one-half arise from the gastrointestinal tract, primarily small intestinal adenocarcinoma and squamous cell carcinoma of the esophagus, mouth and pharynx.[93] The value of screening examinations for the early detection of malignancy and whether or not lifetime adherence to a strict gluten-free diet clearly offers significant protection from malignancy is not known. Patients may respond initially to a gluten-free diet and subsequently relapse despite diet maintenance. Such patients may then be refractory to further dietary therapy. Others are refractory to dietary treatment from its inception and, assuming the validity of their gluten-free diet, may not have celiac disease (unclassified sprue). Collagenous sprue is often regarded as a separate entity from celiac disease. However, subepithelial collagen has been noted in up to 36% of patients with classic celiac disease and in tropical sprue. Even the presence of large amounts of subepithelial collagen has not precluded a successful response to a gluten-free diet in some patients. Finally, ulcerative ileojejunitis is a serious and poorly understood disorder frequently seen in patients with a history of celiac disease. Such patients may have developed a superimposed autoimmune reaction to their intestinal epithelial cells.[95]

TREATMENT

Treatment for celiac disease consists of a gluten-free diet. After gluten restriction, clinical improvement, particularly in children, can be seen within days, and morphologic abnormalities return toward normal in weeks. A life-long gluten-free diet is recommended for all celiac disease patients, regardless of symptoms. How strict should the diet be — absolute, or tailored according to the level of gluten sensitivity of the patient? Because clinical improvement correlates with the strictness of the diet, and because gliadin and related prolamins result in damage to the mucosa, their restriction, in theory, should be complete for all patients. However, celiac disease diets are often individualized according to symptoms and histology. A recent study reported that a low-gluten diet (that is, 2.5 g/per day) resulted in mild lymphocytic infiltration of the jejunal epithelium but did not affect gross jejunal morphology or stimulate a significant serum antigluten antibody response.[96] Based on this limited data, these investigators proposed that celiac disease could be treated with a low-gluten, rather than a gluten-free, diet. However, at present, such a diet does not appear warranted in childhood during normal growth and development or prudent in adults because of suggestive evidence that a gluten-free diet may decrease the incidence of complicating malignancy.[97]

Failure to respond to a gluten-free diet may occur if there is poor dietary compliance, an improperly prescribed diet, an associated or complicating disease, or an incorrect diagnosis of celiac disease as the cause of malabsorption. A recent report suggests that cyclosporine may be an effective treatment in some cases of "atypical celiac disease".[98]

REFERENCES

1. Kagnoff MF: Celiac disease: a model of an immunologically mediated intestinal disease. *Immunol Clin N Am* 8:505–520, 1988.
2. Aretaeus, quoted by Major RH: Classic Descriptions of Disease, ed. 3 Springfield, IL, Charles C Thomas, 1945, pp 600–601.
3. Gee S: On the coeliac affliction. *St Barth Hosp Rep* 24:17P, 1888.
4. Dicke WK, Weijers HA, van de Kamer JH: Coeliac disease. II. The presence in wheat of a factor having a deleterious effect in cases of coeliac disease. *Acta Paediatr* 42:34–42, 1953.
5. van de Kamer H, Weijers HA, Dicke WK: Coeliac disease. IV. An investigation into the injurious constituents of wheat in connection with the action on patients with coeliac disease. *Acta Paediatr* 42:223–231, 1953.
6. Cole SG, Kagnoff MF: Celiac disease In: Annual Review of Nutrition, vol. 5. Palo Alto, Annual Reviews, Inc., 1985, pp 241–266.
7. Strobel S, Busuttil A, Ferguson A: Human intestinal mucosal mast cells: expanded population in untreated coeliac disease. *Gut* 24:222–227, 1983.
8. Sterchi EE, Woodley JF: Peptidases of the human intestinal brush border membrane. In McNicholl B, McCarthy CF, Fottrell PF: *Perspectives in Celiac Disease.* Baltimore, University Park Press, 1978, pp 437–449.
9. Phelan JJ, Stevens FM, McNicholl B, et al: Coeliac disease: the abolition of gliadin toxicity by enzymes from *Aspergillus niger. Clin Sci Mol Med* 53:35–43, 1977.
10. Bernardin JE, Aunders RM, Kasarda DD: Absence of carbohydrate in celiac-toxic A-gliadin. *Cereal Chem* 53:612–614, 1976.
11. Kolberg J, Sollid L: Lectin activity of gluten identified as wheat germ agglutinin. *Biochem Biophys Res Commun* 130:867–872, 1985.
12. Colyer J, Kumar PS, Waldron NM, et al: Gliadin binding to rat and human enterocytes. *Clin Sci* 72:593–598, 1987.
13. Bjarnason I, Peters TJ: In vitro determination of small intestinal permeability: demonstration of a persistent defect in patients with coeliac disease. *Gut* 25:145–150, 1984.
14. Hamilton I, Cobden I, Rothwell J, et al: Intestinal permeability in coeliac disease: the response to gluten withdrawal and single-dose gluten challenge. *Gut* 23:202–210, 1982.
15. Kasarda DD: Toxic proteins and peptides in celiac disease: relations to cereal genetics. In Walcher D, Kretchmer M: *Foods, Nutrition and Evolution.* New York, Masson, 1981, pp 201–216.
16. Kasarda DD, Bernardin JE, Nimmo CC: Wheat proteins. In Pomerancz Y: *Advances in Cereal Science and Technology,* Vol 1. St. Paul, American Association of Cereal Chemists, 1976, pp 158–236.

17. Kasarda DD, Nimmo CC, Bernardin JE: Structural aspects and genetic relationships of gliadins. In Hekkens WTJM, Pena AS: *Proceeding of the Second International Celiac Symposium*. Leiden, H.E. Stenfert Korese, B.V., 1974, pp 25–36.

18. Garcia-Olmeda F, Carbonero P, Jones BL: Chromosomal locations of genes that control wheat endosperm proteins. In Pomerancz Y: *Advances in Cereal Science and Technology*. St. Paul, American Association of Cereal Chemists, 1982, pp 1–47.

19. Kasarda DD, Autran JC, Lew EJL, et al: N-terminal amino acid sequences of ω-gliadins and ω-secalins: implications for the evolution of prolamin genes. *Biochem Biophys Acta*. 747:138:138–150, 1983.

20. Kasarda DD, Bernardin JE, Qualset CO: Relationship of gliadin protein components to chromosomes in hexploid wheats. *Proc Natl Acad Sci USA* 73:3646–3650, 1976.

21. Kasarda DD, Lafiandra D, Morris R, et al: Genetic relationships of wheat gliadin proteins. *Kulturpflanze* 32:533–552, 1984.

22. Ciclitira PJ, Hunter JO, Lennox ES: Clinical testing of bread made from nullisomic 6A wheats in celiac patients. *Lancet* 2:234–236, 1980.

23. Woychik JH, Boudy JA, Dimler RJ: Starch gel electrophoresis of wheat gluten proteins with concentrated urea. *Arch Biochem Biophys* 94:477–482, 1961.

24. Kagnoff MF, Austin RK, Johnson HCL, et al: Celiac sprue: correlation with murine T-cell responses to wheat gliadin components. *J Immunol* 129:2693–2697, 1982.

25. Autran JC, Lew EJL, Nimmo CC, et al: N-terminal amino acid sequencing of prolamins from wheat and related species. *Nature* 282:527–529, 1979.

26. Kasarda DD: Structure and properties of α-gliadins. *Ann Tech Agric* 29:151–173, 1980.

27. Bartels D, Thompson RD: The characterization of cDNA clones coding for wheat storage proteins. *Nucleic Acids Res* 11:2961–2977, 1983.

28. Bietz JA, Juebna FR, Sanderson JE, et al: Wheat gliadin homology revealed through N-terminal amino acid sequence analysis. *Cereal Chem* 54:1070–1083, 1977.

29. Shewry PR, Autran J-C, Nimmo CC, et al: N-terminal amino acid sequence homology of storage protein components from barley and a diploid wheat. *Nature* 286:520–522, 1980.

30. Shewry PR, Lew EJL, Kasarda DD: Structural homology of storage proteins coded by the *Hor-1* locus of barley *(Hordeum vulgare L.)*. *Planta* 153:246–253, 1981.

31. Bernardin JE, Kasarda DD, Mecham DK: Preparation and characterization of α-gliadin. *J Biol Chem* 242:445–450, 1967.

32. Falchuk ZM, Gebhard RL, Sessoms C, et al: An in vitro model of gluten sensitive enteropathy in organ culture. *J Clin Invest* 53:487–500, 1974.

33. Hekkens WTJM, Haex AJC, Willighagen RGJ: Some aspects of gliadin fractionation and testing by a histochemical method. In Booth CC, Dowling RH: *Coeliac Disease*. Edinburgh, Churchill Livingstone, 1970, pp 11–18.

34. Kasarda DD, Okita TW, Bernardin JE, et al: Nucleic acid (cDNA) and amino acid sequences of α-type gliadins from wheat *(Triticum aestivum L.)*. *Proc Natl Acad Sci USA* 81:4712–4716, 1984.

35. Rafalski JA, Scheets K, Metzler M, et al: Developmentally regulated plant genes: the nucleotide sequence of a wheat gliadin genomic clone. *EMBO J* 3:1409–1415, 1984.

36. Kendall MJ, Cox PS, Schneider R, et al: Gluten subfractions in coeliac disease. *Lancet* 2:1065–1067, 1972.

37. Jos J, Charbonnier L, Mougenot JF, et al: Isolation and characterization of the toxic fraction of wheat gliadin in celiac disease. In McNicholl B, McCarthy CF, Fottrell PF: *Perspectives in Celiac Disease*. Baltimore, University Park Press, 1978, pp 75–90.

38. Ciclitira PJ, Evans DJ, Fagg NLK, et al: Clinical testing of gliadin fractions in celiac patients. *Clin Sci* 66:357–364, 1984.

39. Howdle PD, Ciclitira PJ, Simpson FG, et al: Are all gliadins toxic in celiac disease? An in vitro study of α, β, γ and ω gliadins. *Scand J Gastroenterol* 19:41–47, 1984.

40. Jos J, Charbonnier L, Mosse J, et al: The toxic fraction of gliadin digests in coeliac disease. Isolation by chromatography on Biogel P-10. *Clin Chim Acta* 119:263–274, 1982.

41. Kagnoff MF, Austin RK, Hubert JJ, et al: Possible role for a human adenovirus in the pathogenesis of celiac disease. *J Exp Med* 160:1544–1557, 1984.

42. Bos JL, Polder LJ, Bernards R, et al: The 2.2 kb E1b mRNA of human Ad12 and Ad5 codes for two tumor antigens starting at different AUG triplets. *Cell* 27:121–131, 1981.

43. Kimura T, Sawada Y, Shinawawa M, et al: Nucleotide sequence of the transforming early region E1b of adenovirus type 12 DNA: structure and gene organization, and comparison with those of adenovirus type 5 DNA. *Nucleic Acids Res* 9:6571–6589, 1981.

44. Flint SJ: Transformation by adenoviruses. In Tooze J: *Molecular Biology of Tumor Viruses II. DNA Tumor Viruses.* Cold Spring Harbor, NY, Cold Spring Harbor Press 1980, pp 547–576.

45. Middleton PJ: Role of viruses in pediatric gastrointestinal disease and epidemiologic factors. In Tyrrell DAJ, Kapikian AZ: *Virus Infections of the Gastrointestinal Tract.* New York, Marcel Dekker, 1982, pp 211–225.

46. Mak S, Mak I, Smiley JR, et al: Tumorigenicity and viral gene expression in rat cells transformed by Ad12 virions or by the EcoR1 C fragment of Ad12 DNA. *Virology* 98:456–460, 1979.

47. Perricaudet M, le Moullec J-M, Tiollais P, et al: Structure of two adenovirus type 12 transforming polypeptides and their evolutionary implications. *Nature* 288:174–176, 1980.

48. Wilson MC, Fraser NW, Darnell JE: Initiation sites by high doses of UV irradiation: evidence for three independent promoters within the left 11% of the Ad2 genome. *Virology* 94:175–184, 1979.

49. Norrby E, Ankerst J: Biological characterization of structural components of adenovirus type 12. *J Gen Virology* 5:183–194, 1969.

50. Kagnoff MF, Paterson YJ, Kumar PJ, et al: Evidence for the role of a human intestinal adenovirus in the pathogenesis of coeliac disease. *Gut* 28:995–1001, 1987.

51. Kagnoff MF: Celiac disease: pathogenesis and clinical features. In Shaffer E and Thomson ABR: *Modern Concepts in Gastroenterology.* New York, Plenum Press, 1989 2:227–250, 1989.

52. D'Ambrosio E, Del Grosso N, Chicca A, et al: Neutralizing antibodies against 33 human adenoviruses in normal children in Rome. *J Hyg (Camb)* 89:155–166, 1982.

53. Karagiannis JA, Priddle JD, Jewell DP: Cell-mediated immunity to a synthetic gliadin peptide resembling a sequence from adenovirus 12. *Lancet* 2:884–886, 1987.

54. Lydford-Davis H, Karagiannis JA, Priddle JD, et al: Preliminary characterization of leucocyte migration inhibition factor (LIF) produced by lymphocytes from coeliac patients when stimulated with gluten peptides. *Clin Sci* 72:89P, 1987.

55. Katz SI, Hall RP, Lawley TJ, et al: Dermatitis herpetiformis: the skin and the gut. *Ann Intern Med* 93:857–874, 1980.

56. Lawley TJ, Strober W, Yaoita H, et al: Small intestinal biopsies and HLA types in dermatitis herpetiformis patients with granular and linear IgA skin deposits. *J Invest Dermatol* 74:9–12, 1980.

57. Levenson SD, Austin RK, Dietler MD, et al: Specificity of anti-gliadin antibody in celiac disease. *Gastroenterology* 89:1–5, 1985.

58. MacDonald WC, Dobbins WO, Rubin CE: Studies on the familial nature of celiac sprue using biopsy of the small intestine. *N Engl J Med* 272:448–456, 1968.

59. Stenhammer L, Brand A, Wagermark J: A family study of coeliac disease. *Acta Paediatr Scand* 71:625–628, 1982.

60. Polanco I, Biemond I, van Leeuwen A, et al: Gluten-sensitive enteropathy in Spain: genetic and environmental factors. In McConnell RB: *The Genetics of Coeliac Disease.* Lancaster, MTP Press Ltd. 1981, pp 211–231.

61. Alper CA, Fleischnick E, Awdeh Z, et al: Extended major histocompatibility complex haplotypes in patients with gluten-sensitive enteropathy. *J Clin Invest* 79:251–256, 1987.

62. Howell MD, Austin RK, Kelleher D, et al: An HLA-D region restriction fragment length polymorphism associated with celiac disease. *J Exp Med* 164:333–338, 1986.

63. Howell MD, Smith JR, Austin RK, et al: An extended HLA-D region haplotype associated with celiac disease. *Proc Natl Acad Sci USA* 85:222–226, 1988.

64. Kagnoff MF, Harwood JI, Erlich HA: HLA Class II DP subregion genes associated with celiac disease. *Gastroenterology,* 96:A244, 1989.

65. Kagnoff MF, Harwood JI, Erlich HA: Cloning and sequence analysis of the polymorphic HLA class II genes associated with celiac disease. *Gastroenterology,* 96:A243, 1989.

66. Scholz S, Albert E: HLA and diseases: involvement of more than one HLA-linked determinant of disease susceptibility. *Immunol Rev* 70:77–88, 1983.

67. Kagnoff MF: Two genetic loci control the murine immune response to A-gliadin, a wheat protein that activates coeliac sprue. *Nature* 296:158–160, 1982.

68. Kagnoff MF, Weiss JB, Brown RJ, et al: Immunoglobulin allotype markers in gluten-sensitive enteropathy. *Lancet* I:952–953, 1983.

69. Weiss JB, Austin RK, Schanfield MS, et al: Gluten-sensitive enteropathy. Immunoglobulin G heavy-chain (Gm) allotypes and the immune response to wheat gliadins. *J Clin Invest* 72:96–101, 1983.

70. Carbonara AO, DeMarchi M, van Loghem E, et al: Gm markers in celiac disease. *Hum Immunol* 6:91–95, 1983.

71. Trefts PE, Kagnoff MF: Gluten-sensitive enteropathy: the T-dependent anti-A-gliadin antibody response maps to the murine histocompatibility locus. *J Immunol* 126:2249–2252, 1981.

72. Ciclitira PJ, Ellis HJ, Evans DJ: A solid phase radioimmunoassay for measurement of circulating antibody titres to wheat gliadin and its subfractions in patients and adult celiac disease. *J Immunol Methods* 62:231–239, 1983.

73. Scott BB, Boodall A, Stephenson P, et al: Small intestinal plasma cells in coeliac disease. *Gut* 25:41–46, 1984.

74. Ciclitira PJ, Ellis JH, Wood GM, et al: Secretion of gliadin antibody by coeliac jejunal mucosal biopsies cultured in vitro. *Clin Exp Immunol* 64:119–124, 1986.

75. Chorzelksi TP, Beutner EJ, Sulej J, et al: IgA antiendomysium antibody: a new immunological marker of dermatitis herpetiformis and coeliac disease. *Br J Dermatol* 111:395–402, 1984.

76. Maury CPJ, Teppo AM: Demonstration of tissue 90-kD glycoprotein as antigen in circulating IgG immune complexes in dermatitis herpetiformis and coeliac disease. *Lancet* 2:892–894, 1984.

77. Stern M, Bender SW, Gruttner R, et al: Serum antibodies against gliadin and reticulin in a family study of coeliac disease. *Eur J Pediatr* 135:31–36, 1980.

78. Guan R, Rawcliffe PM, Priddle JD, et al: Cellular hypersensitivity to gluten derived peptides in coeliac disease. *Gut* 28:426–434, 1987.

79. Simpson FG, Robertson AF, Howdle PD, et al: Cell-mediated immunity to dietary antigens in coeliac disease. *Scand J Gastroenterol* 17:671–676, 1982.

80. Corazza GR, Rawcliffe PM, Frisoni M, et al: Specificity of leucocyte migration inhibition test in coeliac disease: a reassessment using different gluten subfractions. *Clin Exp Immunol* 60:117–122, 1985.

81. Flores AF, Winter HS, Bhan AK: In vitro model to assess immunoregulatory T-lymphocyte subpopulations in gluten-sensitive enteropathy (GSE). *Gastroenterology* 82:1058 (Abstract), 1982.

82. Malizia G, Trejdosiewicz LK, Wood GM, et al: The microenvironment of coeliac disease: T-cell phenotypes and expression of the T2 T blast antigen by small bowel lymphocytes. *Clin Exp Immunol* 60:437–446, 1985.

83. Griffiths CE, Barrison IG, Leonard JN, et al: Preferential activation of CD4 T lymphocytes in the lamina propria of gluten-sensitive enteropathy. *Clin Exp Immunol* 72:280–283, 1988.

84. Sarles J, Gorvel JP, Olive D, et al: Subcellular localization of class I (A, B, C) and class II (DR and DQ) MHC antigens in jejunal epithelium of children with coeliac disease. *J Pediatr Gastroenterol Nutr* 6:51–56, 1987.

85. Neild GH: Coeliac disease: a graft-versus-host-like reaction localized to the small bowel wall? *Lancet* 1:811–812, 1981.

86. Manson-Smith DF, Bruch RG, Parrott DMV: Villous atrophy and expulsion of intestinal *Trichinella spiralis* are mediated by T cells. *Cell Immunol* 47:285–292, 1979.

87. Shanahan F, McKenna R, McCarthy CF, et al: Coeliac disease and diabetes mellitus: a study of 24 patients with HLA typing. *Q J Med* 51:329–335, 1982.

88. Brocchi E, Corazza GR, Caletti G, et al: Endoscopic demonstration of loss of duodenal folds in the diagnosis of celiac disease. *N Engl J Med* 22:319:741–744, 1988.

89. Holmes GKT, Prior P, Lane MR, et al: Malignancy in coeliac disease-effect of a gluten free diet. *Gut* 30:333–338, 1989.

90. Bode S, Gudmand-Hyer E: The diagnostic value of the D-xylose absorption test in adult coeliac disease. *Scand J Gastroenterol* 22:1217–1222, 1987.

91. Bjarnason I, Peters TJ, Veall N: A persistent defect in intestinal permeability in coeliac disease demonstrated by a ^{51}Cr-labelled EDTA absorption test. *Lancet* 1:323–325, 1983.

92. Fotherby KJ, Wraight EP, Neale G: ^{51}Cr-EDTA/^{14}C-mannitol intestinal permeability test. Clinical use in screening for coeliac disease. *Scand J Gastroenterol* 23:171–177, 1988.

93. Swinson CM, Slavin G, Coles EC, et al: Coeliac disease and malignancy. *Lancet* 1:111–115, 1983.

94. Salter DM, Krajewski AS, Dwar AE: Immunophenotype analysis of malignant histiocytosis of the intestine. *J Clin Pathol* 39:8–15, 1986.

95. Strober W, Falchuk ZM, Rogentine GN, et al: The pathogenesis of gluten-sensitive enteropathy. Ann Intern Med 83:242–256, 1975.

96. Montgomery AMP, Goka AKJ, Kumar PJ, et al: Low gluten diet in the treatment of adult coeliac disease: effect on jejunal morphology and serum anti-gluten antibodies. *Gut* 29:1557–1563, 1988.

97. Juby LD, Rothwell J, Axon AT: Lactulos/mannitol test: an ideal screen for celiac disease. *Gastroenterology* 96:79–85, 1989.

98. Berstein EF, Whitington PF: Successful treatment of atypical sprue in an infant with cyclosporine. *Gastroenterology* 95:199–204, 1988.

CHAPTER 25

Food Allergy

RICHARD H. DUERR

FERGUS SHANAHAN

INTRODUCTION

The concept of food allergy is not new. Hippocrates described urticaria and gastro-intestinal symptoms following milk ingestion more than 2,000 years ago.[1] In 1921, Prausnitz and Küstner described the presence of a reagin in the serum of a fish-allergic individual that could be passively transferred to the skin of a normal individual.[2] Brunner and Walzer, in 1928, reported that wheal and flare reactions occur in the skin of normal individuals if they ingest fish after intradermal injection of serum from fish-allergic individuals.[3] Subsequently, immunologic hypersensitivity to a variety of dietary antigens has been reported.

Unfortunately, confusion and controversy have clouded the subject of food allergy in the past. Some physicians have approached the subject with skepticism and relegated it to the level of food faddism, cultism, and quackery. In part, this is due to failure of some authors to use appropriate terminology and a methodical, objective, unbiased, scientific approach to the investigation of the problem. In addition, the mass media and some quarters of the medical profession have fostered widespread public misconceptions regarding the prevalence, scope, and nature of food allergic disease as exemplified by the following statements from a food allergy "expert" published in the popular press:

> According to current medical estimates, 10 percent of all Americans suffer from food allergies. I believe, though, that the number is much higher and that many food allergy sufferers have not had their problem diagnosed.

In the same article, the author goes on to say:

> In addition to "traditional" allergic reactions, like hives, rashes, hay fever and nausea, certain foods are believed to provoke a series of mental and behavioral reactions which

include depression, anxiety, irritability and compulsive eating and drinking. Food allergies can also be behind headaches, joint and muscle pain, gastrointestinal problems such as cramps, diarrhea, nausea, fatigue — even an unexplained weight gain.[4]

Statements such as these have generated more public concern over the issue than is warranted and have bolstered the public perception that food allergy is a major public health problem.[5] At the same time, such statements have also undermined public confidence in the ability of the medical profession to properly diagnose and treat food allergy.

Fortunately, particularly in the last few decades, a great deal of scientifically sound work has contributed to a growing body of knowledge concerning food allergy. The goals of this chapter are to place the role of *true* food allergy into proper perspective, review our current understanding of the pathophysiology underlying food allergy, and discuss clinical features including clinical manifestations and differential diagnosis of food allergy, evaluation of the patient with suspected food allergy, and treatment/prevention of food allergy.

Terminology

Part of the confusion surrounding the subject of food allergy has been due to the failure of some authors to distinguish between immunologically and nonimmunologically mediated adverse reactions to foods. The terms *food allergy* and *food hypersensitivity* are interchangeable but should be reserved for those adverse reactions to food that have been shown to be immunologically mediated. *Food intolerance* is a term that should be used to describe nonimmunologically mediated adverse reactions to food due to toxic, infectious, or pharmacologic agents, metabolic responses, manifestations of gastrointestinal tract disorders, or responses that are psychogenic in origin (Table 25–1).[6]

Prevalence of Food Allergy

Community surveys have revealed that one-fifth to one-third of the population surveyed report adverse reactions to some food.[5,7,8] However, when double-blind food challenges are used, most complaints of adverse reactions to food cannot be objectively verified.[9–11] The prevalence of true food allergy is not known, but it has been estimated to range from 0.3% to 7.5% in children; it is believed to decrease with age, and it is more common in atopic individuals.[12] Most adverse reactions to food are probably not immunologically mediated.

PATHOPHYSIOLOGY

The Mucosal Barrier

During an average individual's lifetime, the GI tract will handle approximately 100 tons of food, which represents the largest antigenic load confronting the immune system.[13,14] The local mucosal immune system is uniquely adapted to meet this antigenic challenge.[15,16] Together with a variety of nonimmunologic factors, it comprises "the mucosal barrier," which prevents penetration of potentially harmful intraluminal antigenic, toxic, and infectious agents (Fig. 25–1).[6,17–22]

Table 25–1 NONIMMUNOLOGICALLY MEDIATED ADVERSE REACTIONS TO FOODS[a]

Contaminants and additives
  Dyes, flavorings and preservatives
    Tartrazine
    Nitrites and nitrates
    Monosodium glutamate
    Sulfiting agents
    Benzoates
  Toxins
    Bacterial (i.e., *Staphylococcus aureus, Clostridium botulinum*)
    Fungal (i.e., ergot, aflatoxins)
    Seafood-associated (i.e., scombroid poisoning, saxitoxin from shellfish)
  Infectious agents
    Bacteria (i.e., *Salmonella, Shigella, Campylobacter, Yersinia, Escherichia coli*)
    Parasites (i.e., *Giardia* and *Trichinella*)
    Virus (i.e., hepatitis, rotavirus, enterovirus)
  Other contaminants
    Heavy metals
    Pesticides
    Antibiotics
Pharmacologic agents
  Caffeine (i.e., coffee, tea, soft drinks, cocoa)
  Theobromine (i.e., tea, chocolate)
  Histamine (i.e., fish, beer, wine, chocolate)
  Tyramine (i.e., cheeses, banana, avocado)
  Tryptamine (i.e., tomato)
  Serotonin (i.e., banana, tomato, avocado, pineapple)
  Phenylethylamine (i.e., chocolate)
  Alcohol
Gastrointestinal tract disorders
  Structural abnormalities (i.e., hiatal hernia, obstruction)
  Enzyme deficiencies (i.e., lactase deficiency, galactosemia, phenylketonuria)
  Malignancy
  Other diseases (i.e., peptic ulcer disease, cholelithiasis, pancreatic insufficiency)
Psychogenic reactions

[a] This list is intended to be representative of nonimmunologic causes of adverse reactions to foods, but it is not comprehensive.

Nonimmunologic factors contributing to the mucosal barrier include pancreatic and other digestive enzymes, mucus secretion, peristalsis, the indigenous intestinal flora, and the continual renewal of the mucosal epithelial lining. The blind-loop syndrome and mucosal injury due to gastroenteritis are conditions in which nonimmunologic defense mechanisms may be impaired and lead to increased penetration by intraluminal antigen.[6,14,20,22] Gastric acid has been listed as an important factor in many reviews of this subject; however, the finding that adults with achlorhydria have a lower incidence of circulating antibovine serum albumin antibodies than adults with normal or elevated stimulated gastric acid output would argue to the contrary.[23]

The gastrointestinal secretory immune system is an important component of the mucosal barrier. The predominant immunoglobulin in intestinal secretions is

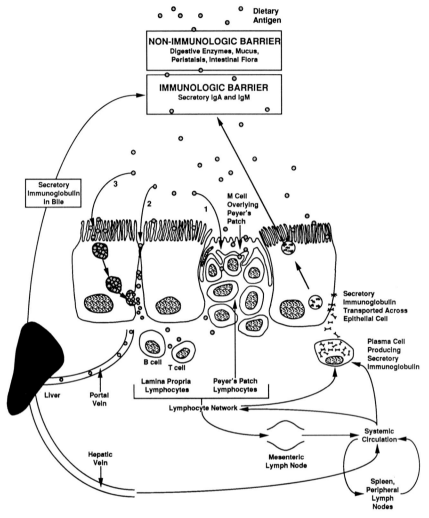

Figure 25–1 An elaborate mucosal barrier guards against penetration of poten-tially harmful agents from the intestinal lumen. However, even under normal circum-stances, small quantities of intact dietary antigens pass through the mucosal barrier and appear in the systemic circulation. Mechanisms of antigen uptake include: 1) uptake by the specialized M cells, which are adapted for sampling of the luminal environment and delivering antigenic material to the underlying lymphoid tissue in Peyer's patches; 2) penetration through the interepithelial tight junctions (increased in states of mucosal inflammation or injury); and 3) passage through the columnar epithelial cells in vesicles. MHC class II molecules expressed on the surfaces of intes-tinal epithelial cells may be involved in selective transcellular transport of antigen. Once antigen has been taken up, it may be processed by the intestinal lymphocyte network, which is in communication with the systemic circulation and peripheral lymphoid tissue. Antigen also passes through the portal vein into the reticuloendo-thelial system of the liver, which probably plays a role in modulation of the immune response to dietary antigen. The net result of all of these interactions is usually oral tolerance, but sensitization to dietary antigen may occur.

secretory IgA (sIgA), an IgA dimer integrally associated with a secretory component that renders stability and resistance to proteolysis.[21] IgA-producing cells comprise approximately 80% and 90%, respectively, of all immunoglobulin-producing cells in the small intestine and the colon.[24] Dimeric IgA produced by these cells diffuses to the basolateral membrane of columnar epithelial cells, where it attaches to secretory component, which is synthesized by the epithelial cells. Secretory IgA is then transported in vesicles across the epithelial cells and secreted into the lumen by exocytosis. sIgA may also enter the intestinal lumen in bile.[25,26] Luminal sIgA is thought to decrease adherence of antigen to epithelial cells and thereby block antigen uptake (immune exclusion).[19,25,27] It has been proposed that immune exclusion may also involve clearance of complexes of environmental antigen and polymeric IgA from the circulation.[25,26] The importance of the phenomenon of immune exclusion may be appreciated by the study of people with selective IgA deficiency. Although most of these people are asymptomatic, many of them have increased levels of circulating immune complexes and precipitins to bovine milk and ruminant serum proteins,[28-31] and there is an increased incidence of atopic, immune-complex-mediated, and autoimmune disease associated with selective IgA deficiency.[31] IgM may also occur in a secretory form and supplement the function of sIgA.[24]

In addition to the local components of the mucosal barrier, it is recognized that the reticuloendothelial system of the liver may act as a "second line of defense" against penetration of potentially harmful agents from the gut. When liver disease impedes this system, symptoms may develop from the escape of these agents into the systemic circulation.[18,20,32]

Many of the nonimmunologic and immunologic components of the mucosal barrier are not fully developed in neonates and infants. Pepsin activity, enterokinase activity, and stimulated secretion of carboxypeptidase B, trypsin, and chymotrypsin are low in neonates and may not reach maturity until several months of age or even the second year of life.[33,34] Neonates have no detectable IgA or IgM in exocrine fluids,[22,35] and maturation of intestinal IgA production may not occur until 1-2 months of age in bottle-fed, healthy infants.[36] Serum β-lactoglobulin concentrations are higher in preterm than in term infants,[37] and mean titers of serum antibodies to proteins of cow's milk- and soy-based formulas are higher in infants fed these formulas since birth than in infants fed these formulas for the first time after 3 months of age.[38] Thus, absorption of intact macromolecules is greatest in early life.

In the neonate and infant with an immature mucosal barrier, ingestion of breast milk may play an important role. sIgA in breast milk may inhibit absorption of antigenic macromolecules, and breast milk contains hormones and growth factors such as epidermal growth factor, which may facilitate maturation of the mucosal barrier.[39-41] Indirect clinical evidence for an enhancing effect of breast milk on the mucosal barrier early in life comes from studies suggesting that breast feeding until 4-6 months of age may prevent the development of food allergies. These studies are discussed later in this chapter.

Antigen Uptake

Despite the presence of an elaborate mucosal barrier, there is convincing evidence that small quantities of intact antigenic macromolecules can penetrate the gastrointestinal mucosa and appear in the systemic circulation under normal circumstances.[3,42-46] As discussed above, macromolecule absorption is greater early in life and in conditions causing disruption of the mucosal barrier.

A variety of mechanisms for antigen uptake exist (Fig. 25–1). The specialized microfold epithelial (M) cells overlying Peyer's patches appear to be specifically adapted for sampling the gastrointestinal luminal environment and delivering small amounts of intact antigenic material to the lymphoid tissue in Peyer's patches.[47] Rat and human intestinal epithelial cells can present antigen in vitro, inducing proliferation of primed T cells, and major histocompatibility complex (MHC) class II molecules expressed on the enterocyte surface appear to be important in the process of antigen presentation, as evidenced by blocking of the stimulatory effect on T cells by antibodies to Ia molecules.[48,49] It has been suggested that MHC class II molecules expressed by intestinal epithelial cells may be involved in selective transcellular transport of antigen.[50] These mechanisms of antigen uptake as well as nonselective uptake of macromolecules through and between the intestinal columnar epithelial cells are discussed more extensively in Chapter 3.

Immune Response to Dietary Antigen

When dietary antigen is presented to the local mucosal immune system, three antigen-specific immunologic responses may occur: a local secretory IgA antibody response may occur; rarely, a systemic immune response may be mounted; or, commonly, a state of immunologic tolerance may develop.[15,26,51]

Oral Tolerance

The phenomenon of systemic hyporesponsiveness to dietary antigen was first suggested in the medical literature in 1829 when Dakin, describing contact sensitivity to poison ivy, commented:

> [Some] say the bane will prove the best antidote, and hence advise the forbidden leaves to be eaten, both as a preventive and cure to the external disease.[52]

Native Americans prevented contact sensitivity to poison ivy by eating the leaves of the plant.[53] Laboratory evidence for immunologic tolerance after ingestion of antigen was reported as early as 1911 when Wells demonstrated that feeding guinea pigs antigen prevented the development of systemic anaphylaxis.[54,55] Subsequently, this phenomenon, sometimes termed the Sulzberger-Chase phenomenon,[56] has been demonstrated in animals for a variety of orally administered antigens including ovalbumin, bovine serum albumin, contact-sensitizing agents, heterologous red cells, and inactivated bacteria or viruses.[57-71] It appears that presentation of thymus-dependent, soluble, nonreplicating antigens to the mucosal immune system preferentially leads to oral tolerance, while presentation of thymus-independent, particulate antigens such as those associated with potentially invasive microorganisms leads to an active immune response.[51,70-74]

IgE-mediated and delayed-type hypersensitivity are the immune mechanisms most easily suppressed after feeding proteins, and the suppression of these immune mechanisms is the most long-lasting.[51] IgE-mediated and delayed-type hypersensitivity are also the immune mechanisms most commonly involved in food allergy, a condition that is tantamount to lack of oral tolerance.

Many complex immunologic pathways are probably involved in the induction of oral tolerance, but the presence or lack of T-cell responsiveness seems to be the principle factor determining whether immunologic tolerance will develop to dietary protein antigens.[51,53,58,72,75-78] Prevention of systemic cell-mediated immunity to dietary proteins appears to be due to activation of specific suppressor T cells.[51,58,77,78] In vitro antigen presentation by MHC class II expressing intestinal epithelial cells has been shown to preferentially stimulate proliferation of lymphocytes that are phenotypically and functionally suppressor T cells.[48,49,79] In contrast, MHC class II-restricted antigen presentation by macrophages, monocytes, dendritic cells, and B cells preferentially induces helper T cells. Perhaps the suppressor T cells induced under the influence of antigen-presenting intestinal epithelial cells are involved in the generation of oral tolerance.[50] Unlike tolerance of systemic cell-mediated immunity, tolerance of systemic humoral immunity does not appear to be secondary to the action of suppressor T cells and may result from helper T-cell unresponsiveness or other additional mechanisms.[51,58,72,76-78] The liver may also play a role in down-regulation of the systemic immune response to certain dietary antigens.[32,80-83]

The subject of oral tolerance is discussed more extensively in Chapter 9.

Food Hypersensitivity

Penetration of the mucosal barrier by food antigen may lead to sensitization, and subsequent absorption of even minute quantities of antigen may result in allergic reactions.[20] As discussed earlier in this chapter, antigen penetration may be increased early in life and in conditions in which the mucosal barrier is disrupted. Failure to develop oral tolerance to food antigens presented early in life or breakdown of oral tolerance may lead to clinical food hypersensitivity.

Food hypersensitivity reactions can be subdivided into *immediate* (IgE-mediated, type I hypersensitivity) and *delayed* (late-phase IgE-mediated, immune complex-mediated, and cell-mediated). Delayed reactions appear to be involved in the pathogenesis of gluten-sensitive enteropathy (discussed extensively in Chapter 24), food-protein enteropathy,[84-87] and possibly eosinophilic gastroenteritis[6,88,89] but immediate (type I, IgE-mediated) hypersensitivity reactions account for the majority of immunologically mediated adverse reactions to foods and will be the focus of this discussion.

The phenomenon of immediate wheal and flare reactions after injection of small amounts of food antigen into the skin of some individuals is well described and demonstrates the presence of IgE on mast cell surfaces that reacts with food antigens.[90] Such reactions occur in normal individuals after intradermal injection of serum from an allergic individual followed by ingestion of the antigen to which the serum donor is allergic.[3,42,43] Similar reactions have been described in human ileal and colonic mucosa after passive sensitization followed by ingestion or direct application of the antigen,[91] and mast cells in passively sensitized human jejunal mucosa specimens have been shown to degranulate in vitro upon challenge with the corresponding antigen.[92] Finally, recent reports that plasma histamine rises significantly in patients with cutaneous, gastrointestinal, or respiratory symptoms elicited by double-blind, placebo-controlled food challenges but not in patients with negative food challenges, while the activated complement components C3a and C5a remain unchanged after positive food challenges, provide further evidence for the involvement of IgE-mediated mast cell or basophil activation in the pathogenesis of food hypersensitivity.[93-95] No differences were found in venous blood basophil number, total histamine content of leukocytes, or spontaneous histamine release in vitro before and at intervals after positive food challenges, suggesting that activation of target tissue mast cells rather than basophils accounts for the rise in plasma histamine after positive food challenge.[94,95]

Mast cells are abundant in the gut and exist in every layer of the gut wall.[96] In the rat, intestinal mucosal mast cells differ morphologically, biochemically, and functionally from those located in the connective tissue of the gut and other sites.[97-100] Evidence for human mast cell heterogeneity is also emerging.[100-107]

If luminal antigen penetrates the mucosa in a sensitized individual, antigen-specific IgE on the surface of mucosal mast cells may be bridged by antigen and trigger activation of the mast cells with degranulation and release of potent mediators (Fig. 25–2). Expected consequences of intestinal anaphylaxis include increased vascular permeability, mucus production, chemotaxis, smooth muscle contraction, and stimulation of pain fibers.[96,100,103,108] In a rat model of intestinal anaphylaxis, altered intestinal myoelectric and motor activity, mucosal damage, decreased net absorption of H_2O, Na^+ and Cl^-, and active Cl^- secretion occur.[109-113]

Local intestinal anaphylaxis allows increased penetration of foreign antigens through the disrupted mucosal barrier, which may result in greater sensitization to dietary antigens, dissemination of such antigens to other sites in the body, and propagation of symptoms.[20,114,115] Increased uptake of nonspecific luminal antigens may stimulate an IgG-mediated response.[20] Systemic uptake of specific antigen may lead to IgE-mediated activation of mast cells in other target organs such as skin and lung, or acute systemic anaphylaxis may occur due to activation of systemic mast cells and basophils. When systemic mast cells and basophils are activated, many potent mediators are released or generated including preformed substances such as histamine, heparin, eosinophil chemotactic factor of anaphylaxis, chondroitin sulfates, and enzymes, and newly generated substances such as prostaglandins, leukotrienes, and platelet-activating factor.[103,116-118] The mediators released by tissue mast cells in immediate IgE-mediated hypersensitivity reactions may stimulate a cellular inflammatory response that is indistinguishable histologically from a type IV cell-mediated response (the late-phase IgE-mediated immune response).[94,95,119,120]

Figures 25–1 and 25–2 summarize our current understanding of the pathophysiology underlying IgE-mediated food allergy.

Food Allergens

A limited number of foods cause most food hypersensitivity reactions. Milk, eggs, peanuts, nuts, fish, shellfish, soybeans, and wheat are the most commonly implicated foods.[90,94,121] The prevalence of allergy to a particular food may depend in part on dietary patterns of the society. For example, rice is a common culprit in Japan but rare in the United States, while peanut hypersensitivity is common in the United States but rare in Sweden, where peanuts and peanut butter are infrequently eaten.[94]

Specific antigens from codfish, shrimp, peanuts, soybeans, and cow's milk responsible for hypersensitivity reactions have been isolated and character-

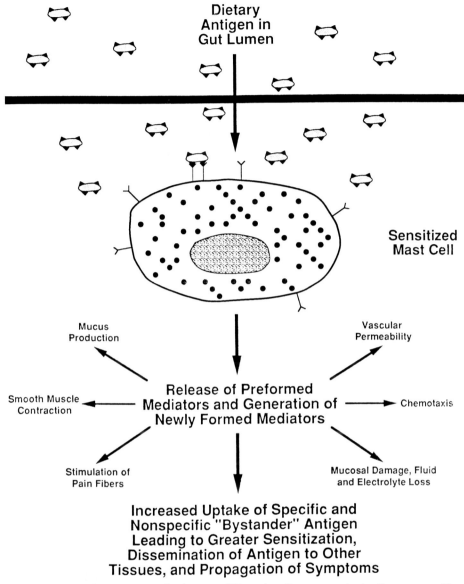

Figure 25 – 2 When even minute quantities of antigen penetrate the mucosal barrier in a sensitized individual, IgE-mediated intestinal anaphylaxis may occur and lead to increased uptake of both specific and nonspecific "bystander" antigens, resulting in dissemination of antigens to other sites in the body where further hypersensitivity reactions may occur.

ized.[122-127] Many food allergens demonstrate heat stability, acid stability, and/or resistance to proteolysis, and most of them have a relatively small molecular weight of 10,000–70,000 daltons. Thus they may retain their immunogenicity through food processing treatments and digestion, and their size may be ideal for bridging two IgE molecules.[127]

CLINICAL FEATURES

Clinical Manifestations of Food Allergy

Food allergy may be manifest by a variety of symptoms and signs encompassing many different organ systems.

Systemic anaphylaxis as a result of food hypersensitivity is the most serious immunologically mediated adverse reaction to food. A recent study of 102 patients with presumed idiopathic anaphylaxis revealed that five patients had positive skin prick tests to one or more food antigens and a positive oral challenge with the incriminated food(s), and two additional patients with positive skin prick tests had no further reactions after elimination of the incriminated food(s).[128] Systemic anaphylaxis may be the first clinical manifestation of food hypersensitivity, or symptoms such as urticaria and abdominal pain on previous exposure to the food may antedate full-blown systemic anaphylaxis.[129] Virtually any organ system may be involved, but predominant symptoms include oral and pharyngeal swelling and pruritus, abdominal pain, vomiting, diarrhea, dyspnea, wheezing, urticaria, angioedema, chest pain, hypotension, and shock. Generally, symptoms occur within minutes after ingestion of the culprit food, but they have been reported to occur hours later.[129,130] Exercise may have a profound effect on the clinical expression of food hypersensitivity as manifest by reports of exercise-induced systemic anaphylaxis or urticaria/angioedema following ingestion of food allergens.[131–134]

Oropharyngeal manifestations range from pruritus, tingling, and oral/perioral urticaria to frank edema of the lips, tongue, buccal mucosa, and pharynx, which may rarely cause airway obstruction. These reactions are usually transient and are not necessarily followed by other symptoms.[14,135] Noncongenital fissuring of the lips, tongue, buccal mucosa, and pharynx associated with food ingestion has been described and is believed to be secondary to release of mediators in IgE-mediated hypersensitivity reactions.[6,136]

Gastrointestinal manifestations of immediate hypersensitivity reactions to foods include nausea, vomiting, diarrhea, abdominal pain, distention, and flatus.[6,94,135] Chronic diarrhea, malabsorption, and hypoproteinemia may be due to delayed hypersensitivity reactions to foods such as in the food-protein enteropathies[84–87] and gluten-sensitive enteropathy (see Chapter 24). In addition to the immediate and delayed reactions described above, cow's milk hypersensitivity in infants may cause occult gastrointestinal bleeding or frank colitis with gross gastrointestinal bleeding.[6,137,138]

Nausea, vomiting, cramping, abdominal pain, diarrhea, malabsorption, protein-losing enteropathy, anemia, intermittent gastric and small bowel obstruction, and eosinophilic ascites are potential manifestations of eosinophilic gastroenteritis, which may be due to food hypersensitivity in some cases.[6,88,89]

Immunologically mediated adverse reactions to food are not the cause of symptoms for the vast majority of patients suffering from the irritable bowel syndrome (IBS), but food hypersensitivity might be considered in a small subset of patients with IBS and a strong history of atopy.[139]

There is no convincing evidence that food hypersensitivity plays a primary role in the pathogenesis of inflammatory bowel disease (IBD). The notion that IBD is due to "bystander" damage from the immune response elicited by an external agent (i.e., dietary, viral, or bacterial) is only theoretical, and the finding of circulating antibodies to food antigens in some patients with Crohn's disease and ulcerative colitis may simply represent a response of the immune system to increased penetration of dietary antigens through the damaged mucosal barrier.[129]

Skin manifestations of food hypersensitivity include urticaria/angioedema, atopic dermatitis, and gluten-sensitive dermatitis herpetiformis.

While most cases of urticaria/angioedema are not due to food hypersensitivity,[140] acute urticaria/angioedema due to food hypersensitivity usually does not pose any diagnostic difficulty as patients usually associate such dramatic symptoms with a specific food. Chronic urticaria, on the other hand, frequently presents a difficult diagnostic dilemma, but it is rarely due to allergy.[6,129,141,142]

Atopic dermatitis is frequently caused by food hypersensitivity. In one recent series, approximately 50% of 160 patients referred for evaluation of severe atopic dermatitis were found to have positive double-blind, placebo-controlled food challenges, and removal of the incriminated food(s) was associated with improvement in the course of the atopic dermatitis in patients who complied with the appropriate elimination diet.[94]

Dermatitis herpetiformis is a pruritic, papulovesicular rash that typically appears on the elbows, knees, and buttocks. Gluten sensitivity clearly plays a role in the etiology of this disorder, which may occur without any clinical or histologic evidence for coincident gluten-sensitive enteropathy.[143]

Respiratory manifestations of food hypersensitivity for which there is good evidence include allergic rhinitis, laryngeal edema, and asthma. Asthma due to food allergy is usually associated with other clinical manifestations (i.e., gastrointestinal or skin manifestations).[144-146] The prevalence of food hypersensitivity as a cause of asthma has been reported to range from 4% to 9% among children with asthma, but the data in adults is quite discordant, with a range from 0.5% to 57%.[144] Cross-reaction between food and inhalant antigens appears to be important in the pathogenesis of some cases of asthma caused by food hypersensitivity.[144]

Neuropsychiatric disorders such as the tension-fatigue syndrome, attention deficit disorder, schizophrenia, depression, and a wide range of other neuropsychiatric symptoms have been attributed to food hypersensitivity without any convincing evidence for these claims. There is no well-defined role for food hypersensitivity in the pathogenesis of these disorders.[6,147] An exception is that migraine headaches may be caused by food hypersensitivity in some individuals.[148]

Differential Diagnosis

Symptoms attributed to food allergy are frequently nonspecific, and adverse reactions to food may be due to many other processes that are not immunologically mediated (Table 25-1). Gastrointestinal structural abnormalities, digestive enzyme deficiencies, peptic ulcer disease, cholelithiasis, or pancreatic disease, and infections with bacteria, parasites, or virus may cause vomiting, diarrhea, or abdominal pain that may be attributed to food ingestion. Adverse reactions to contaminants, additives, and pharmacologic agents in food may mimic immunologically mediated reactions to food. Examples include but are not limited to vomiting and diarrhea after ingestion of food contaminated with toxin producing *Staphylococcus aureus; Salmonella* infection after ingestion of improperly handled poultry; headache, nausea, upper body flushing and warmth, numbness over the back of the neck, chest pain or pressure, and wheezing secondary to ingestion of monosodium glutamate[149,150]; bronchospasm, urticaria, vomiting, flushing, hypotension, and shock after ingestion of metabisulfite[151,152]; nausea, vomiting, abdominal cramps, diarrhea, headache, flushing, urticaria, and tingling in the mouth due to large amounts of histamine and other substances produced by contaminating bacteria in improperly handled tuna and other scombroid fish[153,154]; and reactions to a number of vasoactive amines that may be present in foods such as cheeses, chocolate, and red wine.[6]

Symptoms attributed by patients to food allergy may also have a psychogenic basis. Pearson et al.[11] and Rix et al.[155] studied patients presenting to an allergy clinic with a variety of symptoms attributed to foods; only 4 of 23 were confirmed to have adverse reactions to food substances using double-blind food challenges. Each of these four patients presented with classic atopic symptoms. The remaining 19 patients whose symptoms were not confirmed to be secondary to an adverse reaction to food by objective means presented with many different somatic and psychologic symptoms, and all but one of these patients were found to have a psychiatric disorder, most commonly depression, based on a standardized psychiatric interview scoring system and evaluation by a research psychiatrist. Several of the latter patients were able to eat foods previously believed to cause their symptoms after supportive therapy, treatment of depression, or modification of external stress-provoking factors.

Evaluation of the Patient With Suspected Food Allergy

When encountering a patient who reports symptoms that are food-related or suggestive of food hypersensitivity, the physician is challenged to determine whether the patient belongs to the minority, particularly small among adults, with genuine adverse reactions to specific foods. An objective evaluation is necessary in order to: 1) avoid inappropriate dietary restriction and potentially inadequate nutrition in the majority whose symptoms are not due to adverse reactions to specific food(s); and 2) identify and properly treat the small subset who will be found to have adverse reactions to specific foods.

A careful history and physical examination may yield information that will be helpful in distinguishing immunologically mediated reactions to specific foods from nonimmunologically mediated adverse reactions to foods and psychogenic reactions. The nature and severity of symptoms, frequency of symptoms, temporal relationship to ingestion of food, type(s) of food implicated, method of preparation of the implicated food(s), presence of additives or contaminants, and relationship to exercise may provide clues.

While the history and physical examination may provide information that will direct the course of further evaluation, information from other diagnostic procedures is needed to make a diagnosis of food hypersensitivity. These additional diagnostic procedures include: 1) tests for immunologic reactions to food; 2) controlled oral food challenge; and 3) elimination diet.

Tests for Immunologic Reactions to Food

With the exception of jejunal biopsy, which is required for the diagnosis of gluten-sensitive enteropathy and food-protein enteropathy, there are at present no tests of proven clinical utility for food antigen-immune complex or cell-mediated immunologic mechanisms of food hypersensitivity.[156] Food antigen-antibody complexes can be measured, but they are present in normal individuals as well as in those with food hypersensitivity, and their significance is not well understood.[115,157,158] In vitro lymphocyte blastogenesis in the presence of specific food does not distinguish normal individuals from those with presumed food hypersensitivity.[115] Inhibition of leukocyte migration in vitro upon exposure to food antigen has been reported to distinguish controls from: 1) infants and children with adverse reactions to cow's milk; and 2) children with delayed-onset adverse reactions to milk or corn and negative tests for food-antigen-specific IgE.[115,159–161] The assay is presumed to measure release of a lymphokine, leukocyte migration inhibition factor, during cell-mediated food hypersensitivity reactions, but its clinical utility as a possible marker of cell-mediated hypersensitivity reactions to foods remains to be clarified.

While the presence of non-IgE antibodies to food antigens is seen in normal individuals and is not clinically useful, the detection of IgE specific for food antigen is clinically relevant and serves as a useful screening test for IgE-mediated hypersensitivity reactions to food antigens.[13,156] Tests for the detection of specific IgE include in vivo direct skin testing and in vitro assays such as the radioallergosorbent test (RAST), enzyme-linked immunosorbent assay (ELISA), and the leukocyte histamine release assay.

Direct skin testing involves introduction of small amounts of food antigen extracts and control solutions into different areas of the skin of the forearm or back by prick/puncture (the preferred method), scratch, or intradermal injection techniques. The use of adequately standardized food extracts and controls is essential, but when properly performed, these tests are sensitive and economical for detection of specific, cutaneous, mast-cell bound IgE. Details of skin testing techniques are discussed in references 162–167. Generally, food skin tests that produce wheals 3 mm or greater in diameter than the negative control test are considered positive. While direct skin testing is quite sensitive, it is not nearly as specific for clinical IgE-mediated food hypersensitivity as assessed by double-blind, placebo-controlled food challenges.[90,94,168] Thus food extract skin tests for specific, cutaneous, mast-cell bound IgE tend to have high negative predictive accuracies and low positive predictive accuracies for clinical IgE-mediated food hypersensitivity. They are useful to screen patients for the possibility of IgE-mediated reactions to specific food antigens, but a positive skin test does not necessarily correlate with clinically relevant food hypersensitivity and should generally be followed by challenge with the implicated food. Because of the risk of anaphylaxis, direct skin testing should be performed only by an experienced physician and should not be employed when there has been a history of anaphylaxis related to food ingestion. Extensive skin disease may also prevent its use. Under these circumstances, an in vitro test for the detection of food antigen-specific IgE should be performed in lieu of direct skin testing.

RAST and ELISA for the detection of circulating food antigen-specific IgE are similar in vitro tests that employ covalent binding of food extracts to solid-phase supports such as filter paper disks, agarose particles, or plastic microtiter plate wells. Patient serum is incubated with the bound food antigen, washed, and then exposed to a radiolabeled or enzyme-tagged antibody to human IgE.[164] Proper performance of these tests requires close attention to technical details, and they are time-consuming and expensive. RAST is no more sensitive or specific than direct skin testing, and its use in addition to direct skin testing provides no significant improvement in predictive value for clinical hypersensitivity over direct skin test-ing alone.[168] Therefore, while these in vitro tests are useful research tools, they are preferred over direct skin testing for clinical use only when direct skin testing is contraindicated due to a history of food-related anaphylaxis or when there is extensive skin disease.

The leukocyte histamine release assay is an indirect in vitro test for the presence of basophil-bound specific IgE. In this test, peripheral blood leukocytes are iso-lated, suspended in buffer, and incubated with various concentrations of antigen. Histamine content of the supernatant is then measured.[164] High spontaneous his-tamine release from peripheral blood leukocytes (without addition of antigen to the leukocyte suspension) has been reported in children with food hypersensitiv-ity.[94,169] Like other tests for food antigen-specific IgE, release of histamine from leukocytes may be useful as a screening test to select patients who will require further evaluation, but a positive test alone should not be used to make a diagnosis of food hypersensitivity. The clinical use of this test has been limited due to the requirement for freshly isolated peripheral blood leukocytes.

Controlled Oral Food Challenge

The most reliable and unbiased method to evaluate patients for the possibility of adverse reactions to specific food(s) is the double-blind, placebo-controlled oral food challenge. Details of the procedure are described in references 6, 90, 163, 167, and 170. After elimination of the suspected food and other foods commonly asso-ciated with food hypersensitivity for an arbitrary period (usually 1–2 weeks), the suspected food is reintroduced, disguised in a tolerated food or liquid, or crushed and dried in tartrazine-free opaque gelatin capsules. The challenge food is admin-istered beginning with 10–100 mg and increasing the amount until symptoms are produced or a total of 8 grams is ingested. An observer records clinical symptoms and findings. Placebo preparations are also administered, and neither the patient nor the observer know the content of the preparation that is administered. An unequivocal positive reaction such as asthma or hives in a patient who infrequently has such reactions is sufficient evidence for an adverse reaction to the food, provid-ing that placebo challenge is negative. However, if the patient has a history of frequent symptoms or completely subjective complaints, a statistically significant number of positive challenges along with negative placebo challenges is necessary in order to confirm the diagnosis.[12,14] Because natural ingestion of the suspect food is not exactly mimicked in a blinded food challenge, false-negative challenges are possible.[6,12] A positive result does not distinguish between immunologically and nonimmunologically mediated adverse reactions to food.

Because double-blind, placebo-controlled food challenges are lengthy and ex-pensive procedures, unblinded "open" or single-blind food challenges in the physi-cian's office may be used to identify patients who may then be evaluated by the double-blind, placebo-controlled method.

Like direct skin testing, oral food challenge is contraindicated in patients with a history of food-related anaphylaxis.

Elimination Diet

Systematic elimination of different foods along with a food and symptom diary may be useful in the evaluation of some patients suspected as having adverse reactions to food. An extensive discussion of different elimination diets is provided elsewhere.[6] We recommend the following approach. The patient should keep a detailed food and symptom diary for an arbitrary time period such as 2 weeks before elimination of any food or food group. If no particular food or food group is implicated, one is chosen for elimination according to the probability that it will cause an adverse reaction. If symptoms do not abate after an arbitrary time period, usually 1–2 weeks, the eliminated food or food group is then reinstated into the diet, and another food or food group is selected for elimination. Prolonged, extensive elimination diets are to be avoided. If symptoms resolve during a food elimination trial, rechallenge with the implicated food(s) should be performed before long-term elimination is recommended, provided that there is no history of food-related anaphylaxis. An open challenge with objectively verifiable recurrence of symptoms may suffice when only a single food or a few minor foods are implicated, but double-blind, placebo-controlled challenges should be performed if multiple foods are implicated. The need for supervision by a physician upon reintroduction of the implicated food(s) is underscored by a report of anaphylaxis developing in 4 of 80 patients with atopic dermatitis during food challenge following elimination trials.[171]

Unproven, Controversial Tests

A number of tests have been lauded as being useful for the detection of food hypersensitivity without proof of their efficacy. Leukocytotoxic testing is based on the unsubstantiated claim that addition of antigen to whole blood or a serum leukocyte suspension from a food-allergic individual will cause death and disintegration of the leukocytes. Sublingual provocation and neutralization testing involves sublingual administration of diluted food allergen followed by application of a more dilute solution of the same food allergen extract to "neutralize" symptoms if they develop. These and other controversial, unproven techniques have been critiqued by the American Academy of Allergy, and their clinical use is not recommended.[172]

Recommended Diagnostic Approach

While the approach to evaluation of the patient with suspected food hypersensitivity or other adverse reactions to specific foods should be individualized, taking into consideration factors such as the nature and severity of symptoms, frequency of symptoms, age of the patient, and expected compliance with diagnostic testing procedures, a suggested general guideline is shown in Table 25–2.

Treatment of Food Allergy

The definitive treatment for food allergy is avoidance of the culprit food allergen(s). A dietician's assistance is extremely helpful in outlining a diet that eliminates the unwanted food allergen(s) but is still nutritionally sound. When the patient does develop symptoms after food allergen exposure, the treatment for each specific symptom is no different from the usual treatment for that symptom; for example, acute anaphylaxis, asthma, and urticaria are treated just as if they had been caused by a precipitant other than a food allergen.

Antihistamines may be used to treat urticaria/angioedema and rhinitis due to food hypersensitivity. Combination treatment with H_1 and H_2 receptor antagonists has shown promise in the treatment of chronic urticaria, though the effect on

Table 25-2 GENERAL GUIDELINES TO INVESTIGATION OF PATIENTS WITH SUSPECTED FOOD ALLERGY

History of severe reaction or anaphylaxis
1. Avoid implicated food
2. Do not attempt a skin test or a food challenge
3. Use in vitro test (i.e. RAST)

Less severe reactions with specific food(s) implicated by history
1. Skin test (prick/puncture technique with fresh food or commercial extract if available)

If skin test is positive	*If skin test is negative*
2a. Eliminate implicated food(s) temporarily, then perform open challenge	2b. Immediate hypersensitivity is very unlikely, but if the history is impressive, consider temporary elimination of implicated food(s) followed by open challenge.
If open[a] challenge is negative	*If open[a] challenge is negative*
3a. No food restriction, observe, and repeat challenge if symptoms recur	3b. Same as in 3a
If open challenge is positive	*If open challenge is positive*
4a. Eliminate implicated food, but perform double-blind placebo-controlled oral food challenge if several foods of nutritional importance are involved or if the symptoms elicited by open challenge are not objectively verifiable	4b. Perform double-blind, placebo-controlled oral food challenge

Food allergy claimed but no specific foods or multiple foods are implicated
1. Reassess full clinical picture and consider nonimmunologic causes for symptoms (Table 25-1)
2. If history is impressive, perform skin tests for commonly encountered foods and instruct patient to keep a food diary
3. Temporary elimination diet if specific food(s) are implicated by skin tests or diary, then proceed as in 2a above
4. If specific food(s) are still not implicated and symptoms persist, consider systematic, temporary elimination diets
5. If specific food(s) are implicated by systematic elimination diets, proceed as in 2a above
6. If symptoms persist and specific food(s) are not implicated after systematic elimination diets, consider once again nonimmunologic causes including a psychogenic origin

[a] Depending on the nature of the food and the ease with which it can be camouflaged in other food preparations, a single blind challenge may be performed in preference to open challenge.

urticaria due to food hypersensitivity specifically was not studied.[173] The use of H_1 and H_2 receptor antagonists for prophylaxis and treatment of gastrointestinal food hypersensitivity reactions has been recommended by some experts, but there has been no proof that they are efficacious for these symptoms.[6,174]

Corticosteroids are indicated for the treatment of eosinophilic gastroenteritis, which may be caused by food hypersensitivity in some cases.[6,88,89,174] These drugs have also been generally accepted for short-term use in the treatment of severe allergic gastroenteropathies.[6,174]

Epinephrine is used in the treatment of systemic anaphylaxis secondary to any precipitating agent including food hypersensitivity. When the food allergen is a common ingredient that may be hidden in prepared foods, the patient should carry epinephrine and be instructed in its use.

There is conflicting information in the medical literature regarding the efficacy of cromolyn sodium in the treatment of food hypersensitivity. Many studies have been published, but some of them used patients without clear documentation of food hypersensitivity by the double-blind, placebo-controlled method, and some studies were not adequately designed for proper evaluation of the drug.[174] A recent study of children with atopic dermatitis and egg hypersensitivity, using double-blind, placebo-controlled oral food challenges and positive prick skin tests to egg for documentation of egg hypersensitivity, showed no benefit of cromolyn sodium in a double-blind, placebo-controlled crossover trial.[175]

Ketotifen, a relatively new investigational drug that exhibits antihistaminic and antianaphylactic properties, has been used in a few studies attempting to assess its efficacy in the treatment of food hypersensitivity. These largely uncontrolled or small studies have had conflicting results, and well-designed double-blind, placebo-controlled trials are needed to resolve the question.[174,176-178]

Techniques of immunotherapy such as administration of incremental amounts of antigen subcutaneously or orally, subcutaneous neutralization, and sublingual neutralization have no proven efficacy in the treatment of food hypersensitivity, and any such therapy should be limited to use in well-designed clinical research studies.[6,172]

Fortunately, a significant number of children with food hypersensitivity may become tolerant to the offending food over a period of years, perhaps depending in part on the particular food allergen,[94,179-181] though the longer a food allergy exists, the less likely it is to resolve.[181] Thus, life-long elimination of the culprit food allergen may not be necessary in some young children with food hypersensitivity.

Prevention of Food Allergy

Prevention is the ultimate therapy for any disease. For food hypersensitivity, preventive measures would avoid sensitization to food allergens.

Since a 1936 report of a sevenfold increase in the incidence of eczema in cow's milk-fed compared with breast-fed 9-month-old infants,[182] many prospective infant feeding studies have attempted to assess for the effect of breast feeding and dietary manipulation on the prevention of food allergy. While these studies have many inherent problems such as lack of randomization to breast-fed versus control groups creating potential bias in subject recruitment, lack of blinding, difficulty in documenting compliance, differences in the timing of introduction of solid foods, and in some cases a brief duration of breast feeding, they do suggest that prolonged breast feeding (until 4–6 months of age) and late introduction of solid foods reduces allergic disease.[176,183] Although studies performed in Finland suggest that breast feeding until 6 months of age prevents the development of food allergy in the first year of life, elimination of potential dietary allergens in the first year of life may only postpone and not prevent the development of food allergy.[184,185]

Food allergens may cross the placenta and cause specific IgE sensitization in the prenatal period, though this is an infrequent event.[183,186,187] Food substances consumed by the mother are also transmitted in maternal breast milk and may precipitate sensitization in the breast-fed infant.[44,94,176,183,188-190] Recent information suggests that avoidance of major food allergens by the mother during the second and third trimester of pregnancy and breast feeding may be of more benefit than breast feeding alone in the prevention of food hypersensitivity.[94]

While the role of dietary manipulation for prevention of food allergy in infants has not been completely elucidated, current knowledge would support a recommendation for breast feeding without solid food introduction until 4–6 months of age whenever feasible, particularly when the infant is predisposed to atopic disease (family history or elevated cord IgE). In addition, perhaps the ingestion of major food allergens (i.e., peanuts, fish, eggs, milk) should be limited by mothers of infants at risk for the development of atopy, but this should not be at the expense of proper nutrition.

CONCLUSIONS

Food allergy is a relatively uncommon but definite clinical entity that has been shrouded in confusion and controversy in the past. A number of factors have contributed to the confusion and controversy including failure of some authors to use appropriate terminology and lack of a widely adopted scientific approach to investigation of the problem. In addition, the popular press and some self-proclaimed experts have succeeded in blowing the problem out of proportion, leading to public paranoia and lack of faith in the medical profession's ability to properly diagnose and treat food allergic disease.

Fortunately, a large body of scientifically sound knowledge concerning food allergy has evolved. If we adhere to the appropriate use of a standard terminology and follow an objective and unbiased approach to the evaluation of patients with complaints of adverse reactions to foods, confusion and controversy need no longer cloud the subject of food allergy.[191] Education of the public and efforts to counter unorthodox, scientifically unsubstantiated claims with scientifically sound knowledge should bring the problem back into proper perspective and restore public faith in the ability of the medical profession to deal with the problem.

Though a large body of knowledge regarding food allergy has evolved, much more needs to be learned about the mechanisms involved in modulation of the immune response to dietary antigens and pathogenesis of hypersensitivity reactions to foods, particularly the delayed hypersensitivity reactions. Further research will provide information that will allow us to become more sophisticated in the diagnosis, treatment, and prevention of food allergy.

REFERENCES

1. Bahna SL, Heiner DC: Cow's milk allergy: pathogenesis, manifestations, diagnosis, and management. *Adv Pediatr* 25:1–37, 1978.
2. Prausnitz P, Küstner H: Studien über die VeberempFindlichkeit. *Z Bakt Orig* 86:160–168, 1921.

3. Brunner M, Walzer M: Absorption of undigested proteins in human beings. The absorption of unaltered fish proteins in adults. *Arch Intern Med* 42:172–179, 1928.

4. Berger SM: Mean cuisine: how friendly foods become secret foes. *Mademoiselle* 91(6):170, 1985.

5. Sloan AE, Powers ME: A perspective on popular perceptions of adverse reactions to foods. *J Allergy Clin Immunol* 78:127–133, 1986.

6. Anderson JA, Sogn DD (eds): Adverse reactions to foods. American Academy of Allergy and Immunology Committee on Adverse Reactions to Foods. Bethesda, MD, National Institute of Allergy and Infectious Diseases, National Institutes of Health, NIH Publication No. 84-2442, 1984.

7. Burr ML, Merrett TG: Food intolerance: a community survey. *Br J Nutr* 49:217–219, 1983.

8. Bender AE, Matthews DR: Adverse reactions to foods. *Br J Nutr* 46:403–407, 1981.

9. Bock SA, Martin MM: The incidence of adverse reactions to foods—a continuing study [Abstract]. *J Allergy Clin Immunol* 71:98, 1983.

10. May CD: Food allergy—material and ethereal. *N Engl J Med* 302:1142–1143, 1980.

11. Pearson DJ, Rix KJB, Bentley SJ: Food allergy: how much in the mind? A clinical and psychiatric study of suspected food hypersensitivity. *Lancet* 1:1259–1261, 1983.

12. Metcalfe DD: Food hypersensitivity. *J Allergy Clin Immunol* 73:749–762, 1984.

13. Johansson SGO, Dannaeus A, Lilja G: The relevance of anti-food antibodies for the diagnosis of food allergy. *Ann Allergy* 53:665–670, 1984.

14. Sampson HA, Buckley RH, Metcalfe DD: Food allergy. *JAMA* 258:2886–2890, 1987.

15. Bienenstock J, Befus AD: Mucosal immunology. *Immunology* 41:249–270, 1980.

16. Bienenstock J: The mucosal immunologic network. *Ann Allergy* 53:535–539, 1984.

17. Walker WA: Pathophysiology of intestinal uptake and absorption of antigens in food allergy. *Ann Allergy* 59 (5 Part II):7–16, 1987.

18. Kleinmann RE, Harmatz PR, Walker WA: The gastrointestinal immune barrier: its role in preventing antigen penetration of the intestine. In Shorter RG, Krisner JB: Gastrointestinal Immunity for the Clinician. Orlando, Grune & Stratton, 1985, p 23.

19. Kleinmann RE, Walker WA: Antigen processing and uptake from the intestinal tract. *Clin Rev Allergy* 2:25–37, 1984.

20. Walker WA: Mechanisms of antigen handling by the gut. *Clin Immunol Allergy* 2:15–40, 1982.

21. McNabb PC, Tomasi TB: Host defense mechanisms at mucosal surfaces. *Annu Rev Microbiol* 35:477–496, 1981.

22. Atkins FA, Metcalfe DD: The diagnosis and treatment of food allergy. *Annu Rev Nutr* 4:233–255, 1984.

23. Kraft SC, Rothberg RM, Knauer CM, et al: Gastric acid output and circulating anti-bovine serum albumin in adults. *Clin Exp Immunol* 2:321–330, 1967.

24. Brandtzaeg P, Bjerke K, Kett K, et al: Production and secretion of immunoglobulins in the gastrointestinal tract. *Ann Allergy* 59(5 Part II):21–39, 1987.

25. Bienenstock J, Befus AD: Some thoughts on the biologic role of immunoglobulin A. *Gastroenterology* 84:178–185, 1983.

26. Bienenstock J: Cellular and secretory aspects of the gastrointestinal tract. *Clin Immunol Allergy* 2:5–14, 1982.

27. Walker WA, Isselbacher KJ, Bloch KJ: Intestinal uptake of macromolecules: effect of oral immunization. *Science* 177:608–610, 1972.

28. Cunningham-Rundles C, Brandeis WE, Good RA, et al: Milk precipitins, circulating immune complexes, and IgA deficiency. *Proc Natl Acad Sci USA* 75:3387–3389, 1978.

29. Buckley RH, Dees SC: Correlation of milk precipitins with IgA deficiency. *N Engl J Med* 281:465–469, 1969.

30. Huntley CC, Robbins JB, Lyerly AD, et al: Characterization of precipitating antibodies to ruminant serum and milk proteins in humans with selective IgA deficiency. *N Engl J Med* 284:7–10, 1971.

31. Ammann AJ, Hong R: Selective IgA deficiency: presentation of 30 cases and a review of the literature. *Medicine* 50:223–236, 1971.

32. Triger DR: The liver as an immunologic organ. *Gastroenterology* 71:162–168, 1976.

33. McNeish AS: Enzymatic maturation of the gastrointestinal tract and its relevance to food allergy and intolerance in infancy. *Ann Allergy* 53:643–648, 1984.

34. Antonowicz I, Lebenthal E: Developmental pattern of small intestinal enterokinase and disaccharidase activities in the human fetus. *Gastroenterology* 72:1299–1303, 1977.

35. Selner JC, Merrill MA, Claman HN: Salivary immunoglobulin and albumin: development during the newborn period. *J Pediatr* 72:685–689, 1968.

36. Haneberg B, Aarskog D: Human faecal immunoglobulins in healthy infants and children, and in some with diseases affecting the intestinal tract or the immune system. *Clin Exp Immunol* 22:210–222, 1975.

37. Roberton DM, Paganelli R, Dinwiddie R, et al: Milk antigen absorption in the preterm and term neonate. *Arch Dis Child* 57:369–372, 1982.

38. Eastham EJ, Lichauco T, Grady MI, et al: Antigenicity of infant formulas: role of immature intestine on protein permeability. *J Pediatr* 93:561–564, 1978.

39. Udall JN, Colony P, Fritze L, et al: Development of gastrointestinal mucosal barrier. II. The effect of natural versus artificial feeding on intestinal permeability to macromolecules. *Pediatr Res* 15:245–249, 1981.

40. Sheard NF, Walker WA: The role of breast milk in the development of the gastrointestinal tract. *Nutr Rev* 46:1–8, 1988.

41. Weaver LT, Walker WA: Epidermal growth factor and the developing human gut. *Gastroenterology* 94:845–847, 1988.

42. Ratner B, Gruehl HL: Passage of native proteins through the normal gastro-intestinal wall. *J Clin Invest* 13:517–532, 1934.

43. Wilson SJ, Walzer M: Absorption of undigested proteins in human beings. IV. Absorption of unaltered egg protein in infants and in children. *Am J Dis Child* 50:49–54, 1935.

44. Hemmings WA: First experience of dietary antigen. *Lancet* 1:818, 1980.

45. Paganelli R, Levinsky RJ: Solid phase radioimmunoassay for detection of circulating food protein antigens in human serum. *J Immunol Methods* 37:333–341, 1980.

46. Husby S, Jensenius JC, Svehag S-E: Passage of undegraded dietary antigen into the blood of healthy adults. Quantification, estimation of size distribution, and relation of uptake to levels of specific antibodies. *Scand J Immunol* 22:83–92, 1985.

47. Owen RL: Sequential uptake of horseradish peroxidase by lymphoid follicle epithelium of Peyer's patches in the normal unobstructed mouse intestine: an ultrastructural study. *Gastroenterology* 72:440–451, 1977.

48. Bland PW, Warren LG: Antigen presentation by epithelial cells of the rat small intestine. I. Kinetics, antigen specificity and blocking by anti-Ia antisera. *Immunology* 58:1–7, 1986.

49. Mayer L, Shlien R: Evidence for function of Ia molecules on gut epithelial cells in man. *J Exp Med* 166:1471–1483, 1987.

50. Bland P: MHC class II expression by the gut epithelium. *Immunol Today* 9:174–178, 1988.

51. Mowat AM: The regulation of immune responses to dietary protein antigens. *Immunol Today* 8:93–98, 1987.

52. Dakin R: Remarks on a cutaneous affection, produced by certain poisonous vegetables. *Am J Med Sci* 4:98–100, 1829.

53. Richman LK, Chiller JM, Brown WR, et al: Enterically induced immunologic tolerance. I. Induction of suppressor T lymphocytes by intragastric administration of soluble proteins. *J Immunol* 121:2429–2434, 1978.

54. Wells HG, Osborne TB: The biological reactions of the vegetable proteins. I. Anaphylaxis. *J Infect Dis* 8:66–124, 1911.

55. Wells HG: Studies on the chemistry of anaphylaxis. III. Experiments with isolated proteins, especially those of the hen's egg. *J Infect Dis* 9:147–171, 1911.

56. Chase MW: Inhibition of experimental drug allergy by prior feeding of the sensitizing agent. *Proc Soc Exp Biol Med* 61:257–259, 1946.

57. Hanson DG, Vaz NM, Rawlings LA, et al: Inhibition of specific immune responses by feeding protein antigens. II. Effects of prior passive and active immunization. *J Immunol* 122:2261–2266, 1979.

58. Miller SD, Hanson DG: Inhibition of specific immune responses by feeding protein antigens. IV. Evidence for tolerance and specific active suppression of cell-mediated immune responses to ovalbumin. *J Immunol* 123:2344–2350, 1979.

59. Thomas HC, Parrott DMV: The induction of tolerance to a soluble protein antigen by oral administration. *Immunology* 27:631–639, 1974.

60. Asherson GL, Zembala M, Perera MACC, et al: Production of immunity and unresponsiveness in the mouse by feeding contact sensitizing agents and the role of suppressor cells in the Peyer's patches, mesenteric lymph nodes, and other lymphoid tissues. *Cell Immunol* 33:145–155, 1977.

61. Asherson GL, Perera MACC, Thomas WR: Contact sensitivity and the DNA response in mice to high and low doses of oxazolone: low dose unresponsiveness following painting and feeding and its prevention by pretreatment with cyclophosphamide. *Immunology* 36:449–459, 1979.

62. Newby TJ, Stokes CR, Bourne FJ: Effects of feeding bacterial lipopolysaccharide and dextran sulphate on the development of oral tolerance to contact sensitizing agents. *Immunology* 41:617–621, 1980.

63. Gautam SC, Battistio JR: Orally induced tolerance generates an efferently acting suppressor T cell and an acceptor T cell that together down-regulate contact sensitivity. *J Immunol* 135:2975–2983, 1985.

64. Mattingly JA, Waksman BH: Immunologic suppression after oral administration of antigen. I. Specific suppressor cells formed in rat Peyer's patches after oral administration of sheep erythrocytes and their systemic migration. *J Immunol* 121:1878–1883, 1978.

65. Kagnoff MF: Effects of antigen-feeding on intestinal and systemic immune responses. II. Suppression of delayed-type hypersensitivity reactions. *J Immunol* 120:1509–1513, 1978.

66. Kagnoff MF: Effects of antigen-feeding on intestinal and systemic immune responses. III. Antigen-specific serum-mediated suppression of humoral antibody responses after antigen feeding. *Cell Immunol* 40:186–203, 1978.

67. Kagnoff MF: Effects of antigen-feeding on intestinal and systemic immune responses. IV. Similarity between the suppressor factor in mice after erythrocyte-lysate injection and erythrocyte feeding. *Gastroenterology* 79:54–61, 1980.

68. Kiyono H, McGhee JR, Wannemuehler MJ, et al: Lack of oral tolerance in C3H/HeJ mice. *J Exp Med* 155:605–610, 1982.

69. MacDonald TT: Immunosuppression caused by antigen feeding. II. Suppressor T cells mask Peyer's patch B cell priming to orally administered antigen. *Eur J Immunol* 13:138–142, 1983.

70. Stokes CR, Newby TJ, Huntley JH, et al: The immune response of mice to bacterial antigens given by mouth. *Immunology* 38:497–502, 1979.

71. Rubin D, Weiner HL, Fields BN, et al: Immunologic tolerance after oral administration of reovirus: requirement for two viral gene products for tolerance induction. *J Immunol* 127:1697–1701, 1981.

72. Titus RG, Chiller JM: Orally induced tolerance. Definition at the cellular level. *Int Arch Allergy Appl Immunol* 65:323–338, 1981.

73. Challacombe SJ, Tomasi TB: Systemic tolerance and secretory immunity after oral immunization. *J Exp Med* 152:1459–1472, 1980.

74. Klein JR, Kagnoff MF: Nonspecific recruitment of cytotoxic effector cells in the intestinal mucosa of antigen-primed mice. *J Exp Med* 160:1931–1936, 1984.

75. Ngan J, Kind LS: Suppressor T cells for IgE and IgG in Peyer's patches of mice made tolerant by the oral administration of ovalbumin. *J Immunol* 120:861–865, 1978.

76. Mowat AM, Thomas MJ, MacKenzie S, et al: Divergent effects of bacterial lipopolysaccharide on immunity to orally administered protein and particulate antigens in mice. *Immunology* 58:677–683, 1986.

77. Mowat AM, Strobel S, Drummond HE, et al: Immunological responses to fed protein antigens in mice. I. Reversal of oral tolerance to ovalbumin by cyclophosphamide. *Immunology* 45:105–113, 1982.

78. Mowat AM: Depletion of suppressor T cells by 2'-deoxyguanosine abrogates tolerance in mice fed ovalbumin and permits the induction of intestinal delayed-type hypersensitivity. *Immunology* 58:179–184, 1986.

79. Bland PW, Warren LG: Antigen presentation by epithelial cells of the rat small intestine. II. Selective induction of suppressor T cells. *Immunology* 58:9–14, 1986.

80. Cantor HM, Dumont AE: Hepatic suppression of sensitization to antigen absorbed into the portal system. *Nature* 215:744–745, 1967.

81. Battisto JR, Miller J: Immunological unresponsiveness produced in adult guinea pigs by parenteral introduction of minute quantities of hapten or protein antigen. *Proc Soc Exp Biol Med* 111:111–115, 1962.

82. Qian JH, Hashimoto T, Fujiwara H, et al: Studies on the induction of tolerance to alloantigens. I. The abrogation of potentials for delayed-type-hypersensitivity responses to alloantigens by portal venous inoculation with allogeneic cells. *J Immunol* 134:3656–3661, 1985.

83. Triger DR, Cynamon MH, Wright R: Studies on hepatic uptake of antigen. I. Comparison of inferior vena cava and portal vein routes of immunization. *Immunology* 25:941–950, 1973.

84. Kuitunen P, Visakorpi JK, Savilahti E, et al: Malabsorption syndrome with cow's milk intolerance. Clinical findings and course in 54 cases. *Arch Dis Child* 50:351–356, 1975.

85. Vitoria JC, Camarero C, Sojo A, et al: Enteropathy related to fish, rice, and chicken. *Arch Dis Child* 57:44–48, 1982.

86. Iyngkaran N, Abidin Z, Meng LL, et al: Egg-protein-induced villous atrophy. *J Pediatr Gastroenterol Nutr* 1:29–33, 1982.

87. Van Sickle GJ, Powell GK, McDonald PJ, et al: Milk- and soy protein-induced enterocolitis: evidence for lymphocyte sensitization to specific food proteins. *Gastroenterology* 88:1915–1921, 1985.

88. Cello JP: Eosinophilic gastroenteritis — a complex disease entity. *Am J Med* 67:1097–1104, 1979.

89. Kulczycki A, MacDermott RP: Adverse reactions to food and eosinophilic gastroenteritis. In Shorter RG, Kirsner JB (eds): Gastrointestinal Immunity for the Clinician. Orlando, Grune & Stratton, 1985, p 131.

90. Bock SA, Lee WY, Remigo KL, et al: Studies of hypersensitivity reactions to foods in infants and children. *J Allergy Clin Immunol* 62:327–334, 1978.

91. Gray I, Harten M, Walzer M: Studies in mucous membrane hypersensitiveness. IV. The allergic reaction in the passively sensitized mucous membranes of the ileum and colon in humans. *Ann Intern Med* 13:2050–2056, 1940.

92. Selbekk BH, Aas K, Myren J: In vitro sensitization and mast cell degranulation in human jejunal mucosa. *Scand J Gastroenterol* 13:87–92, 1978.

93. Sampson HA, Jolie PL: Increased plasma histamine concentration after food challenges in children with atopic dermatitis. *N Engl J Med* 311:372–376, 1984.

94. Sampson HA: IgE-mediated food intolerance. *J Allergy Clin Immunol* 81:495–504, 1988.

95. Sampson HA: The role of food allergy and mediator release in atopic dermatitis. *J Allergy Clin Immunol* 81:635–645, 1988.

96. Lemanske RF, Atkins FM, Metcalfe DD: Gastrointestinal mast cells in health and disease. Part 1. *J Pediatr* 103:177–184, 1983.

97. Enerback L: The gut mucosal mast cell. *Monogr Allergy* 17:222–232, 1981.

98. Bienenstock J, Befus AD, Pearce F, et al: Mast cell heterogeneity: derivation and function, with emphasis on the intestine. *J Allergy Clin Immunol* 70:407–412, 1982.

99. Shanahan F, Denburg JA, Bienenstock J, et al: Mast cell heterogeneity. *Can J Physiol Pharmacol* 62:734–737, 1984.

100. Atkins FM: Intestinal mucosal mast cells. *Ann Allergy* 59(5 Part II):44–53, 1987.

101. Befus D, Goodacre R, Dyck N, et al: Mast cell heterogeneity in man. I. Histologic studies of the intestine. *Int Arch Allergy Appl Immunol* 76:232–236, 1985.

102. Irani AA, Schechter NM, Craig SS, et al: Two types of human mast cells that have distinct neutral protease compositions. *Proc Natl Acad Sci USA* 83:4464–4468, 1986.

103. Schwartz LB: Mediators of human mast cells and human mast cell subsets. *Ann Allergy* 58:226–235, 1987.

104. Enerbäck L: Mucosal mast cells in the rat and in man. *Int Arch Allergy Appl Immun* 82:249–255, 1987.

105. Schwartz LB, Bradford TR, Irani AM, et al: The major enzymes of human mast cell secretory granules. *Am Rev Respir Dis* 135:1186–1189, 1987.

106. Barrett KE, Metcalfe DD: Heterogeneity of mast cells in the tissues of the respiratory tract and other organ systems. *Am Rev Respir Dis* 135:1190–1195, 1987.

107. Lowman MA, Rees PH, Benyon RC, et al: Human mast cell heterogeneity: histamine release from mast cells dispersed from skin, lung, adenoids, tonsils, and colon in response to IgE-dependent and nonimmunologic stimuli. *J Allergy Clin Immunol* 81:590–597, 1988.

108. Barrett KE, Metcalfe DD: The mucosal mast cell and its role in gastrointestinal allergic diseases. *Clin Rev Allergy* 2:39–53, 1984.

109. Scott RB, Diamant SC, Gall DG: Motility effects of intestinal anaphylaxis in the rat. *Am J Physiol* 255:G505–G511, 1988.

110. Patrick MK, Dunn IJ, Buret A, et al: Mast cell protease release and mucosal ultrastructure during intestinal anaphylaxis in the rat. *Gastroenterology* 94:1–9, 1988.

111. Perdue MH, Chung M, Gall DG: Effect of intestinal anaphylaxis on gut function in the rat. *Gastroenterology* 86:391–397, 1984.

112. Perdue MH, Forstner JF, Roomi NW, et al: Epithelial response to intestinal anaphy-

laxis in rats: goblet cell secretion and enterocyte damage. *Am J Physiol* 247:G632–G637, 1984.

113. Perdue MH, Gall DG: Intestinal anaphylaxis in the rat: jejunal response to in vitro antigen exposure. *Am J Physiol* G427–G431, 1986.

114. Byars NE, Ferraresi RW: Intestinal anaphylaxis in the rat as a model of food allergy. *Clin Exp Immunol* 24:352–356, 1976.

115. Kniker WT: Immunologically mediated reactions to food: state of the art. *Ann Allergy* 59(5 Part II):60–70, 1987.

116. Peters SP, Schleimer RP, Naclerio RM, et al: The pathophysiology of human mast cells: *in vitro* and *in vivo* function. *Am Rev Respir Dis* 135:1196–1200, 1987.

117. Wasserman SI: Mediators of immediate hypersensitivity. *J Allergy Clin Immunol* 72:101–115, 1983.

118. Serafin WE, Austen KF: Mediators of immediate hypersensitivity reactions. *N Engl J Med* 317:30–34, 1987.

119. Gleich GJ: The late phase of the immunoglobulin E-mediated reaction: a link between anaphylaxis and common allergic disease? *J Allergy Clin Immunol* 70:160–169, 1982.

120. Leiferman KM, Ackerman SJ, Sampson HA, et al: Dermal deposition of eosinophil-granule major basic protein in atopic dermatitis. *N Engl J Med* 313:282–285, 1985.

121. Lessof MH, Wraith DG, Merrett TG, et al: Food allergy and intolerance in 100 patients — local and systemic effects. *Q J Med* 195:259–271, 1980.

122. Elsayed S, Bennich H: The primary structure of allergen M from cod. *Scand J Immunol* 4:203–208, 1975.

123. Hoffman DR, Day ED, Miller JS: The major heat stable allergen of shrimp. *Ann Allergy* 47:17–22, 1981.

124. Sachs MI, Jones RT, Yunginger JW: Isolation and partial characterization of a major peanut allergen. *J Allergy Clin Immunol* 67:27–34, 1981.

125. Moroz LA, Yang WH: Kunitz soybean trypsin inhibitor. A specific allergen in food anaphylaxis. *N Engl J Med* 302:1126–1128, 1980.

126. Goldman AS, Anderson DW, Sellers WA, et al: Milk allergy. I. Oral challenge with milk and isolated milk proteins in allergic children. *Pediatrics* 32:425–443, 1963.

127. Taylor SL, Lemanske RF, Bush RK, et al: Food allergens: structure and immunologic properties. *Ann Allergy* 59(5 Part II):93–99, 1987.

128. Stricker WE, Anorve-Lopez E, Reed CE: Food skin testing in patients with idiopathic anaphylaxis. *J Allergy Clin Immunol* 77:516–519, 1986.

129. Metcalfe DD, Samter M, Condemi JJ: Reactions to foods. In Samter M, Talmage DW, Frank MM, Austen KF, Claman HN (eds): Immunological Diseases, ed. 4. Boston, Little, Brown, 1988, p 1149.

130. Golbert TM, Patterson R, Pruzansky JJ: Systemic allergic reactions to ingested antigens. *J Allergy* 44:96–107, 1969.

131. Maulitz RM, Pratt DS, Schocket AL: Exercise-induced anaphylactic reaction to shellfish. *J Allergy Clin Immunol* 63:433–434, 1979.

132. Buchbinder EM, Bloch KJ, Moss J, et al: Food-dependent, exercise-induced anaphylaxis. *JAMA* 250:2973–2974, 1983.

133. Kidd JM, Cohen SH, Sosman AJ, et al: Food-dependent exercise-induced anaphylaxis. *J Allergy Clin Immunol* 71:407–411, 1983.

134. Kushimoto H, Toshiyuki A: Masked type I wheat allergy. Relation to exercise-induced anaphylaxis. *Arch Dermatol* 121:355–360, 1985.

135. Hutchins P, Walker-Smith JA: The gastrointestinal system. *Clin Immunol Allergy* 2:43–76, 1982.

136. Anderson JA, Jackson CE, Krull EA, et al: Hypersensitive furrowed mouth. *Clin Proc Child Hosp Natl Med Center* 36:269–286, 1980.

137. Bahna SL: Milk allergy in infancy. *Ann Allergy* 59(5 Part II):131–136, 1987.

138. Hill DJ, Ford RPK, Shelton MJ, et al: A study of 100 infants and young children with cow's milk allergy. *Clin Rev Allergy* 2:125–142, 1984.

139. Zwetchkenbaum JF, Burakoff R: Food allergy and the irritable bowel syndrome. *Am J Gastroenterol* 83:901–904, 1988.

140. Champion RH, Roberts SOB, Carpenter RG, et al: Urticaria and angio-oedema. A review of 554 patients. *Br J Dermatol* 81:588–597, 1969.

141. Sampson HA: Immunologically mediated adverse reactions to foods: role of T cells and cutaneous reactions. *Ann Allergy* 53:472–475, 1984.

142. Green GR, Koelsche GA, Kierland RR: Etiology and pathogenesis of chronic urticaria. *Ann Allergy* 23:30–36, 1965.

143. Leonard J, Haffenden G, Tucker W, et al: Gluten challenge in dermatitis herpeti-formis. *N Engl J Med* 308:816–819, 1983.

144. Novembre E, Martino M, Vierucci A: Foods and respiratory allergy. *J Allergy Clin Immunol* 81:1059–1065, 1988.

145. Atkins FM, Steinberg SS, Metcalfe DD: Evaluation of immediate adverse reactions to foods in adult patients. I. Correlation of demographic, laboratory, and prick skin test data with response to controlled oral food challenge. *J Allergy Clin Immunol* 75:348–355, 1985.

146. Wraith DG: Asthma and rhinitis. *Clin Immunol Allergy* 2:101–112, 1982.

147. Pearson DJ, Rix KJB: Allergomimetric reactions to food and pseudofood-allergy. In Dukor P, Kallós P, Schlumberger HD, et al (eds): Pseudo-Allergic Reactions. Involvement of Drugs and Chemicals, vol. 4. Basel, Karger, 1985, p 59.

148. Mansfield LE, Vaughan TR, Waller SF, et al: Food allergy and adult migraine: double-blind and mediator confirmation of an allergic etiology. *Ann Allergy* 55:126–129, 1985.

149. Allen DH, Baker GJ: Chinese-restaurant asthma. *N Engl J Med* 305:1154–1155, 1981.

150. Kwok RHM: Chinese-restaurant syndrome. *N Engl J Med* 278:796, 1968.

151. Stevenson DD, Simon RA: Sensitivity to ingested metabisulfites in asthmatic subjects. *J Allergy Clin Immunol* 68:26–32, 1981.

152. Schwartz HJ: Sensitivity to ingested metabisulfite: variations in clinical presentation. *J Allergy Clin Immunol* 71:487–489, 1983.

153. Merson MH, Baine WB, Gangarosa EJ, et al: Scombroid fish poisoning. Outbreak traced to commercially canned tuna fish. *JAMA* 228:1268–1269, 1974.

154. Taylor SL, Guthertz LS, Leatherwood M, et al: Histamine production by *Klebsiella pneumoniae* and an incident of scombroid fish poisoning. *Appl Environ Microbiol* 37:274–278, 1979.

155. Rix KJB, Pearson DJ, Bentley SJ: A psychiatric study of patients with supposed food allergy. *Br J Psychiatry* 145:121–126, 1984.

156. Björkstén B: New diagnostic methods in food allergy. *Ann Allergy* 59(5 Part II):150–152, 1987.

157. Paganelli R, Quinti I, D'Offizi GP, et al: Immune complexes in food allergy: a critical reappraisal. *Ann Allergy* 59(5 Part II):157–161, 1987.

158. Paganelli R, Matricardi PM, Aiuti F: Interactions of food antigens, antibodies, and antigen-antibody complexes in health and disease. *Clin Rev Allergy* 2:69–78, 1984.

159. Khoshoo V, Bhan MK, Arora NK, et al: Leukocyte migration inhibition in cow's milk protein intolerance. *Acta Pediatr Scand* 75:308–312, 1986.

160. Ashkenazi A, Levin S, Idar D, et al: In vitro cell-mediated immunologic assay for cow's milk allergy. *Pediatrics* 66:399–402, 1980.

161. Minor JD, Tolber SG, Frick OL: Leukocyte inhibition factor in delayed-onset food allergy. *J Allergy Clin Immunol* 66:314–321, 1980.

162. Bernstein LI: Proceedings of the task force on guidelines for standardizing old and new technologies used for the diagnosis and treatment of allergic diseases. *J Allergy Clin Immunol* 82:487–526, 1988.

163. Bock SA, Sampson HA, Atkins FM, et al: Double-blind, placebo-controlled food challenge (DBPCFC) as an office procedure: a manual. *J Allergy Clin Immunol* 82:986–997, 1988.

164. Yunginger JW: Proper application of available laboratory tests for adverse reactions to foods and food additives. *J Allergy Clin Immunol* 78:220–223, 1986.

165. Bock SA, Buckley J, Holst A, et al: Proper use of skin tests with food extracts in diagnosis of hypersensitivity to food in children. *Clin Allergy* 7:375–383, 1977.

166. May CD, Bock SA: A modern clinical approach to food hypersensitivity. *Allergy* 33:166–188, 1978.

167. Bock SA: Food sensitivity. A critical review and practical approach. *Am J Dis Child* 134:973–982, 1980.

168. Sampson HA, Albergo R: Comparison of results of skin tests, RAST, and double-blind, placebo-controlled food challenges in children with atopic dermatitis. *J Allergy Clin Immunol* 74:26–33, 1984.

169. May CD, Remigo L: Observations on high spontaneous release of histamine from leucocytes in vitro. *Clin Allergy* 12:229–241, 1982.

170. May CD: Objective clinical and laboratory studies of immediate hypersensitivity reactions to foods in asthmatic children. *J Allergy Clin Immunol* 58:500–515, 1976.

171. David TJ: Anaphylactic shock during elimination diets for severe atopic eczema. *Arch Dis Child* 59:983–986, 1984.

172. Reisman RE: American Academy of Allergy: Position statements — controversial techniques. *J Allergy Clin Immunol* 67:333–338, 1981.

173. Phanuphak P, Schocket A, Kohler PF: Treatment of chronic idiopathic urticaria with combined H_1 and H_2 blockers. *Clin Allergy* 8:429–433, 1978.

174. Sogn D: Medications and their use in the treatment of adverse reactions to foods. *J Allergy Clin Immunol* 78:238–243, 1986.

175. Burks WA, Sampson HA: Double-blind placebo-controlled trial of oral cromolyn in children with atopic dermatitis and documented food hypersensitivity. *J Allergy Clin Immunol* 81:417–423, 1988.

176. Kjellman N-IM: Food allergy-treatment and prevention. *Ann Allergy* 59(5 Part II):168–174, 1987.

177. Molkhou P, Dupont C: Ketotifen in prevention and therapy of food allergy. *Ann Allergy* 59(5 Part II):187–193, 1987.

178. Boner AL, Richelli C, Antolini I, et al: The efficacy of ketotifen in a controlled double-blind food challenge study in patients with food allergy. *Ann Allergy* 57:61–64, 1986.

179. Buscino L, Benincori N, Cantani A, et al: Chronic diarrhea due to cow's milk allergy. A 4- to 10-year follow-up study. *Ann Allergy* 55:844–847, 1985.

180. Bock SA: Natural history of severe reactions to foods in young children. *J Pediatr* 107:676–680, 1985.

181. Bock SA: The natural history of food sensitivity. *J Allergy Clin Immunol* 69:173–177, 1982.

182. Grulee CG, Sanford HN: The influence of breast and artificial feeding on infantile eczema. *J Pediatr* 9:223–225, 1936.

183. Zeiger RS, Heller S, Mellon M, et al: Effectiveness of dietary manipulation in the prevention of food allergy in infants. *J Allergy Clin Immunol* 78:224–238, 1986.

184. Saarinen UM: Prophylaxis for atopic disease: role of infant feeding. *Clin Rev Allergy* 2:151–167, 1984.

185. Saarinen UM, Kajosaari M: Does dietary elimination in infancy prevent or only postpone a food allergy? A study of fish and citrus allergy in 375 children. *Lancet* 1:166–167, 1980.

186. Kaufman HS: Allergy in the newborn: skin test reactions confirmed by the Prausnitz-Küstner test at birth. *Clin Allergy* 1:363–367, 1971.

187. Buscino L, Cantani A: Prevention of atopy—current concepts and personal experience. *Clin Rev Allergy* 2:107–123, 1984.

188. Shacks SJ, Heiner DC: Allergy to breast milk. *Clin Immunol Allergy* 2:121–136, 1982.

189. Gerrard JW: Allergies in breastfed babies to foods ingested by the mother. *Clin Rev Allergy* 2:143–149, 1984.

190. Jakobsson I, Lindberg T: Cow's milk proteins cause infantile colic in breast-fed infants: a double-blind crossover study. *Pediatrics* 71:268–271, 1983.

191. May CD: Are confusion and controversy about food hypersensitivity really necessary? *J Allergy Clin Immunol* 75:329–333, 1985.

CHAPTER 26

Chronic Gastritis and Pernicious Anemia

ROBERT G. STRICKLAND

INTRODUCTION

The association between gastric autoimmunity and diffuse chronic inflammatory disease of the gastric mucosa was first suggested in 1959, when Taylor identified a serum inhibitor of intrinsic factor (IF) activity in patients with pernicious anemia (PA) not previously treated with oral porcine IF.[1] This observation was quickly confirmed,[2] and identification of the inhibitor as an autoantibody to IF was subsequently established.[3] In 1962, Irvine et al.[4] and Taylor et al.[5] described the presence of parietal cell autoantibody in PA serum, detectable by complement fixation using a saline extract of human gastric mucosa or indirect immunofluorescence on human gastric mucosal tissue sections.

These initial findings set the stage for the extensive and continuing research that has followed concerning the immunology of chronic gastritis and pernicious anemia. The recent isolation of *Campylobacter pylori* from gastric mucosa[6] and the mounting evidence that this organism may be pathogenic in man, leading to some forms of chronic gastritis, has stimulated renewed interest in these disease processes.

CHRONIC GASTRITIS

Chronic gastritis is the commonest pathologic finding encountered in the human stomach. Biopsy studies of the gastric mucosa in randomly selected adult population samples disclose a prevalence of chronic gastritis of 60–70%.[7] In approximately 80% of these subjects, the lesion is graded as chronic superficial or mild atrophic gastritis.[8] The significance of these less severe grades of chronic gastritis is uncertain, since progression to advanced atrophic gastritis is unusual and apparent regression is also observed.[9]

Advanced chronic atrophic gastritis (CAG) affects approximately 10% of adults, according to Finnish population studies.[7,8] An additional morphologic classification in CAG relates to differing patterns of distribution of this pathologic process in the stomach.[8,10,11] Type A refers to a corpus-predominant gastritis with relative sparing of the antral mucosa; type B refers to antral-predominant disease with variable corpus involvement (absent, patchy, mild); type AB refers to generalized or pan-CAG (Fig. 26–1). In a recent population study the frequencies of these three morphologic phenotypes of CAG were type A, 11%; type B, 51%; and type AB, 38%.[8] In general, autoimmune markers are observed with the A phenotype;[10] *C. pylori* colonization, on the other hand, was not observed in type A CAG but was present in 16 of 17 patients with type B CAG and 23 of 32 with type AB CAG.[12]

PERNICIOUS ANEMIA

Pernicious anemia is the commonest cause of vitamin B_{12} deficiency in Western populations, its estimated prevalence being 0.1%. The fundamental abnormality in PA is a severe CAG or gastric atrophy of the corpus mucosa (phenotype A), leading to achlorhydria, intrinsic factor secretory failure, and consequent vitamin B_{12} malabsorption. There is evidence from long-term follow-up studies that PA evolves from pre-existing type A CAG.[10,13]

IMMUNOLOGIC FEATURES

There is no identifiable general disturbance in humoral or cellular immune function in these disorders. An apparent exception to this statement is that patients with the common variable immunodeficiency (CVID) syndrome display a high incidence (50%) of severe CAG and vitamin B_{12} deficiency.[14] However, the gastric lesion in this disorder is of the AB phenotype (uniform pan CAG), plasma cells are lacking in the damaged mucosa, circulating gastric autoantibodies are absent and mechanisms other than IF deficiency appear to contribute to the vitamin B_{12}

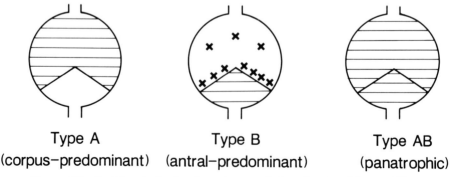

Type A
(corpus–predominant)

Type B
(antral–predominant)

Type AB
(panatrophic)

Figure 26–1 Morphologic phenotypes of chronic atrophic gastritis.

Table 26 – 1   CIRCULATING GASTRIC AUTOANTIBODIES IN PERNICIOUS ANEMIA

Autoantibody	Antigenic Site	% Incidence
Intrinsic factor		
Type I	Vitamin B_{12} binding site	70
Type II	IF, IF-B_{12} complex	35
Parietal cell		
Microsomal	Canalicular microvilli (? membrane H^+, K^+-AT Pase)	90
Surface	Surface membrane of parietal cell	88
Gastrin receptor	Gastrin receptor on parietal cell	30

deficiency in CVID (Table 26 – 1). These observations favor the view that this form of CAG is fundamentally distinct from the gastric lesion of Addisonian PA.

Intrinsic Factor Antibodies

Two types of intrinsic factor antibodies (IFA) have been identified. Type I or blocking IFA reacts with the vitamin B_{12} binding site of intrinsic factor. Type I IFA is detectable in serum of 70% of PA patients using a sensitive radioassay.[15] Type II or binding IFA is directed against both IF and the IF-B_{12} complex and is detectable in 30–40% of PA patients.[15] Type II IFA is rarely, if ever, detected in the absence of type I IF antibody.[15] Serum IFA can be of the IgG or IgA subclass, and a study of light chain distributions disclosed heterogeneity, thus providing evidence against monoclonality of the response.[16] The presence of IF antibodies is almost pathognomonic of the evolving or established gastric lesion of PA.[17] The only exception has been one report of a small group of patients with thyroid disease in whom vitamin B_{12} absorption remained normal over several years despite the persistent presence of IFA.[18]

Parietal Cell Antibodies

Using indirect immunofluorescence, parietal cell antibody is detected in up to 90% of PA sera.[5,15,17] Initial studies disclosed antibody reactivity against gastric parietal cell microsomes. The microsomal antigen appears to be a lipoprotein and can be destroyed by detergents, papain, and trypsin but not by RNAse, phospholipase, or alkalinization.[19,20] An electron microscopic study using horseradish peroxidase-labeled antibody localized the antigen to microvillus membranes of the parietal cell canalicular system.[21] A recent study has indicated that this antibody may be reactive against the H^+ K^+-ATPase of the parietal cell canalicular membrane.[22]

Parietal cell microsomal antibody is cell-specific but not species-specific. The best substrate for use in clinical testing is human gastric corpus mucosa from blood group O patients. In view of the current paucity of such material, mouse stomach provides a satisfactory alternative. However, the use of rat stomach for this purpose is unsatisfactory. This is because human serum may display a heteroantibody reaction against rat parietal cells that can then lead to false-positive test results.[23]

Recently, two additional parietal cell autoantibodies, apparently distinct from that directed against the microsomal (canalicular) antigen, have been described in patients with PA. Parietal cell surface antibody (PCSA) was observed by immuno-fluorescence using isolated viable canine parietal cell-enriched suspensions in 88% of 60 PA sera.[24] PCSA reactivity is abolished following serum absorption with whole viable parietal cells but not by gastric mucosal microsomes. In addition, 73% of the PA sera containing PCSA demonstrated in vitro cytotoxic activity against canine parietal cells in the presence of complement.[25]

The same group of investigators has also described a circulating autoantibody to the gastrin receptor on parietal cells in 6 of 20 patients with PA.[26] For these studies, IgG fractions from serum were used to demonstrate inhibition of specific binding of radiolabeled human G17 to isolated parietal cell-enriched suspensions from rat gastric mucosa. Additionally, all six IgG fractions inhibited gastrin-stimulated but not histamine-stimulated [^{14}C]aminopyrine accumulation in the parietal cell preparations.

There are no reports of PCSA or gastrin receptor antibodies in the absence of PA. However, a considerable literature exists with regard to the occurrence of parietal cell microsomal autoantibody. This is reviewed in detail elsewhere.[27] The microsomal antibody is prevalent (20–30%) in PA relatives and in patients with a variety of endocrine disorders, including thyrotoxicosis, Hashimoto's thyroiditis, hypothyroidism, insulin-dependent diabetes mellitus, idiopathic Addison's disease, idiopathic hypoparathyroidism, and primary gonadal failure. In all these conditions autoantibodies to the involved endocrine cells are also observed, and on further testing those showing the presence of parietal cell antibody will frequently be discovered to have type A CAG. Similar increased prevalence of parietal cell microsomal antibody and type A CAG has been observed in patients with vitiligo or with unexplained chronic iron deficiency.

Parietal cell microsomal antibody is also detectable in apparently healthy members of the population. In an unselected adult population in Australia comprising 3,492 subjects, the prevalence of this antibody was 4.8%.[23] The prevalence rose with advancing age from 2.5% in the third decade to 9.6% in the eighth decade. These observations were carefully controlled to avoid the problem of false-positive results due to heteroantibodies. A recent population study of the relationship between parietal cell antibody and gastric mucosal morphology found that chronic gastritis of varying degree existed in all but one antibody-positive subject and that the distribution of the gastritis was of the A phenotype (antral-sparing) in all subjects.[28]

Gastrin Cell Autoantibodies

In 1979, Vandelli et al. reported the presence of autoantibody to antral gastrin-producing (G) cells in 8 of 106 subjects with CAG phenotype B.[29] However, in the recent population study of Uibo et al.,[28] the presence of G-cell antibodies showed no correlation with antritis. Thus the significance of G-cell antibodies must at this time be regarded as doubtful.

Cellular Immunity to Gastric Antigens

Two in vitro techniques, lymphocyte blast transformation and leukocyte migration inhibition, have been widely applied to the evaluation of cellular immunity to a variety of gastric antigens using peripheral blood leukocytes from patients with PA or CAG. In general, the studies using crude gastric mucosal antigens have provided inconsistent or low-frequency positive results, perhaps due to antigenic impurity. The use of intrinsic factor preparations appears to yield more consistent results.[30] In particular, the study of Weisbart et al. using purified porcine IF and an agarose-leukocyte migration test gave a clear positive result with PA cells and negative results using cells from normal subjects or patients with CAG.[31] Limited studies in patients with type A CAG indicate infrequent cellular immunity to crude gastric antigens and absence of cellular immunity to IF.[30-33]

Gastric Mucosal Immunologic Observations

Early studies of the cell types infiltrating the corpus mucosa in PA focused on the significant increase in immunoglobulin-containing plasma cells (particularly IgG-containing) in the target organ.[33] By contrast, in an extensive study of postgastrectomy chronic gastritis in which neither gastric autoantibodies nor cellular immunity to gastric antigens are observed, IgA cells predominated in the mucosal infiltrate.[34] More recently, T-cell monoclonal antibodies have been used to identify and quantitate T lymphocytes and their major subpopulations (T helper, T suppressor) in PA gastric mucosa.[35] T cells were increased in PA mucosa compared with normal control mucosa; however, the major increase (sixfold over normal mucosa) was in non-T cells, probably representing B cells, although these were not directly identified in this study. No differences in mucosal T-helper to T-suppressor ratios were observed in PA mucosa compared with normal controls.

The plasma cells infiltrating the gastric mucosa of PA patients have been shown to contain parietal cell microsomal antibody and type II intrinsic factor antibody.[36] Gastric autoantibodies are also detectable in gastric secretions in patients with PA. IF antibodies may in fact occur more frequently in gastric secretions than in serum; type I IF antibody can complex with residual IF in these secretions, and it has proved possible to dissociate the complexes, thus revealing previously "hidden" antibody to IF.[37] Indeed, it has been suggested that IF antibodies in gastric secretions may be a critical determinant in reducing IF availability to a point at which vitamin B_{12} absorption can no longer be sustained. Antibody class of gastric juice parietal cell and intrinsic factor antibodies may be either IgG or IgA, and there is no clear correlation between Ig class of these antibodies in serum and gastric juice in individual patients.[38]

In other putative autoimmune processes, cells that are the primary targets for immunologic injury often express HLA-DR antigen on their cell surfaces. No studies of DR expression on surviving parietal cells in PA or autoimmune CAG have been reported. However, DR expression was recently described in CAG without circulating gastric autoantibodies, suggesting that this feature is not restricted to autoimmune gastric mucosal injury.[39]

GENETIC PREDISPOSITION-IMMUNOGENETIC STUDIES

The familial occurrence of PA is well established. Even more striking is the increased prevalence of parietal cell microsomal and intrinsic factor antibodies, of gastric hypofunction, vitamin B_{12} malabsorption, and chronic gastritis in 20–30%

of PA relatives.[40,41] A more recent study has established that the chronic gastritis in PA relatives is frequently severe and of the A phenotype.[42] This is particularly true of first-generation, older relatives. These observations are consistent with inheritance of a specific form of chronic gastritis (type A, associated with gastric autoimmune reactions) as an autosomal dominant characteristic. However, observations of gastric morphology in second-generation, younger PA relatives reveal a less characteristic lesion of diffuse, mild pan-gastritis.[8] This may reflect environmental initiating factors in the mucosal injury, which over many decades evolves into type A CAG in those genetically predisposed to this lesion.[9]

A number of studies have sought associations of histocompatibility genes with PA. In general these results have shown possible, but inconsistent associations of PA with A3 and B7 haplotypes[43,44] and more consistent but not universal associations with DR2 and DR4.[44,45] In addition, differences between subgroups of patients with PA based on the presence or absence of associated endocrinopathies have been suggested.[45] At present, however, there is no strong evidence for the role of specific immunogenetic influences in PA, such as is observed in B27-associated arthropathies.

PATHOGENIC SIGNIFICANCE OF GASTRIC AUTOIMMUNITY

The preceding observations strongly implicate autoimmune mechanisms in the gastric mucosal damage of PA and a small subpopulation of patients with chronic gastritis. Thus these two disorders share a distinctive gastric morphology (phenotype A), and type A chronic gastritis appears to represent a prepernicious anemia state. Gastric autoimmune reactions are highly restricted both in their occurrence (confined to PA and type A gastritis) and their cell specificity (confined to structural and secretory products of the parietal cell). The gastric mucosal immunopathology is consistent with immune-mediated injury, and the recent observations on parietal cell surface antibody provide a possible in vivo mechanism for injury to these specialized cells.

Early Experimental Studies

Chronic gastritis can be induced in experimental animals by immunization with gastric juice or gastric mucosal homogenates. Monkeys and dogs are most susceptible to induction of this "autoallergic gastritis," whereas rats, guinea pigs, and mice appear resistant to this approach. Cellular immune mechanisms appear most relevant in this model, since the onset of mucosal damage corresponds in time more closely to development of cellular immunity to gastric antigens than to appearance of circulating gastric antibodies.[46]

However, other studies have clearly demonstrated significant effects of gastric autoantibodies on gastric structure and function in experimental systems. Inoculation of rats with human IgG fractions of serum containing parietal cell microsomal or intrinsic factor antibodies induces atrophy of the respective target cells — parietal cells or chief cells (the latter being the site of IF secretion in the rat) — and impaired secretion of acid or intrinsic factor.[47,48] Similar biologic effects of gastric autoantibodies have been reported in dogs and in the isolated bullfrog gastric mucosa.[49] Whereas chronic inflammation is prominent in the "autoallergic" model, inoculation of autoantibodies does not result in a gastric mucosal inflammatory response.

It can be concluded from the foregoing that none of these experimental immune manipulations has resulted in a true model of human PA, or type A CAG.

An Animal Model of Type A CAG and PA?

Recently, a group of Japanese investigators have described a possible animal model of human autoimmune gastritis.[50] BALB/C nu/ + mice undergoing neonatal thymectomy 3 days after birth developed chronic gastritis restricted to the corpus mucosa, parietal cell microsomal autoantibodies, decreased intrinsic factor secretion, and vitamin B_{12} absorption over a 12-month period of observation. Autoimmune thyroiditis, oophoritis, or orchitis also occurs in this model, mimicking the endocrinopathies observed in association with human autoimmune gastritis. Effects on acid secretion and intrinsic factor antibodies were not reported in this study, and the animals did not develop anemia over the observation period of 1 year. As in human type A CAG, damage of both parietal cells and chief cells was observed. However, in contrast to the atrophic appearance in the human disease, the corpus mucosa in these mice was macroscopically hypertrophic due to a greatly expanded epithelial and mucous neck cell zone. Whether with extended observation this hypertrophic response would be followed by atrophy is not known at this time.

The immunologic findings included marked mucosal infiltration by T cells (Thy 1.2+, and both Lyt1 and Lyt2) at an early stage (1.5 – 3 months); B-cell infiltration occurred much later (6 months). The gastric lesion could be adoptively transferred to unaffected mice by spleen cells but not by serum. These observations imply a primary role of T cells in the initiation of this form of experimental autoimmune gastritis. The specific T-cell types were not identified; however, delayed-type hypersensitivity (DTH) appeared to be involved. Thus, DTH reactions in mouse footpads were induced by parietal cell-enriched gastric mucosal fractions in those mice developing autoimmune gastritis.

In summary, this animal model represents a promising new approach to a better understanding of the mechanisms involved in autoimmune gastric mucosal injury.

CLINICAL IMPLICATIONS

Diagnosis

Several recent studies have reported on measurements of serum pepsinogens in the diagnosis of chronic gastritis and PA. Immunoreactive pepsinogen I (PG I) is secreted by chief cells of the corpus mucosa. PG II is present in chief cells, antral glands, and mucous neck cells of the entire gastric mucosa. CAG of the corpus mucosa is associated with low PG I levels, since the gastric lesion includes destruction of chief cells. PG II levels are increased in less severe grades of chronic gastritis of the corpus mucosa. Thus it has been proposed that a low PG I/PG II ratio together with an absolute decrease in PG I suggests CAG, whereas a low ratio with normal PG I indicates less advanced forms of chronic gastritis.[51]

Table 26–2 DIFFERENTIAL CHARACTERISTICS OF TYPE A, TYPE B, AND TYPE AB ATROPHIC GASTRITIS

Phenotype	% Frequency[a]	PCA[b]	Gastrin	Pepsinogens	*C. pylori*
A	11	Present	Elevated	PGI, PGI/II↓	Absent
B	51	Absent	Normal	Not studied	Present
AB	38	Infrequent	Normal	PGI, PGI/II↓	Present

[a] Data of Kekki et al.[8]

[b] Parietal cell microsomal antibody.

A second serologic marker of chronic gastritis is the fasting serum gastrin level.[52,53] In the presence of achlorhydria, gastrin levels are greatly elevated in a majority of patients with PA or type A CAG. Antral sparing together with G-cell hyperplasia in antral and corpus mucosa appear to be the underlying mechanisms. With severe antral gastritis (types B or AB), however, gastrin levels are normal despite the presence of acid hyposecretion or achlorhydria, because of G-cell destruction in these forms of gastritis.

Diagnostic suspicion of PA still rests largely on initial hematologic and/or neurologic findings. Among the many possible confirmatory tests, the combination of a high basal serum gastrin level and radioassays for type I intrinsic factor antibody and serum pepsinogen I offers a highly sensitive noninvasive diagnostic panel.

Type A chronic gastritis represents a significant risk factor for eventual evolution to PA.[10,13] It is largely asymptomatic; however, the recognition that certain patient groups are at higher risk for this lesion may result in earlier diagnosis. Such groups include PA relatives and patients with endocrine disease (especially multiple endocrine disorders), chronic unexplained iron deficiency, and vitiligo. In these situations serum PG I and II, serum gastrin, and parietal cell antibody testing will identify a majority of such patients.

The diagnosis of the more prevalent nonautoimmune phenotypes of CAG (B,AB) is more problematic. While nonulcer dyspepsia may result in identification of some patients in these categories, a majority are without symptoms. This is of particular concern in view of the current evidence implicating B and AB phenotypes of CAG as more significant precursors of gastric cancer than PA or type A CAG.[8,10] The recent association of *C. pylori* colonization with types B and AB (but not type A) CAG[12] and the suggested use of serum antibody testing for diagnosis of this infection[54] are of interest, but application of such testing in the clinical setting remains to be defined.

Management

There is no known treatment that will restore to normal the gastric mucosa of patients with PA or type A CAG. Several earlier studies of the effect of corticosteroids revealed some evidence for partial parietal cell regeneration, improved vitamin B_{12} absorption, and decreased serum titers of gastric autoantibodies.[28] The doses required to obtain these effects were substantial, and since replacement therapy with vitamin B_{12} is simple and safe, there is no place for the use of corticosteroids in the treatment of these disorders.

There is much current interest in the therapeutic effects of various antibiotic regimes in the eradication of *C. pylori* in patients colonized with this organism. Early results do suggest significant healing of gastritis in response to such therapy.[55] However, the completeness of such healing is not fully defined (especially the "chronic" component), eradication is particularly difficult (requiring multiple antibiotics), and significant relapse rates are observed following such therapy. For the present, treatment of *C. pylori*-associated chronic gastritis should probably be confined to clinical therapeutic trials.

CONCLUSIONS AND FUTURE DIRECTIONS

Much has been learned about the immunology of PA and chronic gastritis in the 30 years since Taylor first provided us with the initial firm link between the immune system and these disorders.

The available evidence clearly supports the notion that the gastric lesion in PA and a small proportion of patients with chronic gastritis is due to autoimmune tissue injury of the corpus mucosa of the stomach. What remains unclear is the exact mechanism(s) involved in the gastric mucosal injury, particularly the relative importance of cellular and humoral pathways in this process. Also unclear is the potential importance of immunoregulatory mechanisms at the tissue (gastric mucosal) level and the role of perturbations of such mechanisms in immunologic gastric mucosal injury. The development of autoimmunity to IF is likely to be a critical factor in the transition of type A CAG to PA, yet this fact has not been prospectively demonstrated. These questions are difficult to resolve solely by continued investigation of the human disease state. Further study of the recently described animal model of autoimmune gastritis could provide a better definition of the mechanisms underlying the breakdown in self-tolerance to gastric antigens in these disorders.

No clear environmental triggers to autoimmune gastric mucosal injury have yet been identified. Current evidence implicates *C. pylori* as a possible cause of nonautoimmune (B, AB phenotypes) CAG but not of PA or type A CAG.

Finally, the precise nature of the genetic factor in PA and type A CAG remains unknown. In this regard, we can expect that further studies involving a variety of immunogenetic markers in more precisely defined population groups will be forthcoming.

In conclusion, the prospects for a better understanding of PA and autoimmune gastritis in the future are indeed bright. We have much to learn about autoimmune disease processes in general. The disorders discussed in this chapter still have much to teach us about these processes.

REFERENCES

1. Taylor KB: Inhibition of intrinsic factor by pernicious anemia sera. *Lancet* 2:106–108, 1959.
2. Schwartz, M: Intrinsic factor antibody in serum from patients with pernicious anemia. *Lancet* 2:1263–1267, 1960.
3. Jeffries GH, Hoskins DW, Sleisenger MH: Antibody to intrinsic factor in serum from patients with pernicious anemia. *J Clin Invest* 41:1106–115, 1962.

4. Irvine WJ, Davies SH, Delamore IM, et al: Immunological relationship between pernicious anemia and thyroid diseases. *Br Med J* 2:454–456, 1962.

5. Taylor KB, Roitt IM, Doniach D, et al: Autoimmune phenomena in pernicious anemia: gastric antibodies. *Br Med J* 2:1347–1352, 1962.

6. Warren JR, Marshall BJ: Unidentified curved bacilli on gastric epithelium in active chronic gastritis. *Lancet* 1:1273–1275, 1983.

7. Siurala M, Isokoski M, Varis K, et al: Prevalence of gastritis in a rural population. Bioptic study of subjects selected at random. *Scand J Gastroenterol* 3:211–223, 1968.

8. Kekki M, Siurala M, Varis K, et al: Classification principals and genetics of chronic gastritis. *Scand J Gastroenterol* 22(Suppl 141):1–28, 1987.

9. Ihamaki T, Kekki M, Sipponen P, et al: The sequelae and course of chronic gastritis during a 30- to 34-year bioptic follow-up study. *Scand J Gastroenterol* 20:484–491, 1985.

10. Strickland RG, Mackay IR: A reappraisal of the nature and significance of chronic atrophic gastritis. *Am J Dig Dis* 18:426–440, 1973.

11. Glass GBJ, Pitchumoni CS: Atrophic gastritis. *Hum Pathol* 6:219–250, 1975.

12. Siurala M, Sipponen P, Kekki M: *Campylobacter pylori* in a sample of Finnish population: relations to morphology and functions of the gastric mucosa. *Gut* 29:909–915, 1988.

13. Irvine WJ, Cullen DR, Mawhinney H: Natural history of autoimmune achlorhydric atrophic gastritis. A 1–15 year follow-up study. *Lancet* 2:482–485, 1974.

14. Heremans PE, Diax-Buxo JA, Stobo JD: Idiopathic late onset immunoglobulin deficiency. Clinical observations in 50 patients. *Am J Med* 61:221–237, 1976.

15. Samloff IM, Kleinman MS, Turner MD, et al: Blocking and binding antibody to intrinsic factor and parietal cell antibody in pernicious anemia. *Gastroenterology* 55:575–583, 1968.

16. Bernier GM, Hines JD: Immunologic heterogeneity of autoantibodies in patients with pernicious anemia. *New Engl J Med* 277:1386–1391, 1967.

17. Fisher JM, Mackay IR, Taylor KB, et al: An immunologic study of categories of gastritis. *Lancet* 1:176–180, 1967.

18. Rose MS, Chanarin I, Doniach D, et al: Intrinsic factor antibodies in absence of pernicious anemia 3–7 year follow-up. *Lancet* 2:9–12, 1970.

19. Baur S, Roitt IM, Doniach D: Characterization of the human gastric parietal cell autoantigen. *Immunology* 8:62–68, 1965.

20. Ward HA, Nairn RC: Gastric parietal cell autoantigen. Physical, chemical and biologic properties. *Clin Exp Immunol* 10:435–457, 1972.

21. Hoedemaeker PJ, Ito S: Ultrastructural localization of gastric parietal cell antigen with peroxidase-coupled antibody. *Lab Invest* 22:184–188, 1970.

22. Karlsson FA, Burman P, Loof L, et al: Enzyme-linked immunosorbent assay of H^+, K^+-ATPase, the parietal cell antigen. *Clin Exp Immunol* 70:604–610, 1987.

23. Strickland RG, Hooper B: The parietal cell heteroantibody in human sera: prevalence in a normal population and relationship to parietal cell autoantibody. *Pathology* 4:259–263, 1972.

24. De Aizpurua HJ, Toh BH, Ungar B: Parietal cell surface reactive autoantibody in pernicious anemia demonstrated by indirect membrane immunoflurorescence. *Clin Exp Immunol* 52:341–349, 1983.

25. De Aizpurua HJ, Cosgrove LJ, Ungar B, et al: Autoantibodies cytotoxic to gastric parietal cells in serum of patients with pernicious anemia. *N Engl J Med* 309:625–629, 1983.

26. De Aizpurua HJ, Ungar B, Toh BH: Autoantibody to the gastrin receptor in pernicious anemia. *N Engl J Med* 313:479–483, 1985.

27. Strickland RG: Gastritis. *Front Gastrointest Res* 1:12–48, 1975.

28. Uibo R, Krohn K, Villako K, et al: The relationship of parietal cell, gastrin cell, and thyroid autoantibodies to the state of the gastric mucosa in a population sample. *Scand J Gastroenteral* 19:1075–1080, 1984.

29. Vandelli C, Bottazzo GF, Doniach D, et al: Autoantibodies to gastrin-producing cells in antral (type B) chronic gastritis. *N Engl J Med* 300:1406–1410, 1979.

30. James D, Asherson G, Chanarin I, et al: Cell-mediated immunity to intrinsic factor in autoimmune disorders. *Br Med J* 4:494–496, 1974.

31. Weisbart RH, Bluestone R, Goldberg LS: Cellular immunity to intrinsic factor in pernicious anemia. *J Lab Clin Med* 85:87–92, 1975.

32. Goldstone AH, Calder EA, Barnes EW, et al: The effect of gastric antigens on the *in vitro* migration of leucocytes from patients with atrophic gastritis and pernicious anemia. *Clin Exp Immunol* 14:501–508, 1973.

33. Odgers RJ, Wangel AG: Abnormalities in IgA-containing mononuclear cells in the gastric lesion of pernicious anemia. *Lancet* 2:846–849, 1968.

34. Chapel HM, Hoare AM: A study of the aetiology of gastritis following gastric surgery. I. Immunofluorescent studies of the gastric mucosa. *Clin Exp Immunol* 37:441–444, 1979.

35. Kaye MD, Whorwell PJ, Wright R: Gastric mucosal lymphocyte subpopulations in pernicious anemia and in normal stomach. *Clin Immunol Immunopathol* 28:431–440, 1983.

36. Baur S, Fisher JM, Strickland RG, et al: Autoantibody-containing cells in the gastric mucosa in pernicious anemia. *Lancet* 2:887–890, 1968.

37. Rose MS, Chanarin I: Dissociation of intrinsic factor from its antibody. Application to study of pernicious anemia gastric juice specimens. *Br Med J* 1:468–470, 1969.

38. Strickland RG, Baur S, Ashworth LAE, et al: A correlative study of immunological phenomena in pernicious anemia. *Clin Exp Immunol* 8:25–36, 1971.

39. Spencer J, Pugh S, Isaacson PG: HLA-D region antigen expression of stomach epithelium in absence of autoantibodies. *Lancet* 2:983, 1986.

40. Wangel AG, Callender ST, Spray GH, et al: A family study of pernicious anemia. I. Autoantibodies, achlorhydria, serum pepsinogen and vitamin B_{12}. *Br J Haematol* 14:161–181, 1968.

41. Wangel AG, Callender St, Spray GH, et al: A family study of pernicious anemia. II. Intrinsic factor secretion, vitamin B_{12} absorption and genetic aspects of gastric autoimmunity. *Br J Haematol* 14:183–204, 1968.

42. Varis K, Ihamaki T, Harkonen M, et al: Gastric morphology, function and immunology in first-degree relatives of probands with pernicious anemia and controls. *Scand J Gastroenterol* 14:129–139, 1979.

43. Mawhinney H, Lawton JMW, White AG, et al: HL-A3 and HL-A7 in pernicious anemia and autoimmune atrophic gastritis. *Clin Exp Immunol* 22:47–53, 1975.

44. Thomsen M, Jorgensen F, Brandsborg M, et al: Association of pernicious anemia and intrinsic factor antibody with HLA-D. *Tissue Antigens* 17:97–103, 1981.

45. Ungar B, Mathews JD, Tait BD, et al: HLA-DR patterns in pernicious anemia. *Br Med J* 1:768–770, 1981.

46. Krohn KJE, Finlayson NDC: Interrelations of humoral and cellular immune responses in experimental canine gastritis. *Clin Exp Immunol* 14:237–245, 1973.

47. Tanaka N, Glass GBJ: Effect of prolonged administration of parietal cell antibodies from patients with atrophic gastritis and pernicious anemia on the parietal cell mass and hydrochloric acid outputs in rats. *Gastroenterology* 58:482–494, 1970.

48. Inada M, Glass GBJ: Effect of prolonged administration of homologous and heterologous intrinsic factor antibodies on the parietal and peptic cell mass and the secretory function of the rat gastric mucosa. *Gastroenterology* 69:396–408, 1975.

49. Loveridge N, Bitensky L, Chayen J, et al: Inhibition of parietal cell function by human gammoglobulin containing gastric parietal cell antibodies. *Clin Exp Immunol* 41:264–270, 1980.

50. Fukuma K, Sakaguchi S, Kuribayashi K, et al: Immunologic and clinical studies on murine experimental autoimmune gastritis induced by neonatal thymectomy. *Gastroenterology* 94:274–283, 1988.

51. Samloff IM, Varis K, Ihamaki T, et al: Relationships among serum pepsinogen I, serum pepsinogen II and gastric mucosal histology. A study in relatives of patients with pernicious anemia. *Gastroenterology* 83:204–209, 1982.

52. Strickland RG, Bhathal PS, Korman MG, et al: Serum gastrin and the antral muscosa in atrophic gastritis. *Br Med J* 4:451–453, 1971.

53. Varis K, Samloff IM, Ihamaki T, et al: An appraisal of tests for severe atrophic gastritis in relatives of patients with pernicious anemia. *Dig Dis Sci* 24:187–191, 1979.

54. Perez-Perez GI, Dworkin BM, Chodos JE, et al: *Campylobacter pylori* antibodies in humans. *Ann Intern Med* 109:11–17, 1988.

55. Blaser MJ: Gastric *campylobacter*-like organisms, gastritis and peptic ulcer disease. *Gastroenterology* 93:371–383, 1987.

CHAPTER 27

Lymphoproliferative Disorders of the Gastrointestinal Tract

KLAUS J. LEWIN

WAYNE W. GRODY

INTRODUCTION

Considering the extensive lymphoid tissue normally present in the mucosa along its length, it is not surprising that the gastrointestinal tract is a common site for lymphoproliferative disorders. These disorders may be benign (lymphoid hyperplasias) or malignant (lymphomas) and can occur within the confines of the existing lymphoid structure or extend beyond it by direct transmural expansion or drainage to mesenteric lymph nodes.

LYMPHOID HYPERPLASIA

Primary lymphoid hyperplasia occurs in virtually all parts of the gastrointestinal tract and may be either focal or diffuse. Aside from the five most common clinicopathologic groups listed in Table 27–1 and discussed individually below, lymphoid hyperplasia has been described rarely in unusual locations such as the esophagus and colon.[1,2] Lymphoid hyperplasia can also occur as a secondary component in a number of other conditions, including nonerosive gastritis, Crohn's disease, and ulcerative colitis. In some clinical settings, distinguishing primary from secondary forms may be difficult. Even more problematic is the frequent difficulty in distinguishing a benign hyperplasia from malignant lymphoma of the gastrointestinal tract. In this regard we particularly discourage use of the term pseudolymphoma as a synonym for some types of lymphoid hyperplasia, since the latter term more accurately reflects the nature of the pathologic process.

Table 27 – 1   CLASSIFICATION OF GASTROINTESTINAL LYMPHOID HYPERPLASIA

Focal lymphoid hyperplasia of the stomach (gastric pseudolymphoma)
Focal lymphoid hyperplasia of the small intestine
Focal lymphoid hyperplasia of the rectum (benign lymphoid polyp, rectal tonsil)
Focal nodular lymphoid hyperplasia of the terminal ileum and appendix
Diffuse nodular lymphoid hyperplasia

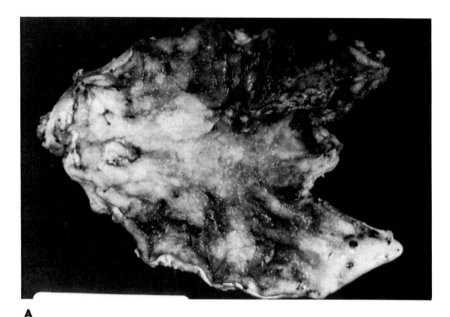

A

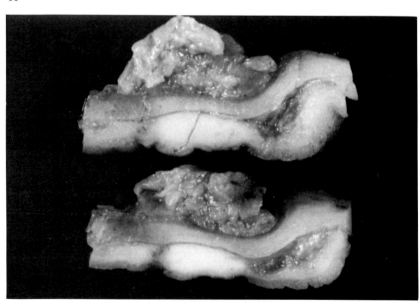

B

Figure 27 – 1   Resection specimens of gastric lymphoid hyperplasia, showing a large ulcer with surrounding thickened, scarred mucosa **(A)** and dense submucosal fibrosis in cross section **(B)**.

548

Focal Lymphoid Hyperplasia of the Stomach

This lesion of adults usually presents with symptoms suggestive of gastric ulcer disease. Both radiologically and endoscopically, the lesion may simulate either a peptic ulcer[3-6] or, more frequently, a malignant neoplasm,[3-14] hence its common designation as gastric pseudolymphoma.

Pathology

The stomach is usually ulcerated in a manner that may mimic tumors because of raised ulcer margins and/or thickened rugal folds (Fig. 27–1). Two architectural patterns have been described.[4,5,7] The most common presentation is as a chronic gastric ulcer with a lymphoid infiltrate at the margins and along the floor (Fig. 27–2). The second variety is marked by gastric thickening and cobblestoning of the mucosa due to lymphocytic infiltration predominantly in the mucosa and submucosa, but ulceration is only superficial or absent (Fig. 27–3). Other presentations are occasionally seen, including exophytic masses or deep ulcerations.

Histologically, lesions typically show mucosal ulceration with underlying fibrosis and a dense inflammatory infiltrate composed predominantly of small mature lymphocytes admixed with lesser numbers of immunoblasts, plasma cells, and eosinophils (Fig. 27–4). Lymphoid follicles with or without obvious germinal centers are scattered throughout the infiltrate, and in our experience are best formed and most abundant superficially in the mucosa and upper mucosa.[4] Single-file columns of lymphocytes may be seen between collagen bundles in the fibrotic areas (Fig. 27–5).[1] Such histologic variants as nodular lymphoid hyperplasia and angiofollicular hyperplasia can also occur in the stomach.[3]

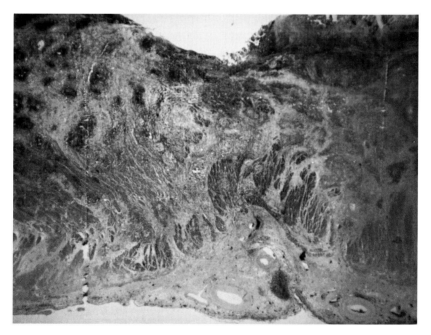

Figure 27–2 Full-thickness section of gastric lymphoid hyperplasia showing appearance of the chronic ulceration, transmural fibrosis, and surrounding lymphoid infiltrate.

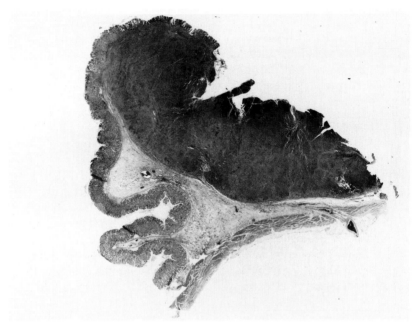

A

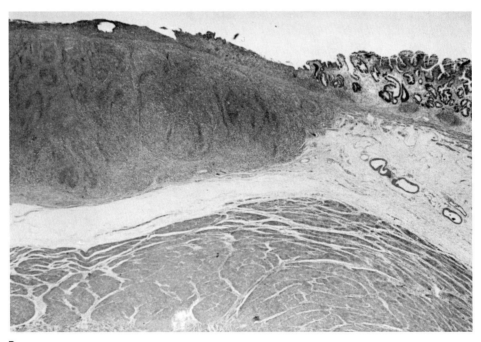

B

Figure 27–3 Presentation of gastric lymphoid hyperplasia as a mass lesion composed of an extensive mucosal and submucosal lymphoid infiltrate with lymphoid nodules visible. The mucosal surface may be intact **(A)** or superficially eroded **(B),** but in either case there is no scarring, as would be seen with a chronic gastric ulcer.

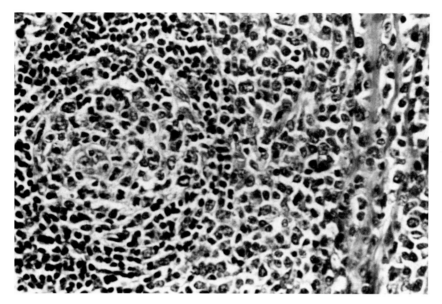

Figure 27–4 Appearance of infiltrate in gastric lymphoid hyperplasia, demonstrating a lymphoid follicle, free mature lymphocytes, and a surrounding admixture of inflammatory cells including immunoblasts, plasma cells, and eosinophils.

Differential Diagnosis
As might be expected, the key issue in differential diagnosis of these lesions is the exclusion of malignant lymphoma. The most important distinguishing features relate to the nature of the lymphoid infiltrate. First, the polymorphous infiltrate of lymphoid hyperplasia can be contrasted with the monomorphous population-obliterating mucosal glands in lymphoma (Fig. 27–6). Second, the lymphoid follicles in hyperplasia are admixed throughout the infiltrate, whereas in lymphoma they are found at the periphery of the lesion. The cytology of the infiltrate also provides a clue, since the large cell "histiocytic" and small cleaved cell types comprising most gastric lymphomas are readily distinguished from the mature cells populating a lymphoid hyperplasia. However, in the rare well-differentiated lymphocytic lymphomas and in suboptimally fixed specimens, distinction from lymphoid hyperplasia may be difficult. Such cases can often be resolved by immunohistochemical studies demonstrating a polyclonal immunoglobulin pattern with prominent T-cell reaction in hyperplastic infiltrates and monoclonal immunophenotyping in malignant ones.[15-17] However, caution is dictated by recent reports of gastric lymphoid hyperplasia exhibiting monotypic cytoplasmic immunoglobulin.[18] Whether these unusual cases represent a prelymphomatous state remains to be determined. Undoubtedly the newer molecular techniques for detecting clonal immunoglobulin gene rearrangements (see below) will be of help in addressing this question.

Also making diagnosis difficult is the large component of inflammatory cells sometimes found in gastrointestinal lymphomas, especially those of the pleomorphic large cell and Mediterranean varieties as well as malignant histiocytosis of the intestine. While these entities rarely involve the stomach, the diagnosis should be suggested by the finding of bizarre atypical lymphocytes scattered within a polymorphous infiltrate.

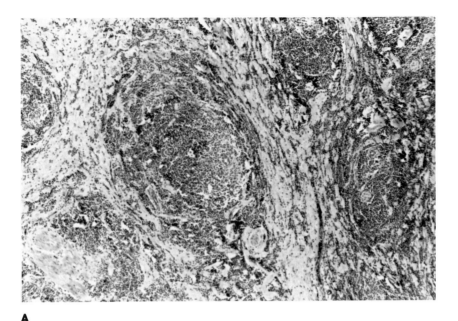

A

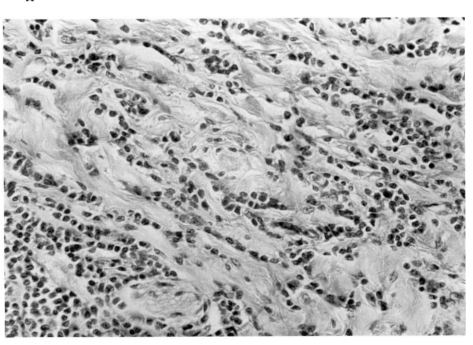

B

Figure 27 – 5 Low- **(A)** and high-power **(B)** histologic architecture of gastric lymphoid hyperplasia, showing abundant lymphoid follicles and intervening collagenous fibrous tissue containing infiltrating lymphocytes in a single-file pattern.

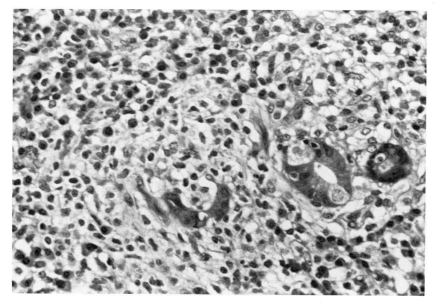

Figure 27 – 6 This monomorphous infiltrate with destruction of gastric glands is characteristic of gastric lymphoma and can be contrasted with the polymorphous infiltrate of gastric lymphoid hyperplasia shown in Figures 27 – 4 and 27 – 5.

General pathologists are most likely to encounter gastric lymphoid hyperplasia as a component at the margins of a typical chronic peptic ulcer. However, on rare occasions gastric lymphoma may have this architectural arrangement, so that careful examination of the lymphoid infiltrate is essential.[4,7]

Malignant Predisposition of Gastric Lymphoid Hyperplasia
While a few cases of gastric lymphoid hyperplasia with an associated lymphoma have been reported,[7,19-21] a definite precursor relationship remains to be established. Significantly, none of the reported cases of lymphoid hyperplasia expressing a monotypic immunoglobulin pattern has thus far developed recurrence or progressed to disseminated lymphoma.[22] Some patients with other so-called pseudo-lymphomas in sites such as lymph nodes, salivary glands, and orbit have subsequently developed lymphoma, and so it is likely that the potential for predisposition exists in gastric lymphoid hyperplasia as well, albeit as a rare event.

Despite the recent introduction of the large particle biopsy forceps to retrieve more abundant material for study, caution is advised in interpretation, since both lymphoid hyperplasia and gastric lymphoma may be superficially ulcerated, and an endoscopic procedure may biopsy only that part. Laparotomy therefore continues to be necessary for diagnosis in a substantial proportion of cases.

Focal Lymphoid Hyperplasia of the Small Intestine

This is an exceedingly uncommon condition with few acceptable cases in the literature that could clearly be distinguished from lymphoma.[4,23] We have seen three cases, one located in the duodenum and two in the mid-small intestine.[24]

Patients usually present with recurrent abdominal pain, and radiologic examination reveals a focal constricting lesion. Grossly there is nodular or circumferential thickening of the mucosa. In contrast to gastric lymphoid hyperplasia, the mucosa is not ulcerated. Histologic and cytologic criteria for distinguishing the lesion from lymphoma are as described for gastric lymphoid hyperplasia.[25]

Focal Lymphoid Hyperplasia of the Rectum

Focal lymphoid hyperplasia of the large intestine appears to be located almost exclusively in the rectum, where it produces symptoms of bleeding, constipation, anal discomfort, prolapse of a rectal mass, and diarrhea.[26-28] Patients frequently have associated anorectal lesions, such as hemorrhoids, anal fissures, and colonic carcinoma. The condition occurs in all age groups but is most common in the second to fifth decades.

Usually the lowermost 10–15 cm of the rectum is affected.[4] Most lesions present as single polyps; when multiple, they usually number less than six. However, the polyps may sometimes be numerous enough to impart a cobblestone appearance to the mucosa.[29] The polyps are most commonly sessile, from a few mm to 5 cm in diameter, with a smooth surface and a pale yellow or white color.[4,26,30]

Microscopically, a heavy lymphoid infiltrate containing large follicles with prominent germinal centers is present in the lamina propria and submucosa (Fig. 27–7). Ulceration is not a typical feature, and low-lying polyps may even be covered by anal squamous epithelium.[4,26,30-32] The lymphoid nodules straddle the mucosa and submucosa and are therefore in a location similar to the solitary lymphoid nodules found in the normal colon. Differentiation from malignant lymphoma is not often an issue, since the latter is exceedingly rare at this site.[33]

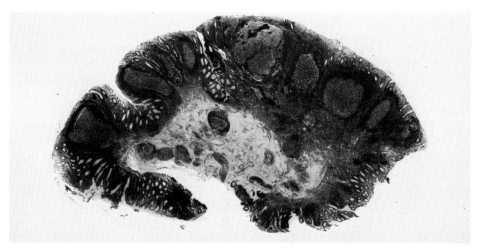

Figure 27–7 Focal lymphoid hyperplasia of the rectum, demonstrating polyploid appearance of the lesion with large lymphoid follicles and intact but attenuated surface epithelium. From Ranchod M, et al: Lymphoid hyperplasia of the gastrointestinal tract: a study of 26 cases and review of the literature. *Am J Surg Path* 2:383–400, 1978, with permission.

Diagnostic excisional biopsy is acceptable treatment for lymphoid polyps of the rectum. If the lesions are multiple and the patient is asymptomatic, complete excision is probably not necessary since these lesions can apparently regress spontaneously, and the incidence of local recurrence is low.[4,30]

Focal Nodular Lymphoid Hyperplasia of the Terminal Ileum and Appendix

Lymphoid hyperplasia of the terminal ileum and appendix may occur either together or separately and is usually found in children or young adults.[34-39] Involvement of the appendix is much less frequently reported,[34,35] possibly because appendices in this age group normally have such active lymphoid tissue that the question arises as to what constitutes abnormal lymphoid proliferation. It is our belief that pathologic features that have the potential for producing symptoms, such as thickening and swelling of the appendix with luminal narrowing, should be seen before a diagnosis of focal lymphoid hyperplasia is made. Patients with ileal or appendiceal involvement usually present with ileocecal intussusception or a clinical syndrome that simulates acute appendicitis.[40-43] Less frequently, hematochezia may be the major complaint.[43]

Gross examination shows that the mucosa of the terminal ileum is thickened and may have a cobblestone appearance. A more distinct mass lesion, which may have a papillary appearance, has also been described. Lymphoid hyperplasia of the appendix results in swelling and thickening of the mucosa and submucosa and luminal obliteration (Fig. 27–8). Histologically, both the terminal ileum and appendix show marked hyperplasia of mucosal and submucosal lymphoid tissue with many lymphoid follicles containing conspicuous germinal centers (Fig. 27–9).

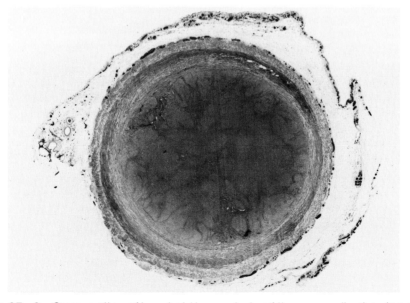

Figure 27 – 8   Cross section of lymphoid hyperplasia of the appendix, showing obliteration of the lumen by mucosal and submucosal lymphoid nodules.

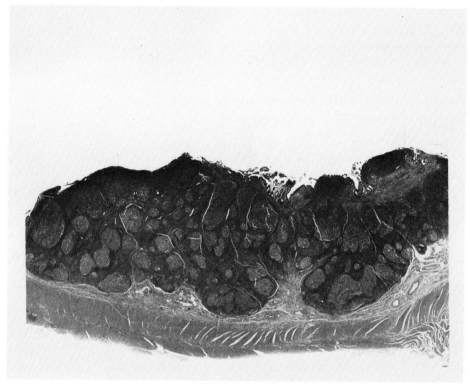

Figure 27–9 Lymphoid hyperplasia of the ileum, demonstrating marked hyperplasia of mucosal and submucosal lymphoid tissue, with abundant lymphoid follicles and germinal centers. From Ranchod M, et al: Lymphoid hyperplasia of the gastrointestinal tract: a study of 26 cases and review of the literature. *Am J Surg Path* 2:383–400, 1978, with permission.

Differentiation from nodular lymphoma may require immunophenotyping or gene rearrangement studies.

Development of intussusception is usually seen in infants who do not have an ileocecal mass lesion due to lymphoid hyperplasia but rather a more modest degree of lymphoid expansion. Possibly the strategic circumferential distribution of the lymphoid tissue in the ileocecal valve[44] may be important in providing the stimulus for intussusception (Fig. 27–10). The recent isolation of various adenovirus strains from patients with ileocecal intussusception[45,46] and the occasional demonstration of adenovirus in intussuscepted tissue[46] suggest that at least some cases of ileocecal lymphoid hyperplasia may have an infectious etiology. Nodular lymphoid hyperplasia of the terminal ileum has also been described in patients with familial polyposis and Gardner's syndrome.[47,48]

Diffuse Nodular Lymphoid Hyperplasia of the Intestine

Diffuse nodular lymphoid hyperplasia is characterized by the presence of numerous small discrete lymphoid nodules involving a variable segment of the small

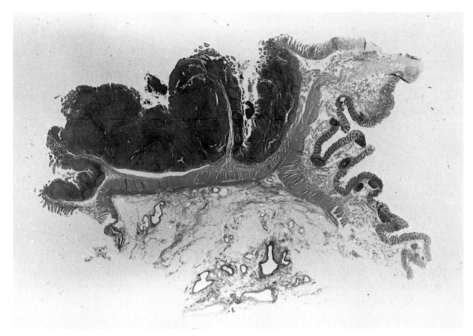

Figure 27 – 10 Lymphoid hyperplasia of the terminal ileum in an infant who presented with intussusception.

intestine, large intestine, or both. It can be divided into two major clinicopathologic groups: those with acquired hypogammaglobulinemia and those without. Use of the term gastrointestinal pseudoleukemia for this condition[49] is confusing and should be abandoned, since it implies a circulating component that does not exist.

With Hypogammaglobulinemia

This form occurs most commonly with late-onset hypogammaglobulinemia and occasionally in isolated IgA deficiency.[50-52] Conversely, however, only a small proportion of patients with late-onset hypogammaglobulinemia develop nodular lymphoid hyperplasia. Most patients present in the second to fifth decades[51] and have decreased serum IgG and normal, decreased, or absent serum IgA and IgM in various combinations, which manifest as recurrent sinopulmonary infections or diarrhea. Giardiasis is commonly present and appears to be responsible for the diarrhea in many but not all patients.[51,53-57] However, even in those patients whose diarrhea responds to Flagyl and antibiotic therapy, there is no corresponding disappearance of the lymphoid nodules.[51] A variety of associated conditions may be encountered, including pernicious anemia, cholelithiasis, thyrotoxicosis, myxedema, diverse skin lesions, arthritis, keratoconjunctivitis, splenomegaly, and sarcoidosis.[58] Most important, however, is the increased risk of developing neoplasms, up to 24% incidence in the series of Hermans et al.,[51] with carcinoma of the gastrointestinal tract being the most frequent.[51,59-61] Lymphomas, including one of gastrointestinal origin, have also been reported.[51]

Nodular lymphoid hyperplasia with hypogammaglobulinemia most commonly affects the small intestine only, but occasionally colonic and rarely gastric involvement may occur.[4,51,54,62] Grossly, the mucosa is studded with sessile or polypoid nodules, measuring up to 5 mm in diameter;[4,51,63] they appear on barium studies as multiple translucencies.[51] Histologically, the lesions are composed of one or several hyperplastic lymphoid nodules. When large, these nodules may produce blunting of the overlying villi, but mucosal ulceration is not seen. The lymphoid nodules are confined to the lamina propria and superficial submucosa (Fig. 27–11), but a similar type of lymphoid hyperplasia is commonly found in mesenteric lymph nodes. A decrease or absence of plasma cells is often noted in the lamina propria. Even those patients who appear to have normal numbers of mucosal plasma cells can be shown by immunoperoxidase staining to have an absence or paucity of IgA-marking cells and compensatory hyperplasia of IgM or IgG isotypes. It has been postulated that the lymphoid hyperplasia that occurs in these patients represents a compensatory proliferation of lymphocytes, which are unable to undergo full maturation to immunoglobulin-secreting cells.[53,55,64]

Without Hypogammaglobulinemia

This form is in fact much more frequent than nodular lymphoid hyperplasia associated with late-onset hypogammaglobulinemia. Robinson et al.,[65] in a study of 1,000 consecutive autopsies, found 30 incidental cases of nodular lymphoid hyperplasia in patients who had died without gastrointestinal symptoms, giardiasis, or hypogammaglobulinemia. They applied the term "enterocolitis lymphofollicularis" to this lesion, but we prefer the term diffuse nodular lymphoid hyperplasia because of its morphologic similarity to that seen in late-onset hypogammaglobulinemia, and because it shows no evidence of a classical "enterocolitis" characterized by inflammation and mucosal destruction. In their series, Robinson et al[65] found that the small intestine alone was involved in 13% of cases, the large intes-

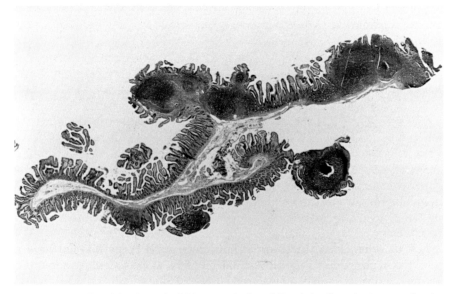

Figure 27–11 Nodular lymphoid hyperplasia of the intestine from a patient with common variable immunodeficiency disease, showing numerous mucosal lymphoid nodules with blunting of overlying intestinal villi.

tine alone in 40%, and the small and large intestine together in 47%. As at autopsy, nodular lymphoid hyperplasia of the colon is a common incidental finding on barium enema, especially in children who are being worked up for a variety of unrelated gastrointestinal complaints.[66-68] Serum immunoglobulin levels are typically normal.[66]

The mucosal nodules in this disorder usually measure up to 0.4 cm in diameter, but rarely they may reach 2 cm in size.[69] Histologic patterns resemble those seen in the hypogammaglobulinemic form, except that the lamina propria contains normal numbers of plasma cells.

It is probable that these lesions represent hyperplasia of the solitary lymphoid follicles normally present in the gastrointestinal tract.[66-69] Support for this concept is provided by the umbilication of the colonic nodules, which Franken[67] and Capitanio and Kirkpatrick[66] consider helpful in making the diagnosis radiologically. This radiologic umbilication has its histologic counterpart in modifications of the mucosal crypts of Lieberkuhn associated with solitary colonic follicles. One or more of the crypts overlying the lymphoid follicle are widened and elongated, allowing trapping of barium to produce the umbilication seen radiologically. In view of this, diffuse nodular lymphoid hyperplasia must be considered in any differential diagnosis of multiple polypoidal lesions seen radiologically in the colon. This is especially important in patients who are being evaluated for familial polyposis, in whom unnecessary colonic resection may be performed.[55,59,70] Since patients with the hypogammaglobulinemic form of nodular lymphoid hyperplasia are asymptomatic, and there are well-documented cases of spontaneous regression,[66-68] resection of these lesions is unnecessary.

Nodular lymphoid hyperplasia must also be distinguished from multiple lymphomatous polyposis of the intestine,[71] which may be difficult if the lymphoma is follicular and lymphocytic in type. It should also be kept in mind that patients with nodular lymphoid hyperplasia without hypogammaglobulinemia do occasionally develop lymphoma.[59,72] Indeed, Matuchansky et al.[59] were able to demonstrate immunohistochemically a transition from hyperplastic lymphoid follicles to neoplastic ones in one case.

MALIGNANT LYMPHOMA

Conditions Associated With an Increased Risk of Lymphoma

A number of gastrointestinal lesions are found in association with or appear to predispose to malignant gastrointestinal lymphomas (Table 27–2). They are discussed individually below.

Celiac Disease
Patients with celiac sprue (with or without dermatitis herpetiformis) have an increased risk of developing gastrointestinal lymphoma and carcinoma, accounting for a major proportion of the mortality in these patients.[73-78] The characteristic clinical setting is that of a known celiac, usually in his fifties, who deteriorates for no apparent reason,[76] although in some cases the associated celiac sprue is clinically occult.[77]

Table 27-2 CONDITIONS PREDISPOSING TO GASTROINTESTINAL LYMPHOMA

Celiac disease including dermatitis herpetiformis
Immunoproliferative small intestinal disease (Mediterranean lymphoma and alpha-chain disease)
Lymphoid hyperplasia of the gastrointestinal tract, especially gastric lymphoid hyperplasia and diffuse nodular lymphoid hyperplasia (with and without hypogammaglobulinemia)
Immunodeficiency disorders of the gastrointestinal tract
Primary, especially common variable immunodeficiency and selective IgA deficiency
Acquired, especially AIDS, and transplantation
Ulcerative colitis and Crohn's disease

Pathology
Lesions may be single or diffuse and involve primarily the small intestine, although occasionally the stomach or mesenteric nodes alone are affected. The diseased bowel is usually thickened and may ulcerate, producing hemorrhage, perforation, or obstruction[74,75,78] and accounting for a tendency in the past to misdiagnose the condition as ulcerative jejunoileitis.

Histologically, both monomorphic (of the diffuse large cell type, Rappaport's "histiocytic" lymphoma), and pleomorphic (with accompanying inflammatory cells and histiocytes) patterns are seen.[78-80] Naturally, the latter are more likely to be misdiagnosed as ulcerative jejunoileitis. The atypical lymphoid cells have large multilobulated, indented, or folded nuclei and prominent nucleoli; they may contain phagocytized erythrocytes, platelets, or cell debris. Reed-Sternberg-like cells are sometimes seen. Initial immunohistochemical studies suggested that these tumors were true histiocytic lymphomas,[78-80] but more recent work indicates that they may be of T-cell origin.[81]

The characteristic polymorphous infiltrate present in endoscopic biopsy material in celiac disease can render the diagnosis of lymphomatous change difficult.[74,82] The finding of a dense inflammatory infiltrate separating the base of the gland crypts from the muscularis mucosa, extending beyond the muscularis mucosa into the submucosa, or containing scattered "atypical lymphocytes" should raise the suspicion of early malignancy.

Treatment
Since lymphoma complicating celiac disease and ulcerative nongranulomatous jejunoileitis may be indistinguishable clinically, and because there is some evidence that the latter may also develop lymphoma,[76] the treatment of both conditions is the same, namely segmental resection and staging. To date there is no evidence that a gluten-free diet protects against the development of lymphoma in celiac disease.[76]

Immunoproliferative Small Intestinal Disease (IPSID)
Many, if not most cases of this indolent lymphoplasmacytic disorder eventually develop an associated lymphoma.[83] The benign and malignant phases of this condition are discussed in detail below.

Lymphoid Hyperplasia of the Gastrointestinal Tract

Evidence concerning the propensity of these lesions to progress to malignant lymphoma has been presented in the discussion of the individual disorders above.

Other Conditions

Immunodeficiency disorders, both congenital and acquired (including AIDS), are associated with an increased risk of lymphoma.[84,85] Lymphoma has also been described in association with ulcerative colitis, Crohn's disease,[86-88] and epithelial neoplasms,[89] although the exact incidence and significance remain unclear.

Lymphoma of the Gastrointestinal Tract and Mesentery

Definition

Primary intestinal lymphomas include those presenting in the gastrointestinal tract with no evidence of liver, spleen, or distal lymph node involvement at the time of presentation. Lymphomas originating in the mesenteric lymph nodes are included as well,[90] by virtue of their similarity in clinical presentation and causal relationship with such prelymphomatous intestinal diseases as celiac sprue and IPSID.[86,91] Questions of definition arise in those cases of lymphoma presenting with gastrointestinal manifestations but that on work-up are found to have microscopic dissemination. Do these represent cases of primary gastrointestinal lymphoma with secondary dissemination (which we know can occur in roughly 50% of cases), or merely nodal lymphoma with intestinal movement? We prefer to regard them as gastrointestinal lymphomas with dissemination, although from a practical point of view the question is somewhat moot, as they need to be managed as disseminated lymphomas.

Etiology and Pathogenesis

Despite the aforementioned clinical association of some cases with predisposing conditions, the etiology and pathogenesis of gastrointestinal lymphomas remains uncertain. Isaacson has noted that these tumors share the specific homing patterns of gut-associated lymphoid tissue, which may account for their characteristic invasion of gastrointestinal glands and tendency to remain localized to the gut for long periods.[92]

The cell of origin of primary gastrointestinal lymphomas has been the subject of controversy for many years. Particularly contentious has been the notion of true histiocytic lymphomas, which some investigators have claimed to be more frequent in the gastrointestinal tract than elsewhere.[93] However, recent immunohistochemical studies, especially when conducted on frozen tissue, have shown that the vast majority of these tumors stain positively for B- or, less often, T-cell markers, indicating that their derivation is in fact from lymphoid cells.[94-96,97] In light of these findings, we feel that true histiocytic lymphomas in the gastrointestinal tract are extremely rare, if they exist at all.

Clinical Presentation

Gastrointestinal lymphoma is a disease of middle age, showing no sex predilection and, with the exception of the Mediterranean lymphomas, no significant racial distribution.[86,98-103] Patients typically present with ulcer symptoms or intestinal obstruction, accompanied by pain and hemorrhage or rarely by perforation and intussusception.[86,90,98,101,102,104,105] Malabsorption is uncommon except in those cases complicating celiac sprue and IPSID.[86]

Pathology

The gastrointestinal tract is the commonest site for primary extranodal lymphomas[86,100,106] and is secondarily involved in about 10% of cases of disseminated nodal lymphoma.[107,108] The most frequent site of involvement is the stomach (50%), followed by the small intestine (37%, usually ileum) and the ileocecal region (13%),[86,101-103,106,109,110] with the remainder of the intestinal tract and mesentery only uncommonly involved.[100,103] At the time of presentation, the lymphoma is confined to the affected viscus in about one-half the cases,[111-113] involves regional nodes in an additional one-third,[86,98,101,103] and has already disseminated more widely in about 20%. These figures, of course, are arrived at only after adequate work-up and staging, since the extent of involvement is not always apparent on initial clinical examination.[86]

Primary gastrointestinal lymphomas are most commonly single. Multiple lesions may occur in up to 20% of intestinal lymphomas and are less common in the stomach.[86,90,102] They usually number from two to six lesions, with diffuse lymphomatous polyposis being a much less common presentation.[90,114,115] The finding of multiple lesions should raise the suspicion of a primary mesenteric lymphoma secondarily involving the gastrointestinal tract.[86]

Gastrointestinal lymphomas usually present at the time of diagnosis as large (average, 7.9 cm) exophytic polypoid masses or infiltrative lesions with a white-yellow appearance on cut section. The infiltrative growths exhibit localized mucosal ulceration and raised margins, and cause either uniform thickening of the bowel or, less commonly, an annular napkin-ring lesion mimicking carcinoma. We have also seen atypical ulcerative lesions without apparent thickening of the bowel wall.

Histologically, gastrointestinal lymphomas are characterized by a monomorphous atypical lymphoid infiltrate causing expansion and thickening of the mucosa, pushing apart and destroying glands and separating muscle fibers (Fig. 27–12). Sometimes the infiltrate may be polymorphous, leading to confusion with the lymphoid hyperplasias.[86,116] Early gastrointestinal lymphoma tends to be limited to the mucosa and superficial submucosa, while more advanced cases are commonly associated with mucosal ulceration and more extensive infiltration of the viscus.

Primary Hodgkin's disease of the gastrointestinal tract is vanishingly rare,[86] and so any overview of gastrointestinal lymphomas falls principally within the non-Hodgkin's group. With the exception of Burkitt's lymphoma and IPSID-associated lymphoma (Mediterranean lymphoma), the histologic types, classified according to the working formulation of the National Cancer Institute,[117] are similar to those encountered in lymph nodes.[86]

Most gastrointestinal lymphomas are diffuse, only 10% being nodular (Fig. 27–13). The majority are of the large cell type (Rappaport's "histiocytic" lymphoma or Luke's large noncleaved follicular center cell lymphoma) (Fig. 27–14).[100] Some of these exhibit a polymorphous infiltrate composed of plasmacytoid cells, atypical immunoblasts, Reed-Sternberg-like cells, and an accompanying inflammatory cell infiltrate composed of mature lymphocytes, plasma cells, histiocytes

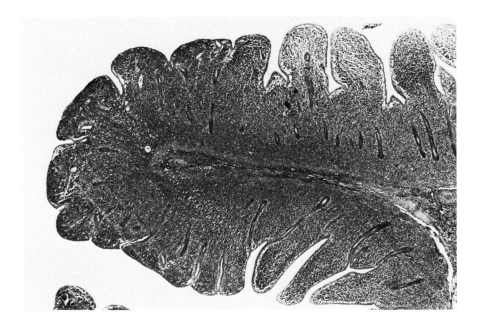

A

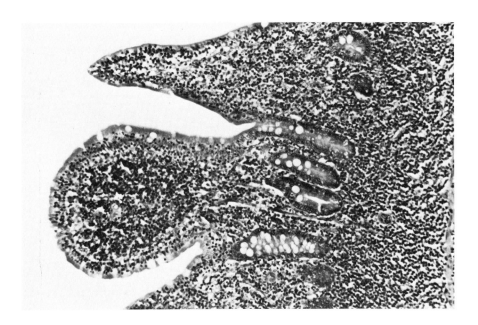

B

Figure 27-12 Malignant lymphoma of the small bowel showing diffuse lymphoid infiltration of the mucosa causing widening of villi and separation of crypt bases from the underlying muscularis mucosa **(A, B)**.

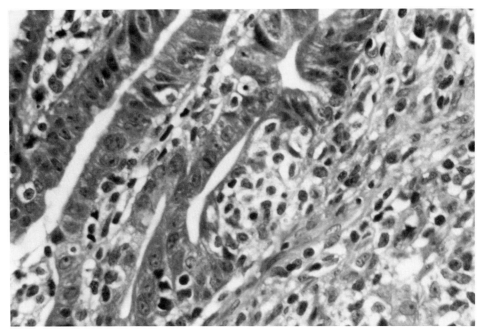

C

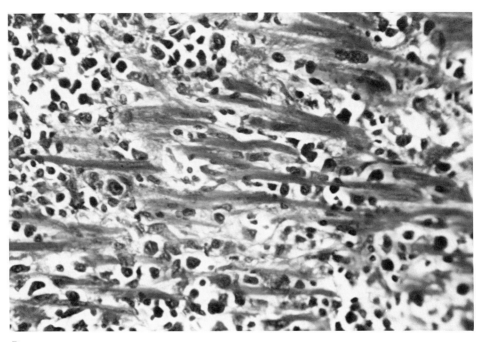

D

Figure 27–12 (cont'd) Infiltration of glandular epithelium **(C)**, and infiltration and separation of muscle fibers within the muscularis mucosa **(D)**.

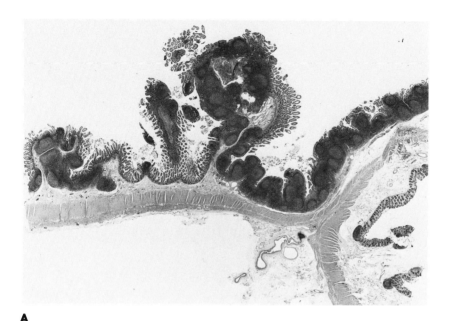

A

B

Figure 27–13 Small intestinal lymphoma of nodular **(A)** and diffuse **(B)** types. The latter exhibits diffuse infiltration of all layers of the bowel wall with adjacent lymph node involvement.

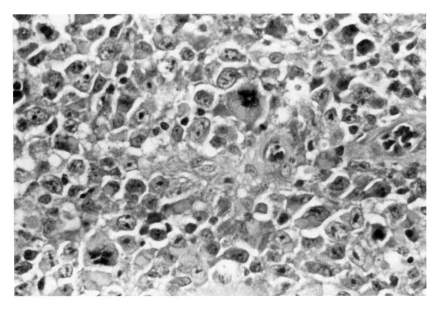

Figure 27–14 Large cell malignant lymphoma (large noncleaved follicular center cell type), characterized by large round vesicular nuclei containing prominent nucleoli and ample cytoplasm.

and sometimes eosinophils, with variable sclerosis;[86] this is equivalent to Rappaport's pleomorphic histiocytic lymphoma or Luke's immunoblastic sarcoma.

The second most common class of gastrointestinal lymphomas are the small cell type, usually cleaved (Rappaport's poorly differentiated lymphocytic lymphoma) (Fig. 27–15). Some of these tumors will show both nodular and diffuse patterns in the same lesion,[118] presumably reflecting evolution from a nodular into a diffuse phase.[119] Recognition of residual nodular areas in these cases may be of important prognostic value. Malignant lymphomas of the small lymphocytic type (well-differentiated lymphocytic lymphoma) are uncommon, and, as is true for these lymphomas elsewhere, one must first exclude a lymphocytic leukemia (Fig. 27–16).

The gastrointestinal tract is one of the sites of predilection for the rare cases of American Burkitt's lymphoma,[86,120,121] primarily in children. They are found most commonly around the ileocecal region and in the mesenteric nodes and usually exhibit a "starry sky" pattern of undifferentiated lymphoid cells, with scant cytoplasm, regular round nuclei, finely dispersed chromatin, and numerous small nucleoli (Fig. 27–17). These tumors may show a nodular pattern,[86] consistent with recent evidence that nonendemic Burkitt's lymphoma is of B-cell origin and may selectively involve B-cell areas such as Peyer's patches and solitary lymphoid follicles.[122] Other histologic patterns occasionally encountered include mixed small and large cell lymphomas, immunoblastic (Fig. 27–18) or signet-ring cell (Fig. 27–19) lymphomas, and composite lymphomas.[86]

Differential Diagnosis
The major problems in diagnosis are encountered in differentiating some lymphomas from lymphoid hyperplasia and poorly differentiated adenocarcinoma,

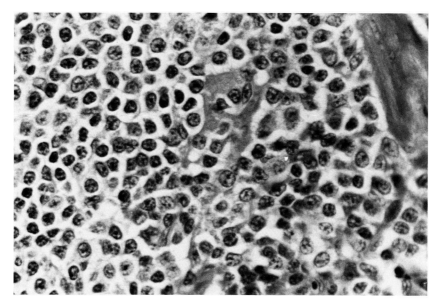

Figure 27–15 Malignant lymphoma, small cleaved cell type (poorly differentiated lymphocytic lymphoma in the Rappaport classification.)

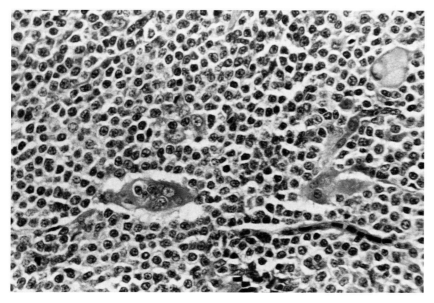

Figure 27–16 Malignant lymphoma, small lymphocytic type (well-differentiated lymphocytic lymphoma). Note the monomorphic population of mature-looking lymphocytes.

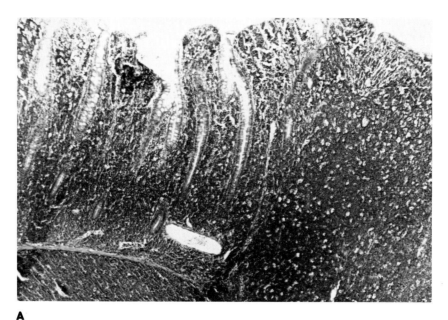

A

B

Figure 27–17 Burkitt's lymphoma, illustrating the classic "starry sky" pattern **(A)** resulting from interspersed macrophages containing phagacytosed nuclear debris **(B)**. The bulk of the infiltrate is composed of lymphocytes with scant cytoplasm, regular round nuclei, and small nucleoli.

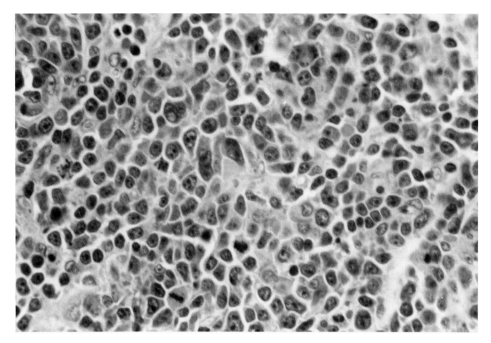

Figure 27–18 Malignant lymphoma, large cell immunoblastic type, showing marked pleomorphism of nuclei.

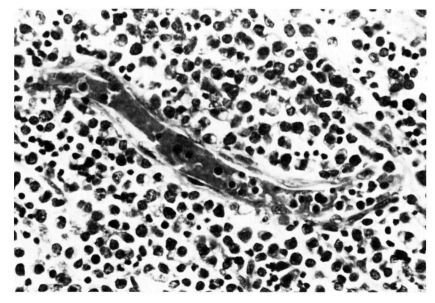

Figure 27–19 Malignant lymphoma, signet-ring cell type, produced by cytoplasmic vacuolization.

especially in the rare cases of malignant lymphoma of the small lymphocytic type (well differentiated) because of the mature nature of the lymphoid infiltrate. At the opposite end of the spectrum are the pleomorphic large cell and the IPSID-associated lymphomas whose polymorphous infiltrates and predominance of inflammatory cells may obscure the atypical lymphoid cells. Immunohistochemistry or gene rearrangement studies may be helpful in these situations.

Poorly differentiated adenocarcinoma can on occasion be almost indistinguishable from lymphoma, especially in the stomach. Multiple sections should be examined for evidence of glandular differentiation, a transition zone of tumor arising from atypical glands, or immunohistochemical staining for keratins and/or carcinoembryonic antigen versus common leukocyte antigen.

The rare cases of multiple lymphomatous polyposis may cause confusion with nodular lymphoid hyperplasia,[86,90,115,123] but only the latter will be comprised of nodules with prominent germinal centers largely confined to the lamina propria.

Progression of Disease and Prognosis
Progression of lymphoma, seen in about 60% of cases[86,99,103,124] occurs by local extension to adjacent soft tissues and by drainage to mesenteric and periaortic lymph nodes. Involvement of other abdominal viscera may also occur.[86,98,103,125] Extra-abdominal spread occurs in up to 50% of cases, involving most commonly the peripheral lymph nodes, lung, brain, and meninges,[86] although virtually all organs are vulnerable.[86,126] There appears to be no correlation between the propensity for extra-abdominal dissemination and the initial site or stage of the tumor.[86] The majority of relapses occur early, and most patients die within 1 year of relapse.

Despite this finding, overall survival with gastrointestinal lymphomas is relatively good, the 5-year survival being about 45%.[86,125-129] Clinical stage at presentation is crucial: 2-year actuarial survival when tumors are localized to the viscus and regional nodes is about 75%, compared with 0% for more widespread dissemination.[86] There is also some evidence that stage 1 lesions (lymphoma confined to the viscus) have a better prognosis than those with accompanying involvement of regional lymph nodes (stage 2), but reports in the literature are conflicting on this point,[86,105,126,128-133] possibly due to variability of the staging procedures employed.[86] The site of the primary tumor may also be of prognostic significance, with gastric and cecal lymphomas registering a more favorable 5-year survival than tumors of the small intestine and rectum.[86,98,101,104,120] Likewise, the histologic subtype may have an influence, as nodular lymphomas and diffuse small (well-differentiated) lymphocytic lymphomas appear to do better than diffuse large cell lymphomas.[123,127-129,134]

Treatment
Patients treated with surgery and postoperative radiotherapy and/or chemotherapy appear to do significantly better than those treated with surgery alone,[126-130,135] and it has even been suggested that resection before definitive radiation therapy is unnecessary.[136] However, we feel strongly that resection of the primary lesion is important in order to achieve local control and prevent the high risk of bleeding and perforation that may complicate radiotherapy. Also, since it has such important implications for prognosis, the full extent of disease should be ascertained by a proper staging procedure,[86,99,125,136] including sampling of mesenteric and para-aortic lymph nodes, biopsy of the liver, careful inspection of the spleen, and exclusion of a nodal lymphoma as the primary source of the intestinal lesion.

Childhood Lymphomas

Gastrointestinal lymphomas in childhood show a number of statistical differences compared with those in adults.[86] The childhood tumors occur almost exclusively in the ileum and ileocecal region, in contrast to the common involvement of other sites, notably the stomach, in adults. The proportion of histopathologic types also differs: while large cell lymphoma is again the most frequent variety, small cell lymphomas are noticeably rare, mirroring the types of childhood lymphomas encountered in other sites.[111] The overall survival figures for children are comparable with those in adults.[86]

Secondary Malignant Lymphomas and Leukemias

While many of the overall clinical features are the same, disseminated lymphoma with secondary gastrointestinal involvement is more likely to produce marked ulcers in the stomach and to involve multiple gastrointestinal sites than primary intestinal lymphoma.[99,136,137] They also have a much poorer survival (3%).

Gastrointestinal complications of leukemia occur in up to 25% of cases[138–144] and include tumorous infiltration of the bowel with ulceration and obstruction, opportunistic infection usually localized to the esophagus and large bowel but sometimes disseminated,[139] and neutropenic enterocolitis, which may result in perforation and gram-negative septicemia.[139,140,143,144]

IPSID and IPSID-Associated Lymphoma (Mediterranean Lymphoma and Alpha-Chain Disease)

IPSID was first described in a group of Oriental Jews and Arabs with primary small bowel lymphoma,[145,146] but subsequently it became apparent that this disease had a more widespread distribution, and it has since been encountered in many parts of the world.[86,91,145–152] Beginning in 1968, cases of IPSID were reported in which an abnormal paraprotein, consisting of alpha-chains devoid of light chains, was secreted into the serum and jejunal juices. These cases were designated as alpha-chain disease.[91,153–159] The amount of heavy-chain secretion varied greatly from case to case, and sometimes could be demonstrated only immunocytochemically within the plasma cell cytoplasm. Confusion surfaced in the literature as to whether all cases of IPSID with or without lymphoma produced the abnormal paraprotein and were really cases of alpha-chain disease. We now know that IPSID can occur ab initio with or without lymphoma,[83,91] that lymphoma does not invariably develop in these cases,[83,160] and that IPSID with or without lymphoma need not necessarily produce a paraprotein. About 30–50% will do so,[160,162] and rarely other abnormal gammaglobulins are produced, such as gamma-heavy-chain.[163,164]

Clinical Presentation
Cases of IPSID with or without alpha-chain production are indistinguishable. Young persons are primarily affected, with no sex predilection. The disorder is characterized by malabsorption, producing symptoms of chronic diarrhea, weight loss, and abdominal pain. Presentation in the form of an acute abdominal crisis due to obstruction or intestinal perforation has been reported.[91,145]

Etiology

The etiology and pathogenesis of IPSID are the subject of much speculation, with both genetic and environmental factors implicated. Most cases have been reported in patients with a low socioeconomic living standard, poor hygiene, malnutrition, and a high rate of intestinal infections.[91,165,166] There is an apparent association with HLA types AW19 and B12.[91,151] Because some patients with plasma cell infiltration apparently remit spontaneously or reportedly respond to antibiotic therapy, and because alpha-heavy-chain is not usually demonstrated in the malignant infiltrate,[79] it has been postulated that plasma cell infiltration is a benign proliferative response to antigenic stimulation, possibly in genetically predisposed individuals, which subsequently undergoes malignant dedifferentiation, perhaps due to some oncogenic agent. However, it is of note that clonal immunoglobulin gene rearrangements have been detected even in the initial plasma cell infiltration stage (prior to histologically overt lymphoma),[167] and so it may be incorrect to consider this strictly a "benign" process. Others have suggested that the antigenic response initiates an immune-deficient state that predisposes patients to lymphomas.

Pathology

The two morphologic stages of IPSID are: 1) a benign-appearing diffuse plasmacytic cell infiltration of the lamina propria (PCI) (Fig. 27–20A); and 2) malignant lymphoma superimposed on the diffuse plasmacytic infiltrate (Fig. 27–20B). The latter stage has been designated IPSID-associated lymphoma (IAL)[160] and also Mediterranean lymphoma. Cases of IPSID are histologically indistinguishable from alpha-chain disease, aside from the immunohistochemical detection of the abnormal paraprotein in the latter.[160,168]

The PCI stage is characterized by diffuse involvement of the jejunum with frequent extension to the ileum but only rarely encompassing the stomach or large bowel. Grossly, the plasmacytic infiltrate causes dilatation of the small bowel and thickening of the mucosal folds. Histologically, an infiltrate composed of mature-appearing plasma cells and, less commonly, mature lymphocytes is seen in the lamina propria, displacing crypts upward away from the muscularis mucosa and causing variable villous blunting (Fig. 27–21).[83,91] Probably in the majority of cases (although it may take many years), the infiltrate becomes progressively atypical and extends beyond the muscularis mucosa (Fig. 27–21, lower left).

The IAL stage may be multifocal and is grossly characterized by diffuse thickening of the viscus.[109,145,150] Ulcerated lesions may also be seen.[91] Microscopically, the infiltrate is usually polymorphous, composed of atypical small lymphoid cells, plasmacytoid cells, and Reed-Sternberg-like cells, admixed with mature plasma cells, lymphocytes, and eosinophils (Fig. 46).[91] However, we and others[160] have also seen cases with a more monomorphous infiltrate resembling diffuse large cell noncleaved lymphoma (Fig. 47). Although the lymphoma usually involves the jejunum, it may spare the small intestine and involve the mesenteric lymph nodes only, usually with preservation of the medullary sinuses.[205]

Diagnosis and Differential Diagnosis

Once IPSID is suspected by finding the characteristic diffuse plasmacytic infiltrate in the lamina propria, it should be determined whether the patient has alpha-chain disease by detection of paraprotein in serum, urine, or jejunal juices and also by

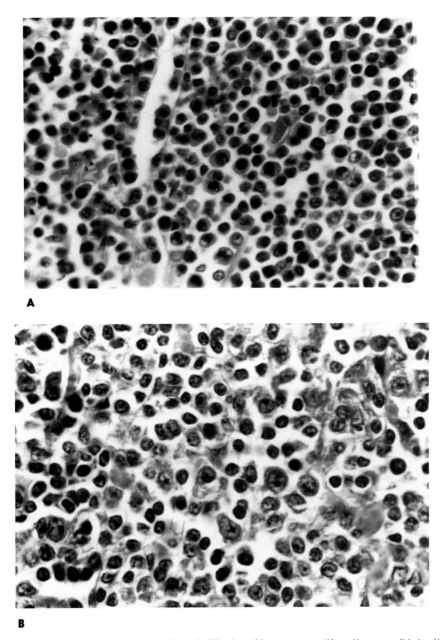

Figure 27 – 20 The monomorphous infiltrate of immunoproliferative small intestinal disease (IPSID), composed of mature-appearing lymphocytes **(A),** contrasted with the polymorphous infiltrate of IPSID-associated lymphoma with its mixture of mature lymphocytes, immunoblasts, and plasmacytoid cells **(B).**

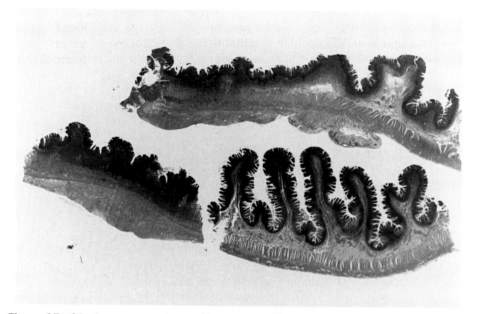

Figure 27–21 Low-power views of immunoproliferative small intestinal disease with dense lymphoid infiltrate confined to the mucosa (lower right tissue fragment), and IPSID-associated lymphoma showing extension of the infiltrate through all layers of the small intestine (left and above).

immunohistochemistry in tissue sections. In many cases the abnormality is not detected by routine immunoelectrophoresis with polyvalent antiserum, and mono-specific antiserum to IgA is required.[145]

Histologically, the disorder must be differentiated from other conditions causing villous blunting and increased plasmacytic infiltration of the lamina propria, such as celiac disease, infectious gastroenteritis, kwashiorkor, and tropical sprue.[91] In IPSID the dominant feature is the dense plasma cell infiltration, whereas in the other disorders it is a secondary phenomenon. The finding of a massive plasmacytic infiltration predominantly in the stomach raises the question of whether this manifestation should be designated as IPSID. The answer is unknown, because although the typical histological features of the disorder are displayed, albeit at an unusual site, the clinical behavior of such gastric lesions remains to be determined.

The usual gastrointestinal lymphomas seen in the USA, the "Western type" lymphomas, will not normally be confused with IPSID-associated lymphomas, since the former involve mainly the stomach and ileum rather than the jejunum; they also lack the massive plasma cell infiltrate in the lamina propria adjacent to the tumor.[91] Occasionally "Western type" lymphomas have been reported to produce alpha-heavy-chain,[169,170] but they lack the other clinicopathologic features of IPSID.

Prognosis and Management
IPSID may persist in an indolent state for years[152] [up to 7 in one report[83]] and may even go into remission on antihelminthic and antibiotic therapy.[160] However, once

the lymphomatous phase supervenes, the prognosis is generally poor, with an average survival of 32 months. Since patients seldom have evidence of disease above the diaphragm, wide-field abdominal radiation has been the recommended treatment,[160] although prior resection of tumor may be necessary to reduce the range of postradiation bowel perforation.[91]

Solitary Plasmacytomas of the Gastrointestinal Tract

These lesions are uncommon, accounting for 4–12% of extramedullary plasmacytomas.[171–174] Clinically they present many of the features characteristic of myelomas, including prevalence in middle-aged and elderly men[172] and not infrequent association with a monoclonal protein spike in the serum or urine.[173,175]

Pathology
The majority are located in the stomach and small bowel,[173,174,176,177] but cases have also been described in the colon.[178] The histologic hallmark is a monomorphous infiltrate of plasma cells, sometimes with extracellular amyloid deposition. The plasma cells may contain crystalline inclusions,[174,179,180] and those cases are invariably associated with a dysproteinemia. Some tumors may display more cellular pleomorphism, and we have seen an unusual case with numerous bizarre Russell's bodies. The differential diagnosis must include localized extramedullary manifestations of multiple myeloma, inflammatory pseudotumors (plasma cell granulomas),[172,178,181–183] and the massive plasmacytic cell infiltration associated with Mediterranean lymphoma and alpha-chain disease.[91] The lack of bone marrow plasmacytosis in multiple aspirations will help to exclude multiple myeloma.[172] Pseudotumors can usually be excluded histologically by demonstrating a monomorphic population of plasma cells with little admixture of inflammatory cells or granulomatous change.[172,178,181] In addition, the neoplastic nature of the lesion can be demonstrated immunohistochemically by detection of a single immunoglobulin in the plasma cells.[177–179,184]

Treatment
Surgery with or without local radiotherapy appears to be the treatment of choice, although some authorities have advocated chemotherapy.[172]

Work-Up of Gastrointestinal Lymphomas

Endoscopic Biopsy
Provided the biopsy is adequate in size, not crushed, and not from a deeply ulcerated area, a diagnosis of malignant lymphoma can frequently be confirmed by endoscopy. Biopsies showing mainly necrosis and a mixed inflammatory infiltrate may be difficult to interpret, since these findings may be seen in superficial biopsies of ulcerated lymphomas and in gastric lymphoid hyperplasia, both of which are commonly associated with peptic ulceration. In these cases it is important to take additional biopsies from multiple sites. The endoscopist should be careful to avoid causing unnecessary crush artifact when removing the tissue from the biopsy forceps. Use of the new large particle forceps now available will often yield superior specimens subject to much less distortion. Finally, separate biopsy material should

be obtained and quickly frozen for subsequent immunohistochemical studies. If repeat biopsies do not resolve the issue of lymphoma versus lymphoid hyperplasia, laparotomy will be necessary.

Laparotomy
It should be stressed that once laparotomy is undertaken, lymphoma staging is essential to determine the extent of the disease. Laparotomy is also a convenient time to obtain adequate amounts of frozen tissue for immunophenotyping or subsequent DNA extraction for gene rearrangement studies.

Special Diagnostic Techniques

Immunohistochemistry
Lymphomas are tumors of transformed lymphocytes whose benign counterparts comprise the major arms of the immune system: T cells, B cells, and their various subsets. Over the last 10–15 years, a wide array of cytoplasmic and cell surface proteins have been identified as specific for one or another lymphocyte subset, or even for a defined stage of maturation within a given subset. Thus, for example, the presence of surface immunoglobulins is a marker of B cells, antigen CD20 is a marker of pre-B cells, antigen T3 is a marker of both mature T cells and pre-T cells, and so on.[185,186] Use of a fluorescent or enzymatically labeled primary or secondary antibody raised against these antigens will allow their detection in tissue sections (immunohistochemistry) or in monodisperse cell suspensions (flow cytometry; see below). When morphologic criteria alone are insufficient or ambiguous, such techniques can be used: 1) to determine whether a poorly differentiated tumor is of lymphoid origin; 2) to ascertain the specific cell type (i.e., B- or T-cell subset); and 3) in the case of B-cell lesions, to determine whether a suspicious infiltrate represents a monoclonal (hence malignant) or polyclonal (e.g., inflammatory or hyperplastic) proliferation. This last distinction is made by applying antibodies specific for surface immunoglobulins and observing uniform expression of one or the other light chain in a lymphoma, in contrast to polyclonal expression of *kappa or lambda* in the normal 2:1 ratio in an inflammatory or hyperplastic lesion[16] (Fig. 27–22).

Immunohistochemistry is a tricky procedure requiring careful quality control and cognizance of potential artifacts resulting from poor tissue fixation or variability in specificity of commercial antibodies. Also, there are some difficult cases in which immunohistochemistry is simply not a powerful enough technique for extracting useful information. In these cases, one of the newer approaches described below may be helpful.

Flow Cytometry
This technique allows for the rapid characterization and statistical analysis of enormous numbers of cells within a lesion, using essentially the same antibody reagents applied to immunohistochemistry.[187,188] Because of the numbers involved and the fact that the fluorescence of each individual cell is determined electronically, results are less prone to the subjective bias of the human eye by light microscopy. Moreover, the sensitivity of the technique is sufficient to pick up small subpopulations of cells and low-intensity antigens that would be undetectable by immunohistochemistry. New developments in multiparameter analysis using double fluorochrome labeling permit the simultaneous quantitation of B cells, mono-

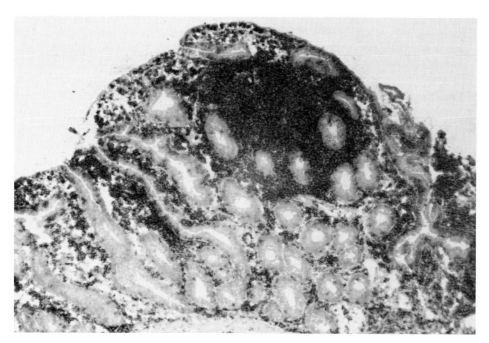

Figure 27–22   Mucosal biopsy of a malignant lymphoma demonstrating monotypic immunoperoxidase staining for kappa-light-chain.

cytes, T-helper cells, T-suppressor cells, and natural killer (NK) cells.[189] However, the general applicability of the technique is still limited by cost considerations, difficulty in obtaining representative monodisperse cell suspensions for analysis, and some of the same problems with reagent specificity that continue to plague immunohistochemistry.

DNA Hybridization
The markers of lymphoid differentiation detected phenotypically by immunohisto-chemistry and flow cytometry can be evaluated earlier, more sensitively, and more precisely by analysis of the lymphoid genotype at the DNA level. This is made possible by the recent dramatic expansion in knowledge about the molecular biology of normal lymphocyte development. It is now known that lymphocytes achieve their incredible degree of immunologic diversity (i.e., the ability to respond to a virtually infinite variety of foreign antigens) by undergoing gene rearrangements of their antigen receptor loci (immunoglobulin genes in the B-cell lineage and T-cell receptor genes in the T-cell lineage).[190] The nature of the rearrangements is so varied and complex that they can be used to determine both clonality and cell of origin of the daughter populations.[191]

   Molecular analysis of these rearrangements for diagnostic purposes is based on two premises, both of which may be somewhat overly simplistic. The first is that lymphoid neoplasia is a clonal process, while nonneoplastic, inflammatory, and hyperplastic disorders are either nonclonal or polyclonal. The second assumption is that any cell that has rearranged its immunoglobulin genes is of B-cell origin, while a cell exhibiting rearrangement of T-cell receptor genes is of T-cell lineage.

Both heavy- and light-chain immunoglobulin subunits, as well as a and a' T-cell receptor subunits, are formed by the rearrangement of germline DNA, which brings initially distant variable (V) region sequences into proximity with joining (J and D) region and constant (C) region sequences. (Actually, the final stage in linking C with V-D-J sequences is via RNA splicing rather than DNA rearrangement.) Depending upon which of a battery of individual V, J, and D genes have been chosen for incorporation within the final receptor molecule by a particular cell (which will be a different combination for each clonal cell halotype), restriction endonuclease cleavage of the rearranged DNA followed by electrophoresis and Southern blot hybridization[192] with a radioactively labeled J-region DNA probe will yield different-sized rearranged fragments.[193] In an inflammatory or hyperplastic reaction containing a polymorphous population of lymphocytes responding to many different antigenic epitopes, countless DNA rearrangements will be represented, yielding a mixture of so many different-sized fragments on the Southern blot that the hybridization pattern will appear as a diffuse smear with only the constant germline band standing out. In a malignant lesion, however, in which all or most of the cells have arisen from a single clone, a clonal rearrangement band will be seen on the Southern blot in a position different from the germline band. The sensitivity of the technique is such that if as few as 1% of the cells in a mixed lesion have arisen from a single clone, a rearranged band will be visible on the blot.[194] This makes possible detection of an incipient lymphoma in a suspicious lesion, or early occult recurrence after therapy, long before its malignant nature would be evident by either routine histology or immunohistochemistry. For example, Smith et al.[167] used such an analysis to detect clonal immunoglobulin gene rearrangements in the plasma cell infiltrative phase of IPSID, demonstrating the true neoplastic nature of this lesion even in its early stages. Indeed, the technique is really the *only* way to establish clonality of T-cell lesions, for which there is no counterpart to the immunohistochemical assay of comparative kappa- and lambda-light-chain expression in B-cell lesions.[195] Also, since the gene rearrangements occur at an early stage of differentiation, prior to the expression of the encoded proteins, the technique can be used to characterize pre-B and pre-T cell lymphomas even when immunophenotyping is negative.

Like the other special diagnostic techniques discussed in this section, gene rearrangement studies are fraught with a number of potential pitfalls. The technique may actually be *too* sensitive for certain purposes, as it is not yet clear whether observation of a faint clonal band at the 1% detection level necessarily indicates malignancy, as opposed to an oligoclonal inflammatory response. Another dilemma arises from reports of overlap in the molecular genetic determination of cell of origin.[191] For example, rearrangement of immunoglobulin heavy-chain genes has been found in some T-cell and myeloid malignancies,[196,197] and, conversely, T-cell receptor gene rearrangements have been found in some pre-B cell lymphomas.[198] Finally, compared with most other techniques in diagnostic pathology, gene rearrangement studies are quite expensive, time-consuming, and technically cumbersome, requiring an attending and support staff well-versed in basic molecular biology. Such resources are not yet available even in many larger centers. Still, despite these problems, molecular analysis of gastrointestinal lymphoproliferative lesions represents an existing new frontier in our further understanding and improved diagnosis of these disorders.

REFERENCES

1. Sheahau DG: Focal lymphoid hyperplasia (pseudolymphoma) of the esophagus. *Am J Surg Path* 9:141–147, 1985.
2. Strodel WE, Cooper R, Eckhauser F, et al: Pseudolymphoma masquerading as colonic malignancy. *Dis Colon Rectum* 26:68–72, 1983.
3. Jacobs DS: Primary gastric malignant lymphoma and pseudolymphoma. *Am J Clin Pathol* 40:379–394, 1963.
4. Ranchod M, Lewin KJ, Dorfman RF: Lymphoid hyperplasia of the gastrointestinal tract: a study of 26 cases and review of the literature. *Am J Surg Path* 2:383–400, 1978.
5. Wright CJE: Pseudolymphoma of the stomach. *Hum Pathol* 4:305–318, 1973.
6. Chiles JT, Platz CE: The radiographic manifestation of pseudolymphoma of the stomach. *Radiology* 116:551–556, 1975.
7. Brooks JJ, Enterline HT: Gastric pseudolymphoma: its three subtypes and relation to lymphoma. *Cancer* 51:476–486, 1983.
8. Buchholz RR, Reid RA: Pseudolymphoma of the stomach. *Surg Clin North Am* 52:485–491, 1972.
9. Perrillo RP, Tedesco FJ. Gastric pseudolymphoma. A spectrum of presenting features and diagnostic considerations. *Am J Gastroenterol* 65:226, 1976.
10. Watson RJ, O'Brien MT: Gastric pseudolymphoma (lymphofollicular gastritis). *Ann Surg* 171:98–106, 1970.
11. Eras P, Winawer SJ: Benign lymphoid hyperplasia of the stomach simulating gastric malignancy. *Am J Dig Dis* 14:510–515, 1969.
12. Faris TD, Saltzstein SL: Gastric lymphoid hyperplasia: a lesion confused with lymphosarcoma. *Cancer* 17:207–212, 1964.
13. Perez CA, Dorfman RF: Benign lymphoid hyperplasia of the stomach and the duodenum. *Radiology* 57:505–510, 1966.
14. Tandon RK, Tandon HD, Singh DS, et al: Benign lymphoid hyperplasia of the stomach mimicking gastric malignancy. *Am J Gastroenterol* 66:36–41, 1976.
15. Mori S, Mohri N, Schimamine T: Reactive lymphoid hyperplasia of the stomach: an immunohistochemical study. *Acta Pathol Jpn* 30:671–680, 1980.
16. Saraga P, Hurlimann J, Ozzello L: Lymphomas and pseudolymphomas of the alimentary tract: an immunohistochemical study with clinicopathologic correlations. *Hum Pathol* 12:713–723, 1981.
17. Barge J, Molas G, Potet I: Lymphoid stromal reaction in gastrointestinal lymphomas: immunohistochemical study of 14 cases. *J Clin Pathol* 40:760–765, 1987.
18. Eimoto T, Futami K, Naito H, et al: Gastric pseudolymphoma with monotypic cytoplasmic immunoglobin. *Cancer* 55:788–793, 1985.
19. Wolf JA, Spjut HJ: Focal lymphoid hyperplasia of the stomach preceding gastric lymphoma: a case report and review of the literature. *Cancer* 48:2518–2523, 1981.
20. Saltzstein SL: Extranodal malignant lymphomas and pseudolymphomas. *Pathol Annu* 4:159–184, 1969.
21. Murayama H, Kikuchi M, Eimoto T, et al: Early lymphoma coexisting with reactive lymphoid hyperplasia of the stomach. *Acta Pathol Jpn* 34:679–686, 1984.
22. Scoazec JY, Brousse N, Potet F, et al: Focal malignant lymphoma in gastric pseudolymphoma: histologic and immunohistochemical study of a case. *Cancer* 57:1330–1336, 1986.
23. Gudjonsson H, Jonas M, Krawilt EL, et al: Pseudolymphoma of the jejunum. *Dig Dis Sci* 32:1314–1318, 1987.

24. Golodner H, Slobodkin M, Ripstein CM: Papillary lymph nodule hyperplasia of the duodenum. *Surgery* 37:409–414, 1955.

25. Rudzik O, Bienenstock J: Isolation and characteristics of gut mucosal lymphocytes. *Lab Invest* 30:260–266, 1974.

26. Helwig EB, Hansen J: Lymphoid polyps (benign lymphoma) and malignant lymphoma of the rectum and anus. *Surg Gynecol Obstet* 92:233–243, 1951.

27. Holtz F, Schmidt LA: Lymphoid polyps (benign lymphoma) of the rectum and anus. *Surg Gynecol Obstet* 106:639–642, 1958.

28. Keeling WM, Beatty GL: Lymphoid polyps of the rectum. Report of three cases in siblings. *Arch Surg* 73:753–756, 1956.

29. Meissner WW: Benign lymphoma of the rectum: review of the literature and report of fifteen additional cases. *J Int Coll Surg* 26:739–749, 1956.

30. Cornes JS, Wallace H, Morson BC: Benign lymphomas of the rectum and anal canal: a study of 100 cases. *J Pathol Bacteriol* 82:371–382, 1961.

31. Sniderman BF: Benign lymphoma of the rectum. *Am J Surg* 82:611–615, 1951.

32. Harwood RA, Abreu FB: Benign lymphoma and diffuse lymphoid hyperplasia: a case report. *Am J Proctol* 26:63–66, 1975.

33. Heule BV, Taylor CR, Terry R, et al: Presentation of malignant lymphoma in the rectum. *Cancer* 49:2602–2607, 1982.

34. Molas G, Potet F, Nogig P: Hyperplasie lymphoide focale (pseudo-lymphome) de l'ileon terminal chez l'adulte. *Gastroenterol Clin Biol* 9:630–633, 1985.

35. Nathans AA, Merenstein H, Brown SS: Lymphoid hyperplasia of the appendix. Clinical study. *Pediatrics* 12:516–524, 1953.

36. Charlesworth D, Fox H, Mainwaring AR: Benign lymphoid hyperplasia of the terminal ileum. *Am J Gastroenterol* 53:579–584, 1970.

37. Cornes JS, Dawson IMP: Papillary lymphoid hyperplasia at the ileocecal valve as a cause of acute intussusception in infancy. *Arch Dis Child* 38:89–91, 1963.

38. Selke AC, Jona JZ, Belin RP: Massive enlargement of the ileocecal valve due to lymphoid hyperplasia. *Am J Roetgenol* 127:518–520, 1976.

39. Stout AP: Isolated lymphoid hyperplasia in the cecum and appendix of children. *Am J Dis Child* 34:797–806, 1927.

40. Fieber SS, Schaefer HJ: Lymphoid hyperplasia of the terminal ileum—a clinical entity? *Gastroenterology* 50:83–98, 1966.

41. Dewar GJ, Lim CNH, Michalynshyn B, et al: Gastrointestinal complications in patients with acute and chronic leukemia. *Can J Surg* 24:67–71, 1981.

42. Sarason EL, Prior JT, Prowda RL: Recurrent intussusception associated with hypertrophy of Peyer's patches: *N Eng J Med* 253:905–908, 1955.

43. Swartley RN, Stayman JW: Lymphoid hyperplasia of the intestinal tract requiring surgical intervention. *Ann Surg* 155:238–240, 1962.

44. Perrin WS, Lindsay EC. Intussusception: a monograph based on 400 cases. *Br J Surg* 9:46–71, 1921–1922.

45. Clark EJ, Phillips IA, Alexander ER: Adenovirus infection in intussusception in children in Taiwan. *JAMA* 208:1671–1674, 1969.

46. Yunis EJ, Hashida Y: Electron microscopic demonstration of adenovirus in appendix veriformis in a case of ileocecal intussusception. *Pediatrics* 51:566–570, 1973.

47. Dorazio RA, Whelan TJ: Lymphoid hyperplasia of the terminal ileum associated with familial polyposis coli. *Ann Surg* 171:300–302, 1970.

48. Gruenberg J, Mackman S. Multiple lymphoid polyps in familial polyposis. *Ann Surg* 175:552–554, 1972.

49. Cosens CG: Gastrointestinal pseudoleukemia: a case report. *Ann Surg* 148:129–133, 1958.

50. Hermans PE, Huizenga KA, Hoffman HN, et al: Dysgammaglobulinemia associated with nodular lymphoid hyperplasia of the small intestine. *Am J Med* 40:78–89, 1966.

51. Hermans PE, Dias-Buxo JA, Stobo JD. Idiopathic late-onset immunoglobulin deficiency: clinical observations in 50 patients. *Am J Med* 61:221–237, 1976.

52. Gryboski JD, Self TW, Clemett A, et al: Selective immunoglobulin A deficiency and intestinal nodular lymphoid hyperplasia: correction of diarrhea with antibiotics and plasma. *Pediatrics* 42:833–836, 1968.

53. Johnson BL, Goldber LS, Pops MA, et al: Clinical and immunological studies in a case of nodular lymphoid hyperplasia of the small bowel. *Gastroenterology* 61:369–374, 1971.

54. Bird DC, Jacobs JB, Silbinger M, Wolff SM. Hypogammaglobulinemia with nodular lymphoid hyperplasia of the intestine. Report of a case with rectosigmoid involvement. *Radiology* 92:1535–1536, 1969.

55. Hodgson JR, Hoffman HN, Huizenga KA: Roentgenologic features of lymphoid hyperplasia of the small intestine associated with dysgammaglobulinemia. *Radiology* 88:883–888, 1967.

56. Ajdukiewiewicz AB, Youngs GR, Bouchier IAD: Nodular lymphoid hyperplasia with hypogammaglobulinemia. *Gut* 13:589–595, 1972.

57. Milano AM, Lawrence LR, Horowitz L: Nodular lymphoid hyperplasia of the small intestine and colon with giardiasis. A case with borderline serum IgA levels. *Am J Dig Dis* 16:735–737, 1971.

58. Davis SD, Eidelmann S, Loop JW. Nodular lymphoid hyperplasia of the small intestine and sarcoidosis. *Arch Intern Med* 126:668–672, 1970.

59. Matuchansky C, Morichau-Beauchant M, Touchard G, et al: Nodular lymphoid hyperplasia of the small bowel associated with primary jejunal malignant lymphoma. *Gastroenterology* 78:1587–1592, 1982.

60. Cornelis BHW, Lamers MD, Wagener T, et al: Jejunal lymphoma in a patient with primary adult-onset hypogammaglobulinemia and nodular lymphoid hyperplasia of the small intestine. *Dig Dis Sci* 25:553–557, 1980.

61. Aguilar FP, Alfonso V, Rivas S, et al: Jejunal malignant lymphoma in a patient with adult-onset hypogammaglobulinemia and nodular lymphoid hyperplasia of the small bowel. *Am J Gastroenterol* 82:472–475, 1987.

62. De Smet AA, Tubergen DG, Martel W: Nodular lymphoid hyperplasia of the colon associated with dysgammaglobulinemia. *Am J Roentgenol* 127:515–517, 1976.

63. Penny R: Nodular lymphoid hyperplasia of the small intestine and hypogammaglobulinemia. *Gastroenterology* 56:982–985, 1969.

64. Waldmann TA, Broder S, Blease RM, et al: Role of suppressive T cells in pathogenesis of common variable hypogammaglobulinemia. *Lancet* 2:609–613, 1974.

65. Robinson MJ, Padron S, Rywlin AM. Enterocolitis lymphofollicularis: morphologic, pathologic, and serum immunoglobulin patterns. *Arch Pathol* 96:311–315, 1973.

66. Capitanio MA, Kirkpatrick JA: Lymphoid hyperplasia of the colon in children. Roentgen observations. *Radiology* 94:323–327, 1970.

67. Franken WA: Lymphoid hyperplasia of the colon. *Radiology* 94:329–334, 1970.

68. Theander G, Tragardh B: Lymphoid hyperplasia of the colon in childhood. *Acta Radiol Diag* 17:631–640, 1976.

69. Louw JH: Polypoid lesions of the large bowel in children with particular reference to benign lymphoid polyposis. *J Pediatr Surg* 3:195–209, 1968.

70. Collins JO, Falk M, Guibone R: Benign lymphoid polyposis of the colon: a case report. *Pediatrics* 38:897–899, 1966.

71. Cornes JS: Multiple lymphomatous polyposis of the gastrointestinal tract. *Cancer* 14:249–257, 1961.

72. Kahn LB, Novis BH: Nodular lymphoid hyperplasia of the small bowel associated with primary small bowel reticulum cell lymphoma. *Cancer* 33:837–844, 1974.

73. Asquith P, Haeney MR: Celiac disease. In Asquith P, ed.: *Immunology Of The Gastrointestinal Tract.* Edinburgh, Churchill Livingston 1979, Vol. 69.

74. Swinson CM, Slavin G, Coles EC, et al: Coeliac disease and malignancy. *Lancet* 1:111–115, 1983.

75. Roehrkasse RL, Roberts IM, Wald A, et al: Celiac sprue complicated by lymphoma presenting with multiple gastric ulcers. *Gastroenterology* 91:740–745, 1986.

76. Cooper BT, Holmes GKT, Ferguson R, et al: Celiac disease and malignancy. *Medicine* 59:249–261, 1980.

77. Freeman HJ, Weinstein WM, Shnitka TK, et al: Primary abdominal lymphoma: presenting manifestation of celiac sprue or complicating dermatitis herpetiformis. *Am J Med* 63:585–594, 1977.

78. Isaacson P, Jones DB, Sworn MJ, et al: Malignant histiocytosis of the intestine: report of three cases with immunological and cytochemical analysis. *J Clin Pathol* 35:510–516, 1982.

79. Isaacson P, Wright DH, Judd MA, et al: Primary gastrointestinal lymphomas: the classification of 66 cases. *Cancer* 43:1805–1819, 1979.

80. Isaacson P: Primary gastrointestinal lymphoma (Editorial). *Virchows Arch (Pathol Anat)* 391:1–8, 1981.

81. Salter DM, Krajewski AS, Dewar AE: Immunophenotype analysis of malignant histiocytosis of the intestine. *J Clin Pathol* 39:8–15, 1986.

82. Klaevman HL, Gebhard RL, Sessoms C, et al: In vitro studies of ulcerative ileojejunitis. *Gastroenterology* 68:572–582, 1975.

83. Gilinsky NH, Novis BH, Mee AS, et al: Immunoproliferative small-intestinal disease: follow-up of an alpha-chain negative, lymphoma-free group. *J Clin Gastroenterol* 5:421–428, 1983.

84. Appleman HD, Hirsch SD, Schnitzer B, et al: Clinicopathologic overview of gastrointestinal lymphomas. *Am J Surg Path* 9:51–71, 1985.

85. Ioachim HL, Weinstein A, Robbins RD, et al: Primary anorectal lymphoma: a new manifestation of the acquired immune deficiency syndrome (AIDS). *Cancer* 60:1449–1453, 1987.

86. Lewin KJ, Ranchod M, Dorfman RF: Lymphomas of the gastrointestinal tract: a study of 117 cases presenting with gastrointestinal disease. *Cancer* 42:693–707, 1978.

87. Loehr WJ, Mujahed Z, Zahn FD, et al: Primary lymphoma of the gastrointestinal tract: review of 100 cases. *Ann Surg* 170:232–238, 1969.

88. Baker D, Chirprut RO, Rimer D, et al: Chronic lymphoma in ulcerative colitis. *J Clin Gastroenterol* 7:379–386, 1985.

89. Falconieri G, Melato M, Bucconi S, et al: Malignant lymphoma arising in an intestinal polyp. *Histopathology* 11:215–216, 1987.

90. Dawson IMP, Cornes JS, Morson BC: Primary malignant lymphoid tumors of the intestinal tract. Report of 37 cases with a study of factors influencing prognosis. *Br J Surg* 49:80–89, 1961.

91. Lewin KJ, Kahn LB, Novis BH: Primary intestinal lymphoma of "Western" and "Mediterranean" type, alpha-chain disease and massive plasma cell infiltration. *Cancer* 38:2511–2528, 1976.

92. Isaacson P, Wright DH: Malignant lymphoma of mucosa-associated lymphoid tissue. A distinctive type of B-cell lymphoma. *Cancer* 52:1410–1416, 1983.

93. Isaacson P, Wright DH, Jones DB: Malignant lymphoma of true histiocytic (monocyte/macrophage) origin. *Cancer* 51:80–91, 1983.

94. Otto HF, Bettman I, Weltzien JV, et al: Primary intestinal lymphomas. *Virchows Arch (Pathol Anat)* 391:9–31, 1981.

95. Yamanaka N, Ishii Y, Hoshiba H, et al. A study of surface markers in gastrointestinal lymphoma. *Gastroenterology* 79:673–677, 1980.

96. Grody WW, Magidson JG, Weiss LM, et al: Gastrointestinal lymphomas: immunohistochemical studies on the cell of origin. *Am J Surg Path* 9:328–337, 1985.

97. Berger F, Coiffier B, Bonneville C, et al: Gastrointestinal lymphomas: immunohistochemical study of 23 cases. *Am J Clin Pathol* 88:707–712, 1987.

98. Azzopardi JG, Menzies T: Primary malignant lymphoma of the alimentary tract. *Br J Surg* 47:358–366, 1960.

99. Gray GM, Rosenbery SA, Cooper AD, et al: Lymphomas involving the gastrointestinal tract. *Gastroenterology* 82:143–152, 1982.

100. Freeman C, Berg JW, Cutler SJ: Occurrence and prognosis of extranodal lymphomas. *Cancer* 29:252–260, 1972.

101. Allen AW, Donaldson G, Sniffen RC, et al: Primary malignant lymphoma of the gastrointestinal tract. *Ann Surg* 140:428–438, 1954.

102. Faulkner JW, Docherty MB: Lymphosarcoma of the small intestine. *Surg Gynecol Obstet* 95:76–84, 1952.

103. Frazer JW: Malignant lymphomas of the gastrointestinal tract. *Surg Gynecol Obstet* 108:182–190, 1959.

104. Burman SO, van Wyke FAK: Lymphomas of the small intestine and cecum. *Ann Surg* 143:349–359, 1956.

105. Lim FE, Hartman AS, Tan EGC, et al: Factors in the prognosis of gastric lymphoma. *Cancer* 39:1715–1720, 1977.

106. Bush RS: Primary lymphoma of the gastrointestinal tract. *JAMA* 228:1291–1294, 1974.

107. Goffinet DR, Warnke R, Dunnick NR, et al: Clinical and surgical (laparotomy) evaluation of patients with non-Hodgkin's lymphomas. *Cancer Treat Rep* 61(6):981–992, 1977.

108. Hande KR, Fisher RI, DeVita VT, et al: Diffuse histiocytic lymphoma involving the gastrointestinal tract. *Cancer* 41:1984–1989, 1978.

109. Vanden Heule B, Taylor CR, Terry R, et al: Presentation of malignant lymphoma in the rectum. *Cancer* 49:2602–2607, 1982.

110. Joseph JI, Lattes R: Gastric lymphosarcoma: clinicopathologic analysis of 71 cases and its relation to disseminated lymphosarcoma. *Am J Clin Path* 45:653–669, 1966.

111. Buckley RH, Whismant JK, Schiff RI, et al: Corrections of severe combined immunodeficiency by fetal liver cells. *N Engl J Med* 294:1076–1081, 1976.

112. Beschorner WE, Tutschka PJ, Santos GW: Sequential morphology of graft-versus-host disease in the rat radiation chimera. *Clin Immunol Immunopathol* 22:203–224, 1982.

113. Epstein RJ, McDonald GB, Sale GE, et al: The diagnostic accuracy of the rectal biopsy in acute graft-versus-host disease: a prospective study of thirteen patients. *Gastroenterol* 78:764–771, 1980.

114. Cornes JS: Multiple lymphomatous polyposis of the gastrointestinal tract. *Cancer* 14:249–257, 1961.

115. Ruppert GB, Smith VM: Multiple lymphomatous polyposis of the gastrointestinal tract. *Gastrointest Endosc* 25:67–79, 1979.

116. Shepherd NA, Blackshaw AJ, Hall PA, et al: Malignant lymphoma with eosinophilia of the gastrointestinal tract. *Histopathology* 11:115–130, 1987.

117. Rosenberg SA, Berard CW, Brown BW, et al: National Cancer Institute sponsored study of classifications of non-Hodgkin's lymphomas: summary and description of a working formulation for clinical usage. The non-Hodgkin's lymphoma pathologic classification project. *Cancer* 49:2112–2135, 1982.

118. Warnke RA, Kim H, Fuks Z, et al: The coexistence of nodular and diffuse patterns in nodular non-Hodgkin's lymphomas: significance and clinicopathologic correlation. *Cancer* 40:1229–1233, 1977.

119. Rappaport H, Winter WJ, Hicks EB, et al: Follicular lymphoma: a reevaluation of its position in the scheme of malignant lymphoma based on a survey of 253 cases. *Cancer* 9:792–821, 1956.

120. Usher FC, Dixon CF: Lymphosarcoma of the intestines. *Gastroenterology* 1:160–178, 1943.

121. Levine PH, Kamaraja LS, Connelly RR, et al: The American Burkitt's Lymphoma Registry: eight years' experience. *Cancer* 49:1016–1022, 1982.

122. Mann RB, Jaffe ES, Braylan RC, et al: Nonendemic Burkitt's lymphoma: a B-cell tumor related to germinal centers. *N Engl J Med* 295:685–691, 1976.

123. Sheehan DG, Martin F, Bagkinsky S, et al: Multiple lymphomatous polyposis of the gastro-intestinal tract. *Cancer* 28:408–425, 1971.

124. Issacson P, Wright D: Extranodal malignant lymphoma arising from mucosa associated lymphoid tissue. *Cancer* 53:2515–2524, 1984.

125. Weingrad DN, Decosse JJ, Sherlock P, et al: Primary gastrointestinal lymphoma: a thirty year review. *Cancer* 49:1258–1265, 1982.

126. Cox JD: Prognostic factors in malignant lymphoreticular tumors of the small bowel and ileocecal region: a review of 50 case histories. *Int J Radiation Oncology Bio Phys* 5:185–1909, 1979.

127. Shimm DS, Dosoretz DE, Anderson T, et al: Primary gastric lymphoma: an analysis with emphasis on prognostic factors and radiation therapy. *Cancer* 52:2044–2048, 1983.

128. Filippa DA, Lieberman PH, Weingrad DN, et al: Primary lymphomas of the gastrointestinal tract: analysis of prognostic factors with emphasis on histological type. *Am J Surg Pathol* 7:363–372, 1983.

129. Dworkin B, Lightdale CJ, Weingrad DN, et al: Primary gastric lymphoma: a review of 50 cases. *Dig Dis Sci* 27:986–992, 1982.

130. Naqvi MS, Burrows L, Kark AE: Lymphosarcoma of the gastrointestinal tract: prognostic guides based on 162 cases. *Ann Surg* 170:221–231, 1969.

131. Dragosics B, Bauer P, Radaszkiewicz T: Primary gastrointestinal non-Hodgkin's lymphomas. A retrospective clinicopathologic study of 150 cases. *Cancer* 55(5):1060–1073, 1985.

132. Maor MH, Maddux B, Osbourne BM, et al: Stages IE and IIE non-Hodgkin's lymphoma of the stomach: comparison of treatment modalities. *Cancer* 54:2330–2337, 1984.

133. Jones RE, Willis S, Inne DJ, et al: Primary gastric lymphoma: problems in staging and management. *Am J Surg* 55:118–123, 1988.

134. Aozasa K, Ueda T, Jurata A, et al: Prognostic value of histologic and clinical factors in 56 patients with gastrointestinal lymphomas. *Cancer* 61:304–315, 1988.

135. Nelson DF, Cassady JR, Traggis D, et al: The role of radiation therapy in localized respectable intestinal non-Hodgkin's lymphoma in children. *Cancer* 39:89–97, 1977.

136. Hermann R, Panahon AM, Barcos MP, et al: Gastrointestinal involvement in non-Hodgkin's lymphoma. *Cancer* 46:215–222, 1980.

137. Rosenfelt F, Rosenberg SA: Diffuse histiocytic lymphoma presenting with gastrointestinal tract lesions: the Stanford experience. *Cancer* 45:2188–2193, 1980.

138. Cornes JS, Gwynfor T, Fisher GB: Leukaemic lesions of the gastrointestinal tract. *J Clin Path* 15:305–313, 1962.

139. Prolla JC, Kirsner JB: The gastrointestinal lesions and complications of the leukemias. *Ann Intern Med* 61:1084–1103, 1964.

140. Moir DH, Bale PM: Necropsy findings in childhood leukaemia emphasizing neutropenic enterocolitis and cerebral calcification. *Pathology* 8:247–258, 1976.

141. O'Sullivan WD, Child CG: Illeocecal intussusception caused by lymphoid hyperplasia. *J Pediatr* 38:320–324, 1951.

142. Sherman NJ, Williams K, Woolley MM: Surgical complications in the patient with leukemia. *J Pediatr Surg* 8:235–244, 1973.

143. Kies MS, Leudke DW, Boyd JF, et al: Neutropenic enterocolitis. *Cancer* 43:730–734, 1979.

144. McCarthy D, Holland I, Lavender JP, et al: Pneumatosis coli in adult acute myeloid leukaemia. *Clin Radiol* 30:175–178, 1979.

145. Alpha-chain disease and related small intestinal lymphoma. Report of a WHO meeting of investigators. *Arch Fr Mal App Dig* 65:591–607, 1976.

146. Seijffers MJ, Levy M, Hermann G: Intractable watery diarrhea, hypokalemia and malabsorption in a patient with Mediterranean type of abdominal lymphoma. *Gastroenterology* 55:118–124, 1968.

147. Eidelman S, Parkins RA, Rubin CE: Abdominal lymphoma presenting as malabsorption: a clinicopathologic study of nine cases in Israel and a review of the literature. *Medicine* 45:111–137, 1966.

148. Ramot B, Shahin N, Bubis JJ: Malabsorption syndrome in lymphoma of the small bowel. *Isr J Med Sci* 1:221–226, 1965.

149. Al-Saleem T, Al-Bahrani Z: Malignant lymphoma of the small intestine in Iraq (Middle East lymphoma). *Cancer* 31:291–294, 1973.

150. Nasr K, Haghighi P, Bakhashandeh K, et al: Primary lymphoma of the upper small intestine. *Gut* 11:673–678, 1970.

151. Novis BH, Banks S, Marks IN, et al: Abdominal lymphoma presenting with malabsorption. *Quart J Med* 40:521–540, 1971.

152. Asselah F, Slavin G, Sowter G, et al: Immunoproliferative small intestinal disease in Algerians: light microscopic and immunochemical studies. *Cancer* 52:227–237, 1983.

153. Rambaud JC, Bognel C, Prost A, et al: Clinicopathological study of a patient with "Mediterranean" type of abdominal lymphoma and a new type of IgA abnormality ("alpha chain disease"). *Digestion* 1:321–336, 1968.

154. Rambaud JC, Matuchansky C: Alpha-chain disease pathogenesis and relation to Mediterranean lymphoma. *Lancet* 1:1430–1432, 1973.

155. Issacson P: Middle East lymphoma and alpha-chain disease: an immunohistochemical study. *Am J Surg Pathol* 3:431–441, 1979.

156. Seligmann M, Mihaesco E, Hurez D, et al: Immunochemical studies in 4 cases of alpha chain disease. *J Clin Invest* 48:2374–2389, 1968.

157. Seligmann M: Immunochemical, clinical and pathological features of alpha-chain disease. *Arch Intern Med* 135:78–82, 1975.

158. Seligmann M, Mihaesco E: Studies on alpha-chain disease. *Ann NY Acad Sci* 190:487–500, 1971.

159. Shahid MJ, Alami SY, Nassar VH, et al: Primary intestinal lymphoma with paraproteinemia. *Cancer* 35:848–858, 1975.

160. Gilinsky NH, Chaimowitz G, Van Standen ML: Immunoproliferative small-intestinal disease with lymphoma. Diagnostic difficulties and pitfalls. *S Afr Med J* 69:260–262, 1986.

161. Monges H, Aubert L, Chamlian A, et al: Maladie des chaines alpha a forme intestinale. Presentation d'un cas traite par antibiotherapie avec remission clinique, histiologique et immunologique. *Arch Fr Mal App Dig* 64:223–231, 1975.

162. Ramot B, Shalin N, Bubis JJ: Malabsorption syndrome in lymphoma of the small intestine. A study of 13 cases. *Isr J Med Sci* 1:221–226, 1965.

163. Bender SW, Danon F, Preud'homme JL, et al: Gamma heavy chain disease stimulating alpha chain disease. *Gut* 19:1148–1152, 1978.

164. Papac RJ, Rosenstein RW, Richards F, et al: Gamma heavy chain disease seen initially as gastric neoplasm. *Arch Int Med* 138:1151–1153, 1978.

165. Doe WF: Alpha chain disease and related small intestinal lymphomas. In Asquith P: *Immunology of the gastrointestinal tract,* Edinburgh: Churchill Livingston, 1974, 366, Vol. 366.

166. Roge J, Druet P, March C: Lymphome Mediterraneen avec maladie des chaines alpha: triple remission clinique, anatomique at immunologique. *Pathol Biol* 18:851–858, 1970.

167. Smith WJ, Price SK, Isaacson PG: Immunoglobulin gene rearrangement in immunoproliferative small intestinal disease (IPSID). *J Clin Pathol* 40:1291–1297, 1987.

168. Coulbois J, Galian P, Galian A, et al: Gastric form of alpha-chain disease. *Gut* 27:719–725, 1986.

169. Tungebar MF: Gastric signet-ring cell lymphoma with alpha heavy chains. *Histopathology* 10:725–733, 1986.

170. Cho C, Linscheer WG, Bell R, et al: Colonic lymphoma producing alpha-chain disease protein. *Gastroenterology* 83:121–126, 1982.

171. Isaacson P, Buchanan R, Mepham BL: Plasma cell granuloma of the stomach. *Human Pathol* 9:355–358, 1978.

172. Wiltshaw E: The natural history of extramedullary plasmacytoma and its relation to solitary myeloma of bone and myelomatosis. *Medicine* 55:217–238, 1976.

173. Nahanishi I, Kajikawa K, Migita S, et al: Gastric plasmacytoma. An immunologic and immuno-histochemical study. *Cancer* 49:2025–2028, 1982.

174. Ferrer-Roca O: Primary gastric plasmacytoma with massive intracytoplasmic crystalline inclusions. A case report. *Cancer* 50:755–759, 1982.

175. Douglas HO, Sika JV, LeVenn HH: Plasmacytoma: a not so rare tumor of the small intestine. *Cancer* 28:456–460, 1971.

176. Asselah F, Crow J, Slavin G, et al: Solitary plasmacytoma of the intestine. *Histo-pathology* 6:631–645, 1982.

177. Rygaard-Olsen C, Boedker A, Emus HC, et al: Extramedullary plasmacytoma of the small intestine. A case report studied with electron microscopy and immunoperoxidase technique. *Cancer* 50:573–576, 1982.

178. Gleason TH, Hammar SP: Plasmacytoma of the colon. *Cancer* 50:130–133, 1982.

179. Funakoshi N, Kanoh T, Kobayashi Y, et al: IgM-producing gastric plasmacytoma. *Cancer* 54:638–643, 1984.

180. Remigio PA, Klaum A: Extramedullary plasmacytoma of stomach. *Cancer* 27:562–568, 1971.

181. McCaffrey J, Kingston CW, Hasker WE: Extramedullary plasmacytoma of the gastrointestinal tract. *Aust NZ J Surg* 41:351–353, 1972.

182. Sharma KD, Shrivastav JD: Extramedullary plasmacytoma of gastrointestinal tract. With a case report of plasmacytoma of the rectum and a review of the literature. *Arch Pathol* 71:229–233, 1961.

183. Soga J, Saito K, Suzuki N, et al: Plasma cell granuloma of the stomach. A report of a case and review of the literature. *Cancer* 25:618–625, 1970.

184. Scott FET, Dupont PA, Webb J: Plasmacytoma of the stomach: diagnosis with the aid of immunoperoxidase technique. *Cancer* 41:675–681, 1978.

185. Stashenko P, Nadler LM, Hardy R, et al: Characterization of a new B lymphocyte-specific antigen in man. *J Immunol* 125:1678–1685, 1980.

186. Weiss A, Stobo JD: Requirement for the coexpression of T3 and the T cell antigen receptor on a malignant human T cell line. *J Exp Med* 160:1284–1299, 1984.

187. Coon JS, Landay AL, Weinstein RS: Advances in flow cytometry for diagnostic pathology. *Lab Invest* 57:453–479, 1987.

188. Frierson HF: Flow cytometric analysis of ploidy in solid neoplasms: comparison of fresh tissues with formalin-fixed paraffin-embedded specimens. *Hum Pathol* 19:290–294, 1988.

189. Horan PK, Slezak S, Poste G: Improved flow cytometric analysis of leukocyte subsets: simultaneous identification of five cell subsets using two-color immunofluorescence. *Proc Natl Acad Sci USA* 83:8361–8365, 1986.

190. Tonegawa S: Somatic generation of antibody diversity. *Nature* 302:575–581, 1983.

191. Cossman J, Uppenkamp M, Sundeen J, et al: Molecular genetics and the diagnosis of lymphoma. *Arch Pathol Lab Med* 112:117–127, 1988.

192. Southern EM: Detection of specific sequences among DNA fragments separated by gel electrophoresis. *J Mol Biol* 98:503–510, 1975.

193. Sklar JL, Weiss LM, Cleary ML: Diagnostic molecular biology of non-Hodgkin's lymphomas. In Berard CW, Dorfman RF, Kaurman N: *Malignant Lymphoma, IAP Monographs in Pathology,* Baltimore: Williams & Wilkins, 1984:204–224, Vol. 29.

194. Cleary ML, Chao J, Waruke R, et al: Immunoglobulin gene rearrangement as a diagnostic criterion of B cell lymphoma. *Proc Natl Acad Sci USA* 81:593–597, 1984.

195. Knowles DM, Pelicci P-G, Dall-Favera R: T-cell receptor beta chain gene rearrangements: genetic markers of T-cell lineage and clonality. *Hum Pathol* 17:546–551, 1986.

196. Ha K, Minden M, Hozumi N, et al: Immunoglobulin μ-chain gene rearrangement in a patient with T cell acute lymphoblastic leukemia. *J Clin Invest* 73:1232–1236, 1984.

197. Ha K, Minden M, Hozumi N, et al: Immunoglobin gene rearrangement in acute myelogenous leukemia. *Cancer Res* 44:4658–4660, 1984.

198. Pelicci P-G, Knowles DM, Dalla-Favera R: Lymphoid tumors displaying rearrangements of both immunoglobulin and T cell receptor genes. *J Exp Med* 162:1015–1024, 1985.

CHAPTER 28

Intestinal and Hepatic Manifestations of Graft-Versus-Host Disease

WILLIAM E. BESCHORNER

RONALD P. TURNICKY

INTRODUCTION

Bone marrow transplantation has gained wide acceptance for the treatment for hematopoietic malignancies, severe plastic anemia, and congenital immune and enzyme deficiencies.[1-3] Initially, numerous posttransplant complications limited the success of transplants, including nonmarrow toxicity from total body irradiation and aggressive chemotherapy, infection, relapse of malignancy, and acute and chronic graft-versus-host disease (GVHD).[4] Numerous improvements in the procedure, including use of prophylactic agents such as Cyclosporine have lessened the incidence of GVHD and significantly increased the disease-free survival.[5-7] Still, acute and chronic GVHD presents a significant challenge for many recipients.[7-9]

Although cutaneous GVHD is the best understood aspect, the involvement of the intestinal tract and the liver frequently determines the clinical outcome of the transplant. The erythematous rash of acute GVHD is often accompanied by profuse secretory diarrhea and elevation of liver transaminases and bilirubin. Patients frequently die of intestinal hemorrhage and sepsis from related intestinal pathogens.[10-12] While the injury to the liver is not as dramatic, those with cutaneous and hepatic GVHD do more poorly than with cutaneous GVHD alone.[10,11,13]

This chapter will briefly introduce the pathology and immunopathology of these two systems, the possible pathogenetic mechanisms of injury, and some areas where additional research is indicated. Many relevant articles have regrettably been omitted due to space, and the emphasis here reflects our own personal experience and bias.

This work was supported in part by grants from the U.S. Department of Health and Human Services (CA15396, CA28701, and DK40618).

Graft-Versus-Host Disease

After World War II, bone marrow transplantation was initially explored as a response to exposure to lethal irradiation. Jacobson demonstrated that rodents could be protected from lethal irradiation by either shielding the spleen with lead or injecting splenocytes into the irradiated animal.[14,15] When other outbred animals were used as donors, the recipients survived the initial phase but later developed a lethal runting syndrome with ruffled fur, weight loss, and diarrhea.[16,17]

Billingham and Simonson demonstrated that this secondary disease actually resulted from an immunologic attack of the donor immune system against the host, terming it graft-versus-host reaction and graft-versus-host disease.[18,19] This conclusion was based on the observations that the "secondary disease" was achieved only if the donor graft was immunocompetent, recognized an antigen on the host, and could not be rejected by the host. Sequential pathologic studies characterized an early lymphoid proliferation followed by a later phase of injury to the common target tissues including the skin, liver, and intestinal tract.[4,20,21] Very simply put, GVHD appeared to parallel the mixed lymphocyte reaction with an early lymphocyte proliferative phase, responding to the host antigens, and a later cytotoxic phase with aggressor or cytotoxic lymphocytes emigrating to and injuring the target tissues.

While GVHD still represents an immunologic reaction against the host, the pathogenesis is not that straightforward. Host factors as well as immunologic variables mitigate the severity as well as the pathologic pattern of GVHD. Different animal models appear to have different pathogeneses.

The essential component is the engraftment of histoincompatible donor lymphocytes. While these cells must recognize the host, they cannot be rejected by the host. Two basic models can achieve this. First, in the semiallogeneic model, parental lymphocytes are injected into an F1 hybrid. While the parental cells recognize the host as foreign, the host accepts the parental cells as self. Second, the host immune system can simply be destroyed by lethal total body irradiation or high-dose chemotherapy. This model is referred to here as the *irradiation chimera* model.

While both approaches elicit GVHD, there are significant immunopathologic differences. Host lymphocytes are recruited into the immune reaction of the semiallogeneic model, producing a more vigorous lymphoproliferative reaction. The effector cells responsible for tissue injury could also be recruited from the host. The irradiation chimera model reflects principally the donor cells responding to the host antigen stimulation. Although the host initially contains radioresistant leukocytes, including histiocytes, mast cells, plasma cells, and some small lymphocytes, most of these cells disappear shortly after engraftment.[22] On the other hand, the reaction reflects an immature immune system.[23–25] Because our interests center on understanding clinical GVHD in human radiation chimeras, the results from this model will be emphasized.

Acute GVHD presents at 2 weeks to 3 months posttransplant with the sudden, often simultaneous, development of erythema, abnormal hepatic chemistries, and secretory diarrhea. The skin pathology is characterized by a mild lymphocytic infiltrate in the epidermis and associated necrotic dyskeratotic cells.[4,20,21,26]

Chronic GVHD, in contrast, presents insidiously at 3 months to 1 year with manifestations that resemble different autoimmune diseases including lichen planus, scleroderma, Sjögren's syndrome, dermatomyositis, myasthenia gravis, and primary biliary cirrhosis.[27-32] The histology differs from acute GVHD, with a mixed, more intense infiltrate of lymphocytes, histiocytes, and frequently eosinophils.[30,33] In the later stages, the tissues are fibrotic. As with acute GVHD, chronic GVHD occurs principally in allogeneic recipients, particularly if they have had previous acute GVHD.[34,35] Nonetheless, there is evidence that the injury in the peripheral tissues is mediated by autoreactive lymphocytes (demonstrating anti-donor reactivity).[36] At the target tissue, then, chronic GVHD may be a true autoimmune disease. An abnormal thymic environment is usually associated with chronic GVHD.[37-39] Quite possibly the allogeneic reaction alters the thymic environment, leading to a loss of self-tolerance.

GRAFT-VERSUS-HOST DISEASE OF THE INTESTINAL TRACT

Intestinal Acute GVHD

Acute GVHD usually starts with an erythematous, sensitive rash. Within a few days, crampy abdominal pain and watery diarrhea ensue.[40,41] In severe cases of intestinal GVHD, sheets of mucosa slough into the stool. Often the GVHD progresses to life-threatening intestinal hemorrhage. The intestinal complications, however, often are difficult to diagnose and treat. Diarrhea can be due to toxicity or primary infection. The onset of diarrhea can precede the characteristic rash, and it often persists after the cutaneous GVHD is successfully treated.

X-ray films and computerized tomography of the abdomen show diffuse edema of the wall. This, however, is not specific for GVHD and is also seen with viral enteritis.[42,43]

Endoscopy observations during the early part of GVHD are often unremarkable or may only show erythema.[44,45] These findings are often at variance with remarkable crypt injury observed histologically. As the GVHD progresses, the gross appearance may show ulceration or diffuse sloughing. Autopsy studies of intestinal involvement show relative sparing of the gastric mucosa, moderate injury to the duodenal, and jejunal mucosa, with the most severe injury observed in the terminal ileum.[4,40] The rectal mucosa is usually less severely injured. In the more severe cases, the entire small and large bowel mucosa is sloughed (Fig. 28–1).

In early and mild episodes the villi are shortened and widened. Multiple apoptotic lesions are seen in the crypts. These consist of round vacuoles within the crypt basement membrane containing cellular and nuclear debris (Fig. 28–2). The lamina propria contain greater numbers of lymphocytes, but there is a marked decrease in the number of plasma cells, particularly those containing IgA and IgM. The apoptotic lesions are most frequently seen at the base of the crypts.[4,9,20,40,44-47]

Later the villous structure is lost, and the surface epithelium is replaced with a regenerative low cuboidal epithelium or fibrinopurulent membrane. There is marked dropout of the crypts.

The injury in rodent models is rarely as severe as in primates. Descriptions of semiallogeneic models, in the absence of irradiation, emphasize villous blunting, crypt hyperplasia, increased mitotic figures, and increased intraepithelial lymphocytes.[48-50]

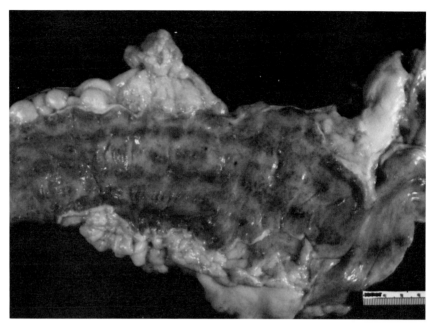

Figure 28–1 Fresh autopsy specimen of the ileal-cecal region from a patient with severe acute GVHD. The mucosa has been sloughed in entirety. Histologic section reveals only regenerative epithelium.

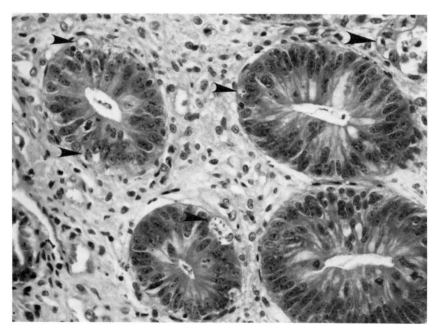

Figure 28–2 Rectal biopsy with early acute graft-versus-host disease. Multiple apoptotic lesions are present within the crypts (small arrows). One crypt is undergoing severe degeneration (large arrow). Note also the paucity of plasma cells within the lamina propria. H and E, ×250.

More severe injury is observed in irradiation models with numerous apoptotic lesions and crypt dropout.[21,40]

Any discussion of the pathogenesis of intestinal injury must address not only the epithelial injury but also the effect of GVHD on intestinal immunity and the role of the microflora. Although these three components are clearly interrelated, the relevant observations will be initially discussed separately.

The most direct evidence suggesting *cell-mediated injury to the epithelium* are the fine structure observations of lymphocytes in intimate contact with injured epithelial cells.[51] The lymphocyte cell membrane manifests broad-based contact with the epithelial cells as well as protruding into the epithelium at multiple points. The Golgi apparatus and membrane-bound granules are polarized to the region of contact.[52] Light microscopy demonstrates increased lamina propria lymphocytes. These are often focally increased near the crypts. The number of intraepithelial lymphocytes, however, does not correlate well with the number of apoptotic lesions in the irradiation model. The number of intraepithelial lymphocytes in the unirradiated semiallogeneic model is increased with GVHD. In this model, however, apoptotic lesions are not apparent.

The nature of the intraepithelial lymphocytes is unclear. Phenotypic and functional analysis of the semiallogeneic model suggest that the IEL are natural killer (NK) cells. In human radiation chimeras, GVHD was associated with increased CD8+ T lymphocytes in the lamina propria and epithelium. There was no increase in phenotypic NK cells or macrophages.[53] Most studies of radiation chimeras indicate that circulating and cutaneous lymphocytes are antigen-specific cytotoxic T lymphocytes.[54,55]

Mowat et al. have compared the intraepithelial lymphocytes of the unirradiated semiallogeneic model to radiation chimera of the same strains.[56] In the unirradiated semiallogeneic chimeras, splenic NK cells are increased, corresponding with increased intestinal IEL and epithelial proliferation. In their radiation chimeras, however, the NK cells peak at day 3 posttransplant. On day 4 the NK cells disappear coincident with the appearance of cytotoxic T lymphocytes capable of lysing host cells.

Regardless of the nature of the effector cell immediately responsible for epithelial injury, T lymphocytes are clearly required for the development of GVHD. Eliminating donor T lymphocytes in either of the animal models or in human transplant settings essentially eliminates development of GVHD.[57-59] While T cells may develop directly into the responsible effector cells, they also could have indirect effects. For example, they could produce a thymic dysplasia leading to abnormal T-cell ontogeny and interfering with the development of tolerance to the host.[60-62] Within the target tissue, donor T cells could influence the epithelial injury through the release of lymphokines such as immune interferon.[63] These lymphokines induce expression of epithelial histocompatibility antigens and stimulate other lymphocytes, including NK cells.[64,65]

Phenotype studies of irradiation models report a predominance of CD8+ lymphocytes in human intestinal biopsies.[66] Clones of CD8+ and CD4+ lymphocytes react with targets bearing class I and II antigens respectively.[67] In murine transplants, class I or class II mismatches lead to GVHD, but the GVHD and enteropathy appears more severe with class II antigen discrepancies.[50,68] Radiation murine chimeras (semiallogeneic) with class I antigen mismatches develop primarily CD8+ infiltrates, while those varying only at the class II loci demonstrate a mixture of CD4+ and CD8+ cells.[50] The predominance of CD8+ lymphocytes within the gut may not simply be a function of the histocompatibility mismatch. CD8+ lymphoblasts from the thoracic duct demonstrated a greater homing ability for the gut than did CD4+ lymphoblasts.

Because the diarrhea often coincides with the development of cutaneous and hepatic GVHD, it is tempting to consider the gut as just another end-stage target tissue. It is quite possible, however, that the responsible lymphocytes are derived from the host Peyer's patches (PP). Lymphocytes isolated from the PP will induce a strong GVHD.[69] Furthermore, local irradiation to the host PP markedly reduces the observed intestinal injury.[50]

The intestinal epithelium normally expresses only low levels of class I antigen and undetectable levels of class II histocompatibility antigens. With acute GVHD, however, the mucosal epithelium displays high levels of class II histocompatibility antigens.[70,71] This expression could stimulate the donor antihost immune reaction. The T-cell receptor and helper lymphocytes require the recognition not only of the antigen but also the class II protein. Epithelial cells with induced class II antigen could therefore better present other histocompatibility or external antigens more effectively to the donor immune system. With a class II antigen mismatch, the induced expression serves both functions of antigen presentation and antigen.

Theory aside, is the induced expression essential for target injury? A sequential study of cutaneous GVHD suggests that in most patients the induced expression is a secondary phenomena following the onset of GVHD.[72] The induced expression may therefore simply be the result of the infiltrating lymphocytes, which may release lymphokines such as immune interferon and interleukin-4.[73-75] In contrast to most rodent studies, it should be remembered that human marrow transplants are generally performed with sibling donors matched at the classes I and II loci.

Quite possibly, even the intestinal epithelium might not be an essential antigen or cellular target. If parental strain intestine is transplanted at the same time as marrow and spleen cells into an F1 host, the pathology is the same in the transplanted parental intestine as in the F1 host.[56,76] Initially this was thought to demonstrate an "innocent bystander effect," with donor lymphocytes reacting to host leukocytes that had recirculated into the parental graft. Soluble mediators released would secondarily injure the epithelium. Alternately, this could also reflect an autoimmune reaction.[77,78] These intestinal studies have emphasized epithelial proliferation rather than apoptoses and thus may represent the epithelial response rather than injury per se.

One of the earliest observations was the significance of the intestinal flora. While mismatched transplants commonly lead to severe diarrhea and high mortality, mismatched (even xenogeneic) transplants in gnotobiotic recipients are not associated with diarrhea or high mortality.[79,80] Selective recontamination of the gnotobiotic recipients leads to diarrhea and fatal GVHD with gram-negative organisms.[81] Conversely, decontamination of recipients with nonabsorbable antibiotics appears to provide some protection against GVHD in small studies.[82,83]

At the simplest level, the flora could be superinfecting an intestinal lesion created by an immune reaction. Autopsy observations of bacterial enteritis and associated sepsis suggests that invasion and penetration by flora is common with GVHD.[47]

The flora, however, most likely contributes indirectly as well. Van Bekkum observed that the flora also exacerbated the *cutaneous* lesions of GVHD and proposed that the flora stimulated a cross-reaction with normal epithelial components.[82] Endotoxin from gram-negative bacilli furthermore enhances the immune reaction. Injection of small doses of endotoxin into chimeras enhanced not only the intestinal GVHD but also cutaneous GVHD.[84] Antibodies to endotoxin have a protective effect against GVHD.[85,86] If endotoxin penetrated into the lamina propria, it could stimulate the immune reaction against the host by stimulating the release of multiple cytokines from T cells and macrophages, including interleukin (IL-1), immune interferon, and tumor necrosis factor alpha (TNF-α).[87-90] The IL-1 would activate regional lymphocytes. TNF-α released by macrophages could directly injure the epithelium.[91] Repeated injections of endotoxin into neonatal mice produces a runting syndrome similar to GVHD.[92] Treatment of murine radiation chimeras with monoclonal antibody to TNF-α blocks the usual lesions of intestinal and cutaneous GVHD.[93]

The flora could also alter the targets. The lamina propria leukocytes can themselves be antigenic and serve as the targets of GVHD, even after lethal irradiation. While a host exposed to the normal flora would have numerous such cells, they would be relatively sparse in gnotobiotic recipients. This could explain in part the reduced severity of GVHD in newborn chimeras.

GVHD induces a severe and prolonged immune deficiency. This is often not recognized in humans because of the immunosuppressive agents used in treatment. Delayed reconstitution of the immune system is seen, however, in animal models. Acute GVHD creates a thymic dysplasia through the destruction of the thymic epithelium, delaying reconstitution of peripheral immunity.[60,94]

Within the intestinal lamina propria, GVHD is associated with a marked loss of IgA- and IgM-containing plasma cells in the lamina propria.[47] These cells, or their precursors, are relatively radio-resistant and are present in near normal numbers in human recipients with graft failure, so this most likely is a function of the immune reaction of GVHD rather than the ablative preparatory protocol. Salivary IgA is also markedly reduced in patients with chronic GVHD (most with a history of acute GVHD).[95] These abnormalities could account for the increased sepsis by associated enteric pathogens and, later, the numerous caries.

Presumably, GVHD also enhances the immune deficiency by depleting antigen-presenting cells, including the relatively radio-resistant host dendritic cells and the M cells overlying the Peyer's patches.[96,97]

Any pathogenetic explanation of the severe intestinal injury seen in radiation chimeras must incorporate the factors that are essential. They should also include observations consistently observed and probably essential. The first essential component is the engraftment of T lymphocytes reactive to the host antigens. When the donor T lymphocytes are depleted, GVHD rarely develops. While some have described increased intraepithelial NK cells, we are not aware of any depletion studies in which the absence of NK cells has prevented GVHD. The other essential factor is the presence of gram-negative bacteria. Directly related is the release of endotoxin and TNF-α. GVHD can be prevented at any of these three points by utilizing a sterile host, or antibodies to endotoxin or TNF-α.

Three components *consistently* observed with severe injury in the *radiation* chimera include extraintestinal GVHD, apoptotic lesions within the crypts, and a deficiency of the mucosal immunity. Cutaneous GVHD usually coincides with the onset of diarrhea. This finding indicates clearly that GVHD-generated effector cells capable of injuring host targets *are* in circulation at the onset of the intestinal component. Apoptotic lesions are also an early observation present in biopsies taken at the onset of diarrhea. The immune deficiency, defined by absence of IgA and IgM plasma cells may occur slightly later.

The initial event is most likely a cellular immune reaction against the intestine facilitating invasion of gram-negative bacteria or endotoxin. The surface epithelium appears intact at this point without significant increase in the IEL. Possibly the immune reaction eliminates dendritic cells or other components critical to the barrier against endotoxins. The immune reaction can lead to other sequelae, which, although not essential, contribute to the injury, such as the proliferation of the epithelium, Ia antigen induction, and increase in mast cells.

The lamina propria histiocytes release TNF-α. The release could be induced by endotoxin or could result from lysis by the donor immune system.[98] TNF-α was initially recognized for its ability to kill tumor cells.[99] The crypt epithelium possibly resembles the tumors, with its rapid epithelial proliferation. The mechanism of injury is unclear but may involve a direct interaction with the epithelium or could injure the endothelial cells in the vessels nurturing the crypts.[91,100-102] If sufficiently extensive it would interfere with the regeneration by depleting the epithelial stem cells.

The injury has features in common with radiation enteritis, including the penetration of endotoxin and the presence of numerous apoptotic lesions. Sequential studies indicate that GVHD is not simply a continuation or exacerbation of radiation enteritis[20,21,46] since radiation injury is repaired prior to the onset of GVHD. Nonetheless, we wonder why radiation enteritis is rapidly repaired in these patients, while GVHD-associated injury progresses to severe mucosal sloughing.

A sustained immune reaction against the epithelium could account for the progressive injury. While the leukocytes would be depleted after the initial phase of the GVHD, the reaction against the epithelium could be enhanced as greater injury leads to more lymphocyte stimulation by endotoxin. If the epithelial expression of class II antigen is a secondary reaction, this latter expression could also enhance the antigenicity of the epithelium.

The progressive injury could also result from an inadequate mucosal immunity. Once the residual host immunity is eliminated, it may be months before the intestinal immune system is reconstituted with donor cells. Besides the obvious problems of luminal pathogens entering the lamina propria and circulation, recipients would be unable to develop an immune response to new oral antigens. Nor could they develop tolerance to ingested antigens. The significance of the immune deficiency is implicated by two observations. Occasional recipients have developed an acute-type GVHD in the late posttransplant period. Presumably by this time the host cells have been eliminated and the mucosa repopulated with donor cells. Although apoptotic lesions are observed, these rarely progress to a generalized mucosal sloughing. Second, while the cutaneous GVHD frequently responds to immunosuppressive agents, the severe diarrhea and epithelial injury of the gut typically persists. Assuming that the cutaneous GVHD reflects the immune reaction against the host, the persistent gut involvement most likely results from secondary reactions and infections.

Oral and Intestinal Chronic GVHD

The intestinal aspects of *chronic* GVHD are neither as life-threatening nor as well characterized as acute GVHD. Nonetheless, they are responsible for considerable morbidity. The immunopathology has potentially important implications for our understanding of intestinal immune deficiency and oral tolerance.

Often recipients present with a sicca syndrome, with profound dryness of their mouth and eyes.[29,30,103,104] Not only is the flow of saliva decreased, secretory IgA within the saliva is also decreased. Notably, these patients may have numerous caries.[95,105] They do not have significant titers of antisalivary gland duct antibodies.[106]

The histopathology of the salivary glands resembles that of Sjögren's syndrome.[30,107,108] Examination of the minor salivary glands seen in lip biopsies are usually helpful in diagnosing chronic GVHD. The ducts have an intraepithelial infiltrate of lymphocytes, while the interstitial regions have a mixture of lymphocytes, macrophages, and plasma cells. In advanced cases, there is dropout of the acini, and the gland is fibrotic.

In the rat model of chronic GVHD, the tongue has a very striking and characteristic picture.[33,109] In the early stages, there is a marked submucosal infiltrate of lymphocytes and histiocytes. This develops into a myositis with injury to the muscle and later dropout of the muscle. In the later phases, the muscle is replaced with dense fibrosis. During the chronic GVHD, the mast cells are quite prominent.

Esophageal involvement with chronic GVHD leads to dysphagia, aspiration, and weight loss. The esophagus, particularly the upper two thirds, is characterized by epithelial desquamation, strictures, webs, and dense mucosal fibrosis.[27,30,33,108,110,111] Although the fibrosis resembles scleroderma, there is generally little atrophy of the muscularis externa.

The watery secretory diarrhea associated with acute GVHD is not commonly observed with chronic GVHD. Rather, such patients have variable problems, including abdominal pain, malabsorption, and bacterial overgrowth of the upper intestinal tract.[11]

During the early years of human marrow transplantation, chronic GVHD was often not recognized or adequately treated until the later stages. Sections of the stomach, intestine, and colon from these patients had fibrosis of the lamina propria and submucosal regions.[30] Today, with earlier recognition and better treatment, the fibrosis is not as prominent. The histologic changes are of a nonspecific nature, with crypt distortion and mild fibrosis.

These problems most likely result from both immune reactions (including autoimmune) against the host and a prolonged immune deficiency. The destruction of the ducts and glands of the salivary glands resembles that seen in the lacrimal glands, the cutaneous eccrine glands, and to some extent the hepatic bile ducts. The myositis described in the tongue is also described in the skeletal muscle of some human recipients with chronic GVHD.[31] Thus the abnormal thymic microenvironment and other factors leading to loss of self-tolerance and systemic autoimmune reactions most likely also produce the intestinal pathology.

A principle predictive factor for chronic GVHD is a previous episode of *acute* GVHD.[34,35] The deficiency of local immunity observed with chronic GVHD most likely begins with acute GVHD.[47,94] The prolonged deficiency as well as the simple destruction of salivary glands would certainly put these patients at greater risk for developing dental caries and bacterial overgrowth of the upper intestinal tract.

While most of us assume that the intestinal tract is an end-stage target of chronic GVHD, one fascinating observation suggests that the intestinal microenvironment might play a primary role. One patient with chronic GVHD was observed to have an apparent reaction to milk, specifically casein.[112] The *cutaneous* manifestations correlated with the oral ingestion of casein. In a systematic study, recipients with GVHD frequently had circulating complexes to bovine casein.[113] This suggests that in this patient at least there was a breakdown of the usual dichotomous reaction, with intestinal antibodies and systemic tolerance to orally ingested antigens.

GRAFT-VERSUS-HOST DISEASE OF THE LIVER

Hepatic Aspects of Acute GVHD

While hepatic GVHD is not as life-threatening as intestinal GVHD, the liver is a major target tissue. Its involvement is usually a harbinger of severe systemic GVHD, associated with greater mortality.[8,9,45]

Acute hepatic GVHD is readily recognized when the hepatic dysfunction follows the onset of the characteristic rash and diarrhea. There is a moderate initial elevation of the alkaline phosphatase and aspartate aminotransferase, followed by a rise in the bilirubin and often hepatomegaly. Overt hepatic failure is unusual, although persistent acute GVHD can lead to prolonged jaundice.

Often, however, hepatic GVHD can be difficult to diagnose. The onset may precede cutaneous and enteric GVHD. Hepatic GVHD must also be differentiated from other complications, including veno-occlusive disease (VOD),[13,114,115] virus infections (including cytomegalovirus, adenovirus, hepatitis B, and non-A, non-B hepatitis),[116,117] and relapse of leukemia with infiltration of the liver. VOD is frequently observed in the early posttransplant period, accompanied by hyperbilirubinemia, weight gain, hepatomegaly, and ascites. Virus infections should be seriously considered if the liver enzymes are markedly elevated.

Histologic examination reveals a progression of injury as a function of posttransplant interval.[4,13,20,21,118-121] When GVHD occurs during the first month posttransplant, the injury is principally lobular, consisting of small foci of necrotic, acidophilic cells and accompanying mild lymphocytic infiltrate. At this stage, the bile ducts may appear unremarkable. Next, there is an infiltrate of the bile duct epithelium by small lymphocytes. This coincides with epithelial injury: vacuolization, cellular debris, and nuclear atypia (Fig. 28–3). The bile duct injury is usually more severe in the smaller ducts and can extend into the periductal glands and into the ducts of Hering.[4,122] The bile ducts may respond by undergoing proliferation. However, if the GVHD is severe or persistent, the bile ducts are lost from the smaller triads. After cutaneous GVHD responds to therapy, the bilirubin often continues to rise. Biopsies during this period will show epithelial atypia but no significant lymphocytic infiltrate. In marrow recipients, repair of the ductal epithelium is delayed. It is important to distinguish the jaundice of the resulting *residual* GVHD from an *active* GVHD.

A third target within the liver may be the vascular endothelium.[119] In a systematic review of marrow transplant liver biopsies, 8 of 32 demonstrated attachment of lymphocytes to the portal or central vein endothelium ("endothelialitis"). Endothelialitis is characteristic in liver allograft rejection.[123] The infiltrates with hepatic GVHD, however, are considerably less than hepatic allograft rejection and therefore more difficult to recognize.

The pathogenesis of hepatic GVHD has not been studied as extensively as cutaneous or enteric GVHD. Most assessments address the duct epithelial injury.

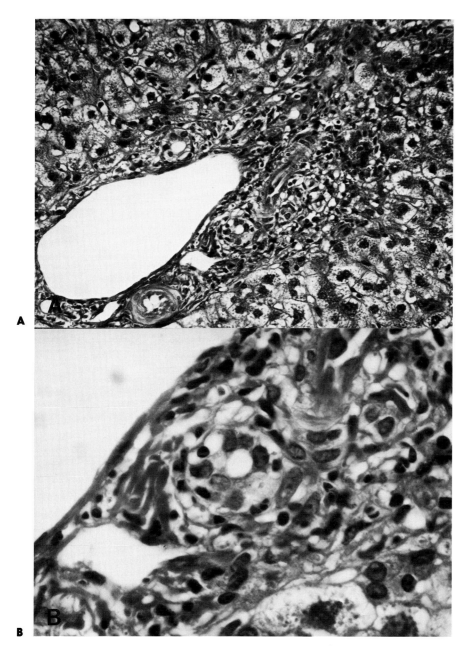

Figure 28 – 3   Liver biopsy with acute GVHD. **A**: The portal triads have a mild infiltrate of lymphocytes. **B**: The bile ducts have lymphocytes within the basement membrane associated with epithelial injury, including vacuolization. H and E; A, ×250; B, ×500.

Ultrastructure descriptions note an intimate contact between infiltrating lymphocytes and the duct epithelial cells.[124] Point contact was observed with the degenerating epithelial cells similar to that described in other tissues with GVHD and suggests a cell-mediated injury to the bile ducts.[51,52]

Generally, acute GVHD is associated with an increase of CD8+ lymphocytes in the portal triads compared with recipients without GVHD.[120,125,126] One study also observed an increase in NK cells.[126] The lymphocytes within the duct basement membrane were not specifically described, however. The effect of histoincompatibility on the phenotype of the infiltrating lymphocytes has not been addressed. Human recipients show predominantly minor histocompatibility differences, while rate studies generally represent differences in both class I and class II MHC antigens.

In the normal liver, the bile duct epithelium expresses minimal class I and no significant class II MHC antigen.[127,128] With GVHD, however, both antigens are intensely expressed.[126,129,130] Similarly, Kupffer cells normally express only focal class II antigen, but with GVHD they demonstrate diffuse class II antigen. The endothelium lining the sinusoids shows an increase in class I antigen with GVHD.[129,130] Since Kupffer cells and possibly endothelial cells originate from circulating cells, it is unclear whether the induced antigen is host or donor in origin.[22,131]

Most of the elements involved in the pathogenesis of intestinal tract GVHD also pertain to the liver. The electron microscopy observations and phenotype studies are consistent with a direct, cell-mediated injury to the duct epithelium. The destruction of host Kupffer cells could certainly contribute to the initial hepatocellular injury by an innocent bystander mechanism. Presumably there is a deficiency of biliary secretory IgA. The liver, therefore, would be more susceptible to the effects of infection and the immune stimulatory effects of endotoxin.

Hepatic Manifestations of Chronic GVHD

The liver is adversely affected in most recipients with chronic GVHD.[30,34] The hepatic dysfunction can be part of a systemic chronic GVHD or the predominant feature. Patients with a more limited hepatic chronic GVHD generally have a better prognosis.[132] There is a variable elevation of the bilirubin, but alkaline phosphatase level is generally elevated.

Biopsies at this stage typically exhibit expanded portal triads, with a mixed infiltrate of lymphocytes, histiocytes, and often eosinophils (Fig. 28–4).[30,119] The infiltrate extends into the periportal region. There is usually increased portal fibrosis, occasionally progressing to cirrhosis.[133,134] The bile ducts are infiltrated with lymphocytes and show injury and bile stasis. In some there is bile duct replication, while in others there is severe duct dropout. These recipients are persistently and strikingly jaundiced.

The overall pathogenesis of chronic graft-versus-host disease was discussed above. Currently there are few systematic descriptions of the immunopathology in the liver. In long-term rat chimeras with chronic GVHD, the sinusoidal and portal infiltrate consisted predominantly of CD4+ T lymphocytes.[125] While few intraepithelial lymphocytes were observed, most of them were CD8+. Most of the portal lymphocytes in a murine model of chronic GVHD were T lymphocytes, with a noted paucity of CD8+ cells.[135] In this study, the bile duct epithelium expressed strong I-A antigen. Immunoelectron microscopy demonstrated the strongest I-A expression along the basilar basement membrane, with minimal expression observed in the apices.[136]

Chronic hepatic GVHD is often compared with primary biliary cirrhosis (PBC).[137,138] Indeed, the similarities provide support for an immune mechanism for

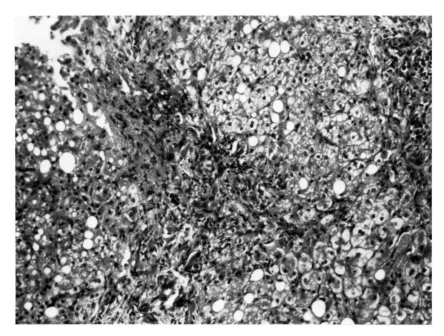

Figure 28–4 Liver biopsy with chronic GVHD. The portal triads are expanded, with increased fibrosis and a mixed cellular infiltrate of lymphocytes and histiocytes. This specimen shows proliferation of the bile ducts. In many patients, however, there is bile duct atresia. Masson trichrome, ×150.

PBC. Both entities represent "dry gland" syndromes with injury not only to the bile ducts but also the salivary and lacrimal glands. While the titers are not as great as PBC, some patients with chronic GVHD do have antimitochondrial antibodies.[30,132] The histology of chronic GVHD resembles the early stages of PBC with bile duct infiltration and necrosis, portal infiltrates, and fibrosis. Granulomatous inflammation is unusual in human recipients and some animal models but have been observed in two murine models.[110,139] The fine structure of the lymphocyte-associated bile duct injury has been related to human chronic GVHD.[140] Finally, the immunopathology of PBC resembles that described with chronic GVHD.[141,142]

This comparison has proved useful in supporting an immune basis for PBC and for establishing readily inducible animal models to further study both entities. The similarities, however, should not lull us into a false sense of understanding. Both remain complex, poorly understood problems. The hepatic lesions of chronic GVHD do not simply represent an immune reaction against the bile duct epithelium. Rather, it is more likely the result of processes occurring elsewhere, such as the loss of self-tolerance normally maintained by the thymus. There are major differences between the two entities, such as the very strong association with anti-mitochondrial antibodies and sex predilection of PBC. Quite possibly, therefore, the initiating events are totally different, and the two simply share a final common pathway. The induced class II antigen on the bile ducts and the infiltrate of CD4+ lymphocytes have been related because of the requirement of CD4+ lymphocytes to recognize class II antigen on the targets.[67] The lymphokines from

CD4+ lymphocytes, however, can themselves induce class II antigen.[63,73] The cause and effect relationship between the lymphocytes and the induced antigen remains unclear. Indeed, lymphocytes cloned from liver biopsies with PBC are predominantly CD8+ cytotoxic cells.[143]

FUTURE DIRECTIONS

Following the classic descriptions of GVHD, many of us were comfortable in our understanding of enteric and hepatic GVHD. Simply put, they represented an alloimmune reaction against the host intestinal and bile duct epithelium. Today, few if any of us feel comfortable with the pathogenesis. Multiple immune processes are reacting against various cellular and molecular targets, some still undefined. GVHD is more than a set of immune reactions. It induces a severe immune deficiency. The resulting opportunistic infections, as well as the systemic circulation of ingested antigens and factors such as endotoxin, can significantly alter these immune reactions. A clear understanding is furthermore hampered by diverse paraphenomena that are often consistently associated with the lesions of GVHD.

In the study of acute GVHD, the sequence of critical immune events leading to epithelial injury must be defined, including both systemic and tissue reactions. The mechanism of the severe deficiency of local immunity must be determined. The specific relationship between infectious agents, the immune reactions of GVHD, and the epithelial injury should be further explored. Progress will come from additional animal studies in which more of the variables are controlled, combined with immunopathology and tissue explant experiments of animal and human tissues.

With improvements in the marrow transplant procedure, patients are surviving longer, which in turn has led to more marrow transplant units opening in recent years and the treatment of older recipients. These three factors have combined to make chronic GVHD a primary clinical challenge. At this point, a better pathologic and immunopathologic description of intestinal chronic GVHD is needed. Hepatic chronic GVHD must also be better defined. The pathogenetic significance of the observed immunopathologic abnormalities has yet to be established.

As the critical variables are better defined and controlled, GVHD may prove quite helpful in understanding similar lesions outside the marrow transplant setting. For example, it is increasingly recognized that the acquired immune deficiency syndrome is not simply a severe immune deficiency with resulting opportunistic infection. Rather, there appears to be an interrelationship between immune deficiency, infection, and immune reactions against the host. More specifically, AIDS complications of enteritis and sclerosing cholangitis share similarities with the enteric and hepatic GVHD. Our understanding of these complications is currently at the descriptive stage. An evolving insight into enteric and hepatic GVHD will most likely provide greater insight into these complications as well.

REFERENCES

1. Bortin MM, Rimm AA: Increasing utilization of bone marrow transplantation. *Transplantation* 42:229–234, 1986.
2. Santos GW: History of bone marrow transplantation. *Clin Haematol* 12:611–39, 1983.

3. Thomas ED: High-dose therapy and bone marrow transplantation. *Semin Oncol* 12(Suppl 6):15–20, 1985.

4. Slavin RE, Woodruff JM: The pathology of bone marrow transplantation. *Pathol Annu* 9:291–344, 1974.

5. Santos GW, Tutschka PJ, Brookmeyer R, et al: Marrow transplantation for acute nonlymphocytic leukemia after treatment with busulfan and cyclophosphamide. *N Engl J Med* 309:1347–53, 1983.

6. Deeg HJ, Storb R, Thomas ED, et al: Cyclosporine as prophylaxis for graft-versus-host disease: a randomized study in patients undergoing marrow transplantation for acute nonlymphoblastic leukemia. *Blood* 65:1325–34, 1985.

7. Santos GW, Tutschka PJ, Brookmeyer R, et al: Cyclosporine plus methylprednisolone as prophylaxis for graft-versus-host disease: a randomized double blind study in patients undergoing allogeneic marrow transplantation. *Clin Transplant* 1:21–8, 1987.

8. Wagner JE, Vogelsang GB, Beschorner WE: The pathology of graft-versus-host disease. *J Pediatr Hematol Oncol* 11:196–212, 1989.

9. Sale GE: Pathology and recent pathogenetic studies in human graft-versus-host disease. *Surv Synth Pathol Res* 3:235, 1984.

10. McDonald GB, Shulman HM, Sullivan KM, et al: Intestinal and hepatic complications of human bone marrow transplantation, part I. *Gastroenterology* 90:460–77, 1986.

11. McDonald GB, Shulman HM, Sullivan KM, et al: Intestinal and hepatic complications of human bone marrow transplantation, part II. *Gastroenterology* 90:770–84, 1986.

12. Beschorner WE: Destruction of the intestinal mucosa after bone marrow transplantation and graft-versus-host disease. *Surv Synth Pathol Res* 3:264–74, 1984.

13. Beschorner WE, Pino J, Boitnott JK, et al: Pathology of the liver with bone marrow transplantation. Effects of busulfan, carmustine, acute graft-versus-host disease, and cytomegalovirus infection. *Am J Pathol* 99:369–85, 1980.

14. Jacobson O, Marks EK, Gaston EO, et al: Effect of spleen protection on mortality following x-irradiation. *J Lab Clin Med,* 34:1538–43, 1949.

15. Jacobson LO, Simmons EL, Marks EK, et al: Recovery from radiation injury. *Science* 113:510–11.

16. Barnes DWH, Loutit JF: Spleen protection: the cellular hypothesis. In Bacq ZM: *Radiobiology Symposium.* London, Butterworths, 1955, pp 134–5.

17. Medawar PB: Introduction; definition of the immunologically competent cell. *Ciba Found Study Group* 16:1–4, 1963.

18. Billingham RE: The biology of graft-versus-host reactions. *Harvey Lect* 62:21–78, 1966.

19. Simonsen M: Graft versus host reactions. Their natural history and applicability as tools of research. *Prog Allergy* 6:349–467, 1962.

20. Woodruff JM, Eltringham JR, Casey HW: Early secondary disease in the rhesus monkey. I. A comparative histopathologic study. *Lab Invest* 20:499–511, 1969.

21. Beschorner WE, Tutschka PJ, Santos GW: The sequential morphology of acute graft-versus-host disease in the rat radiation chimera. *Clin Immunol Immunopathol* 22:203–24, 1982.

22. Gale RP, Sparkes RS, Golde DW: Bone marrow origin of hepatic macrophages (Kupffer cells) in humans. *Science* 201:937–8, 1978.

23. Witherspoon R, Lum L, Storb R: Immunologic reconstitution after human marrow grafting. *Semin Hematol* 21:2–10, 1984.

24. Ault KA, Antin JH, Ginsburg D, et al: Phenotype of recovering lymphoid cell populations after marrow transplantation. *J Exp Med* 161:1483–502, 1985.

25. Elfenbein GJ, Ashkenazi YJ, Barth KC: Further phenotypic characterization of T cells

after human allogeneic bone marrow transplantation. *Transplantation* 39:97–102, 1985.

26. Sale GE, Lerner KG, Barker EA, et al: The skin biopsy in the diagnosis of acute graft-versus-host disease in man. *Am J Pathol* 89:621–35, 1977.

27. Simes MA, Johansson E, Rapola J: Scleroderma-like graft-versus-host disease as late consequence of bone marrow grafting. *Lancet* 2:831–832, 1977.

28. Saurat JH, Didier JL, Gluckman E, et al: Graft-versus-host reaction and lichen planus-like eruption in man. *Br J Dermatol* 92:591–592, 1975.

29. Graze PR, Gale RP: Chronic graft-versus-host disease: a syndrome of disordered immunity. *Am J Med* 66:611–620, 1979.

30. Shulman HM, Sullivan KM, Weiden PL, et al: Chronic graft-versus-host syndrome in man: a long-term clinicopathological study of 20 Seattle patients. *Am J Med* 69:204–217, 1980.

31. Reyes MG, Noronha P, Thomas W Jr, et al: Myositis of chronic graft versus host disease. *Neurology* 33:1222–4, 1983.

32. Bolger GB, Sullivan KM, Spence AM: Myasthenia gravis after allogeneic bone marrow transplantation: relationship to chronic graft-versus-host disease. *Neurology* 36:1087–91, 1986.

33. Beschorner WE, Tutschka PJ, Santos GW: Chronic graft-versus-host disease in the rat radiation chimera. I. Clinical presentation, hematology, histology, and immunopathology in long term chimera. *Transplantation* 33:393–97, 1982.

34. Storb R, Prentice RL, Sullivan KM, et al: Predictive factors in chronic graft-versus-host disease in patients with aplastic anemia treated by marrow transplantation from HLA-identical siblings. *Ann Intern Med* 98:461–466, 1983.

35. Ringden O, Paulin T, Lonnqvist B, et al: An analysis of factors predisposing to chronic graft-versus-host disease. *Exp Hematol* 13:1062–1067, 1985.

36. Parkman R: Clonal analysis of murine graft-vs-host disease. I. Phenotypic and functional analysis of T lymphocyte clones. *J Immunol* 136:3543–8, 1986.

37. Seddik M, Seemayer TA, Kongshavn P, et al: Thymic epithelial functional deficit in chronic graft-versus-host reactions. *Transplant Proc* 11:967–969, 1979.

38. Atkinson K, Incefy GS, Storb R, et al: Low serum thymic hormone levels in patients with chronic graft-versus-host disease. *Blood* 59:1073–1077, 1982.

39. Beschorner WE, Hess AD, Shinn CA, et al: Transfer of cyclosporin A associated syngeneic graft-vs-host disease (GVHD) by thymocytes. Resemblance to chronic GVHD. *Transplantation* 45:209–15, 1988.

40. van Bekkum DW, de Vries JJ: Pathology of the radiation chimera. In: *Radiation Chimeras*. London, Logos, 1967, pp 127–165.

41. Glucksberg H, Storb R, Fefer A, et al: Clinical manifestations of graft-vs.-host disease in human recipients of marrow from HL-A-matched sibling donors. *Transplantation* 18:295–304, 1974.

42. Rosenberg HK, Serota FT, Koch P, et al: Radiographic features of gastrointestinal graft-vs-host disease. *Radiology* 138:371–4, 1981.

43. Jones B, Kramer SS, Saral R, et al: Gastrointestinal inflammation after bone marrow transplantation: graft-versus-host disease or opportunistic infection? *AJR* 150:277–81, 1988.

44. Kruger GRF, Berard CW, DeLellis RA, et al: Graft-versus-host disease: morphologic variation and differential diagnosis in eight cases of HLA-matched bone marrow transplantation. *Am J Pathol* 63:179–85, 1971.

45. Lerner KG, Kao GF, Storb R, et al: Histopathology of graft-vs.-host reaction (GvHR) in human recipients of marrow from HL-A-matched sibling donors. *Transplant Proc* 6:367–71, 1974.

46. Sale GE, Shulman HM, McDonald GB, et al: Gastrointestinal graft-versus-host disease in man. A clinicopathologic study of the rectal biopsy. *Am J Surg Pathol* 3:291–9, 1979.

47. Beschorner WE, Yardley JH, Tutschka PJ, et al: Deficiency of intestinal immunity with graft-vs.-host disease in humans. *J Infect Dis* 144:38–46, 1981.

48. McDonald TT, Ferguson A: Hypersensitivity reactions in the small intestine. III. The effects of allograft rejection and of graft-versus-host disease on epithelial cell kinetics. *Cell Tissue Kinet* 10:301–12, 1977.

49. Mowat AMcI, Ferguson A: Intraepithelial lymphocyte count and crypt hyperplasia measure the mucosal component of the graft-versus-host reaction in mouse small intestine. *Gastroenterology* 83:417–23, 1982.

50. Guy-Grand D, Vassalli P: Gut injury in mouse graft-versus-host reaction. Study of its occurrence and mechanisms. *J Clin Invest* 77:1584–95, 1986.

51. Gallucci BB, Sale GE, McDonald GB, et al: The fine structure of human rectal epithelium in acute graft-versus-host disease. *Am J Surg Pathol* 6:293–305, 1982.

52. Sale GE, Gallucci BB, Schubert MM, et al: Direct ultrastructural evidence of target-directed polarization by cytotoxic lymphocytes in lesions of human graft-vs-host disease. *Arch Pathol Lab Med* 111:333–6, 1987.

53. Dilly SA, Sloane JP: Changes in rectal leucocytes after allogeneic bone marrow transplantation. *Clin Exp Immunol* 67:151–8, 1987.

54. Muto M, Sado T, Aizawa S, et al: Bone marrow transplantation across the major histocompatibility barrier in specific-pathogen-free mice: effects of intact versus T cell depleted bone marrow on the expression of anti-host reaction in the recipient spleens. *J Immunol* 127:2421–5, 1981.

55. Reinsmoen NL, Kersey JH, Bach FH: Detection of HLA restricted anti-minor histocompatibility antigen(s) reactive cells from skin GVHD lesions. *Hum Immunol* 11:P249–57, 1984.

56. Mowat AMcI, Felstein MV, Borland A, et al: Experimental studies of immunologically mediated enteropathy. Development of cell mediated immunity and intestinal pathology during a graft-versus-host reaction in irradiated mice. *Gut* 29:949–56, 1988.

57. Rodt H, Kolb HJ, Netzel B, et al: Effect of anti-T-cell globulin on GVHD in leukemic patients treated with BMT. *Transplant Proc* 13:257–61, 1981.

58. Mason DW: Subsets of T cells in the rat mediating lethal graft versus-host disease. *Transplantation* 32:222–6, 1981.

59. Prentice HG: OKT3 incubation of donor marrow for prophylaxis of acute graft-vs.-host disease (GvHD) in allogeneic bone marrow transplantation. *J Clin Immunol* 2:148S–153S, 1982.

60. Seemayer TA, Lapp WS, Bolande RP: Thymic epithelial injury in graft-versus-host reactions following adrenalectomy. *Am J Pathol* 93:325–38, 1978.

61. Jordan RK, Robinson JH, Hopkinson NA, et al: Thymic epithelium and the induction of transplantation tolerance in nude mice. *Nature* 314:454–6, 1985.

62. Morrissey PJ, Bradley D, Sharrow SO, et al: T cell tolerance to non-H-2-encoded stimulatory alloantigens is induced intrathymically but not prethymically. *J Exp Med* 158:365–77, 1983.

63. Abb J, Abb H, Deinhardt F: Characterization of human interferon gamma-producing leukocytes with monoclonal antileukocyte antibodies. *Med Microbiol Immunol (Berl)* 171:215–23, 1983.

64. Reynolds CW, Timonen TT, Holden HT, et al: Natural killer cell activity in the rat. Analysis of effector cell morphology and effects of interferon on natural killer cell function in the athymic (nude) rat. *Eur J Immunol* 12:577–82, 1982.

65. Holda JH, Maier T, Claman HN: Natural suppressor activity in graft-vs-host spleen

and normal bone marrow is augmented by IL 2 and interferon-gamma. *J Immunol* 137:3538–43, 1986.

66. Dilly SA, Sloane JP: Changes in rectal leucocytes after allogeneic bone marrow transplantation. *Clin Exp Immunol* 67:151–8, 1987.

67. Meuer SC, Schlossman SF, Reinherz EL: Clonal analysis of human cytotoxic T lymphocytes: T4+ and T8+ effector T cells recognize products of different major histocompatibility complex regions. *Proc Natl Acad Sci USA* 79:4395–9, 1982.

68. Piguet P-F: GVHR elicited by products of class I or class I loci of the MHC: analysis of the response of mouse T lymphocytes to products of class I and class II loci of the MHC in correlation with GVHR-induced mortality, medullary aplasia, and enteropathy. *J Immunol* 135:1637–43, 1985.

69. MacDonald TT, Carter PB: Mouse Peyer's patches contain T cells capable of inducing the graft-versus-host reaction (GVHR). *Transplantation* 26:162–5, 1978.

70. Barclay AN, Mason DW: Induction of Ia antigen in rat epidermal cells and gut epithelium by immunological stimuli. *J Exp Med* 156:1665–76, 1982.

71. Sviland L, Pearson AD, Eastham EJ, et al: Class II antigen expression by keratinocytes and enterocytes—an early feature of graft-versus-host-disease. *Transplantation* 46:402–6, 1988.

72. Beschorner WE, Farmer ER, Saral R, et al: Epithelial class II antigen expression in cutaneous GVHD. *Transplantation* 44:237–43, 1987.

73. Pober JS, Gimbrone MA, Cotran RS, et al: Ia expression by vascular endothelium is inducible by activated T cells and by human interferon-gamma. *J Exp Med* 157:1339–1353, 1983.

74. Basham TY, Merigan TC: Recombinant interferon-γ increases HLA-DR synthesis and expression. *J Immunol* 130:1492–1494, 1983.

75. Stuart PM, Zlotnik A, Woodward JG: Induction of class I and class II MHC antigen expression on murine bone marrow-derived macrophages by IL-4 (B cell stimulatory factor 1). *J Immunol* 140:1542–7, 1988.

76. Elson CO, Reilly RW, Rosenberg IH: Small intestinal injury in the graft-versus-host reaction: an innocent bystander phenomenon. *Gastroenterology* 72:886–889, 1977.

77. Hess AD, Vogelsang GB, Silanskis M, et al: Syngeneic graft-versus-host disease after allogeneic bone marrow transplantation and cyclosporine treatment. *Transplant Proc* 20(Suppl 3):487–92, 1988.

78. Havele C, Wegmann TG, Longenecker BM: Tolerance and autoimmunity to erythroid differentiation (B-G) major histocompatibility complex alloantigens of the chicken. *J Exp Med* 156:321–36, 1982.

79. van Bekkum DW, Waay D, De Vries MJ: Evidence of secondary disease in germ free heterologous radiation chimeras. *Exp Hematol* 8:3–5, 1965.

80. Jones JM, Wilson R, Bealmear PM: Mortality and gross pathology of secondary disease in germfree mouse radiation chimeras. *Radiation Res* 45:577–88, 1971.

81. Pollard M, Chang CF, Srivastava KK: The role of microflora in development of graft-versus-host disease. *Transplant Proc* 8:533–6, 1976.

82. van Bekkum DW, Roodenburg J, Heidt PJ, et al: Mitigation of secondary disease of allogeneic mouse radiation chimeras by modification of the intestinal microflora. *J Natl Cancer Inst* 52:401–4, 1974.

83. Mahmoud HK, Schaefer UW, Schuning F, et al: Laminar air flow versus barrier nursing in marrow transplant recipients. *Blut* 49:375–81, 1984.

84. Lampert IA, Moore RH, Huby R, et al: Observations on the role of endotoxin in graft-versus-host disease. In Levin J, Büller HR, ten Cate JW, et al: *Bacterial Endo-*

toxins: *Pathophysiological Effects, Clinical Significance, and Pharmacological Control.* Alan R Liss, 1988, pp 351–9.

85. Faulkner L, Rapson N, Moore R, et al: The influence of the gut flora on graft versus host disease (GvHD) following allogeneic bone marrow transplantation — experimental observations and possible mechanisms. In Levin J, Büller HR, ten Cate JW, et al: *Bacterial Endotoxins: Pathophysiological Effects, Clinical Significance, and Pharmacological Control.* Alan R Liss, 1988, pp 195–206.

86. Cohen J, Moore RH, al Hashimi S, et al: Antibody titres to a rough mutant strain of *Escherichia coli* in patients undergoing allogeneic bone marrow transplantation. Evidence of a protective effect against graft-versus-host disease. *Lancet* 1:8–11, 1987.

87. Rosenstreich DL, Glode LM, Mergenhagen SE: Action of endotoxin on lymphoid cells. *J Infect Dis* 136:S239–45, 1977.

88. Friedman H, Klein TW, Nowotny A, et al: Lipopolysaccharide induction of gamma interferon production. *J Immunol Immunopharmacol* 6:76–7, 1986.

89. Movat HZ, Cybulsky MI, Colditz IG, et al: Acute inflammation in gram-negative infection: endotoxin, interleukin 1, tumor necrosis factor, and neutrophils. *Fed Proc* 46:97–104, 1987.

90. Haeffner-Cavaillon N, Cavaillon JM, Moreau M, et al: Interleukin 1 secretion by human monocytes stimulated by the isolated polysaccharide region of the *Bordetella pertussis* endotoxin. *Mol Immunol* 21:389–95, 1984.

91. Laster SM, Wood JG, Gooding LR: Tumor necrosis factor can induce both apoptic and necrotic forms of cell lysis. *J Immunol* 141:2629–34, 1988.

92. Keast D, Walters MN-I: The pathology of murine runting and its modification by neomycin sulphate gavages. *Immunology* 15:247–62, 1968.

93. Piguet PF, Grau GE, Allet B, et al: Tumor necrosis factor/cachectin is an effector of skin and gut lesions of the acute phase of graft-vs.-host disease. *J Exp Med* 166:1280–9, 1987.

94. Lapp WS, Ghayur T, Mendes M, et al: The functional and histological basis for graft-versus-host-induced immunosuppression. *Immunol Rev* 88:107–33, 1985.

95. Izutsu KT, Sullivan KM, Schubert MM, et al: Disordered salivary immunoglobulin secretion and sodium transport in human chronic graft-versus-host disease. *Transplantation* 35:441–6, 1983.

96. Ermak TH, Owen RL: Differential distribution of lymphocytes and accessory cells in mouse Peyer's patches. *Anat Rec* 215:144–52, 1986.

97. Mayrhofer G, Pugh CW, Barclay AN: The distribution, ontogeny and origin in the rat of Ia-positive cells with dendritic morphology and of Ia antigen in epithelia, with special reference to the intestine. *Eur J Immunol* 13:112–22, 1983.

98. Chen AR, McKinnon KP, Koren HS: Lipopolysaccharide (LPS) stimulates fresh human monocytes to lyse actinomycin D-treated WEHI-164 target cells via increased secretion of a monokine similar to tumor necrosis factor. *J Immunol* 135:3978–87, 1985.

99. Carswell EA, Old LJ, Kassel RL, et al: An endotoxin-induced serum factor that causes necrosis of tumors. *Proc Natl Acad Sci USA* 72:3666–70, 1975.

100. Darzynkiewicz Z, Williamson B, Carswell EA, et al: Cell cycle-specific effects of tumor necrosis factor. *Cancer Res* 44:83–90, 1984.

101. Nawroth PP, Stern DM: Tumor necrosis factor/cachectin-induced modulation of endothelial cell hemostatic properties. *Onkologie* 10:254–8, 1987.

102. Pober JS: Effects of tumour necrosis factor and related cytokines on vascular endothelial cells. *Ciba Found Symp* 131:170–84, 1987.

103. Prause JU, Manthorpe R, Oxholm P, et al: Definition and criteria for Sjogren's syn-

drome used by the contributors to the First International Seminar on Sjogren's syndrome — 1986. *Scand J Rheumatol* 61:17–8, 1986.

104. Gratwohl AA, Moutsopoulos HM, Chused TM, et al: Sjogren-type syndrome after allogeneic bone-marrow transplantation. *Ann Intern Med* 87:703–6, 1977.

105. Schubert MM, Sullivan KM, Morton TH, et al: Oral manifestations of chronic graft-v-host disease. *Arch Intern Med* 144:1591–5, 1984.

106. Rouquette-Gally AM, Boyeldieu D, Prost AC, et al: Autoimmunity after allogeneic bone marrow transplantation. A study of 53 long-term-surviving patients. *Transplantation* 46:238–40, 1988.

107. Janin-Mercier A, Devergie A, Arrago JP, et al: Systemic evaluation of Sjogren-like syndrome after bone marrow transplantation in man. *Transplantation* 43:677–9, 1987.

108. Lawley TJ, Peck GL, Moutsopoulos HM, et al: Scleroderma, Sjogren-like syndrome, and chronic graft-versus-host disease. *Ann Intern Med* 87:707–9, 1977.

109. Beschorner WE, Shinn CA, Fischer AC, et al: Cyclosporine (CsA) induced pseudo graft-versus-host disease (CIPGVHD) in the early post CsA period. *Transplantation* 46:112S–7S, 1988.

110. McDonald GB, Sullivan KM, Plumley TF: Radiographic features of esophageal involvement in chronic graft-vs.-host disease. *AJR* 142:501–6, 1984.

111. Rappaport H, Khalil A, Halle-Pannenko O, et al: Histopathologic sequence of events in adult mice undergoing lethal graft-versus-host reaction developed across H-2 and/or non-H-2 histocompatibility barriers. *Am J Pathol* 96:121–42, 1979.

112. Cunningham-Rundles C, Brandeis WE, Safai B, et al: Selective IgA deficiency and circulating immune complexes containing bovine proteins in a child with chronic graft versus host disease. *Am J Med* 67:883–90, 1979.

113. Cunningham-Rundles C, O'Reilly R: Association of circulating immune complexes containing bovine proteins and graft-versus-host disease. *Clin Exp Immunol* 64:323–9, 1986.

114. Jones RJ, Lee KS, Beschorner WE, et al: Veno-occlusive disease of the liver following bone marrow transplantation. *Transplantation* 44:778–83, 1987.

115. Shulman HM, McDonald GB, Mathews D, et al: An analysis of hepatic veno-occlusive disease and centrilobular hepatocyte degeneration following bone marrow transplantation. *Gastroenterology* 79:1178–91, 1980.

116. Armitage JO, Burns CP, Kent T: Liver disease complicating the management of acute leukemia during remission. *Cancer* 41:737–42, 1978.

117. Locasciulli A, Santamaria M, Masera G, et al: Hepatitis B virus markers in children with acute leukemia: the effect of chemotherapy. *J Med Virol* 15:29–33, 1985.

118. Sale GE, Storb R, Kolb H: Histopathology of hepatic acute graft-versus-host disease in the dog. A double blind study confirms the specificity of small bile duct lesions. *Transplantation* 26:103–6, 1978.

119. Snover DC, Weisdorf SA, Ramsay NK, et al: Hepatic graft versus host disease: a study of the predictive value of liver biopsy in diagnosis. *Hepatology* 4:123–30, 1984.

120. Leszczynski D, Renkonen R, Hayry P: Bone marrow transplantation in the rat. III. Structure of the liver inflammatory lesion in acute graft-versus-host disease. *Am J Pathol* 120:316–22, 1985.

121. Shulman HM, Sharma P, Amos D: A coded histologic study of hepatic graft-versus-host disease after human bone marrow transplantation. *Hepatology* 8:463–70, 1988.

122. Nakanuma Y, Terada T, Ohtake S: Intrahepatic periductal glands in graft-versus-host disease. *Acta Pathol Jpn* 38:281–9, 1988.

123. Fisher ER, Fisher B: Histopathologic and ultrastructural study of allogeneic hepatic transplantation in isogenic rats. *Lab Invest* 23:318–26, 1970.

124. Nonomura A, Kono N, Yoshida K, et al: Histological changes of bile duct in experimen-

tal graft-versus-host disease across minor histocompatibility barriers. II. Electron microscopic observations. *Liver* 8:32–41, 1988.

125. Beschorner WE, Tutschka PJ, Santos GW: Characterization of T lymphocyte subsets in target tissues with acute and chronic graft-versus-host disease (GVHD). *Fed Proc* 41:620a, 1982.

126. Dilly SA, Sloane JP: An immunohistological study of human hepatic graft-versus-host disease. *Clin Exp Immunol* 62:545–53, 1985.

127. Lautenschlager I: Distribution of the major histocompatibility antigens on different components of human liver. *Cell Immunol* 85:191–200, 1984.

128. Settaf A, Milton A: Donor class I and class II major histocompatibility complex antigen expression following liver allografting in rejecting and nonrejecting rat strain combinations. *Transplantation* 46:32–40, 1988.

129. Stet RJ, Thomas C, Koudstaal J, et al: Graft-versus-host disease in the rat: cellular changes and major histocompatibility complex antigen expression in the liver. *Scand J Immunol* 23:81–9, 1986.

130. Suitters AJ, Lampert IA: Class II antigen induction in the liver of rats with graft-versus-host disease. *Transplantation* 38:194–6, 1984.

131. Williams GM, Krajewski CA, Dagher FJ, et al: Host repopulation of endothelium. *Transplant Proc* 3:869–72, 1971.

132. Sullivan KM, Shulman HM, Storb R, et al: Chronic graft-versus-host disease in 52 patients: adverse natural course and successful treatment with combination immunosuppression. *Blood* 57:267–76, 1981.

133. Yau JC, Zander AR, Srigley JR, et al: Chronic graft-versus-host disease complicated by micronodular cirrhosis and esophageal varices. *Transplantation* 41:129–30, 1986.

134. Knapp AB, Crawford JM, Rappepart JM, Gollan JL: Cirrhosis as a consequence of graft-versus-host disease. *Gastroenterology* 92:513–9, 1987.

135. Nonomura A, Koizumi H, Yoshida K, Ohta G: Histological changes of bile duct in experimental graft-versus-host disease across minor histocompatibility barriers. I. Light microscopic and immunocytochemical observations. *Acta Pathol Jpn* 37:763–73, 1987.

136. Nonomura A, Yoshida K, Kono N, et al: Histological changes of bile duct in experimental graft-versus-host disease across minor histocompatibility barriers. III. Immuno-electron microscopic observations. *Acta Pathol Jpn* 38:269–80, 1988.

137. Epstein O, Thomas HC, Sherlock S: Primary biliary cirrhosis is a dry gland syndrome with features of chronic graft-versus-host disease. *Lancet* 1:1166–8, 1980.

138. Epstein O: The pathogenesis of primary biliary cirrhosis. *Mol Aspects Med* 8:293–305, 1985.

139. Saitoh T, Fujiwara M, Nomoto M, et al: Hepatic lesions induced by graft-versus-host reaction across MHC class II antigens: an implication for animal model of primary biliary cirrhosis. *Clin Immunol Immunopathol* 49:166–72, 1988.

140. Bernuau D, Feldmann G, Degott C, Gisselbrecht C: Ultrastructural lesions of bile ducts in primary biliary cirrhosis. *Hum Pathol* 12:782–93, 1981.

141. Si L, Whiteside TL, Schade RR, et al: T-lymphocyte subsets in liver tissues of patients with primary biliary cirrhosis (PBC), patients with primary sclerosing cholangitis (PSC), and normal controls. *J Clin Immunol* 4:262–72, 1984.

142. Colucci G, Schaffner F, Paronetto F: *In situ* characterization of the cell-surface antigens of the mononuclear cell infiltrate and bile duct epithelium in primary biliary cirrhosis. *Clin Immunol Immunopathol* 41:35–42, 1986.

143. Meuer SC, Moebius U, Manns MM, et al: Clonal analysis of human T lymphocytes infiltrating the liver in chronic active hepatitis B and primary biliary cirrhosis. *Eur J Immunol* 18:1447–52, 1988.

CHAPTER 29

Immunologic Aspects of Small Bowel Transplantation

WOLFGANG H. SCHRAUT

INTRODUCTION

Intestinal transplantation is a logical solution to the problem of short bowel syndrome. This syndrome constitutes a state of malabsorption and malnutrition after a major resection or loss of the small intestine, and possibly some or all of the large intestine. Short gut syndrome can result from diverse causes, which vary in their incidence with the age of the patients. Infants may lose a major portion of their intestine because of necrotizing enterocolitis or volvulus, whereas older children may incur intestinal loss because of a variety of acquired conditions or due to trauma. In adults, a common cause of short gut syndrome is Crohn's disease, and in elderly patients, loss of intestinal absorptive capacity most commonly results from mesenteric vascular disease.

Increasing numbers of patients afflicted with short gut syndrome as a consequence of a variety of crippling intestinal disorders are surviving at present because of the availability of total parenteral nutrition (TPN) programs. This form of treatment has achieved unparalleled success for these patients, but it is by no means without problems. Although TPN is life-saving, it fails to restore the patient's normal intestinal function, is time-consuming, and requires the ability to handle the rather sophisticated home TPN equipment. In addition, it is expensive and prone to a number of serious complications such as catheter-related problems, difficulties with venous access sites, sepsis, and long-term disturbances of hepatic and bone metabolism.[1-5] Despite these potential risks and complications of TPN, the patients survive for longer periods and live productive lives. However, renewed interest in the potential of small bowel transplantation, which would obviate the difficulties of TPN, has evolved. Just as renal transplantation freed many renal failure patients from external support and has, for the most part, been cost-effec-

611

tive, one would expect intestinal transplantation to have the potential to accomplish the same result for patients with short bowel syndrome.

Recent advances in immunosuppression, particularly the introduction of cyclosporin A (CsA), have brought dramatic changes to the field of transplantation in general, and, paralleling these advances, interest in small bowel transplantation has surged. This positive climate has resulted in a large number of experimental studies on small bowel transplantation and has culminated in several isolated clinical trials.

The small intestine is unusual among solid organs considered for transplantation because of the large quantity of lymphoid tissue present in the Peyer's patches, in the lymph nodes of the accompanying mesentery, and in the mucosa and submucosa. The lymphoid tissues are a potent antigenic stimulus that results in a vigorous rejection response. Moreover, they are capable of inducing a response against the host, i.e., they are capable of causing graft-versus-host disease (GVHD). Also, the small intestine is unique among organ grafts in being exposed to the exterior; therefore, just like the intestinal tract of a healthy person, a graft must provide the recipient with a barrier function against bacteria, toxic substances, and foreign proteins. Small bowel transplantation can ultimately be successful only when provisions are made for the control of graft rejection and graft-versus-host disease, while the mucosal barrier remains intact against the exterior and while the absorptive function of the graft is kept unimpaired by any aspects of the transplantation procedure or by immunosuppressive therapy.

EXPERIMENTAL MODELS

Attempts at experimental small bowel transplantation date back to the beginning of the century. In 1901, E. Ullmann reported to the Viennese Medical Society on his experiments with transplantation of intestinal segments,[6] and in 1902, Alexis Carrel, who later received the Nobel Prize for medicine, published his studies in dogs.[7] Major advances in small bowel transplantation were achieved in the early 1960s when numerous investigators, foremost among them Lillehei, documented the technical feasibility of small bowel transplantation in several animal models.[8-11] Lillehei and his colleagues[9] were the first to describe a technique for functional bowel transplantation in the dog. These investigators replaced the entire small intestine of the recipient with a pedicle intestinal graft that required vascular anastomoses between the superior mesenteric artery and vein of the graft and the aorta and inferior vena cava of the recipient. The recipients of orthotopic autografts survived indefinitely, whereas allografts were rejected within several days.

The effectiveness of various immunosuppressive regimens was evaluated in dog models involving transplantation of a small intestinal segment as a Thiery-Vella loop in the neck or abdomen, with anastomosis of the intestinal vessels either to the carotid artery and jugular vein or to the external iliac vessels, depending on the site of placement.[10-12] Similar studies were undertaken on pigs[13-17] and rats.[18-20]

Over the past few years in particular, inbred rat models have been employed for investigation of many different aspects of small bowel transplantation. The rat model lends itself to this task because investigators can expand their studies by utilizing the vast knowledge gained on the rat models of general transplantation biology and of intestinal physiology and metabolism.

The rat model of small bowel transplantation was pioneered by Monchik and Russell,[18] who transplanted the entire small intestine as a Thiery-Vella loop (heterotopic accessory graft) in inbred rats. Kort et al.[19] described a method for orthotopic total small bowel transplantation in which the recipient's own small intestine was replaced. They employed vascular anastomoses between the mesenteric artery and abdominal aorta and the portal vein of the graft and that of the recipient. Both heterotopic placement of the graft as a Thiery-Vella loop and orthotopic (placement in gastrointestinal continuity) transplantation of the graft have their advantages and drawbacks; which method is more suitable depends on the scientific questions asked. Heterotopic placement provides accessibility to the graft, an advantage if repeated biopsy and histologic evaluation are to be done. Also, it is a useful method for the study of intestinal preservation, because recovery from the ischemic insult and, ultimately, survival of the graft are the pre-eminent considerations, whereas functional performance in the host is of secondary and subsequent concern. In contrast, investigations employing orthotopic small bowel transplantation are more pertinent to the clinical situation because recipient survival is dependent on an intact, functioning intestinal graft. Studies involving the functional performance of the intestinal graft, the integrity of the mucosal barrier, and protocols investigating aspects of chronic rejection are conducted with greater reliability with orthotopic graft placement.[20]

Several investigators[21-23] evaluated the fate of fetal intestinal allografts placed in a subcutaneous location in adult rat recipients, thereby avoiding the need for vascular anastomoses. Graft acceptance, as expected, required institution of immunosuppressive therapy. The course of rejection was the same as that seen with vascularized grafts. The development and growth of a fetal graft into an architecturally correct and functional small bowel has not been reported, although some functional capacity could be detected.[24,25] The importance of the model in which a free, nonvascularized small bowel graft is used is lessened by the success achieved with study models in which vascularized bowel grafts have been employed, and by the assumption that the use of fetal grafts is not a likely or successful approach to clinical small bowel transplantation.

COURSE OF REJECTION

Transplant Morphology

Histologic evaluation of transplanted tissues obtained either as biopsy specimens or at autopsy forms the standard for the diagnosis of rejection in organ transplantation. The evolution of rejection has been delineated histologically for several models of experimental small bowel transplantation. The well-known indicators of rejection (progressive infiltration of the mucosa and submucosa by lymphoid cells, culminating in destruction of organ architecture, perivascular infiltration, and endothelial injury) are common to all models of experimental small bowel transplantation.[26-29]

The course of the rejection of small bowel grafts has been described in greatest detail in the rat model.[28,29] Histologic changes in the intestinal graft caused by operative handling and ischemia do not persist beyond the third postoperative day and therefore do not result in confusion with the rejection process. Studies on dogs and pigs have yielded the same results.[30,31]

Minor histologic alterations in the epithelium that are attributable to rejection (rare, sporadic crypt cell damage, with increased numbers of lymphoid cells in the adjacent lamina propria) are seen in the rat as early as 3 days after transplantation. These rare mucosal lesions form in parallel with endothelial cell vacuolization and swelling of the adjacent arterioles and venules in the lamina propria.[28] It appears that the crypt epithelium and the microvascular endothelium are the initial sites of rejection.

It has been proposed that the histologic sequence of rejection of small bowel transplants should be discussed in terms of phases rather than in terms of days after transplantation, because it is the phase or stage of rejection of the allograft, and not the time after transplantation, according to which immunosuppressive manipulations must be adjusted.[29]

In phase I, the early stage of rejection, changes seen histologically are confined to the mucosa and submucosa. This phase is defined as infiltration of the lamina propria by lymphocytes and plasma cells of recipient origin,[32] without distortion of the villous architecture of the mucosa, but with villus shortening and rare, focal cellular damage. These prominent histologic changes in the mucosa and submucosa commence on the fifth to sixth day after transplantation in every transplantation model involving major histocompatibility barriers, unless immunosuppressive therapy is employed. As rejection progresses, the infiltrate becomes more prominent and diffuse and, upon examination of cross sections, is distinct from Peyer's patches and from the occasional focal mucosal concentrations of lymphocytes seen in the normal small bowel (Fig. 29–1B). In this phase, the microvascular lesions (endothelial swelling with partial luminal occlusion, intravascular and perivascular lymphoid infiltration) are becoming increasingly prominent.[28,33] Phase I rejection is associated with minimal or absent functional impairment.[28,34] The mesenteric lymph nodes and Peyer's patches show moderate lymphocyte depletion. When the fully allogeneic BN→LEW rat strain is used, a lymph follicle of normal cellularity with prominent lymphoblasts is encountered occasionally, indicating stimulation of donor lymphocytes, i.e., a graft-versus-host (GvH) reaction.[35,36] With prompt adjustment of immunosuppressive therapy, phase I is likely to be completely reversible.

Phase II is an intermediate histologic stage of rejection that develops gradually and has no clear starting point. It is characterized by intense mucosal and submucosal infiltration of lymphoid cells; the infiltrate extends into the muscularis propria of the allograft and is associated with shortening and blunting of the villi and with scattered epithelial sloughing (Fig. 29–1C). The microvascular injury described previously is most obvious in areas of prominent mucosal injury. The lymphoid tissues of the graft exhibit progressive lymphocyte depletion. Functional impairment is seen when the maltose absorption test is employed,[34] and active epithelial ion transport is impaired as well.[28] Complete reversal of advanced phase II rejection may not be achievable with present immunosuppressive regimens, and thus phase II should be considered a harbinger of the graft loss that occurs in the subsequent phase III.

Phase III differs histologically in the acute and chronic rejection models in rats, but in both it indicates end-stage, nonreversible rejection and a nonfunctional allograft. In acutely rejected allografts, there is complete mucosal destruction, with islands of flattened mucosa interspersed; this is accompanied by heavy transmural cellular infiltration, notably by lymphocytes and polymorphonuclear leukocytes

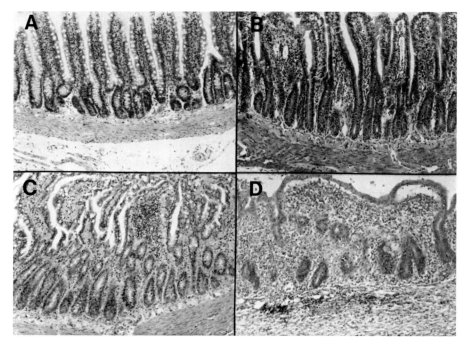

Figure 29–1 Small-bowel allografts undergoing acute rejection. **A:** Normal small bowel. **B:** Phase I rejection. **C:** Phase II rejection. **D:** Phase III rejection. (Hematoxylin-eosin stain, ×100)

(Figs. 29–1D and 29–2A). Gram stain demonstrates bacterial invasion. This process is accompanied by an intense serosal and subserosal cellular infiltrate that is consistent with peritonitis. Culturing of lymph nodes harvested when the recipient's death due to rejection was imminent has failed (in rats) to disclose bacterial invasion/translocation (Schraut and Stangl, unpublished observation). Occlusive microvascular injury is extensive. Phase III of the chronic rejection process is distinguished histologically by mucosal and transmural cellular infiltration. The submucosa and muscularis propria are thickened and fibrosed, but intact (Fig. 29–2B). The lymphoid tissues show decreased cellularity, as well as fibrosis and loss of the normal architecture.

Histologic evaluation of biopsy material has been criticized as an inaccurate and inconsistent method for assessing the status of intestinal allografts, primarily because rejection was thought to be a spotty or patchy process that could be misjudged in a random biopsy of the allograft mucosa. Concerns were raised mainly by investigators who used the dog as the experimental animal.[26,37] Millard et al.[37] contend that the course of rejection is not reflected by progressive histologic impairment at the mucosal level. They found great variability in mucosal changes, whereas vascular changes (cuffing, endothelial thickening) were more consistent and pathognomonic of rejection and were thought to be the primary lesions leading, in turn, to the classical histologic mucosal alterations. By using circumferential cross sections, Rosemurgy et al.[29] and others[27,28,31] found that allograft rejection is quite uniform histologically and that there is a defined and predictable sequence of

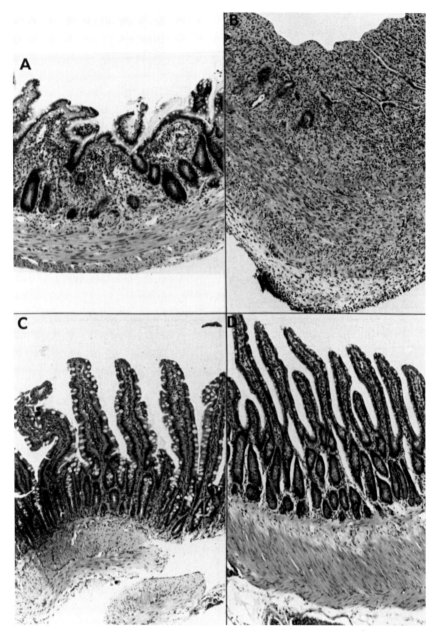

Figure 29–2 Histologic appearance of orthotopic small-bowel allografts. **A:** Small-bowel allograft showing acute rejection with severe mucosal destruction and thinning of the bowel wall (no cyclosporine treatment). **B:** Chronic rejection of an allograft from an animal receiving a short course of cyclosporine demonstrating loss of mucosa, submucosal fibrosis, and bowel wall thickening. **C:** Biopsy specimen obtained 6 months after transplantation from a long-term survivor that received an extended course of cyclosporine showing preservation of mucosa with slight villous blunting. **D:** Orthotopic Lewis isograft 6 months after transplantation demonstrating a normal histologic appearance. (Hematoxylin-eosin stain, ×100)

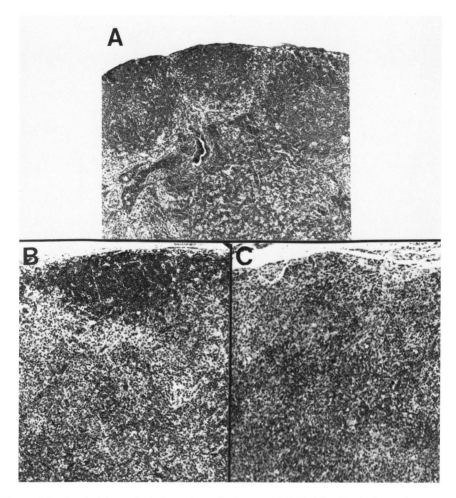

Figure 29–3 **A:** Mesenteric lymph node from a LBN-F1 intestinal allograft rejected by the LEW host: lymphopenia and loss of nodal architecture are striking. **B:** Mesenteric lymph node of the LEW host: normal cellularity and enlarged lymph follicles are evident. **C:** Spleen of the LEW recipient of a LBN-F1 intestinal allograft: normal architecture with prominent lymph follicles is apparent. (×100)

changes that provides a sensitive and specific assessment of the status of intestinal allograft rejection regardless of the particular animal model used.

Evaluation of the lymphoid tissues of the graft (Peyer's patches, mesenteric lymph nodes) undergoing rejection shows progressive lymphocyte depletion and eventual loss of nodal architecture, with hyaline necrosis (Fig. 29–3A). If fully allogeneic donor-recipient pairs are used (e.g., the BN→LEW rat strain combination), a temporary histologic picture featuring simultaneous lymphoid depletion and lymphoid stimulation (with appearance of immunoblasts) can be detected in the lymphoid tissues of the allograft.[36] As long as rejection predominates, the lymphoid tissues of the recipient have normal cellularity and architecture.

In contrast to the immunopathologic findings after small bowel transplantation in the rat or pig model, those for total orthotopic small bowel transplantation in the outbred dog model appear variable, with a spectrum of histologic and clinical events reported to occur.[37,38]

In morphologic studies of canine intestinal grafts with and without the use of immunosuppression, three types of immune reaction have been recognized. When the entire small intestine or a major portion of it is transplanted, some investigators report that there are no changes in the graft; however, the animals die in 7 – 10 days, with histologic evidence of GVHD.[9,38,39,40] When short segment grafts,[10-12] irradiated grafts,[39] or grafts without mesenteric lymph nodes[41] are transplanted, or when immunosuppressive therapy (insufficient to avert rejection) is given to the recipient, then, according to most investigators,[10-13,42-44] graft rejection invariably predominates and follows the classical histologic course.

After total small bowel transplantation in dogs, an "atypical" form of rejection devoid of the usual histologic features has been noted in some of the animals. This was thought to be caused by simultaneous GVHD and rejection.[38] This form of rejection is characterized histologically by blunting of villi, cellular irregularities within the crypts, and sporadic mucosal destruction with sparse cellular infiltration. Vascular changes (fibrinoid necrosis and thrombosis) are seen frequently, and the host lymphoid tissues exhibit lymphocyte depletion, which is highly suggestive of GVHD.

This potential for a variable fate of canine intestinal grafts and thus for variable graft histology has an immunologic basis. In dogs, the intestinal lymphoid tissues probably constitute the major portion of the immune system; consequently, their transplantation with the intestinal allograft can lead to GVHD by overcoming the host's immune system in some dogs, can influence or impair the recipient's immune competence and cause the picture of an "atypical" rejection in others, or, in some animals, can have a minimal impact, but eventually lead to classical graft rejection. With respect to graft histology, a spectrum of findings must be expected when groups of dogs are studied, with the findings in each intestinal graft and host determined by the predominating immune reaction. For example, GVHD may lead to the recipient's death from sepsis before the histologic changes of a simultaneously occurring rejection of the small bowel allograft are recognizable. Under these circumstances, a mucosal biopsy would be inconclusive with regard to identification of the rejection process or GVHD. However, GVHD can be diagnosed from a lymph node or skin biopsy.

Such variability is not expected to arise in future clinical small bowel transplantations, because combination immunosuppressive therapy should suppress GVHD and obviate graft rejection. Furthermore, in humans, a small bowel graft may not elicit GVHD as readily as happens in the dog, and thus rejection may predominate, as is the case in rat and pig models.

Recipient Response

A small intestinal allograft, like any other organ graft, induces an immunologic response in its host that culminates in graft rejection. Host-derived lymphoid cells infiltrate the graft,[32] antidonor antibodies develop,[36,45] and monocyte procoagulant activity increases,[46] to mention just a few measurable host responses.

Extensive histopathologic studies have failed to demonstrate any enlargement of lymph nodes or spleen in the host, as long as GVHD was absent[47] (Fig. 29 – 3B, C). After small bowel transplantation, graft-derived lymphocytes (passenger leukocytes) originating mainly in the mesenteric lymph nodes, migrate into the native small bowel and lymphoid tissues of the host, as was demonstrated with the use of indium-labeled lympho/leukocytes.[48] Furthermore, donor lymphocytes are detected by immune histochemical staining[30] or in mixed lymphocyte cultures of spleen tissue when the spleens of the recipients of fully allogeneic small bowel grafts are harvested several days prior to complete graft rejection (Stangl and Schraut, unpublished data). This response in mixed lymphocyte culture is seen with and without immunosuppressive treatment with CsA. Arnand-Battandier et al.[49] studied lymphoid populations in the transplanted gut of swine 10–12 months after engraftment and demonstrated that the mesenteric lymph nodes of the graft were populated by lymphocytes of recipient origin, whereas within the mucosa a mixed population of recipient and donor origin was encountered; the latter, however, was probably a contamination of mucosal cells (carrying donor antigens) rather than donor-type lymphocytes.

MONITORING OF REJECTION

The central problem in small bowel transplantation, just as in any other form of tissue allotransplantation, continues to be that of graft rejection and the appropriate approaches to its suppression. Integral to the solution of this problem is the need for reliable methods for monitoring graft integrity. Such monitoring should reveal reliably and consistently any early, minor impairment of the morphologic and functional integrity of the allograft, so that immunosuppressive therapy can be adjusted, being either increased for treatment of rejection or decreased for reduction of the complications of immunosuppression (most notably infection).

As with other transplanted organs, such as the kidney or pancreas, the histology of the small bowel allograft is the standard to which other methods of detection and monitoring of rejection are compared. The sequence of histologic changes seen by light microscopy during intestinal allograft rejection has been described repeatedly for various animal models, and, if one accepts its limitations, it is evident that transplant histology can be relied upon for monitoring graft integrity.

The histologic evaluation of intestinal allografts poses several problems. Although full-thickness biopsy specimens provide conclusive information as to the severity of rejection, it may be difficult or impossible to obtain such specimens from a graft placed in gastrointestinal continuity. In such cases, histologic graft assessment becomes possible only by study of mucosal biopsy specimens obtained with a suction apparatus. Such specimens are often superficial, and their histologic evaluation may be inconclusive because involvement of the graft by rejection is not always uniform, or because the rejection process may not become evident by exhibiting the classical histopathologic mucosal changes. Millard et al.[37] have indicated that mucosal biopsy specimens, even when obtained with inclusion of the deep submucosa, were quite variable histologically during rejection, a concern also raised by Rosemurgy et al.[29] for superficial mucosal biopsies on rat small bowel allografts. However, the majority of investigators found sequential deep mucosal biopsies to be reliable and useful monitors of small bowel grafts.[11,15,27,31,35,41,42] The problem of obtaining potentially misleading information from a superficial specimen obtained by suction biopsy can be circumvented by construction of a subcutaneous pouch that is separate from the graft and accessible by an enterostoma.[31,42]

This pouch reflects the changes that occur in the intra-abdominal graft and is readily available for biopsy, even deep biopsy, with a greatly reduced risk of clinically significant bowel perforation.

An inevitable shortcoming of histologic monitoring of intestinal allografts is that histologic findings do not provide a direct measure of allograft function. In phase III, signaling complete allograft rejection, the intestinal graft is devoid of any functional component, i.e., the destruction seen histologically equals functional loss. In phases I and II, however, the histologic appearance allows only an estimate of the functional capacity of the allograft. Functional testing should, therefore, be an integral part of allograft monitoring. Function tests that can be repeated frequently and that reflect the functional and morphologic status of the allograft have been sought. In this search, the integrity of carbohydrate absorption following small intestinal transplantation has been studied by many investigators. The results of function tests involving the absorption of glucose,[22,23,50] alpha-D-glucose,[24,51] ^{14}C-labeled glucose,[43,52,53] maltose,[34,54-56] and xylose[13] have been correlated with the findings on transplant histology. The serial measurement of serum glucose levels after an oral glucose load demonstrated impaired function as rejection progressed; however, it did not allow the detection of impending or early rejection at a time when morphologic changes were still minor and potentially reversible. Furthermore, Holmes et al.[57,58] found glucose absorption to be erratic in the presence of infection or of minor histologic changes in the small bowel allograft. Therefore they proposed utilizing a combination of light-microscopic examination of biopsy material and a glucose absorption test as a better way of monitoring the integrity of an intestinal allograft. Absorption of ^{14}C-labeled glucose is considered a sensitive predictor of early graft rejection by Cohen et al.[52] and Nordgren et al.,[53] who found that reduced absorption coincided with the early histologic changes of rejection (mucosal infiltration by lymphoid cells, shortening of villi).

A method for evaluating the performance of the intestinal *mucosa* is available in the maltose absorption test.[34] This test is based on the functional integrity of the mucosal brush border; specifically, the test requires the brush border disaccharidase maltase, which splits maltose into its monosaccharide moieties, glucose. The glucose is then absorbed actively and, if the maltose load is sufficient, raises the serum glucose level. Several groups of experimenters have found the maltose absorption test to be a reliable indicator of the functional competence of the intestinal graft.[55,56,59] Early in the course of rejection, the peak of the bell-shaped curve (absorption versus time) is diminished, and with progressive rejection the peak is delayed. When rejection becomes clinically evident as diarrhea, inanition, and malabsorption, the curve flattens out. The progression of functional impairment is paralleled by progressive destruction of the architecture of the bowel, as seen on light microscopy (Fig. 29–4).

Other markers of intestinal function, such as serum hexosaminidase levels[60] and other absorption tests like glycine absorption[22] and the absorption and/or excretion of fatty acids,[61] as well as quantitative histochemical measurements of brush border enzyme activity,[62] have been proposed.

Grant et al.[63] found ^{51}Cr-EDTA, a marker of gut permeability, useful in predicting allograft rejection that causes impairment of the mucosal barrier. If one discounts the disadvantage of using an isotope marker, this test appears promising both in concept and in reliability. Schiller et al.[64] and Dennison et al.[65] evaluated allograft motility and myoelectric activity as further potential monitors of rejection. Both groups found that impairment of motility became evident only when

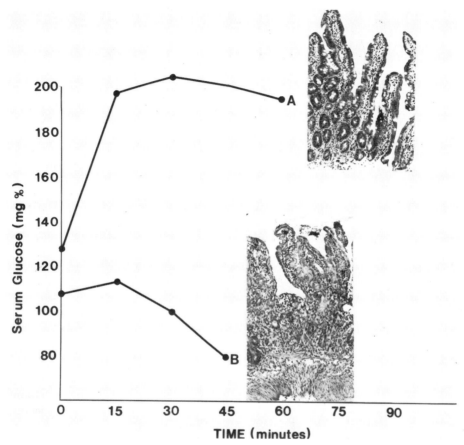

Figure 29-4 Maltose absorption in an orthotopic allograft on the fifth **(A)** and eighth **(B)** postoperative days. Absorption is normal on the fifth and impaired on the eighth day. The simultaneous biopsy on the fifth day shows normal, intact intestinal architecture and, on the eighth day, cellular infiltration, with villus shortening and superficial erosion at the tips of the villi.

graft failure and necrosis were imminent. In a recent report, Vane et al.[66] noted that electrical activity (BER) was depressed and that myoelectric complex potentials were absent until the 11th postoperative day. However, these studies were performed in a heterotopic transplantation model in rats, a model known to engender clinically noticeable motility disorders.[45] Using the orthotopic transplantation model, we did not encounter any clinical indications of a motility disorder, and resumed enteral feedings successfully on the second posttransplantation day.[59]

A different approach to monitoring the rejection process is the study and detection of immunologic responses by the host, rather than awaiting impairment of organ graft morphology or function. Many efforts have been made to find a simple, reliable immunologic marker or test that would indicate the onset or progression of the host's immune response to the allograft. Such a test is yet to be found. Silverman et al.[46] evaluated monocyte procoagulant activity, an index of monocyte immune activation, and noted that increased procoagulant activity paralleled early histologic evidence of rejection. Thus they suggested that this marker may be useful for monitoring.

Hammer et al.,[67] who studied cardiac allografts, found an effective method of detecting the immunologic response of a human host at its inception. Acute rejection was characterized by a significant rise in the content of T lymphocytes and lymphoblasts in peripheral blood. Such changes were not seen with infectious complications, thus allowing appropriate adjustments of the immunosuppressive therapy even at an early stage of rejection. It remains to be seen whether this approach is useful for monitoring intestinal transplants.

Morphologic and functional evaluations have become established as reliable parameters for intestinal allograft surveillance. Their ultimate validation will come when small bowel transplantation is used clinically. An array of function tests for the study of gastrointestinal dysfunction is available in clinical practice; some of these tests may prove useful in small bowel transplantation.

CONTROL OF REJECTION

The main obstacle to small bowel transplantation — and to tissue allotransplantation in general — is allograft rejection and the difficult problem of preventing it.

Small bowel allografts induce a vigorous rejection reaction in their respective hosts. Depending on the size of the graft and its location and whether or not it is placed in continuity with the recipient's own gastrointestinal tract, the rejection reaction can cause graft resorption and fibrosis without severely impairing the recipient's well-being,[11] or it can lead to graft necrosis and the death of the recipient.[9]

Studies in dogs,[68] rats,[35,69] and pigs[15] demonstrated that the rapidity of rejection is governed by the immunologic disparity between donor and host. Better matching, i.e., a lesser degree of histoincompatibility is associated with a less vigorous rejection reaction.

When studied in donor-recipient combinations of inbred rat strains, the rejection of small bowel grafts occurs in approximately the same time span as does rejection of other organ grafts, in spite of the vast amount of immunogenic lymphoid tissue transferred with an intestinal graft. Rejection of intestinal grafts ($\sim$10 days) occurs about as rapidly as that of kidneys ($\sim$9 days), heart ($\sim$8 days), and pancreas ($\sim$9 days) in the LBN-F-1 hybrid → Lewis rat strain combination without the use of immunosuppression. It is likely that the immune response of the recipient is at a maximum even in the presence of small amounts of lymphoid tissue (such as those in the kidney or heart), and that the greater amount of lymphoid tissue (passenger leukocytes, lymphocytes) within intestinal grafts does not accelerate the rejection process. Perhaps complete removal of *all* lymphoid tissues from a small bowel graft would decrease rejection (as is seen for renal and cardiac grafts); however, data in support of such a claim have not appeared. A partial reduction in the amount of lymphoid tissue by the use of segmental allografts does not appear to be sufficient for mitigation of rejection.[70,71]

Effect of Portal Venous Drainage

Many different approaches, other than immunologic matching of donor and recipient, to postponement or control of the rejection of small bowel allografts have been evaluated experimentally. In 1973, Kort et al.[19] noted in a rat strain combination of major histoincompatibility that, when they used orthotopic total small bowel allografts with porto-portal venous anastomosis, thereby conveying the venous outflow of the graft through the liver, the animals enjoyed unusually long survival times. They postulated an immunosuppressive role of the liver and proposed two possible mechanisms of rejection:

1. Antigens detached from the graft or alloreactive cells are degraded or altered during their passage through the liver.[72] Mandel et al.[73] suggested the presence of a cytoplasmic liver enzyme that is capable of degrading transplantation antigens.
2. Circulating antigen-reacting cells, after passage through the graft, are modified in the liver, which prevents or slows their differentiation and division.[74]

In a systematic study of this potential benefit of portal venous drainage of small bowel grafts, we found that heterotopic (accessory) grafts with portal venous drainage were subject to a delayed, chronic form of rejection, whereas grafts with caval venous drainage were rejected acutely.[45] This effect was noted in a semiallogeneic (LBN-F1 → LEW) rat strain combination, but not in the fully allogeneic BN → LEW combination.[36] Furthermore, this advantage of portal over caval venous drainage could not be elicited with orthotopic graft placement when either the semiallogeneic or a fully allogeneic rat strain combination (BN → LEW) was used.[20] We must assume that the immunologic benefits of portal drainage are minor and thus fail to become discernible when donor-recipient combinations of greater immunogenic disparity (BN → LEW versus LBN-F1 → LEW) are used. Portal venous drainage may still be preferable, however, because it avoids any of the metabolic sequelae of caval drainage, which is equivalent to a partial porto-caval shunt.[75,76]

Recipient Splenectomy

Another approach aimed at mitigation of the recipient's immune response to a small bowel graft could be the use of splenectomy. The influence of splenectomy upon the recipient's response to a vascularized allograft has been variable, and therefore this form of therapy remains controversial. Fabre and Batchelor[77] reported that pretransplantation splenectomy suppressed the lymphocytotoxic antibody response to the graft and markedly prolonged the survival of F1 hybrid renal allografts. In contrast, Souther et al.[78] failed to elicit such an effect of pretransplantation splenectomy in a study of cardiac allograft survival in the homozygous Lewis → BN combination.

In our experience, splenectomy associated with porto-caval anastomosis led to prolongation of the recipient's survival and induced a chronic rather than an acute rejection reaction.[45] The addition of splenectomy to porto-portal anastomosis failed to prolong allograft survival in an additive fashion. This might have been expected, since porto-portal anastomosis reduces the immunogenicity of the allograft by operating at the efferent arm of the immune response. It is quite likely that porto-portal anastomosis, which delays, but does not prevent antigenic sensitization, and splenectomy, which also delays without preventing the afferent immunologic response, are not additive, because their primary actions occur in parallel and not sequentially. In addition, even though the studies noted above[45] were performed in an F1 hybrid system, the immunogenic disparity between host and donor rats may have been too great to allow the effects of porto-portal anastomosis and splenectomy to find expression in a discernible, additive prolongation of survival.

Recipient splenectomy may confer at best a moderate immunologic benefit and delay graft rejection. There may be, however, a real contraindication to performing a splenectomy in conjunction with small bowel transplantation. The immune competence of the splenectomized host may be reduced to such a degree that it would allow the induction of GVHD by the intestinal allograft. The experiments on dogs by Cohen et al.,[39] involving small bowel transplantation in conjunction with splenectomy, offer suggestive evidence of such a result, and Bitter-Suermann[79] demonstrated the possibility of such a development by transplanting the spleen into immune-compromised recipients. Whether GVHD develops after transplantation of the small intestine or even of the spleen is dependent on the immune competence of the recipient, the size of the allogeneic inoculum, and the immunogenic disparity between donor and recipient. For example, when transplanting the small bowel from a presensitized BN rat into a LEW rat that underwent a simultaneous splenectomy, we noted unmitigated graft rejection without clinical or histologic evidence of GVHD. Whether recipient splenectomy would put the clinical patient receiving an intestinal allograft at an increased risk of GVHD is unknown. Splenectomy has not, however, mitigated the rejection of other organ grafts and is thus unlikely to exert such an effect in small bowel transplantation.

Enhancement Protocols

Several approaches can be used for modulation of the recipient's immune response aside from immunosuppressive drug regimens (vide infra). According to Hardy et al.,[80] these include enhancement,[81] the use of antibodies,[82,83] donor-specific transfusions,[56,84-86] short-term treatment with CsA,[87] and methods of total lymphoid tissue irradiation.

Experimental attempts to achieve specific suppression of allograft rejection with donor antigen (active enhancement) or antidonor antiserum (passive enhancement), or both, have been successful for renal allografts in rats. Stuart et al.[88] were able to produce specific immunologic enhancement of rat renal allografts by intravenous administration of donor antigen and antidonor antibody 11 and 10 days prior to transplantation, i.e., they combined active and passive enhancement. With this protocol, they prevented the appearance of cell-mediated immunity and blocked the acquisition of immunologic memory by the recipient.[89] It is unclear whether this approach could be applied with the same success to intestinal transplantation; if so, it could be used only in situations in which a living related donor is available. Also, there is evidence[90] that different organ grafts elicit varying immunologic responses when they are transplanted across similar immunogenetic barriers. This is further demonstrated by the studies of Telford and Cory,[91] who attempted passive enhancement alone (administration of antidonor antibody) to prolong the survival of segmental jejunal allografts but who were not successful, whereas Stuart et al.,[88] following the same protocol in the same rat strain combination, succeeded in extending the functional survival of renal allografts.

Martinelli et al.[56] used rats to evaluate the effects of an enhancement protocol consisting of donor-specific blood transfusion prior to small bowel transplantation and concomitant CsA therapy, a combination that had previously been found effective for renal[85] and skin grafts.[86] They were able to achieve long-term survival of functional small bowel allografts in recipients conditioned in this manner and given low doses of CsA. However, this approach is feasible only if a living donor is available, unless pretreatment can be carried out successfully in the immediate perioperative period.

It is apparent that the various methods and protocols available for achieving tolerance of organ grafts[81] have not yet been evaluated sufficiently for intestinal transplantation and that we cannot expect them to replace current clinical methods of immunosuppressive therapy in the near future. However, the ever advancing development and availability of monoclonal antibodies directed against various transplantation antigens, mediators such as interleukin (IL)-2, and of specific cell types may create renewed interest in enhancement protocols.

Treatment With Immunosuppressive Drugs

At present, the major emphasis in rejection control is on nonspecific suppression of the host's immune response to an allograft by means of various drugs and other agents. The initial investigations on mitigating the rejection of intestinal allografts were undertaken in 1959 by Lillehei and colleagues,[8] who launched a systematic experimental study on the feasibility of orthotopic total small bowel transplantation in dogs. Control of rejection with the methods of immunosuppressive therapy available at that time and during the ensuing years [administration of azathioprine, prednisone, and xenogeneic antilymphocyte serum (ALS)] was not possible, although prolonged survival of recipients of small bowel allografts was achieved by Lillehei[9] and others.[10-14] Invariably, recipients of intestinal graft placed in gastrointestinal continuity died from the sequelae of acute rejection (necrosis, sepsis) or of chronic graft rejection (malnutrition due to functional deterioration of the fibrosing graft, culminating in graft necrosis, peritonitis, and generalized sepsis). When heterotopic grafts (in a cervical or intra-abdominal position) were used, the recipient's survival remained unaffected by rejection, while the graft became fibrotic, encapsulated, and partially or completely absorbed.[11,30]

Aside from being insufficient to control the rejection of intestinal allografts, azathioprine and prednisone interfere with enterocyte turnover, and it is thus feared that they impair intestinal barrier function, i.e., that they may precipitate side effects in the intestinal graft.[92] Therefore other drugs or agents that would replace these drugs or allow their dose to be reduced have been evaluated for control of rejection. Antilymphocyte serum was utilized by Deutsch et al.[93] in LEW recipients of fetal LBN-F1 grafts. The median survival time of free, subcutaneously located grafts could be extended from 8 days (without treatment) to 78 days (with biweekly injections of ALS). It is important to realize that the fetal intestine is much less immunogenic than is the adult intestine, in part because of the lack of immunocompetent lymphoid tissues, and that its rejection is therefore less vigorous. Quint et al.[94] were unable to achieve extended survival times for canine jejunal grafts by administering ALS before and after transplantation. Thus monotherapy with ALS, although beneficial, is insufficient for control of rejection of an intestinal allograft.

With the discovery of CsA as an effective immunosuppressive agent by Borel et al.[95] in 1977 and its introduction into clinical practice, graft survival in patients undergoing kidney, heart, and liver transplantation increased significantly. Numerous experimental studies were undertaken with small bowel transplantation in rats, dogs, and pigs. Cyclosporin A proved to be highly effective in preventing the rejection of small bowel allografts in rats.[51,59,96,97] Several studies in various rat strains proved conclusively that CsA (5–15 mg/kg given for 1–4 weeks after transplantation) averts rejection and allows the development of a state of systemic, strain-specific tolerance[59,98] (Fig. 29–2C).

Cyclosporin A used as monotherapy has been less effective in large-animal models of small bowel transplantation. Most investigators using dog[38,42]; or pig models[44,99–101] detected a significant prolongation of graft survival in such animals, but the number of long-term survivors was often only a fraction of the large number of overall attempts because of high technical and immunologic failure rates. The first reported study on the canine model of orthotopic small bowel transplantation, by Craddock et al.,[102] produced 3 long-term survivors among a starting population of 25 dogs. These results could not be improved upon by other investigators, who used CsA in various doses.[44,103,104] The addition of prednisone, azathioprine, and antilymphocyte globulin (ALG)[44,103,105] brought either no benefit or only modest prolongation of graft survival.

Paralleling the experience in canine small bowel transplantation, the experimental studies in the pig model failed to demonstrate any consistent efficacy of immunosuppressive therapy with CsA for averting rejection.[44,99–101] The best results were achieved when CsA was given parenterally to dogs and pigs during the early postoperative weeks. Specific studies[106–108] demonstrated that absorption of this lipophilic drug through the transplanted intestine is suboptimal. Close monitoring of serum drug levels is important so that the CsA dosage can be adjusted. Levels of CsA must be kept in the therapeutic range, primarily for control of rejection, but also for avoidance of mesenteric vascular spasm and the threat of graft ischemia and loss,[109] which is a potential complication when very high drug levels are employed.

It is evident from these data that CsA alone will not consistently prevent rejection in the two large-animal models of small bowel transplantation. Nevertheless, prolongation of graft survival, with long-term survivors, can be demonstrated, particularly when CsA is administered parenterally. It is expected that combination therapy with CsA, azathioprine, antithymocyte globulin, prednisone, and, in addition, monoclonal antibodies (OKT3) will allow further improvement in the control of rejection. It may be necessary to evaluate such combination therapy, which has been found effective in the control of rejection of pancreatoduodenal grafts in the clinical setting,[110,111] by studying small bowel transplantation in a large-animal model, possibly in primates.

Graft/Donor Pretreatment (Reduction of Graft Immunogenicity)

Current efforts and methods of suppression of allograft rejection are centered mainly on the use of a variety of agents that are immunologically nonspecific and that alter the immune response of the recipient to the allograft. The disadvantage of this approach rests in the impairment of the recipient's immune competence, with all of the inherent complications and problems, while the possibility of graft rejection remains. These problems might be circumvented or mitigated if the immunogenicity of the organ graft is reduced. This approach offers no risk to the transplant recipient and is a potential alternative or an adjuvant to nonspecific immunosuppression. For a small bowel allograft, graft immune modulation serves an additional purpose, namely, it prevents the allograft from inducing GVHD.

The immunogenicity of intestinal grafts must be considered particularly strong because the intestine contains a large amount of lymphoid tissue (passenger leukocytes). The passenger leukocytes, which include approximately 90% small peripheral lymphocytes, are thought to contribute significantly to the aggregate immunogenicity of grafted tissues.[112] Reduction of the amount of lymphoid tissue (lymphocytes) by pretreatment of the graft with radiation,[18,113] with antilymphocyte serum,[114] by use of short-segment small bowel grafts,[115] or by resection of graft mesenteric lymph nodes[116] was shown to moderate or even abolish[113] the capacity to induce GVHD in the unidirectional LEW → LBN-F1 rat transplantation model.

The experimental evidence for the effectiveness of these approaches to lessening the immunogenicity of a graft by reducing its lymphocyte content, and thus eliciting a less vigorous rejection reaction, is far less convincing. Kimura et al.[117] and Deltz et al.[70] reported on a relationship between recipient survival time and the length of the transplanted small bowel allograft: shorter (jejunal) grafts were rejected less readily (i.e., the recipients survived) than were longer or entire small bowel grafts (i.e., the recipients died). However, their studies were performed with heterotopic accessory intestinal allografts that were not in gastrointestinal continuity and thus did not contribute to or interfere with the nutritional survival of the recipient. Thus, when using this experimental model, one cannot equate recipient survival with graft survival.[20]

A study by Stangl et al.[118] did not provide any evidence that segmental grafts confer an immunologic advantage over grafts of the entire bowel. Orthotopically placed segmental intestinal grafts were rejected as rapidly as were entire allografts. Furthermore, a short course of treatment with CsA, although effective in prolonging the survival of the recipients of any type or length of intestinal allograft, did not lead to longer survival for the recipients of jejunal grafts than for those of ileal grafts. These findings are in agreement with those of a pathohistologic study by Kimura et al.,[119] who found the course of rejection of short segmental grafts to be the same as that for entire bowel grafts.

Stangl et al.[118] evaluated two immunologic parameters as well as histologic changes as indicators of graft rejection. The measurement of recipient antidonor hemagglutinin titers, which provide a well-defined humoral parameter that is related to the immunologic events taking place in the recipient, failed to demonstrate any difference among ileal, jejunal, and entire allografts, regardless of whether CsA was administered or withheld. Furthermore, when they employed the one-way mixed lymphocyte culture (MLC) assay, lymphocytes, irrespective of their origin from jejunal, ileal, or entire bowel grafts, were equally stimulatory for LEW lymphocytes. Finally, histologic evaluation of biopsy specimens and autopsy material failed to demonstrate any difference in the processes of rejection of the bowel grafts among the groups.

The report by Stangl et al.[118] indicates that the reduction in the amount of lymphoid tissue achievable with use of a jejunal versus an ileal allograft is not sufficient to be reflected in prolonged survival of graft and recipient or in a less pronounced alteration of immunologic parameters. The fact that renal and cardiac allografts transplanted within the same donor-recipient rat strain combination are rejected at between 9 and 13 days, as are intestinal grafts, seems to indicate that the immunogenicity of organ grafts, even those with a minimal amount of lymphoid tissue, is sufficient to induce their rapid rejection. It appears that the immunogenicity of the organ graft itself, aided by a small number of passenger leukocytes, stimulates the recipient's immune processes to a maximum degree. A reduction in the immunogenicity of organ grafts cannot be achieved merely by reduction of their load of lymphoid tissue unless such a reduction is complete or nearly complete. It is quite possible that, in addition to removal of the lymphoid tissues, other immunogenic properties of the intestinal allograft (class I and II antigens) must be altered or eliminated before graft rejection can be mitigated.

Direct irradiation of allografts prior to transplantation, yet another potential approach to reducing graft immunogenicity, was followed by prolonged survival of heart and kidney allografts in rat models.[120] In a study on dogs by Cohen et al.[39] ex vivo irradiation of small-bowel grafts combined with recipient splenectomy resulted in only a moderate extension of graft and host survival. In contrast, in a recent report on a similar experimental study,[121] the authors claim that irradiation of the intestinal graft prior to transplantation, combined with CsA therapy, is more effective in averting rejection than is CsA therapy alone. However, the experimental design of this study and the data themselves do not totally support the claimed effectiveness of pretransplantation radiotherapy. We performed a similar study in rats by using semiallogeneic (LBN-F1 → LEW) and fully allogeneic (BN → LEW) rat strains but failed to detect any effect of graft irradiation in vitro (1,000 rad) upon graft rejection.[122] Experiments by Grant et al.[123] using piglets had the same results, i.e., graft pretreatment with irradiation failed to affect the course of graft rejection.

Several investigators[120,124,125] examined the effect of reducing the amount of immunocompetent lymphoid tissue (passenger leukocytes) in the allograft by using graft/donor pretreatment. Donor pretreatment with ALS, total body irradiation, and cytotoxic drugs was shown to be effective in improving the functional survival of renal and cardiac allografts inasmuch as it caused a marked global leukopenia in the donor. Improved allograft survival was correlated with the degree of leukopenia of the donor at the time of graft harvest. It seems reasonable to expect that such pretreatment will have a major beneficial effect in small bowel transplantation.

Graft/donor pretreatment with ALS given directly into the mesenteric artery one day prior to harvesting and transplantation into a fully allogeneic recipient (BN → LEW rat strain combination) brought moderate prolongation of graft and recipient survival, from 10.1 ± 0.9 days (control, no treatment) to 13.8 ± 1.1 days (Stangl and Schraut, unpublished data). We also evaluated the efficacy of lethal total body irradiation (1,000 rad) of the donor 4 days prior to harvesting the graft, at a time when the donor was severely leukopenic. We were unable to demonstrate prolonged survival for BN allografts transplanted into LEW recipients. Histologic study of these irradiated intestinal allografts showed a marked leuko/lymphopenia but not a complete absence of these cells in the intestinal allograft, thereby, we assume, providing a sufficient immunologic stimulus to the recipient to mount a vigorous rejection reaction.[122] It appears that, for intestinal allografts at least, complete, if not near complete, removal of all passenger leukocytes including dendritic cells is required before a marked prolongation of allograft survival can be expected. The failure of total body irradiation to alter the outcome after small bowel transplantation may also be due to the radioresistance of graft macrophages and dendritic cells, which thus retain their normal antigen-presenting capability and can precipitate an immune response by the recipient.[126]

A mere reduction in the number of lymphocytes in the intestinal graft fails to mitigate the rejection process, as noted before; however, complete removal of the lymphoid tissues and antigen-presenting cells immediately preceding transplantation might provide for a less vigorous rejection process. Complete removal may be achieved if the intestinal graft is preserved by perfusion after harvesting, with the addition of cytotoxic drugs, ALS, or monoclonal antibodies to the perfusate. An approach that is not specifically directed or limited to the removal of passenger lympho/leukocytes, such as the administration of monoclonal antibodies against class II antigens, promises still greater effectiveness.[127] Pretreatment of pancreatic allografts by short-term (3 hours) perfusion with monoclonal antibodies against class II antigens was reported to postpone rejection, probably by delaying antigen presentation.[128] Even a single perfusion of canine renal allografts with monoclonal antibodies effected prolonged survival of the grafts.[129] This technique has become one of our major laboratory goals as we try to develop conditions that are conducive to the depletion of dendritic cells and that can be incorporated readily in a preservation protocol that includes short-term perfusion. If effective, this approach should allow for reduction of immunosuppressive therapy for the recipient, at least in the early posttransplantation period, when the risk of septic complications must be considered highest. In spite of these promising possibilities for immune modulation, the problem of rejection is probably best addressed by a multipronged approach in which immune modulation of the graft is combined with multidrug immunosuppressive therapy of the recipient.

CONTROL OF GRAFT-VERSUS-HOST-DISEASE

By virtue of its large content of lymphoid tissues, an intestinal graft, more than allografts of any other organ except for bone marrow and spleen, can cause GVHD, in addition to inducing a vigorous rejection reaction.[9,18,39,47,96,116,130,131] It has been demonstrated repeatedly that the large number of immunologically competent lymphocytes situated in the mucosa, submucosa, Peyer's patches, and mesenteric lymph nodes, which are transferred with the intestinal allograft can, under certain immunologically defined conditions, precipitate lethal GVHD in the recipient.

Clinical Course and Pathohistology of GVHD

The development of GVHD after small bowel transplantation has been studied most extensively in inbred rats, in experiments in which parental grafts were transplanted into F1 hybrid recipients. Most investigators have used the LBN-F1 → LEW rat strain combination.[18,47,70,96,132] Parental strain allografts have the capacity to induce GVHD because they reside in recipients that are genetically incapable of rejecting the graft.

The first signs of GVHD appear between the 9th and 11th days of transplantation and consist of redness and swelling of the ears, snout, and paws, and of the area around the eyes. Over the ensuing days, the skin becomes dry and scaly, with some loss of hair. In the terminal stage (11th to 16th postoperative day), the rats become emaciated, cold, and listless. This course is associated with progressive weight loss, which, in the last few days of life, becomes precipitous. The same sequence is seen both in animals with an accessory allograft and in those with the allograft placed in gastrointestinal continuity.[113]

In rats that die of GVHD, the most conspicuous finding is a marked enlargement of the lymph nodes and, in some cases, of the spleen. The wall of the lower two-thirds of the small intestine and colon becomes attenuated, and there is evidence of peritonitis.

From the 5th through the 11th postoperative day, animals subject to GVHD have lymph node enlargement and a progressive increase in the relative spleen weight (Fig. 29–5). At the time of death from GVHD, however, the spleen weight

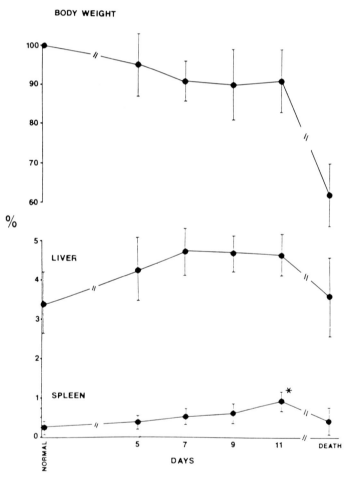

Figure 29–5 Total body weight and relative spleen and liver weight (as percentage of the preoperative weight) during GVHD after heterotopic small-bowel transplantation. The spleen weight increases progressively after transplantation until sudden splenic atrophy occurs on the 12th–13th postoperative day. Splenic atrophy is accompanied by a marked reduction of the total body weight and of the relative liver weight. *, significant increase in relative spleen weight on the 11th postoperative day above the normal spleen weight; day 11: 0.93 ± 0.25; normal: 0.26 ± 0.13, $P <$ 0.05).

has, with few exceptions, become markedly lower; paralleling the development of splenomegaly, a moderate increase in the relative liver weight occurs, which persists up to the 11th postoperative day and then decreases. These are probably agonal reductions.

Rats that die of GVHD have obvious enteritis (reduction of villus height, sloughing of tips of villi, and marked polymorphonuclear cell infiltration of the mucosa and submucosa) that involves their own small bowel and colorectum, whereas the allograft, either orthotopic or heterotopic, has a normal appearance on microscopic inspection.

The lymphatic tissues of a Lewis graft (Peyer's patches and mesenteric lymph nodes) undergo progressive lymphoid depletion beginning on the 5th postoperative day. Initially, this depletion is accompanied by proliferation of histiocytoid cells and immunoblasts in the paracortical area. These immunoblasts disappear over the ensuing days, giving way to progressive lymphopenia, with disappearance of germinal centers and loss of the distinction between the cortex and medulla (Fig. 29–6).

The lymphatic tissues (lymph nodes and spleen) of the LBN-F1 host undergo a similar course of progressive lymphoid depletion and loss of the normal follicular architecture. Histologic changes in the thymus, which are evident after the 7th to the 9th days, consist of progressive cortical thinning and attenuation of the medulla.

In addition to the changes in the lymphoid tissues, a periportal lymphocytic infiltrate is occasionally noted in the livers of rats dying of GVHD. Otherwise, the liver, pancreas, and kidneys are unremarkable. In animals with fulminant GVHD, and in those dying of GVHD, the epidermis is thickened, and the dermis and subcutaneous tissues of the face and feet are infiltrated by mononuclear and polymorphonuclear cells. The progressive histologic changes are paralleled by increasing antihost T-cell activity in the lymphoid tissues of the host.[116] In the dog, GVHD after total small bowel transplantation follows the same histopathologic course and is also marked by progressive destruction of lymphoid tissues.

Prevalence in Animal Models

Whether GVHD will develop depends on the immunogenic disparity between donor and recipient, the size of the allogeneic cell inoculum, and probably the animal species used. The immunologic interactions between the graft and the host range from lethal GVHD to mere stimulation of a small number of allogeneic lymphocytes without clinical consequences. One must clearly distinguish between GVHD, which is a clinical entity, and a GvH reaction, i.e., laboratory evidence that the alloreactive immunocompetent cells are present and stimulated in the graft and host after transplantation. In all of the models of small bowel transplantation, a GvH reaction,[36,38,39,133] when searched for, can be detected.

The severity of GVHD or of a GvH reaction is determined by the number of lymphocytes transferred and the status of the recipient's immune competence. Transplantation of the entire small bowel in the dog, for example, can induce fatal GVHD,[9,131] whereas segmental intestinal allografts containing a lesser quantity of lymphocytes are always rejected without clinical evidence of GVHD.[10-12] Nevertheless, segmental grafts elicit a GvH reaction by releasing immunoblasts into the host's circulation, as shown by Olszewski et al.[133] Furthermore, Deltz et al.,[115] who

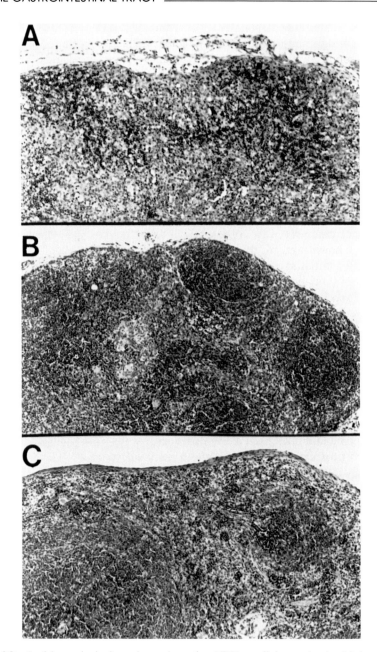

Figure 29–6 Mesenteric lymph nodes of a LEW graft transplanted into a LBN-F1 hybrid recipient (GVHD model). **A:** Normal rat lymph node. **B:** Mesenteric lymph node obtained from the LEW graft 5 days after transplantation shows mild lymphopenia and preserved nodal architecture. **C:** Extensive lymphopenia with loss of germinal centers and nodal architecture ("empty" lymph node) characterizes this mesenteric node from a LEW graft (14th postoperative day; × 100).

used the rat model of accessory small bowel transplantation, demonstrated that GVHD following transplantation of one-half of the small bowel was less intense than that seen after transplantation of the entire small intestine.

As noted, GVHD is an inevitable development in the parental F1 hybrid rat strain combination. When fully allogeneic donor-recipient combinations of rats are studied,[35,36,59,69,96,134,135] rejection rather than fulminant GVHD is prevalent. Nevertheless, there is evidence that the immunocompetent allogeneic lymphocytes of the intestinal graft show a reaction;[35] (Stangl and Schraut, unpublished data). Furthermore, immunocompetent lymphocytes of donor origin can be detected in the lymphoid tissues of the host up to the time when graft rejection is imminent.[118] In the pig model of small bowel transplantation, GVHD has not been reported to be a problem. In the dog, a spectrum of immunologic events following small bowel transplantation, one of these being GVHD, has been demonstrated.

To what degree, if at all, a GvH reaction or GVHD is to be expected in future human small bowel transplantations remains unknown. In humans, the intensity of this reaction will also depend on the number of immunocompetent cells present in the graft, i.e., ultimately on graft size and on the immune competence of the recipient. With fully allogeneic donor-recipient pairs, graft rejection rather than GVHD is anticipated as the predominant immunologic event (the limited clinical experience to date supports this hypothesis). Of course, the recipient will receive immunosuppressive therapy, which should also, inasmuch as it controls rejection, interfere with the expression of GVHD. However, one of the two long-term human survivors of small intestinal grafts[136] was thought, on the basis of clinical signs, to have had an episode of GVHD (with GVHD the possible cause of death), while being treated with ALS, prednisone, and azathioprine. Recently Cohen et al.[137] reported on another clinical attempt at small bowel transplantation in which GVHD may have contributed to an unsuccessful outcome. These experiences, although not providing conclusive evidence for the occurrence of GVHD in clinical small bowel transplantation, emphasize the need for evaluation of this potential problem.

There are three scenarios in which GVHD may become a complicating factor, given a graft-host combination that is expected to engender only a rejection reaction, for example, in the BN → LEW rat strain combination or in future clinical small bowel transplantation.

First, donor lymphocytes might predominate, and GVHD might arise because of profound, pre-existing immunosuppression of the host. This possibility has not been evaluated specifically in a small bowel transplantation model. However, evidence for this possibility comes in a report by Bitter-Suerman,[80] who was able to induce GVHD by transplanting a spleen into an immune-compromised host; further evidence is contained in the clinical experience with bone marrow transplants, which frequently induce GVHD. Adequate recipient preparation and donor/graft pretreatment for inactivation of the alloreactive lymphocytes should obviate this cause of the development of GVHD.

Second, GVHD might develop because of an immunologically induced prevalence of donor lymphocytes resulting from prior, unsuspected sensitization of the donor against the recipient. We evaluated the possible induction of GVHD in the rat model by using the BN → LEW rat strain combination. Small bowel grafts from presensitized donors were rejected without evidence of GVHD; the same rejection occurred even when splenectomy of the recipient was added. Only when the recipients were pretreated with immunosuppressive drugs for four days prior to organ harvesting (in addition to undergoing splenectomy) and then received a small bowel graft from a presensitized donor could we induce GVHD in four of nine recipients (Schraut and Stangl, unpublished data). It appears that an intestinal graft from a sensitized donor is unlikely to induce GVHD, at least in the BN → LEW rat strain combination. Marni et al.[135] reported similar results in a different strain of rats.

Third, GVHD may evolve as a result of immunosuppressive therapy of the recipient, whose immune competence may be impaired to a relatively greater degree than is the immune reactivity of the transferred allogeneic lymphocytes. Experimental evidence for this last possibility is available in the reports by Kirkman et al.[96] and Deltz et al.,[116] who found that, in rats (parent → F1 hybrid combination), CsA treatment limited to 1 or 2 weeks or discontinued 44 days after transplantation failed to be reliable in preventing GVHD. Recently Diflo et al.,[134] who used a rat model with fully allogeneic donor-recipient pairs and employed short-term CsA therapy, demonstrated the development of nonlethal GVHD 3 to 4 weeks later. This mild degree of GVHD, in effect a GvH reaction with a clinical component, disappeared; most of the animals developed tolerance of the intestinal allograft and survived indefinitely.

By using the same rat strain model (BN → LEW) and administering CsA for 28 days, we noted no GVHD or any clinical evidence of a GvH reaction.[59,118] With the same model, when CsA was given for 6 days, we saw only rejection of the graft. However, a unidirectional mixed lymphocyte culture demonstrated allogeneic active (BN) lymphocytes in the lymph nodes of the graft (which was harvested a few days before the recipient's death from rejection). This indicated that the capacity of the cells to mount a GvH reaction still existed in the recipient a few days before complete graft rejection.

Deltz et al.[116] studied antihost T-cell cytotoxicity within several lymphatic compartments of LBN-F1 rats subject to GVHD. Cytotoxicity was high in all compartments (lymph nodes, spleen, blood) unless CsA was given. The drug abrogated antihost activity in surviving rats with the exception of the Peyer's patches of the host's own intestine. An explanation for this "locking in" phenomenon is not available.

In future clinical small bowel transplantation, immunosuppressive treatment is likely to be continued indefinitely and to involve combination drug therapy. Thus the last circumstance described above is unlikely to come to pass.

Diagnosis and Control of GVHD

With the assumption that GVHD may develop after small bowel transplantation in fully allogeneic donor-recipient combinations, methods have to be devised that will allow a distinction between a rejection reaction and GVHD, because both can arise at the same time.[38,134,135] A differential diagnostic strategy has to be developed in which the clinical and histopathologic courses of these two immunologic reactions are compared. Most of the clinical signs and symptoms of the two processes are similar. Dermatitis, diarrhea, generalized lymphadenopathy and enlargement of lymphoid tissue, splenomegaly, and fever are the signs and symptoms of severe GVHD. Diarrhea and fever are also likely to be signs and symptoms of rejection, and dermatitis may arise unrelated to the rejection process as a drug reaction. This leaves rejection to be differentiated from GVHD by the absence of lymphadenopathy and splenomegaly. However, these findings may arise late in the development of GVHD, and even then splenomegaly may not be easily ascertainable by physical examination until marked splenic enlargement has occurred. In clinical bone marrow transplantation, a skin biopsy has been found to be a useful approach for confirming the suspicion of GVHD.[138] The histopathologic findings referable to GVHD have been described as lymphocytic infiltration at the dermal-epidermal junction, together with basal cell degeneration. It has been our experience in the laboratory, however, that the early dermal changes observed clinically are difficult to substantiate by skin biopsy. Only in the presence of fulminant GVHD are the dermatitis and enteritis of the host's native bowel histologically prominent. A graft biopsy would certainly be undertaken if the patient's condition after small bowel transplantation should deteriorate. If the graft biopsy is equivocal and a biopsy of the host's remaining small bowel is inconclusive or unavailable, then biopsy of a peripheral lymph node of the recipient will allow a definitive distinction between a GvH reaction or GVHD and a rejection episode. The histopathologic changes seen in the host's lymphatic tissues are characteristic of GVHD (lymphocyte depletion associated with blurring of the follicular architecture or even complete loss of nodal architecture). Such changes are not seen with a rejection episode[45] (Figs. 29–3 and 29–6).

After small bowel transplantation, a course of treatment of GVHD, either alone or in conjunction with graft rejection, needs to be delineated. Experimental studies by Silvers and Billingham[139] indicate that established GVHD can be alleviated by administration of ALG. Furthermore, in clinical bone marrow transplantation, GVHD has been prevented by prolonged CsA therapy.[140] It thus appears that aggressive immunosuppressive therapy with increased doses of CsA and/or with antilymphocyte serum or monoclonal antibodies directed against T lymphocytes would prevent the progression of a GvH reaction to GVHD. The best possible approach to the problem of GVHD in small bowel transplantation would be to pre-empt its development from the outset by rendering the graft lymphocytes immunologically inactive.

GVHD can be pre-empted by several approaches to graft or donor pretreatment. Lee et al.[113] demonstrated clearly that irradiation of intestinal allografts in vitro before transplantation averts the development of GVHD. The radiation dose that is effective, 1,000 rad, has been shown to cause pyknotic changes in rat lymphocytes, suggesting that graft irradiation destroys or functionally impairs the donor lymphocytes that mediate the GVHD. The concern that such a radiation dose might induce radiation injury is unfounded.[113,123] Pretreatment of the donor with ALS has also been shown to be effective in preventing GVHD.[114] In order to be effective, ALS must be administered prior to or at the time of transplantation; the intraperitoneal has proved to be more effective than the subcutaneous route. Intravenous administration of ALS has not been evaluated. One would expect the use of monoclonal antibodies directed against T lymphocytes to be as effective as ALS in leading to prevention of GVHD after small bowel transplantation.

FUNCTIONAL PERFORMANCE

Multiple studies have been performed for assessment of the functional capacity of the transplanted bowel to absorb nutrients and also to maintain a barrier function against the exterior. The experiments of Kocandrle et al.[141] on dogs demonstrated that isografts have a functional impairment in terms of carbohydrate and fat absorption for several months. However, the functional reserve of the small bowel permitted nutritional balance and eventual weight gain. In the rat model, global nutritional balance (reflected by recipient weight and by normal levels of hemoglobin and albumin) was maintained when total or segmental small bowel grafts were transplanted.[59,142]

For pediatric recipients of small intestinal allografts, the question arises whether normal growth and maturation of the recipients could be achieved. An experimental study on rats indicated that young, immature recipients of small bowel transplants consisting of either the entire small intestine or a segment (ileum or jejunum) grew normally.[142] Irrespective of the use of a segmental or an entire allograft, the caloric nutritional balance of the recipients was maintained, as shown by the fact that all gained weight at a normal rate. As expected, however, nutritional deficits (hypovitaminosis, reduced serum triglyceride levels) developed in recipients of either a jejunal or an ileal allograft when the rats were compared with normal, unoperated controls or with the recipients of an isograft or allograft consisting of the entire small intestine. Such deficits must be viewed as being inherent in the use of a segmental graft and not as resulting from the transplantation procedure. None of the animals in this study exhibited any impairment of gastrointestinal function that could be attributed to the use of cyclosporine as an immunosuppressive agent, or to the fact that the grafts were allogeneic and therefore subject to immunologic processes that could cause functional impairment without leading to graft rejection.

Clearly, transplantation of the entire small bowel would be the best possible solution in the future for the treatment of patients with short gut syndrome by transplantation. However, it is more realistic to envision transplantation of a segmental bowel graft — of course, as long a segment as can be fitted into the recipient's abdominal cavity, which is likely to be partially obliterated and contracted.[143] An ileal or distal small bowel graft would be preferable to a jejunal proximal graft because of its greater absorptive capacity and reserve. Experimental data indicate that, within the limitations of their respective absorptive capacities, segmental small bowel allografts perform as well as allografts or isografts involving the entire small bowel.

In our studies of the rat model of small bowel transplantation, we noted a persistently high level of fecal excretion of fat in all recipients of allografts or isografts.[142] This indicates that impairment of fat absorption is a result of the transplantation procedure, which requires denervation and interruption of the lymphatic drainage. Several studies[59,138,141,144-146] have demonstrated that lymphatic drainage between the intestinal graft and the recipient's retroperitoneal lymphatic system is re-established anatomically. Thus lymphatic interruption may not be the sole determinant of this persistent impairment of fat absorption. When Ballinger et al.[145] studied the effects of isotransplantation in dogs, they also encountered impaired fat absorption, and they proposed that denervation was the main cause of steatorrhea after small bowel transplantation. Their studies indicate that the effects of denervation (which does not cause any change in intestinal motility) and of interruption of the lymphatic system (which is reversed anatomically, but may remain functionally compromised[143,147]) are not completely reversible if they are, as we assume, the cause of this persistent impairment of fat absorption.

It also must be considered that CsA is a fat-soluble substance, and that its absorption, like that of fat, may be compromised. We[107] and others[105,106,108] found that absorption of CsA from intestinal grafts is reduced significantly compared with its absorption from the normal intestine. Thus, if effective serum levels of CsA are to be achieved, it appears necessary in future clinical practice to administer the drug parenterally.

Studies on the rat model of small bowel transplantation demonstrated to us that the type of rejection episode that occurs (with successful control) in renal transplantation is much more serious and life-threatening in intestinal transplantation. The barrier function of the intestinal mucosa, which prevents toxins and bacteria from crossing, is maintained in the early stage of rejection, as has been shown by Arnaud-Battandier et al.[49] However, if rejection progresses, the bowel loses this barrier function, and infection is superimposed upon the rejection process. The recipient of a small bowel graft thus requires close, careful monitoring of allograft integrity and a very diligently applied, preventive form of immunosuppression. Severe mucosal/submucosal infiltration and sporadic mucosal sloughing as a consequence of rejection may not be reversed by adjustment of immunosuppressive therapy but may warrant removal of the transplant. Even if the recipient were to survive such an advanced stage of transplant rejection and the accompanying septic events (which is rare in the rat model of small bowel transplantation), graft fibrosis and obstruction would develop, leading to malnutrition and eventual loss of the graft. Rejection must therefore be detected and avoided at an early stage.

CLINICAL SMALL BOWEL TRANSPLANTATION

As indicated above, rejection has proved the major obstacle to successful human small bowel transplantation. Two children were the first to receive a small bowel graft, in 1964. Both attempts failed because of technical complications.[148] Lillehei et al.[131] and Okumura et al.[149] each performed a cadaver donor transplant, but their patients died after 12 days (from sepsis and rejection) and 12 hours (from graft necrosis), respectively.

The first technically successful intestinal transplant (small bowel and right colon) by Olivier[150] failed because of irreversible rejection, and the patient died after 26 days. Immunosuppressive therapy consisted of administration of azathioprine, steroids, and ALG. Alican et al.[151] transplanted an ileal segment into a 10-year-old child. The graft was removed 10 days later because of necrosis. In 1972, Fortner et al.[136] transferred a 1.7-meter intestinal segment from an HLA-identical donor. Azathioprine, steroids, and ALG were used for immunosuppression; uncontrollable rejection and sepsis, possibly compounded by GVHD, led to the recipient's death after 76 days.

Since CsA became available, at least nine patients, including four children with multivisceral grafts, have received small bowel transplants. Six patients have died, three of them due to sepsis, two because of hemorrhage, and one of unknown causes. In three of the cases, the graft was removed because of rejection. The immunosuppressive regimens used included CsA, steroids, azathioprine, antithymocyte globulin (ATG), and OKT3, given in various doses. Prolonged survival (6–16 months) was achieved by Pellerin at the Hôpital Necker in Paris[153] and by

Starzl's group in Pittsburgh; however, graft acceptance over longer time periods has yet to be realized.

Specific clinical experience with segmental small bowel transplantation has been gained in transplantation of the pancreas together with a segment of duodenum; this segment is anastomosed to the recipient's jejunum or urinary bladder so as to provide for drainage of the exocrine pancreatic secretions. At several centers, a duodenal segment has been transplanted successfully in conjunction with the pancreas.[110,111,152]

Corry et al., at the University of Iowa,[111] reported on more than 20 patients with pancreatoduodenal allografts who were treated with CsA, azathioprine, and prednisone. These patients have been followed for 1–2 years, and the duodenal stump has been viewed repeatedly by cystoscopy in those patients who had a duodenocystostomy. The duodenal graft was found not to be more prone to rejection than was the pancreatic graft. The University of Iowa experience clearly indicates that the rejection of intestinal (duodenal) grafts can be prevented by present day immunosuppressive therapy, and that these grafts remain morphologically intact.

Further clinical experience with small bowel transplantation is evolving through visceral multiorgan transplantation. Starzl and associates at the University of Pittsburgh are developing the simultaneous transplantation of liver, stomach, duodenum, pancreas, and variable lengths of small bowel and colon for pediatric patients in need of such extensive visceral organ replacement.[154] This and similar programs at other institutions are too recent in their inception to allow comments on their impact and future.

Clinical trials of small bowel transplantation will continue, with combination drug therapy used for the control of rejection. Graft/donor pretreatment for the prevention of GVHD may also provide an immunologic advantage in mitigating rejection, although experimental proof of such beneficial effects is still needed. Monitoring of graft integrity is possible with a maltose test, or any other function test, in combination with graft biopsy. A method for safe, short-term preservation of cadaver grafts is available. Paralleling clinical trials, investigative work on small bowel transplantation now being conducted at a number of laboratories will expand our knowledge and understanding of the immunologic, physiologic, and metabolic events in the intestinal graft.

Given effective control of rejection, small bowel transplantation can become an ethical and humanitarian form of treatment. At the start of clinical trials, only patients who would otherwise be definitively and permanently dependent on total parenteral nutrition, who have suffered its severe side effects (recurrent episodes of sepsis, loss of venous access sites, liver failure, severely impaired bone metabolism), and who would therefore have a grave prognosis, should be candidates for intestinal transplants.

REFERENCES

1. Wateska LP, Sattler LL, Steiger E: Cost of a home parenteral nutrition program. *JAMA* 244:2303–4, 1980.
2. Wolfe BM, Beer WH, Hayashi JT, et al: Experience with home hyperalimentation. *Am J Surg* 146:7–14, 1983.
3. Steiger E, Srp F: Morbidity and mortality related to home parenteral nutrition in patients with gut failure. *Am J Surg* 145:102–5, 1983.

4. Seligman JU, Basi SS, Dietel M, et al: Metabolic bone disease in a patient on long-term parenteral nutrition: a case report and review of the literature. *J Parenter Enteral Nutr* 8:722–7, 1984.

5. Bowyer BA, Fleming CR, Ludwig BA, et al: Does long-term parenteral nutrition in adult patients cause chronic liver disease? *J Parenter Enteral Nutr* 9:11–7, 1985.

6. Ullman E: Mikroskopische Praeparate über die Transplantation von verschiedenen Abschnitten des Verdauungstraktes. *Wien Klin Wochenschr* p 599, 1901.

7. Carrel A: The surgery of blood vessels, etc. *Johns Hopkins Hosp Bull* 18:18–28, 1907.

8. Lillehei RC, Goott B, Miller FA: The physiological response of the small bowel of the dog to ischemia including prolonged in vitro preservation of the bowel with successful replacement and survival. *Ann Surg* 150:543–60, 1959.

9. Lillehei RC, Goott B, Miller FA: Homografts of the small bowel. *Surg Forum* 10:197–9, 1959.

10. Taylor RMR, Watson JW, Walker FC, et al: Prolongation of survival of jejunal homografts in dogs treated with azathioprine (Imuran). *Br J Surg* 53:134–8, 1966.

11. Preston FW, Macalalad F, Wachowski TJ, et al: Survival of homografts of the intestine with and without immunosuppression. *Surgery* 60:1203–10, 1966.

12. Hardy MA, Quint J, State D: Effect of antilymphocyte serum and other immunosuppressive agents on canine jejunal allografts. *Ann Surg* 171:51–60, 1970.

13. Keaveny TV, Aglubart F, Belzer FO: Porcine small bowel allotransplantation. *Ir J Med Sc* 3:483–87, 1970.

14. Ruiz JO, Uchida H, Schultz LS, et al: Problems in absorption and immunosuppression after entire intestinal allotransplantation. *Am J Surg* 123:297–303, 1972.

15. Hay JM, Fagniez PL, Parc R, et al: Résultats de l'allotransplantation orthotopique de l'intestine grêle chez le porc. *Ann Chir* 28:1063–67, 1974.

16. Kunlin A, Hay J-M, Hay P-L, et al: Technique de la transplantation orthotopique de l'intestin grêle chez le porc. *Ann Chir* 26:505–10, 1972.

17. Stauffer UG, Becker M, Hirsig J, et al: The risks of small intestinal transplantation for the recipient: experimental results in young minipigs. *J Pediatr Surg* 13:465–7, 1978.

18. Monchik GJ, Russell PS: Transplantation of small bowel in the rat: technical and immunological considerations. *Surgery* 70:693–702, 1971.

19. Kort WJ, Westbroeck DL, MacDicken I, et al: Orthotopic total small-bowel transplantation in the rat. *Eur Surg Res* 5:81–89, 1973.

20. Lee KKW, Schraut WH: Small-bowel transplantation in the rat. Graft survival with heterotopic vs. orthotopic position. In Deltz E, Thiede A, Hamelmann H: *Small Bowel Transplantation. Experimental and Clinical Fundamentals,* Heidelberg, Springer-Verlag, 1986, p 7–13.

21. Zinzar SN, Leitina BI, Tumyan BC, et al: Large organ-like structures formed by syngeneic foetal alimentary tract transplanted as a whole or in parts. *Rev Eur Etudes Clin Biol* 16:455–9, 1971.

22. Leapman SB, Deutsch AA, Grand RJ, et al: Transplantation of fetal intestine: survival and function in a subcutaneous location in adult animals. *Ann Surg* 75:496–502, 1974.

23. Deutsch AA, Leapman SB, Arensman R, et al: Anastomosis of transplanted fetal rat intestine to the normal intestine of the host. *J Surg Res* 15:176–81, 1973.

24. Bass BL, Schweitzer EJ, Harmon JW, et al: Anatomic and physiologic characteristics of transplanted fetal rat intestine. *Ann Surg* 200:734–41, 1984.

25. Schwartz MZ, Flye MW, Storozuk RB: Growth and function of transplanted fetal rat intestine: effect of cyclosporin A. *Surgery* 97:481–6, 1985.

26. Holmes JT, Yeh SDJ, Winawer SJ, et al: New concepts in structure and function of dog jejunal allografts. *Surg Forum* 21:334–6, 1970.

27. Stauffer UG, Mona D, Shmerline DH: Monitoring of small bowel transplants by sequential mucosal suction biopsies. *Z Kinderchir Grenzgeb* 16:32–7, 1975.

28. Madara JL, Kirkman RL: Structural and functional evolution of jejunal allograft rejection in rats and the ameliorating effects of cyclosporine therapy. *J Clin Invest* 75:502–12, 1985.

29. Rosemurgy AS, Schraut WH: Small bowel allografts: sequence of histologic changes in acute and chronic rejection. *Am J Surg* 151:470–75, 1986.

30. Chomette G, Lerf M, Hay JM, et al: Autotransplantation expérimentale de l'intestine grêle chez le porc. *Ann Anat Pathol (Paris)* 20:343–56, 1975.

31. Lossing A, Nordgren S, Cohen Z, et al: Histologic monitoring of rejection in small intestinal transplantation. *Transplant Proc* 14:643–5, 1982.

32. Lear PA, Cunningham AJ, Crane PW, Wood RFM: Lymphocyte migration patterns in small bowel transplants. *Transplant Proc* 21:2881–2, 1989.

33. Crane PW, Lear PA, Sowter C, et al: Early microvascular changes in small intestinal allografts. *Transplant Proc* 21:2906, 1989.

34. Billiar TR, Garberoglio C, Schraut WH: Maltose absorption as an indicator of small intestinal allograft rejection. *J Surg Res* 37:75–82, 1984.

35. Thiede A, Deltz E: Morphological reaction in transplanted small intestine using immunogenetically defined rat strain combinations. *Langenbecks Arch Chir* 346:119–27, 1978.

36. Schraut WH, Abraham VS, Lee KKW: Portal versus systemic venous drainage for small-bowel allografts. *Surgery* 98:579–85, 1985.

37. Millard PR, Dennison A, Hughes DA, et al: Morphology of intestinal allograft rejection and the inadequacy of mucosal biopsy in its recognition. *Br J Exp Pathol* 67:687–98, 1986.

38. Fujiwara H, Raju S, Grogan JB, et al: Total orthotopic small bowel allotransplantation in the dog. *Transplantation* 44:747–53, 1987.

39. Cohen Z, Macgregor AB, Moore KTH, et al: Canine small bowel transplantation: a study of the immunological responses. *Arch Surg* 111:248–53, 1976.

40. Garrido H, Lucea C, Ruiperez S, Gomez-Acebo J: Homotransplant of the small intestine and the graft-versus-host reaction. *Rev Eur Etudes Clin Biol* 15:547–51, 1970.

41. Cohen Z, Nordgren S, Lossing A, et al: Morphological studies of intestinal allograft rejection. Immunosuppression with cyclosporine. *Dis Colon Rectum* 27:228–234, 1984.

42. Kunlin A, Gaston JP, Shiu MH, et al: The isolated allograft pouch: a useful method for monitoring of small bowel allografts. *Surg Forum* 22:237–39, 1971.

43. Reznick RK, Craddock GN, Langer B, et al: Structure and function of small bowel allografts in the dog: immunosuppression with cyclosporin A. *Can J Surg* 25:51–5, 1982.

44. Pritchard TJ, Kirkman RL: Small bowel transplantation. *World J Surg* 9:860–7, 1985.

45. Schraut WH, Rosemurgy AS, Riddel RM: Prolongation of intestinal allograft survival without immunosuppressive drug therapy. *J Surg Res* 34:597–60, 1983.

46. Silverman R, Cohen Z, Levy G, et al: Immune response in small intestinal transplantation in the rat: correlation of histopathology and monocyte procoagulant activity. *Surgery* 102:395–401, 1987.

47. Schraut WH, Lee KKW: Clinicopathologic differentiation of rejection and graft-vs-host disease following small-bowel transplantation. In Deltz E, Thiede A, Hamelmann H: *Small Bowel Transplantation. Experimental and Clinical Fundamentals,* Heidelberg, Springer-Verlag, 1986, p 98–108.

48. Hardy Iga C, Satake K, et al: Migration of donor passenger cells during rat cardiac and intestinal allograft rejection. In Thiede A, Deltz E, Engemann R, et al: *Microsurgical*

Models in Rats for Transplantation Research. Heidelberg, Springer-Verlag, 1985, p 135–44.

49. Arnaud-Battandier F, Salmon H, Aynaud JM, et al: In vitro and in vivo studies of the mucosal immune barrier after long-term small-bowel allotransplantation in pigs using cyclosporine. In Deltz E, Thiede A, Hamelmann H: *Small Bowel Transplantation. Experimental and Clinical Fundamentals.* Heidelberg, Springer-Verlag, 1986, p 39.

50. Holmes JT, Yeh SDJ, Winawer SJ, et al: New concepts in structure and function of dog jejunal allografts. *Surg Forum* 21:334–6, 1970.

51. Hatcher PA, Deaton DH, Bollinger RR: Transplantation of the entire small bowel in inbred rats using cyclosporine. *Transplantation* 43:478–84, 1987.

52. Cohen WB, Hardy MA, Quint J, et al: Absorptive function in canine jejunal autografts and allografts. *Surgery* 65:440–6, 1969.

53. Nordgren S, Cohen Z, Mackenzie R, et al: Functional monitors of rejection in small intestinal transplants. *Am J Surg* 147:152–8, 1984.

54. Seifert F, Deltz E: In Deltz E, Thiede A, Hamelmann H: *Small Bowel Transplantation. Experimental and Clinical Fundamentals,* Heidelberg, Springer-Verlag, 1986, p 79.

55. Maeda K, Oki K, Nakamura K, et al: Small intestine transplantation: a logical solution for short bowel syndrome? *J Pediatr Surg* 23:10–15, 1988.

56. Martinelli GP, Knight RK, Kaplan S, et al: Small bowel transplantation in the rat. *Transplantation* 45:1021–26, 1988.

57. Holmes JT, Yeh SDJ, Winawer SJ, et al: Absorption studies in canine jejunal allografts. *Ann Surg* 174:101–8, 1971.

58. Holmes JT, Klein MS, Winawer SJ, et al: Morphological studies of rejection in canine jejunal allografts. *Gastroenterology* 61:693, 1971.

59. Lee KKW, Schraut WH: Structure and function of orthotopic small-bowel allografts in rats with cyclosporin A. *Am J Surg* 151:55–60, 1986.

60. Maeda J, Schwartz MZ, Bamberger MH, et al: A possible serum marker for rejection after small intestine transplantation. *Am J Surg* 153:68–74, 1987.

61. Stamford WP, Hardy MA: Fatty acid absorption in jejunal allograft and autograft. *Surgery* 75:496–502, 1974.

62. Schroeder P, Sandforth F, Deltz E: Glucose absorption after heterotopic small bowel transplantation. In Deltz E, Thiede A, Hamelmann H: *Small Bowel Transplantation. Experimental and Clinical Fundamentals.* Heidelberg, Springer-Verlag, 1986, p 74.

63. Grant D, Lamont D, Zhong R, et al: Cr-EDTA: A marker of early intestinal rejection in the rat. *J Surg Res* 46:507–14, 1989.

64. Schiller WR, Suriyapa C, Mutcheler JHW, et al: Motility changes associated with canine intestinal allografting. *J Surg Res* 15:379–84, 1973.

65. Dennison AR, Collin J, Watkins RM, et al: Segmental small intestinal allografts in the dog. I. Morphological and functional indices of rejection. *Transplantation* 44:474–78, 1987.

66. Vane DW, Grosfeld JL, Moore W, et al: Impaired motility following small intestinal transplantation. Presented at the annual meeting of the Association for Academic Surgery, Salt Lake City, 1988.

67. Hammer C, Ertel W, Reichenspurner H, Brendel W: Immunologic reactions following heart transplantation and their detection. *Fortschr Med* 101:2041–3, 1983.

68. Westbroek DL, Rothengatter C, Vriesendorp et al: Histocompatibility and heterotopic segmental small-bowel allograft survival in dogs. *Eur Surg Res* 2:401–7, 1970.

69. Lee MD, Kunz HW, Gill TJ, et al: Transplantation of the small bowel across MHC and non-MHC disparities in the rat. *Transplantation* 42:235–8, 1986.

70. Deltz E: Die allogene Dünndarmtransplantation. Funktionelle und morphologische

Untersuchungen der Abstoβungs und der Transplant gegen-Wirt Reaktion (GVHR) im Rattenmodell. München, Zuckerschwerdt, 1984.

71. Stangl MJ, Schraut WH, Moynihan HL, et al: Rejection of ileal versus jejunal allografts. *Transplantation* 47:424–7, 1989.

72. Frey JR, Geleick M, DeWeck A: Immunological tolerance induced in animals previously sensitized to single chemical compounds. *Science* 144:153–5, 1964.

73. Mandel MA, Monaco AP, Russell PS: Destruction of splenic transplantation antigens by a factor present in the liver. *J Immunol* 95:673–82, 1965.

74. Sakai A: Role of the liver in kidney allograft rejection in the rat. *Transplantation* 9:333–4, 1970.

75. Schraut WH, Abraham VS, Lee KKW: Portal versus caval venous drainage for small-bowel allografts. Technical and metabolic consequences. *Surgery* 99:193–8, 1986.

76. Koltun WA, Madara JL, Smith RJ, et al: Metabolic aspects of small bowel transplantation in inbred rats. *J Surg Res* 42:341–7, 1987.

77. Fabre JW, Batchelor JR: The role of the spleen in the rejection and enhancement of renal allografts in the rat. *Transplantation* 20:219–26, 1975.

78. Souther SG, Morris RJ, Vistnes LM: Prolongation of rat cardiac allograft survival by splenectomy following transplantation. *Transplantation* 17:317–9, 1974.

79. Bitter-Suermann H: Induction of lethal graft versus host disease in rats by spleen grafting. *J Surg Res* 34:597–607, 1983.

80. Hardy MA, Chabot J, Tannenbaum G, et al: Graft acceptance: modification of immunogenicity of the donor or the donor organ with or without host immunosuppression. In Deltz E, Thiede A, Hamelmann H: *Small Bowel Transplantation. Experimental and Clinical Fundamentals,* Heidelberg, Springer-Verlag, 1986, p 135–52.

81. Hall BM: Mechanism of specific unresponsiveness to allografts. *Transplant Proc* 16:938–43, 1984.

82. Perry LL, Williams IR: Regulation of transplantation immunity in vivo by monoclonal antibodies recognizing host class II restriction elements. *J Immunol* 134:2935–41, 1985.

83. Cobbold SP, Jayasuriya A, Nash E, et al: Therapy with monoclonal antibodies by elimination of T cell subsets in vivo. *Nature* 312:548–51, 1984.

84. Marquet RL, Heysteck GA: Induction of suppressor cells by donor specific blood transfusion and heart transplantation in rats. *Transplantation* 31:272–9, 1981.

85. Homan NT, Williams KA, Millard PR, et al: Prolongation of renal allograft survival in the rat by pretreatment with donor antigen and cyclosporine A. *Transplantation* 31:423–7, 1981.

86. King HP, Clunie GJA, Dumbli LJ: Pretransplant transfusion and cyclosporin A induced enhancement of rabbit skin allografts. Donor specific versus third party blood. *Transplantation* 37:418–9, 1984.

87. Yoshimura N, Kahan BD: Nature of the suppressor cells mediating prolonged graft survival after administration of extracted histocompatibility antigen and cyclosporin A. *Transplantation* 39:162–8, 1985.

88. Stuart FP, Saitoh T, Fitch FW, et al: Immunologic enhancement of renal allografts in the rat. *Surgery* 64:17–24, 1968.

89. Weiss A, Fitch FW, McKearn TJ, et al: Immunologic memory is regulated in the enhanced rat renal allograft recipient. *Nature* 273:662–4, 1978.

90. Nash JR, Peters M, Bell PRF: Comparative survival of pancreatic islets, heart, kidney and skin allografts in rats with and without enhancement. *Transplantation* 24:70–3, 1977.

91. Telford GL, Corry RJ: Immunological enhancement of rat small intestinal allografts. *Arch Surg* 113:615–7, 1978.

92. Wall AJ, Peters TJ: Changes in structure and peptidase activity of rat small intestine induced by prednisolone. *Gut* 12:445–8, 1971.

93. Deutsch A, Arensman R, Levey R, et al: The effect of antilymphocyte serum on fetal rat intestine transplanted as free subcutaneous homografts. *J Pediatr Surg* 9:29–34, 1974.

94. Quint J, Hardy MA, State D: Effects of antilymphocyte serum on absorptive function and survival of dog intestinal allografts. *Surg Forum* 19:184–6, 1968.

95. Borel JF, Feurer C, Magnel C, et al: Effects of the new antilymphocyte polypeptide cyclosporin A in animals. *Immunology* 33:1017–25, 1977.

96. Kirkman RL, Lear PA, Madara JL, et al: Small intestine transplantation in the rat — immunology and function. *Surgery* 96:280–7, 1984.

97. Harmel RP Jr, Stanley M: Improved survival after allogeneic small intestinal transplantation in the rat using cyclosporine immunosuppression. *J Pediatr Surg* 21:214–7, 1986.

98. Harmel RP, Tutschka P, Sonnino RE, et al: Immune tolerance of intestinal allografts in the rat. Presented at the XII Congress of the International Transplantation Society, Sidney, Australia, 1988.

99. Ricour C, Revillon Y, Arnaud-Battandier F, et al: Successful small bowel allografts in piglets using cyclosporine. *Transplant Proc* 15:3019–26, 1983.

100. Pritchard TJ, Madara JL, Tapper D, et al: Failure of cyclosporine to prevent small bowel allograft rejection in pigs. *J Surg Res* 38:553–58, 1985.

101. Grant D, Duff J, Zhong R, et al: Successful intestinal transplantation in pigs treated with cyclosporine. *Transplantation* 45:279–284, 1988.

102. Craddock GN, Resnick RK, Gilas T, et al: Structure and function of small bowel allografts treated with cyclosporin A. *Surg Forum* 32:350–5, 1981.

103. Aeder MI, Payne WD, Jeng LB, et al: Use of cyclosporine for small intestinal allo-transplantation in dogs. *Surg Forum* 35:387–90, 1984.

104. Raju S, Didlake RH, Cayirli M, et al: Experimental small bowel transplantation utilizing cyclosporine. *Transplantation* 38:561–566, 1984.

105. Diliz-Perez HS, McClure J, Bedetti C, et al: Successful small bowel allotranplantation in dogs with cyclosporine and prednisone. *Transplantation* 37:126–9, 1984.

106. Wassef R, Cohen Z, Nordgren S, Langer B: Cyclosporine absorption in intestinal transplantation. *Transplantation* 39:496–9, 1985.

107. Lee KKW, Hurst R, Schraut WH: Enteral absorption of cyclosporine following small bowel transplantation. *Curr Surg* 45:205–8, 1988.

108. Leimenstoll G, Preissner WCH, Loske G, et al: Different modes of cyclosporin A administration in experimental small bowel transplantation. In Deltz E, Thiede A, Hamelmann H: *Small Bowel Transplantation. Experimental and Clinical Fundamentals.* Heidelberg, Springer-Verlag, 1986, p 166.

109. Crane PW, Davies RL, Sowter C, et al: The effect of cyclosporin on small intestinal vasculature. Presented at the 7th Tripartite Meeting (SRS, SUS, ESSR) Bristol, UK, 1988.

110. Sollinger HW, Stratta RJ, Kalayoglu M, et al: Forty consecutive pancreas transplantation with pancreatico-cystostomy and quadruple immunosuppression. *Surgery* 102:674–9, 1987.

111. Corry RJ, Nghiem DD, Schanbacher B, et al: Critical analysis of mortality and graft loss following simultaneous renal-pancreatic duodenal transplantation. *Transplant Proc* 19:2294–9, 1987.

112. Guttmann RD, Lindquist RR, Ockner SA: Renal transplantation in the inbred rat. Hematopoietic origin of an immunogenic stimulus of rejection. *Transplantation* 8:472–84, 1969.

113. Lee KKW, Schraut WH: In vitro allograft irradiation prevents graft-versus-host disease in small-bowel transplantation. *J Surg Res* 38:364–72, 1985.

114. Shaffer D, Maki T, DeMichele SJ, et al: Studies in small bowel transplantation. Prevention of graft-versus-host disease with preservation of allograft function by donor pretreatment with antilymphocyte serum. *Transplantation* 45:262–9, 1988.

115. Deltz E, Müller-Hermelink HK, Ulrichs K, et al: Development of graft-versus-host reaction in various target organs after small intestine transplantation. *Transplant Proc* 13:1215–16, 1981.

116. Deltz E, Ulrichs K, Schack T, et al: Graft-versus-host reaction in small bowel transplantation and possibilities for its circumvention. *Am J Surg* 151:379–86, 1986.

117. Kimura K, Money SR, Jaffe BM: The effects of cyclosporine on varying segments of small-bowel grafts in the rat. *Surgery* 104:64–69, 1988.

118. Stangl MJ, Schraut WH, Moynihan HL, et al: Effect of cyclosporine therapy in controlling the rejection of ileal versus jejunal allografts. Submitted to *Transplantation*

119. Kimura K, Money SR, Jaffe BA: Short segment orthotopic intestinal isografts and allografts in enterectomized rats. *Transplantation* 44:579–82, 1987.

120. Steinmuller D, Warden G, Coleman M, et al: Prolonged survival of rat heart and kidney allografts irradiated in vitro. *Transplantation* 12:153–6, 1971.

121. Williams JW, McClellan T, Peters TG, et al: Effect of pretransplant graft irradiation on canine intestinal transplantation. *Surg Gynecol Obstet* 167:197–204, 1988.

122. Stangl M, Moynihan HL, Lee TK, et al: Influence of the lymphocyte content of small-bowel allografts upon their rejection. Presented at the 7th Tripartite meeting (SRS, SUS, ESSR) Bristol, UK, 1988.

123. Grant DR, Duff J, Zhong R, et al: Effect of ex vivo allograft irradiation combined with cyclosporine therapy in a pig intestinal transplant model. *Transplant Proc* 21:2879–80, 1989.

124. Guttmann RE, Lindquist RR: Renal transplantation in the inbred rat. Reduction of allograft immunogenicity by cytotoxic drug pretreatment of donors. *Transplantation* 8:490–5, 1969.

125. Freeman JS, Chamberlain EC, Reemtsma K, et al: Prolongation of rat heart allografts by donor pretreatment with immunosuppressive agents. *Transplant Proc* 3:580–2, 1971.

126. Chestnut RW, Grey HM: Antigen presenting cells and mechanisms of antigen presentation. *CRC Crit Rev Immunol* 5:263–316, 1985.

127. Faustman D, Hamptfeld B, Lacey PE: Prolongation of murine islet allograft survival by pretreatment of islets with antibody directed to Ia determinants. *Proc Natl Acad Sci USA* 78:5156, 1981.

128. Lloyd DM, Gaber AO, Buckingham M, et al: Prolonged survival of rat pancreas allografts by ex-vivo perfusion with monoclonal antibodies specific for class II major histocompatibility antigens. *Surg Forum* 38:375–7, 1987.

129. Yanamoto K, Watanabe T, Ohtsubo O, et al: Prolonged survival of dog kidney allografts induced by a monoclonal anti-Ia antibody. *Transplantation* 37:419–20, 1984.

130. Schraut WH, Lee KKW, Dawson PJ, et al: Graft-versus-host disease induced by small bowel allografts. *Transplantation* 41:286–290, 1986.

131. Lillehei RC, Idezuki Y, Feemster JA, et al: Transplantation of stomach, intestine and pancreas; experimental and clinical observations. *Surgery* 62:721–41, 1967.

132. Pomposelli F, Maki T, Kiyoizumi T, et al: Induction of graft-versus-host disease by small intestinal allotransplantation in rats. *Transplantation* 40:343–47, 1985.

133. Olszewski W, Plucinski S: Collection of lymph from dog jejunal allotransplant. *Eur Surg Res* 5:311–19, 1973.

134. Diflo T, Monaco AP, Balogh K, et al: The existence of graft-versus-host disease in long

term surviving fully allogeneic rat small bowel transplant recipients. *Transplant Proc* 21:2875–6, 1989.

135. Marni A, Ferrero ME, Tiengo M, Gaja G: Graft-versus-host and host-versus-graft reactions after small intestinal allografts in hyperimmunized rats: effect of cyclosporine treatment. *Transplant Proc* 19:1207–11, 1987.

136. Fortner JG, Sichuk G, Litwin SD, et al: Immunological response to an intestinal allograft with HLA-identical donor-recipient. *Transplantation* 14:531–5, 1972.

137. Cohen Z, Silverman: Clinical small-bowel transplantation. *Transplant Proc* 19:2588–90, 1987.

138. Slavin RE, Santos GE: The graft-versus-host reaction in man after bone marrow transplantation: pathology, pathogenesis, clinical features and implications. *Clin Immunol Immunopathol* 1:472–98, 1973.

139. Silvers WK, Billingham RE: Studies on the immunotherapy of runt disease in rats. *J Exp Med* 129:647–61, 1969.

140. Powels RL, Clink HM, Spence D: Cyclosporin A to prevent graft-versus-host disease in man after allogeneic bone-marrow transplantation. *Lancet* i:327–9, 1980.

141. Kocandrle V, Houttuin HE, Prohaska JV: Regeneration of the lymphatics after autotransplantation and homotransplantation of entire small intestine. *Surg Gynecol Obstet* 122:587–92, 1966.

142. Schraut WH, Lee KKW, Sitrin M: Recipient growth and nutritional status following transplantation of segmental small-bowel allografts. *J Surg Res* 43:1–9, 1987.

143. Schraut WH, Lee KKW: Procurement of intestinal allografts from living related and from cadaver donors. In Deltz E, Thiede A, Hamelmann H: *Small Bowel Transplantation. Experimental and Clinical Fundamentals.* Heidelberg, Springer-Verlag, 1986, p 203.

144. Goott B, Lillehei RC, Miller FA: Mesenteric lymphatic regeneration after autografts of small bowel in dogs. *Surgery* 48:571–5, 1960.

145. Ballinger WF, Christy MG, Ashby WB: Autotransplantation of the small intestine: the effect of denervation. *Surgery* 52:151–64, 1962.

146. Rotman N, Michot F, Hay JM, et al: Lymphatic regeneration following intestinal transplantation in the pig. In Deltz E, Thiede A, Hamelmann H: *Small Bowel Transplantation. Experimental and Clinical Fundamentals.* Heidelberg: Springer-Verlag, 1986.

147. Clark E, Ferguson MK, Moynihan HL, et al: Mesenteric lymphatic function following total small-bowel transplantation in rats. *Curr Surg* 46:115–117, 1988.

148. Kirkman R: Small bowel transplantation. *Transplantation* 37:429–33, 1984.

149. Okumura M, Fujimara I, Ferrari AA, et al: Transplante del intestino delgrado; apresentacao de un caso. *Rev Hosp Clin Fac Med Sao Paulo* 24:39, 1969.

150. Olivier CL, Retrorri R, Olivier CH, et al: Homotransplantation orthotopique de l'intestin grêle et des côlons droit et transverse chez l'homme. *J Chir (Paris)* 98:323–30, 1969.

151. Alican F, Hardy JD, Cayirli M, et al: Intestinal transplantation: laboratory experience and report of a clinical case. *Am J Surg* 121:150–9, 1971.

152. Prieto M, Sutherland DER, Goetz FC, et al: Pancreas transplant results according to the technique of duct management: bladder versus enteric drainage. *Surgery* 102:680–91, 1987.

153. Goulet O, Revillon Y, Nezelof C, et al: Intestinal transplantation in children. *Arch Fr Pediatr* 45:735–739, 1988.

154. Starzl TE, Todu S, Tzakis A: Abdominal organ cluster transplantation for the treatment of upper abdominal malignancies. Presented at the annual meeting of the American Surgical Association, Colorado Springs, Co 1989.

Index

646